Advances in
PARASITOLOGY

VOLUME **72**

Important Helminth Infections in Southeast Asia: Diversity and Potential for Control and Elimination, Part A

Advances in **PARASITOLOGY**

VOLUME **72**

Important Helminth Infections in Southeast Asia: Diversity and Potential for Control and Elimination, Part A

Edited by

XIAO-NONG ZHOU
National Institute of Parasitic Diseases
Chinese Center for Disease Control and Prevention
Shanghai, People's Republic of China

ROBERT BERGQUIST
Ingerod, Brastad, Sweden

REMIGIO OLVEDA
Department of Health, Research Institute of Tropical Medicine (RITM), Muntinlupa, Manila, Philippines

JÜRG UTZINGER
Department of Epidemiology and Public Health
Swiss Tropical and Public Health Institute
Basel, Switzerland

ELSEVIER

AMSTERDAM • BOSTON • HEIDELBERG • LONDON
NEW YORK • OXFORD • PARIS • SAN DIEGO
SAN FRANCISCO • SINGAPORE • SYDNEY • TOKYO
Academic Press is an imprint of Elsevier

Academic Press is an imprint of Elsevier

32 Jamestown Road, London, NW1 7BY, UK
525 B Street, Suite 1900, San Diego, CA 92101-4495, USA
30 Corporate Drive, Suite 400, Burlington, MA 01803, USA
Radarweg 29, PO Box 211, 1000 AE Amsterdam, The Netherlands

First edition 2010

ISBN: 978-0-12-381513-2
ISSN: 0065-308X

For information on all Academic Press publications
visit our website at www.elsevierdirect.com

Printed and bound in UK
10 11 12   10 9 8 7 6 5 4 3 2 1

CONTENTS

CONTRIBUTORS

Robert Bergquist
Ingerod, Brastad, Sweden

Paul J. Brindley
Department of Microbiology, Immunology and Tropical Medicine, The George Washington University Medical Center, Washington, District of Columbia, USA

Sombat Chayabejara
Chairman, Southeast Asian Regional Program Review Group (RPRG), Suanluang, Bangkok, Thailand

James Conlan
National Animal Health Centre, Department of Livestock and Fisheries, Ministry of Agriculture and Forestry, Luangprabang Road, Vientiane, Lao People's Democratic Republic; World Health Organization Collaborating Centre for the Molecular Epidemiology of Parasitic Infections, School of Veterinary and Biomedical Sciences, Murdoch University, Murdoch, WA, Australia

Socheat Duong
National Centre for Parasitology, Entomology and Malaria Control, Phnom Penh, Cambodia

John P. Ehrenberg
World Health Organization, Regional Office for the Western Pacific, Malaria, Vector-borne and other Parasitic Diseases, Manila, Philippines

Nicole M. Fox
World Health Organization, Regional Office for the Western Pacific, Malaria, Vector-borne and other Parasitic Diseases, Manila, Philippines

Mackenzie K. Henderson
World Health Organization, Regional Office for the Western Pacific, Malaria, Vector-borne and other Parasitic Diseases, Manila, Philippines

Leda Hernandez
Infectious Disease Office, National Center for Disease Prevention and Control, Department of Health, Manila, Philippines

Peter J. Hotez
Department of Microbiology, Immunology, and Tropical Medicine, George Washington University; and Sabin Vaccine Institute, Washington, District of Columbia, USA

Pewpan M. Intapan
Department of Parasitology, Faculty of Medicine, Khon Kaen University, Thailand

Sasithorn Kaewkes
Department of Parasitology, Faculty of Medicine, Khon Kaen University, Thailand

Tuan Le Anh
World Health Organization, Regional Office for the Western Pacific, Malaria, Vector-borne and other Parasitic Diseases, Manila, Philippines

Lydia Leonardo
Department of Parasitology, College of Public Health, University of the Philippines, Manila, Philippines

Shan Lv
Department of Epidemiology and Public Health, Swiss Tropical and Public Health Institute, and University of Basel, Basel, Switzerland; and National Institute of Parasitic Diseases, Chinese Center for Disease Control and Prevention, Shanghai, People's Republic of China

Wanchai Maleewong
Department of Parasitology, Faculty of Medicine, Khon Kaen University, Thailand

Donald P. McManus
Molecular Parasitology Laboratory, Queensland Institute of Medical Research, Brisbane, Australia

Raymond Mendoza
World Health Organization, Regional Office for the Western Pacific, Malaria, Vector-borne and other Parasitic Diseases, Manila, Philippines

Sinuon Muth
National Centre for Parasitology, Entomology and Malaria Control, Phnom Penh, Cambodia

Sophie Odermatt-Biays
Department of Epidemiology and Public Health, Swiss Tropical and Public Health Institute, and University of Basel, Basel, Switzerland

Peter Odermatt
Department of Epidemiology and Public Health, Swiss Tropical and Public Health Institute, and University of Basel, Basel, Switzerland

Remigio Olveda
Department of Health, Research Institute for Tropical Medicine (RITM), Muntinlupa, Manila, Philippines

Samlane Phompida
Centre for Malariology, Parasitology and Entomology, Vientiane, Lao People's Democratic Republic

Martha Fernanda Pineda
World Health Organization, Regional Office for the Western Pacific, Malaria, Vector-borne and other Parasitic Diseases, Manila, Philippines

Liberty G. Reforma
World Health Organization, Regional Office for the Western Pacific, Malaria, Vector-borne and other Parasitic Diseases, Manila, Philippines

Fadjar Satrija
Department of Animal Diseases and Veterinary Public Health, Faculty of Veterinary Medicine, Bogor Agricultural University, Jl. Agatis Kampus IPB Darmaga, Bogor, Indonesia

Somphou Sayasone
Department of Epidemiology and Public Health, Swiss Tropical and Public Health Institute, and University of Basel, Basel, Switzerland; and National Institute of Public Health, Ministry of Health, Vientiane, Lao People's Democratic Republic

Alexander Schratz
World Health Organization, Regional Office for the Western Pacific, Malaria, Vector-borne and other Parasitic Diseases, Manila, Philippines

Banchob Sripa
Tropical Disease Research Laboratory (TDR), Department of Pathology, Faculty of Medicine, Khon Kaen University, Thailand

Peter Steinmann
National Institute of Parasitic Diseases, Chinese Center for Disease Control and Prevention, Shanghai, People's Republic of China; Department of Epidemiology and Public Health, Swiss Tropical and Public Health Institute, and University of Basel, Basel, Switzerland

Mohammad Sudomo
Ecology and Health Status Research and Development Centre, National Institute of Health Research and Development, Ministry of Health, Jakarta, Indonesia

Marcel Tanner
Department of Epidemiology and Public Health, Swiss Tropical and Public Health Institute, and University of Basel, Basel, Switzerland

Ah Sian Tee
World Health Organization, Regional Office for the Western Pacific, Malaria, Vector-borne and other Parasitic Diseases, Manila, Philippines

L. Tommaso Cavalli-Sforza
World Health Organization, Regional Office for the Western Pacific, Malaria, Vector-borne and other Parasitic Diseases, Manila, Philippines

Jürg Utzinger
Department of Epidemiology and Public Health, Swiss Tropical and Public Health Institute, and University of Basel, Basel, Switzerland

A. Lee Willingham III
WHO/FAO Collaborating Center for Research and Training on Neglected and Other Parasitic Zoonoses, Section for Parasitology, Health and Development, Department of Veterinary Disease Biology, Faculty of Life Sciences, University of Copenhagen, Frederiksberg C, Denmark

Hai-Wei Wu
Department of Pathogen Biology, Nanjing Medical University, Nanjing, Jiangsu Province, People's Republic of China; Center for International Health Research, Rhode Island Hospital, Providence, Rhode Island, USA

Wei-Ping Wu
National Institute of Parasitic Diseases, Chinese Center for Disease Control and Prevention, Shanghai, People's Republic of China

Guo-Jing Yang
Jiangsu Institute of Parasitic Diseases, Wuxi, People's Republic of China

Kun Yang
Jiangsu Institute of Parasitic Diseases, Wuxi, People's Republic of China

Yi Zhang
National Institute of Parasitic Diseases, Chinese Center for Disease Control and Prevention, Shanghai, People's Republic of China

Feng Zheng
National Institute of Parasitic Diseases, Chinese Center for Disease Control and Prevention, Shanghai, People's Republic of China

Xiao-Nong Zhou
National Institute of Parasitic Diseases, Chinese Center for Disease Control and Prevention, Shanghai, People's Republic of China

FOREWORD

Based on the high level of both current research and control activity, we decided to dedicate two special volumes of *Advances in Parasitology* to helminth infections of Southeast Asia. Our aim has been to provide an authoritative overview of the current situation and most importantly to identify areas that need greater effort. Our highly motivated guest editors, Xiao-Nong Zhou (National Institute of Parasitic Diseases, Chinese Center for Disease Control and Prevention, Shanghai, People's Republic of China), Robert Bergquist (Ingerod, Brastad, Sweden), Remigio Olveda (Department of Health, Research Institute of Tropical Medicine, Manila, Philippines) and Jürg Utzinger (Department of Epidemiology and Public Health, Swiss Tropical and Public Health Institute, Basel, Switzerland), have used their considerable skills and knowledge to ensure that these volumes provide an exceptional insight into the current situation. By bringing together a panel of international experts and leaders in research and control, they have succeeded in providing a comprehensive information source for this important topic. We very much hope that the two volumes will further stimulate others to participate and help control some of these very debilitating parasitic infections.

David Rollinson and Simon I. Hay

PREFACE

These two volumes of *Advances in Parasitology* cover the major parasitic helminths in Southeast Asia and the People's Republic of China (P.R. China). The reasons for publishing these volumes, I believe, are the remarkable importance of these parasites in almost every country of the region, and the great progress achieved in the past few decades on research and control of the diseases in some of the countries.

It is well recognised that health bears a critical contribution to the social and economic well-beings of individuals and communities. Numerous examples reveal that poverty and ill-health interact with each other both as a cause and as an effect, which is why Southeast Asia has been one of a few most important endemic regions for the helminths and accounts for a large proportion of the global disease burden.

Referred to in the volumes are helminthiases, which are either water-borne, food-borne, mosquito-borne or soil-transmitted. They have had, and continue to have, a dramatic impact on the health of the people and of livestock. The chapters provide updated information on disease epidemiology, pathogenesis and control, and they also highlight insights of particular concern. For instance, the socioeconomically marginalised population groups in Southeast Asia and southern P.R. China are often ethnic minorities, whose characteristic cultural, social and behavioural risk factors are contributory to the prevalence of the diseases. Drug development, vaccine research and application of geospatial health techniques are comprehensively reviewed. The health metrics issue in parasitic infections is also discussed, as the measurement of the morbidity has long been an unsolved issue due to their chronic, insidious and frequently asymptomatic features. Application of biotechnology in the research of genomics, proteomics, transcriptomics and metabonomics is providing extraordinary approaches to a better understanding of the biology of the helminths and their interactions with their hosts. People expect further development of novel tools for control interventions based on the "–omics" information. Knowledge gaps are highlighted and research needs are described in a number of chapters.

Partnership plays an essential role in combating these diseases regionally and internationally. The Regional Network on Asian Schistosomiasis and Other Helminth Zoonoses ($RNAS^+$) are excellent examples for establishing regional collaboration in research management, capacity building and possible coordination of control activities such as in the Mekong subregion.

In the last few years, the World Health Organization (WHO) and the international community have paid special attention to the neglected tropical diseases including these helminthiases. Even though the conditions are still challenging, this is the time to take action in combating these diseases because we now have the powerful and cost-effective tools and tested strategies for most of the infections. Furthermore, the socioeconomic development, including poverty alleviation in the poor populations, is improving access to safe water, better sanitation and housing, which are conducive to prevent the infections. It is indeed encouraging that the neglected tropical diseases are back in policy focus after decades of substantial neglect.

As a huge public health problem in P.R. China, lymphatic filariasis was rampant in most of the populated provinces. Due to the strenuous efforts over the past five decades, the country has declared the national elimination of the disease with WHO's certification in 2008. Therefore, we have reasons to believe that with a dedicated political commitment and available resources in all the countries, people will be able to effectively control the diseases, if not eliminate them in a foreseeable period of time.

Yu Sen-Hai

CHAPTER 1

Important Helminth Infections in Southeast Asia: Diversity, Potential for Control and Prospects for Elimination

Jürg Utzinger,[*,†] **Robert Bergquist,**[‡] **Remigio Olveda,**[§] and **Xiao-Nong Zhou**[¶]

Contents

* Department of Epidemiology and Public Health, Swiss Tropical and Public Health Institute, Basel, Switzerland
† University of Basel, Basel, Switzerland
‡ Ingerod, Brastad, Sweden
§ Department of Health, Research Institute for Tropical Medicine (RITM), Muntinlupa, Manila, Philippines
¶ National Institute of Parasitic Diseases, Chinese Center for Disease Control and Prevention, Shanghai, People's Republic of China

Advances in Parasitology, Volume 72
ISSN 0065-308X, DOI: 10.1016/S0065-308X(10)72001-7

Abstract

Besides the 'big three'—HIV/AIDS, malaria and tuberculosis—there are a host of diseases that, by comparison, are truly neglected. These so-called neglected tropical diseases (NTDs), many of which caused by helminths, are intimately linked with poverty and are rampant where housing is poor; access to clean water and adequate sanitation is lacking; hygiene and nutrition is substandard and populations are marginalised and vulnerable. More than a billion people are affected by NTDs, mainly in remote rural and deprived urban settings of the developing world. An overview of papers published in two special thematic volumes of the *Advances in Parasitology* is provided here under the umbrella of current status of research and control of important helminth infections. A total of 25 comprehensive reviews are presented, which summarise the latest available data pertaining to the diagnosis, epidemiology, pathogenesis, prevention, treatment, control and eventual elimination of NTDs in Southeast Asia and neighbourhood countries. The focus of the first volume provides the current regional status of schistosomiasis, lymphatic filariasis, food-borne trematodiases, echinococcosis and cysticercosis/taeniasis, less common parasitic diseases that can cause epidemic outbreaks and helminth infections affecting the central nervous system. The second volume deals with the tools and strategies for control, including diagnostics, drugs, vaccines and cutting-edge basic research (e.g. the '–omics' sciences). Moreover, cross-cutting themes such as multiparasitism, social sciences, capacity strengthening, geospatial health technologies, health metrics and modelling the potential impact of climate change on helminthic diseases are discussed. Hopefully, these two volumes will become useful for researchers and, most importantly, disease control managers for integrated and sustainable control, rigorous monitoring and eventual elimination of NTDs in Southeast Asia and elsewhere.

1.1. INTRODUCTION

Over the past 15 years, the world has witnessed growing awareness, unprecedented local commitment and political will, the formation of numerous public–private partnerships and the forging of strategic alliances which, together, provide the necessary human, financial and technical means to combat the 'big three', that is HIV/AIDS, malaria and tuberculosis. For example, in the latest report from the Global Fund to Fight AIDS, Tuberculosis and Malaria (the Global Fund in short), it is estimated that, since its establishment in 2002 until the end of 2009, a total of 4.9 million lives have been saved through programmes with a financial envelope of US $ 19.2 billion (The Global Fund to Fight AIDS, Tuberculosis and Malaria, 2010). Indeed, the human population is not only larger than ever before but, on average, also healthier (e.g. measured by average life expectancy) and new ambitious goals have been articulated, for example the eradication of malaria (Anonymous, 2007; Greenwood et al., 2008; Hall and Fauci, 2009). Yet, more work remains to be done, particularly with regard to the prevention, control, local elimination and eventual eradication of the so-called neglected tropical diseases (NTDs). Approximately 16% of the world's population suffers from one or more of these NTDs which, in the words of Dr. Margaret Chan, Director-General of the World Health Organization (WHO), during her 2007 David E. Barmes Global Health Lecture in Bethesda, USA, is "...ancient debilitating diseases strongly associated with poverty. They thrive in areas where water supply and sanitation are inadequate, vectors proliferate, housing is substandard, nutrition is poor and populations are illiterate. These diseases sap the productivity and curtail the human potential of at least one billion people who are the poorest of the poor" (Chan, 2007).

Recent estimates suggest that the NTDs are responsible for over half a million deaths every year and a global burden in excess of 50 million disability-adjusted life years (DALYs) lost annually (Hotez et al., 2006). Awareness of the intimate connection between NTDs and poverty has a long history. For example, a century ago, the Rockefeller Sanitary Commission embarked on the elimination of hookworm disease in the southern parts of the United States (Anonymous, 1909), in an effort to boost the country's regional economic, political and cultural developments (Brown, 1976). After decades of neglect, finally, there is growing interest in the control of NTDs on a local, regional and global scale, not only because of economic, social and human developments, but also because of human rights and equity considerations (Brady et al., 2006; Daar et al., 2007; Hotez, 2008; Hotez et al., 2009; King, 2010a; Lammie et al., 2006; Maudlin et al., 2009; Miguel and Kremer, 2004; Morel et al., 2005; Yaïch, 2009). For example, progress towards achieving the millennium development goals (MDGs) crucially depends on advances made in the prevention, control and eventual elimination of the NTDs as public health problems (May, 2007; Molyneux, 2008). Thanks to the growing awareness of the global burden of NTDs being grossly underestimated and mounting advocacy, the prospects for their control are finally changing for the better, although these changes have yet to be fully translated into political will and commitment with adequate human and financial resources and technical means for prevention, control and elimination (Fenwick, 2006; Hotez et al., 2006, 2007; Lammie et al., 2006; Singer and Castro, 2007; Utzinger et al., 2009). It is in this connection important to further our understanding of the epidemiology of the NTDs, so that multi-pronged, setting-specific and integrated approaches can be deployed to make a durable impact against them, which, in turn, would improve health, equity and well-being.

Here, an overview is provided of two special thematic volumes of the *Advances in Parasitology* pertaining to the epidemiology and control of

NTDs in Southeast Asia and neighbourhood countries. Short prefaces are setting the scene for each volume leading up to the centre piece of 25 comprehensive reviews. These reviews summarise the latest available information on the diagnosis, epidemiology, pathogenesis, prevention, treatment, control and elimination of NTDs. Particular consideration has been given to schistosomiasis, lymphatic filariasis, food-borne trematodiases, echinococcosis and cysticercosis/taeniasis. Less common parasitic diseases that can cause epidemic outbreaks (e.g. capillariasis and trichinellosis), helminth infections affecting the central nervous system (e.g. angiostrongyliasis and gnathostomiasis) and the issue of multi-parasitism are also discussed. The cutting-edge '-omics' sciences are reviewed, including genomics, proteomics, transcriptomics and metabonomics. Several chapters focus on cross-cutting themes, such as capacity strengthening through existing networks, for example Regional Network of Asian Schistosomiasis and other Zoonotic Helminthiasis (RNAS$^+$), exploring links between the NTDs and ethnic minority groups, discussing the role of the social sciences, current challenges in estimating the regional and global NTD burden, development and application of geospatial health technologies and modelling a potential impact of climate change on helminthic diseases. Given the importance of an accurate diagnosis, adequate patient management and large-scale control of helminthiases by means of preventive chemotherapy, separate reviews pertaining to diagnosis and drugs have been prepared. It seems, at least for some of the NTDs discussed here, that vaccines are needed along with other preventive and curative measures to ultimately achieve local elimination, and hence a separate vaccine review is presented. The 25 chapters have been prepared by 69 experts, the majority of whom based in Asia. Most of the chapters are multi-authored, demonstrating the breath and depth of the existing partnerships between universities, research institutions and disease control managers in disease-endemic countries of Southeast Asia and abroad.

1.2. TWO THEMATIC VOLUMES OF THE *ADVANCES IN PARASITOLOGY*

1.2.1. An idea originating in the ancient city of Lijiang

The original idea of this project stems from two meetings, held back-to-back, in September 2007 in the ancient city of Lijiang, Yunnan province, People's Republic of China (P.R. China). Summary reports are available both for the 7th RNAS$^+$ meeting (Zhou et al., 2008a) and the 1st International Symposium on Geospatial Health (Zhou et al., 2009). Six oral presentations from these two meetings were selected for publication in a special section of *Parasitology International*:

- Leonardo et al. (2008) summarising results from a prevalence survey of *Schistosoma japonicum* in two areas of the Philippines, where control of schistosomiasis proved particularly challenging;
- Wu et al. (2008) pursuing a retrospective analysis of the effect of floods on the transmission of *S. japonicum* in the Yangtze River valley of P.R. China;
- Garjito et al. (2008) describing the past and current epidemiological situations of schistosomiasis in Indonesia;
- Lin et al. (2008) performing an in-depth investigation of the diagnostic accuracy of the widely used Kato-Katz technique, concluding that single thick smears considerably under-estimate the prevalence of *S. japonicum* in settings characterised by low-infection intensity;
- Attwood et al. (2008) presenting phylogenetic data of *Neotricula aperta*, the only intermediate host snail of *Schistosoma mekongi*, to understand the past, present and potential future distributions of schistosomiasis in Cambodia and Lao People's Democratic Republic (Lao PDR); and
- Conlan et al. (2008) reviewing the scarce data currently available regarding taeniasis and cysticercosis in Lao PDR, and calling for new research, including standardised community-based surveys.

Additionally, three oral presentations focusing on the spatial distribution of *S. japonicum* and its intermediate host snail *Oncomelania hupensis* within a single county (i.e. Eryuan in Yunnan province) and the spatio-temporal distribution and changing patterns of both human and bovine schistosomiasis japonica across P.R. China were published (Steinmann et al., 2007; Wu et al., 2007; Yang et al., 2009).

The two meetings convened in Lijiang were attended by over 100 scientists and disease control managers primarily from Asia, but collaborators from Australia, Europe and North America and invited guests from Africa also participated. It was the largest RNAS$^+$ meeting held thus far, which shows the increasingly important role of the network in strengthening local and regional co-operations and facilitating exchange of expertise and experiences pertaining to the epidemiology and control of NTDs in Southeast Asia and neighbourhood countries. The African colleagues were invited to stimulate their thinking about how to render the recently established Research Network for Schistosomiasis in Africa (RNSA) more visible and vibrant.

1.2.2. Action towards collaboration and partnership in an enabling environment

When contacted in October 2008, Drs David Rollinson and Simon Hay, the editors-in-chief of the *Advances in Parasitology*, were open to our proposal of producing a major piece pertaining to the NTDs in Southeast Asia.

Their colleagues at Elsevier, Narmada Thangavelu, the development editor, and Lisa Tickner, the publisher, agreed to go along with this idea. Once the depth and breath of the 25 chapters became obvious (e.g. two of the submitted manuscripts were 100+ double-spaced DIN A4 pages long), it was clear that our endeavour needed to be split into two separate volumes.

Before summarising the structure and main thrust of these two volumes, we must firmly acknowledge Drs Rollinson and Hay and their colleagues at Elsevier for their tireless efforts in moving the project along and for keeping us on track with regard to content as well as time. We also highly appreciate the editors and production staffs' patience, as the ultimate delivery of this umbrella piece was delayed by a few weeks. We express our deep gratitude to the many external referees who provided peer-review comments in a timely and constructive fashion. The huge scientific freedom, coupled with a lean, yet highly efficient, publishing environment and the existing collaboration and partnership were the key features that kept us motivated throughout this 18-month project. A big THANKS to all parties involved!

1.2.3. Nuts and bolts

Figure 1.1 provides 'an umbrella view' of the 25 chapters covered in volumes 72 and 73 of the *Advances in Parasitology*, which, together form an understanding of the epidemiology and control of NTDs with particular emphasis on Southeast Asia and neighbourhood countries. Each volume consists of a short preface; the first by Dr. Yu Sen-Hai, a former director of the National Institute of Parasitic Diseases (IPD), Chinese Center for Disease Control and Prevention (China CDC) in Shanghai, and the second by Dr. Robert Ridley, the current director of the Special Programme for Research and Training in Tropical Diseases (TDR). The 25 comprehensive reviews cover a vast territory reflecting the principles of 'translational medicine' as they describe the move from the bench to the field and clinical medicine, from the molecular to the spatial and systemic, and from basic science to operational research and integrated control. The most important results are summarised in Section 1.3 along with implications for the control and elimination of NTDs at a local, regional and global scale.

Three chapters are single-authored pieces (Attwood, 2010; King, 2010b; McManus, 2010), but the remaining 22 chapters underscore the collaborative approach with two contributions prepared by 11 authors each (Schratz et al., 2010; Yang et al., 2010) (Fig. 1.2A). Interestingly, almost four out of five chapters (76.9%) were prepared by scientists and disease control managers from Asia in partnership with authors from the industrialized countries in Europe, the United States and Australia

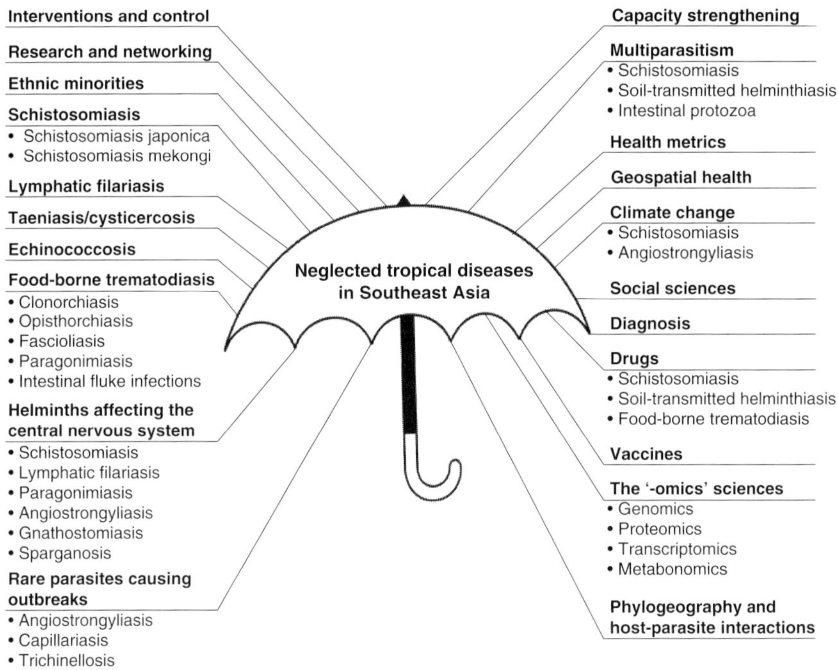

FIGURE 1.1 Umbrella showing the overall structure and main topics covered in two special thematic volumes of the *Advances in Parasitology* pertaining to the NTDs in Southeast Asia and neighbourhood countries (volume 72, left-hand side; volume 73, right-hand side).

(Fig. 1.2B). These collaborations and partnerships have partially been facilitated by the RNAS$^+$ network established in the late 1990s and involved in corralling the expertise needed to produce the present two volumes (Leonardo and Bergquist, 2002; Zhou et al., 2002, 2008a). Gender stratification reveals that 26 of the contributing authors (37.7%) are females (Fig. 1.2C). This percentage is considerably higher than that found in a 2003 analysis of gender composition of editorial boards of six leading general-medicine journals, which reported only 23% females (Keiser et al., 2003).

Figure 1.3 shows the results of a geographical analysis according to author affiliation. Two-thirds of the contributing authors are affiliated with universities, research institutions and disease-control organizations in Southeast Asia and neighbourhood countries. P.R. China represents the highest number of contributing authors ($n = 21.5$, i.e. 31.2%; of note, if an author is affiliated with two different countries, each country counts as half, which explains the figure 21.5), followed by the Philippines ($n = 13$, i.e. 18.8%). In most cases, the lead was taken by a colleague based in Asia and the majority of the senior authors are affiliated to universities,

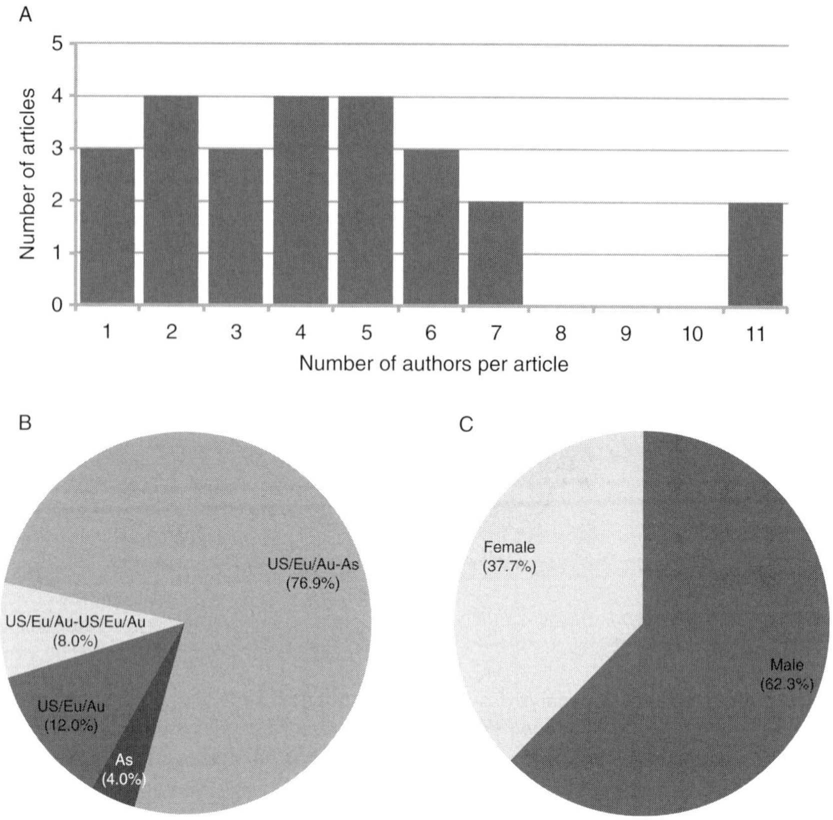

FIGURE 1.2 Bibliometric analysis of 25 reviews published in two special thematic volumes of the *Advances in Parasitology* pertaining to the NTDs in Southeast Asia. Depicted are (A) the number of articles according to the number of authors in each chapter, (B) collaboration and research partnerships stratified by different regions of the world (key: As = Asia, Au = Australia, Eu = Europe, US = United States of America) and (C) gender composition of the 69 contributing authors.

research institutions and disease control organizations in Asia. Many of the reviews represent long-standing research partnerships as the contributing authors have been collaborating for years within institutions that bridge the North–South gap. This is in contrast to findings obtained after an analysis of 2348 full-length articles, published between 2000 and 2002 in six leading tropical-medicine journals, where 48.1% of the contributing authors had affiliations in countries with a high human development index, whereas only 13.7% of the authors came from countries with a low human development index (Keiser et al., 2004). However, the articles of three previous, similar special issues of core parasitology and

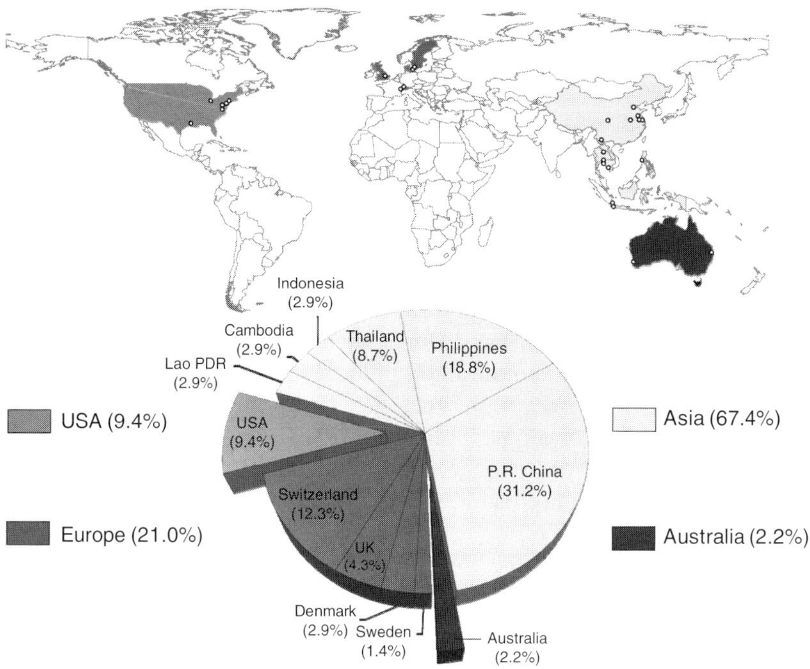

FIGURE 1.3 Geographical analysis, stratifying the 69 authors contributing one or several chapters to these two volumes of the *Advances in Parasitology* by their affiliations. Countries are highlighted with different grey shades to differentiate between Asia, Australia, Europe and the United States. The towns of the contributing authors' affiliations are highlighted with white dots. Of note, if an author is affiliated to two different countries (e.g. P.R. China and Switzerland), each country is counted half.

tropical-medicine journals also show a high representation of authors from the developing world, for example the overview of the control of schistosomiasis in P.R. China, published in *Acta Tropica* (Utzinger et al., 2005), the commemoration of 100 years of research and control of schistosomiasis in Brazil also put forth in *Acta Tropica* (Bergquist, 2008) and, most recently, a special issue of *Parasitology* reviewing and updating the epidemiology and control of schistosomiasis in sub-Saharan Africa (Stothard et al., 2009).

1.3. PROGRESS MADE IN RESEARCH AND CONTROL OF NTDs

1.3.1. The global landscape

Notable progress in the field of NTD control is multi-factorial with the Internet, public–private partnerships built around drug donation programmes and scientific networks as the more prominent new facets

(Hotez et al., 2007; Moran, 2005; Moran et al., 2009; Morel et al., 2005, 2009). When the 'World Wide Web' was launched in 1989, it marked the beginning of the 'world wide use' of the Internet that had so far been of limited service. However, Berners-Lee, then working at CERN, saw it as the solution to the need for information sharing across time and space (see http://www.ted.com/talks/tim_berners_lee_on_the_next_web.html). Although the approach first seemed to amount to putting the carriage before the horse as this need was neither widely perceived nor pronounced, but Berners-Lee foresaw its enormous potential and it is now obvious that without the 'Web', practical applications would have continued to lag common needs in spite of an ever increasing rate of scientific advances. Still, the difficulty of locating and managing the wealth of scientific articles is frustrating and today's searching, analysing, organizing and sharing new findings, bibliographic management in short, underline the importance of management and linking of data as well as translating scientific breakthroughs into policy briefs, so that they become of practical use.

If the 'Web' was the key for connection and information exchange, public–private partnerships play a seminal role for funding, advocacy and fostering control efforts (Maudlin et al., 2009; Molyneux, 2006; Savioli et al., 2002; Widdus, 2005). In retrospect, the collaboration between Merck & Co, the Mectizan Donation Program, WHO and the African Programme for Onchocerciasis Control (APOC) for the control of onchocerciasis in the late 1980s did not only help people with, and those at risk for, onchocerciasis, but also ushered in the very idea of public–private partnerships (Peters and Phillips, 2004; Sékétéli et al., 2002). This way of thinking led to increased integration with regard to NTD control (Brady et al., 2006; Fenwick, 2006; Lammie et al., 2006). As a consequence, control approaches are becoming less vertical, although integration of NTD control programmes, thus far, heavily rely on specific, preventive chemotherapy (Anonymous, 2004; Hotez et al., 2006, 2007, 2009; Reddy et al., 2007; Smits, 2009; WHO, 2006a). However, in order to achieve sustainable control of the NTDs, more integrated approaches are necessary, for example by further strengthening existing health systems and fostering inter-sectoral collaboration between, among others, the health, agriculture, education, financial and water resources sectors (Ehrenberg and Ault, 2005; Holveck et al., 2007; Singer and Castro, 2007; Utzinger and de Savigny, 2006; Utzinger et al., 2003; 2009). This is no news, rather good public health sense, backed up by historical evidence. Charles W. Stiles, for example, who was instrumental during the Rockefeller Sanitary Commission-led efforts against hookworms in the southern United States, concluded that the elimination of hookworm disease should be based on "20% thymol and Epsom salts [treatment] combined with 80% sanitation [prevention]" (Stiles, 1939). This conclusion, we believe, is as important today as it was many decades ago, and it is in this connection that we welcome thinking and action beyond deworming (Anonymous, 2004; Utzinger et al., 2009; Wang et al., 2009a,b).

International donor agencies now find it useful to work directly with pharmaceutical companies and private foundations as mentioned by Bergquist and Tanner (2010). This trend is growing and the last decade has seen the establishment of numerous global partnerships in the public health sector that address challenges such as the 'big three' (The Global Fund to Fight AIDS, Tuberculosis and Malaria, 2010), as well as deficiencies with respect to child and maternal health, nutrition and access to clean water and improved sanitation (Wahlqvist and Kuo, 2009; WHO and UNICEF, 2010). These new partnerships have not only raised the profile of health in general, but also generated unprecedented, financial resources now spilling over into the field of the NTDs. However, formidable challenges remain, as a result of the lack of readily available rapid assessment techniques for mapping the co-endemicity of multiple NTDs, as well as the diversity of disease control approaches and governance structures (Brooker et al., 2009; Kolaczinski et al., 2007; Liese et al., 2010; Sturrock et al., 2009; Utzinger and de Savigny, 2006). Of particular note is the *Global Network for Neglected Tropical Diseases (the Global Network in short; http://globalnetwork.org/).*

1.3.2. Regional advances: Southeast Asia and neighbourhood countries

1.3.2.1. Epidemiology and control of worms: then and now

Not only does Southeast Asia harbour all cases of schistosomiasis japonica (Zhou et al., 2010a), schistosomiasis mekongi (Muth et al., 2010) and the majority of food-borne trematode infections (Keiser and Utzinger, 2009; Sripa et al., 2010), but also one-third of the world's intestinal helminthiases (Hotez and Ehrenberg, 2010), a quarter of the global burden of lymphatic filariasis (Sudomo et al., 2010), and a multitude of less common parasitic infections that can produce outbreaks (Odermatt et al., 2010) or invade the central nervous system (Lv et al., 2010). Moreover, multiparasitism is the norm rather than the exception, although detailed investigations on the epidemiology, risk factors and clinical implications of multiple species helminth and intestinal protozoa infections are lacking (Ezeamama et al., 2005; Pullan and Brooker, 2008; Steinmann et al., 2008, 2010). Considering that Southeast Asia and the Western Pacific Region is also home to a very large number of marginalised, vulnerable population groups, control activities are a priority (Schratz et al., 2010). The epidemiology of many parasitic helminths is different from that of most other infections. For example, the risk an infected person (or animal reservoir host) carries for others is a direct function of the number of worms present in the definitive host, that is the intensity of infection (Anderson and May, 1985). This important issue, highlighted by a family of life cycles collected at the back of volume 1, is the key to unravel our 'wormy world' and has important ramifications for control.

We have moved a long way since 'this wormy world' was first minted in the late 1940s (Stoll, 1947), or have we? In fact, it must be stated that, in spite of vast amounts of new knowledge coming from the development and application of mathematical modelling, molecular biology and the '-omics' sciences, the old appraisal of the wormy world still stands and the various helminth infections still exist much as they did more than 60 years ago when Norman R. Stoll delivered his keynote address to the American Society of Parasitologists (Bethony et al., 2006; Brooker and Utzinger, 2007; Bundy and de Silva, 1998; Crompton, 1999; Hotez and Ehrenberg, 2010; Keiser and Utzinger, 2010). Stoll (1947) did not mince his words when calling for parasitic diseases to be brought under control. However, the task is far from straightforward, since behavioural, cultural, demographic, ecologic, economic, environmental, political, scientific and social factors have derailed efforts until the present time. The elimination of lymphatic filariasis from P.R. China (Lammie et al., 2007; WHO, 2006b) may be the turning point the scientific community and public health experts have been waiting for.

In paying tribute to Stoll's seminal piece, two important papers published in the late 1990s (Bundy and de Silva, 1998; Crompton, 1999) pointed out that the public health significance of helminth infections is far greater than generally acknowledged. Along with the availability of inexpensive, safe and efficacious anthelminthic drugs that can be administered by non-health personnel after minimal training (Savioli et al., 2002; WHO 2006a), this contributed more than anything else to pave the way for the current large-scale control programmes. As mentioned before, international agencies are joining forces with private foundations and industry to manage human helminth infections targeting all the major helminthiases. Apart from the Mectizan Donation Program and APOC, the Bill and Melinda Gates Foundation (BMGF; http://www.gatesfoundation.org), the United States Agency for International Development (USAID; http://www.usaid.gov) and other aid organizations are working in union supporting specialized programmes as for example the Schistosomiasis Control Initiative (SCI; http://www.sci-ntds.org/) and the Global Network to realize the MDGs (http://www.un.org/millenniumgoals/) of sustainable poverty reduction. These activities are now becoming more integrated, targeting several diseases concurrently in many countries (Fenwick, 2006; Fenwick et al., 2009; Lammie et al., 2006; Smits, 2009; Utzinger et al., 2009). Thus, optimism over the prospects for control is no longer misplaced and the new movements in 'this wormy world' of ours remind us of the need to tackle the 'unremittingly corrosive' burden of helminth infections (Stoll, 1947).

Hence, an important issue of volumes 72 and 73 of the *Advances in Parasitology* is to boost interest in research on, and concerted control efforts against, helminth infections that dominate the disease spectrum in many parts of Southeast Asia and other parts of the world (Bethony et al., 2006; Hotez and Ehrenberg, 2010; Hotez et al., 2008). Much space has been devoted to the epidemiology and control of Asian schistosomiasis (Attwood, 2010; Bergquist and Tanner, 2010; Muth et al., 2010; Xiao et al., 2010; Zhou et al., 2010a), which makes sense from public health and economic points of view. Additionally, after lymphatic filariasis, *S. japonicum* may become the second major parasite infection to be eliminated in P.R. China (Wang et al., 2009a). Historically, judging from the absolute numbers of infected people, the schistosomiasis problem seems to have been worse in P.R. China than in the Philippines (Bergquist and Tanner, 2010). The big difference in cross-country, average prevalence that can be calculated (2% in P.R. China versus 8.6% in the Philippines) does not say more than that a comparatively smaller part of the latter country was endemic than the former. In the first decade of the new millennium, we find that the situation still holds, but the figures have changed even more to the advantage of P.R. China (<0.1% versus 0.6% in the Philippines). Although this again may mainly reflect that the former country has managed to reduce the extent of the endemic areas more than the latter, the bottom line is that both countries have reduced the number of people infected with *S. japonicum*, even in the face of strong population growth.

The analysis by Zhou et al. (2010a) not only reveals the importance of integrated control approaches for sustaining the advances achieved in schistosomiasis control to date, but also the need for flexible control approaches and innovation. It is in this connection more than just interesting to learn that Chinese farmers are spearheading the march into the industrial society by exchanging tractors for their water buffaloes (Wang et al., 2009a). Since it has been shown that domestic animals contribute more to sustain transmission than humans (Gray et al., 2009; Wang et al., 2005), this move will lower the risk of transmission of schistosomiasis, at the same time as it on balance might reduce the release of greenhouse gases (Zhou et al., 2008b). However, the current biggest hurdle for further progress are remaining pockets of high transmission, and compliance for repeated preventive chemotherapy (Guo et al., 2005) critically depends on a deeper understanding of people's perception and beliefs of schistosomiasis and practises to prevent and control the disease (Vandemark et al., 2010), a better appreciation of the 'true' burden of schistosomiasis (King, 2010b) and more sensitive diagnostics (Johansen et al., 2010) and rigorous surveillance.

Apart from the presence of *S. japonicum* in P.R. China, the Philippines and in limited foci in Indonesia (Zhou et al., 2010a), *S. mekongi* in Cambodia and Lao PDR should be noted, as this type of schistosomiasis is particularly aggressive with severe organ involvement and a high mortality rate if left untreated (Muth et al., 2010). Prior to 1999, transmission of *S. mekongi* was thought to be restricted to a 300 km section of the Mekong River between Khong Island in Lao PDR and Kratié in Cambodia. The range of both the parasites and its intermediate host snail *N. aperta* are now known to be much larger, with the snail found across central Lao PDR and eastern Cambodia and the parasites also occurring in two additional river systems of eastern Cambodia (Attwood, 2010; Attwood et al., 2004). The distribution of *N. aperta* outside the specific conditions of Mekong River has already raised the estimated population at risk by more than a factor 10 (Attwood et al., 2008), but its wider tolerance indicates that the new figure of 1.5 million might still be an underestimation. Indeed, Attwood (2010) argues that the current absence of *S. mekongi* from most of Lao PDR can be due to reasons other than any ecological barrier. If he is correct, it is conceivable that the invasion of much of Lao PDR by *S. mekongi* is just a question of time. Major water resources development and management (i.e. construction of large hydroelectric dams and expansion of irrigation systems) might further exacerbate the risk of *S. mekongi* in Lao PDR (Erlanger et al., 2008).

No discussion on trematode infections would be complete without examining the food-borne trematodiases, particularly as many of these infections only occur in Southeast Asia (Keiser and Utzinger, 2009). *Clonorchis sinensis*, with an estimated 35 million infections, is the predominant species and clonorchiasis is considered as an emerging infectious disease (Lun et al., 2005; Keiser and Utzinger, 2005, 2009). The estimated number of infections with *Paragonimus* spp. and *Opisthorchis viverrini* are 20.7 million and 10 million, respectively (Keiser and Utzinger, 2009). There are a host of intestinal flukes such as *Fasciolopsis buski*, the echinostomes and the *Heterophyidae*, which are among the most neglected of the NTDs, although some of these infections are fatal (Sripa et al., 2010).

Fifteen million people with lymphatic filariasis live in Southeast Asia. This disease is not only interesting from a scientific point of view but also, in particular, it represents a parasitic disease that has recently been eliminated in P.R. China. When Dr. Chan, Director-General of WHO, in a ceremony in early October 2008 in Beijing congratulated P.R. China for its success in having eliminated this parasitic disease as a public health problem, it was a turning point, not only in the fight against lymphatic filariasis but also for all major parasitic diseases. Dr. Chan noted the crucially important role of the Global Alliance to Eliminate Lymphatic Filariasis (GAELF), which was established as a result of the 1997 World Health Assembly (WHA) resolution 50.29, calling for worldwide elimination of lymphatic filariasis as a public health problem by 2020. It is of interest to be able to follow the activities of the Chinese lymphatic filariasis control project, which started 60 years ago and chronicled in considerable depth by Sudomo et al. (2010). It is encouraging to note that the elimination activities in the surrounding countries where lymphatic filariasis is still endemic are also registering major progress (WHO, 2006b, 2009) and 2020, the target year for its final elimination, seems realistic.

Neurocysticercosis, the most serious form of *Taenia solium* infection, is considered the most preventable cause of epilepsy in the developing world (Lv et al., 2010; Sinha and Sharma, 2009; Willingham and Engels, 2006; Willingham et al., 2010). Although theoretically easy to control, there is a lack of information on the burden and transmission of the disease, partially explained by the unavailability of high-quality diagnostic tools in field-applicable formats. The presence, distribution, public health importance and economic relevance of cysticercosis need to be better documented in Southeast Asia in order to bring it to the attention of affected communities, decision makers and funding bodies alike.

1.3.2.2. DALYs and QALYs

During the September 2007 RNAS$^+$ meeting, held in Lijiang, P.R. China, a training workshop focussing on general and region-specific issues of disease burdens was part of the agenda (Zhou et al., 2008a). This issue is at the heart of elimination discussions and the most recent RNAS$^+$ meeting, which took place in October 2009 in Vientiane, Lao PDR, called attention for concerted efforts to estimate the global burden of food-borne trematodiasis. Indeed, no burden estimates are currently available for the major food-borne trematode infections (Hotez et al., 2006; Keiser and Utzinger, 2009). This is all the more surprising as the causative agents of *opisthorchiasis (i.e. O. viverrini*) and clonorchiasis (i.e. *C. sinensis*) are established risk factors for cholangiocarcinoma (Keiser and Utzinger, 2009; Sripa, 2008; Sripa et al., 2007, 2010). The burden of NTDs is vastly higher in Southeast Asia than previously recognised, but the impact of these diseases is difficult to pin down as it includes parameters above the simple number of people infected by a particular infection. Although the DALY metrics (Murray and Lopez, 1996) was a huge step forward from simple mortality figures, weaknesses of this approach have been pointed out (King, 2010a; King and Bertino, 2008; King et al., 2005). It is emphasised here that the DALY metrics is not always helpful, particularly not with regard to chronic diseases such as schistosomiasis and multiple species helminth infections (King, 2010b). Moreover, disability weights, as employed in the initial global burden of disease (GBD) studies by Murray and Lopez (1996), were based on expert opinion. With regard to schistosomiasis, very low disability weights were assigned, that is 0.005–0.006 on a scale from 0 (i.e. perfect health) to 1 (i.e. death). Recent investigations challenge these disability weights and speculate that the actual disabilities due to chronic schistosomiasis japonica are more than one or even two orders of magnitude higher (Finkelstein et al., 2008; Jia et al., 2007).

The quality-adjusted life year (QALY) seems to better capture the impact of helminthic infections that are characterised by subtle morbidities and long-term chronicity. First experiences with standardised, self-rated quality of life questionnaires have been presented for echinococcosis on the Tibetan Plateau (Budke et al., 2005) and chronic schistosomiasis japonica in P.R. China (Jia et al., 2007). However, there is controversy about how accurately QALYs reflect preferences for health care in other situations, for example in industrialised countries. The debate regarding the use of QALYs in countries at various levels of development has been reviewed (Neumann and Greenberg, 2009). Although this discussion may appear academic, the appreciation of the link between long-term, parasite-mediated inflammation, impact on the course and outcomes of pregnancy, impaired physical and cognitive development during childhood and poor work performance at older age is critical. For example, the QALY highlights evidence of great importance for decision makers such as choosing preventive over curative intervention. Health metrics is gaining in importance and occupies today, together with diagnostics, which strongly influences the appreciation of the 'true' burden of disease (Johansen et al., 2010), a decisive position how to proceed with regard to the diseases at hand.

1.3.2.3. Diagnostics, drugs and vaccines

Chemotherapy-based control programmes significantly reduce the prevalence and intensity of infection and NTD-related morbidity. Hence, preventive chemotherapy is promoted as a rapid impact strategy and has been suggested as a highly cost-effective public health intervention (Hotez et al., 2006, 2007, 2009; Molyneux et al., 2005; WHO, 2006a). Whilst progress in morbidity control due to NTDs through large-scale administration of drugs is laudable, some authors have argued that this success hindered progress in research and development of new drugs, diagnostics and vaccines (Bergquist et al., 2009; Caffrey, 2007; Cioli, 1998; Keiser and Utzinger, 2007; Utzinger et al., 2007). Preventive chemotherapy not only runs the risk of having to be continued indefinitely, but also of inducing drug resistance without the long-term protection a vaccine can offer as complementary intervention (Bergquist et al., 2005; 2008; McManus and Loukas, 2008; Utzinger et al., 2009). Facing the problem that long-term drug treatment represents a continuous expense and risk for drug resistance development, a new goal of vaccine development has been proposed (Bergquist et al., 2005; Bergquist and Lustigman, 2010), that is the integrated drug–vaccine approach. This aims at reposting vaccines from stand-alone tools to adjuncts to chemotherapy. Thus, rather than inducing sterilizing immunity, the new role of vaccination would be to introduce a long-term component into control programmes, thus reducing the likelihood of transmission and re-infection, and lowering the risk of drug resistance development and spread.

By considering the fact that sustained work on vaccine development over many years, notably in the fields of hookworm infection, leishmaniasis, malaria, onchocerciasis and schistosomiasis, effective vaccines are becoming more credible, particularly as experiments in animal models have shown strong promise and several prototype anti-parasite vaccines are entering clinical trials. Additionally, the transmission-blocking approach, that is vaccination of reservoir host animals, has been successful even up to the point of provisional registration of a pig vaccine aiming at breaking the transmission of cysticercosis in humans (Rickard et al., 1995). Several other vaccines also mark a promising step in the whole progress of vaccine development, for example, the immunological control of *Fasciola* in sheep and cattle is within reach and this might have spill-over effects on human schistosomiasis (Tendler and Simpson, 2008). In addition, highly effective, recombinant vaccines have already been developed for the prevention of *Taenia ovis* in sheep, *T. saginata* in cattle, *T. solium* in pigs and *Echinococcus granulosus* in livestock (Lightowlers, 2006). Indeed, transmission-blocking *S. japonicum* vaccines are already in field trials and have shown good results (Da'dara et al., 2008; McManus et al., 2009, 2010). The current accumulation of molecular data and expansion of parasite sequence databases are providing a fresh start by permitting a more rational approach to vaccine discovery and development. Therefore, it is likely that a range of new vaccines can be expected during the next few years. A strong move forward in this field would be facilitated if international donor organizations and private foundations could agree on a joint, major NTD vaccine initiative (Bergquist and Lustigman, 2010).

The global strategy for the control of helminth infections have two, not mutually exclusive and sequential goals, that is morbidity control, followed by elimination as a threat to public health. Clearly, over the past decade, particularly so in areas where helminthiases are highly endemic, the focus has been on the former (WHO, 2006a), but we are now turning to the latter in some parts of the world as new drugs and optimised administration of old ones have worked together to significantly reduce morbidity (Bergquist et al., 2009). The definitive review of anti-schistosomal drugs in P.R. China is presented by Xiao et al. (2010) who summarise the past 60 years of research and development in this field. Whilst praziquantel remains the drug of choice against schistosomiasis, the artemisinins and related compounds have been developed for 'chemoprophylaxis', because these drugs—best know for their anti-malarial properties—are able to prevent the development of egg-laying patent schistosome infections. A second comprehensive review focuses on the current drugs against soil-transmitted helminthiases and food-borne trematodiases and discusses the latest findings with the cyclooctadepsipeptides, monepantel, nitazoxandide and tribendimidine, which might become the next generation of anthelminthic drugs (Keiser and Utzinger, 2010).

In any event, while regular administration of anthelminthic drugs to school-aged children and other people at high risk of morbidity serves as the backbone of interventions in the endemic areas, development of new diagnostics and vaccines has been somewhat put on the backburner due to the excellent efficacy and safety profiles of drug treatment (Bergquist and Lustigman, 2010). However, not only should we think about the need for concerted efforts to discover, develop and deploy the next generation of anthelminthic drugs, but also think how vaccine development can be brought to the fore and how a strategy based on integrated approaches can be forged.

1.3.2.4. The '–omics' sciences

Huge progress has been made over the past 20+ years in the area of the '–omics' sciences, including genomics, proteomics, transcriptomics and metabolic profiling in this wormy world, as reviewed for the *Advances in Parasitology* by Ju et al. (2010) and Wang et al. (2010). For example, we now dispose of the full genome sequences of multiple helminth species, including *S. japonicum* (*Schistosoma japonicum* Genome Sequencing and Functional Analysis Consortium, 2009). Moreover, the global metabolic responses of the hamster to an experimental infection with *S. japonicum*, the hookworm species *Necator americanus* and a co-infection with both parasites concurrently have been characterised (Wang et al., 2006, 2009c; Wu et al., 2010). Results obtained from the '–omics' sciences offer new insights into early events in the evolution of animals and co-evolution of host–parasite systems, will guide a more rationale approach for drug and vaccines target identification, and hence assist the research community in the development of new tools and strategies for the control and elimination of NTDs (Berriman et al., 2009; *Schistosoma japonicum* Genome Sequencing and Functional Analysis Consortium, 2009).

1.3.2.5. Geospatial health technologies

The development of geographical information systems (GIS) together with remote sensing and spatially-explicit risk mapping and prediction provides powerful tools to further our understanding of the frequency and transmission patterns of NTDs, which, in turn, can improve the efficiency of interventions and integrated disease control (Bergquist and Rinaldi, 2010; Clements et al., 2008; Simoonga et al., 2009; Yang et al., 2005).

Geospatial health technologies are also crucial for surveillance, particularly for disease control programmes as they shift the emphasis from morbidity control to transmission control and ultimately elimination. Malone et al. (2010) show the strengths of using a GIS approach for collating, storing and queering of data and displaying disease risk maps, which can be used for several purposes, such as identifying epidemiological risk factors and detection of 'hot spots' for disease transmission. The potential impact of climate change on helminth infections, with two case studies pertaining to angiostrongyliasis and schistosomiasis in P.R. China, is discussed by Yang et al. (2010). The authors employed biology-based models and speculate that predictive capabilities might be further enhanced by expanding these biology-based models to include also ecological and socio-cultural aspects, similar to recent experiences made with dengue (Arunachalam et al., 2010).

Spatially-explicit modelling of helminth infections has not only opened the door for improving forecasting regarding transmission patterns, but also provided predictive maps on how to improve communication between different stakeholders, decision makers and the public. Thus far, however, no organization on a national level has stepped to the forefront with a comprehensive response that provides for an integrated reporting structure that enables timely data collection and assessment, and promotes rapid communication with key organizations and the public. On the other hand, the thematic guide to social science applications of remote sensing, published by the Center for International Earth Science Information Network (CIESIN), shows that the utility of remote sensing can be broadened to include also the social sciences (de Sherbinin et al., 2002).

1.3.2.6. Capability strengthening, teaching and training

In order to successfully deal with the current challenges in Southeast Asia and neighbourhood countries with respect to the NTDs and to prioritise research and control efforts, it is important to understand the role of scientific networks. This issue is discussed by Olveda et al. (2010) who present the RNAS$^+$ as a model for other similar initiatives. The potential of network analysis has also been emphasised for the strategic planning, implementation and management of a programme pertaining to research, development and capacity building of NTDs in Brazil (Morel et al., 2009). The process of successfully embedding research into the health systems of developing countries calls for input from international research institutions and the participation of competent national scientists with local experience and expertise. The role of applied social sciences as a resource for capacity strengthening, teaching and training for research and control of NTDs discussed by Vandemark et al. (2010) complements recent reviews on the social sciences for an enhanced understanding of the epidemiology and control of NTDs (Aagaard-Hansen et al., 2009; Huang and Manderson, 2005).

The infrastructure to improve the control programme of helminthiases is presented by Zhou et al. (2010b) and Malone et al. (2010) in terms of capability strengthening, training and teaching in epidemiology. These papers emphasise that not only the choice of model for research capacity building is an issue of the resources needed but it is also obvious that the results depend on the level of maturity of the national disease control programmes. Three models were proposed to be used in capacity strengthening in the region through (i) existing networks, (ii) international partnership and (iii) current infrastructure of operational research. Apart from RNAS^{+}, the two existing networks in Southeast Asia in the field of tropical medicine are the TROPMED Network of the Southeast Asian Ministers of Education Organization (SAMEO) and the Asian Collaborative Training Network for Malaria (ACTMalaria). International partners in the region are encouraged to integrate their activities with regard to existing programmes as this would facilitate and improve efficiency, effectiveness and delivery in the capacity building as well as health interventions. This is the trend of a new type of collaboration in which international donor agencies work together with commercial, pharmaceutical companies and private foundations, such as the BMGF (Hotez et al., 2007).

TDR' new strategy to deal with challenges arising from the impact on health of NTDs, emerging and re-emerging infectious diseases and climate change has translated into the idea of fostering an effective global research effort on infectious diseases of poverty. Stakeholder consultation in disease-endemic countries is an integral part to govern and prioritise the research agenda. Support for the development of networks that can be sustained in accelerating critical research and management skills in disease-endemic countries is emphasised in the quest to strengthen the capacity of endemic countries for research. For example, implementation of a geospatial health infrastructure in Southeast Asia will mainly depend on robust training programmes for health workers active in different institutions, for example Ministries of Health (MoH), non-governmental organizations (NGOs) and other health organizations involved in research and geospatial health operational applications (Leonardo et al., 2007). Under the auspices of the Global Network for Geospatial Health, a 'training node' entitled the 'International School of Geospatial Health', has been established to offer standardised short courses at IPD in Shanghai. Similar units at the Research Institute for Tropical Medicine (RITM) in the Philippines, the University of the Philippines and the Mekong Institute in Khon Kaen, Thailand have been established for training health workers who are in need of geospatial health technologies for disease risk mapping and surveillance of control programmes. At the same time, training courses on zoonotic helminthiases in the region have been arranged, often in connection with RNAS$^+$ meetings, to take advantage of the availability of regional and international experts (Zhou et al., 2010b).

1.3.2.7. Regional and international collaboration

Rapid and reliable communication between national and international public health agencies is essential to promptly mount an effective response to the threat of infectious diseases. In zoonotic tropical diseases, communication between public health and veterinary communities—including those dealing with domestic animals, wildlife and other animals such as zoo animals—is often weak, which hinders tracking of emerging infectious diseases. Current systems neither allow nor facilitate rapid communication. Moreover, information on disease outbreaks is not directly shared between countries, federal agencies, states or laboratories, whether on the local, provincial or regional level, and the private sector has no vehicle for sharing information with human health or veterinary professionals.

Networking can be defined as a process framework for empowering stakeholders not only to share and apply new knowledge but also to identify and prioritise problems systematically and to participate in the development of appropriate solutions. Olveda et al. (2010) summarise how a small bid for research on schistosomiasis japonica a decade ago eventually developed into a major regional network (i.e. RNAS$^+$). This network led to a new vision not only for the general strengthening of research capabilities in the sub-region, but also for furthering efforts to close the gap between research and control, and hence fostering integrated and inter-sectoral collaboration and disease control efforts.

1.4. CONCLUDING REMARKS

The regional progress noted in the 'war on the worms' and other NTDs in the latest decade cannot only be credited to the current economic upswing in many of the Southeast Asian countries. It is to a large part due to the activity of local and regional networks that have not only been able to raise unprecedented funding by tapping emerging public–private partnerships, now joining forces to roll back 'this wormy world', but also to make good use of this new funding. The financial support issuing from the new collaboration between international donor agencies, private foundations and pharmaceutical companies is big enough to make a clear difference for control activities.

It is important to appreciate that the regional networks have contributed strongly to the advances through furthering collaboration between the research community and disease control managers. These networks have also played an important role in analysis for strategic planning, implementation and capacity building. The success in embedding research into the endemic countries' health systems can be ascribed to input from international research institutions and the participation of competent scientists with local experience and expertise. Indeed, the authorship configurations of the 25 reviews in these two thematic volumes of the *Advances in Parasitology* attest to the collaborations forged between the North and the South as well as between the West and the East.

Chemotherapy-based morbidity control dominates the fight against helminth infections and, in the case of lymphatic filariasis, it seems credible that success can largely be achieved by mass drug administration alone. In other cases, for example schistosomiasis, the integration between various control tools and inter-sectoral collaboration is needed to achieve elimination. The strong progress of the national schistosomiasis control programme in P.R. China relies as much on snail control as on chemotherapy and it is plausible that the high level of re-infection in the remaining endemic areas in P.R. China and elsewhere requires an integrated approach that includes a vaccine. While praziquantel can be relied on for cure of infection, snail control and transmission-blocking vaccines are needed to reduce the risk of re-infection.

Above all, the recent elimination of lymphatic filariasis from P.R. China is a turning point in the 'war on the worms'. However, this advance does not only support the likelihood that the achievement can be repeated in other countries but it also raises the hope that other NTDs can be eliminated as a public health problem in the foreseeable future. This is therefore not the time to rest on the laurels but to step up vigilance to root out remaining problems and then focus on surveillance to counteract any re-emergence and to deal with post-transmission squeals of chronic diseases that will be with us long after the infections have been eliminated.

ACKNOWLEDGEMENTS

We are grateful to Drs David Rollinson and Simon Hay, editors-in-chief of the *Advances in Parasitology*, Mrs. Narmada Thangavelu, development editor at Elsevier, Mrs. Lisa Tickner, publisher at Elsevier, and Mr. Vijayaraj Purush and Mr. Ezhilvijayan Balakrishna, project managers at Elsevier, for their willingness to engage with us in the current project. Their expertise, encouragement, patience and leadership were crucial to keep us on track. We thank all the contributing authors and external referees for their contributions. We are indebted to Mr. Benjamin Speich and Mrs. Kathrin Ziegelbauer from the Swiss Tropical and Public Health Institute for their help in preparing Figs. 1.1–1.3. J. Utzinger acknowledges financial support from the Swiss National Science Foundation (project no. PPOOB-102883, PPOOB-119129) and X.N. Zhou from the Chinese Important Scientific Research Project on Infectious Diseases (grant no. 2008ZX10004-011).

REFERENCES

Aagaard-Hansen, J., Mwanga, J.R., Bruun, B., 2009. Social science perspectives on schistosomiasis control in Africa: past trends and future directions. Parasitology 136, 1747–1758.

Anderson, R.M., May, R.M., 1985. Helminth infections of humans: mathematical models, population dynamics, and control. Adv. Parasitol. 24, 1–101.

Anonymous, 1909. The Rockefeller commission for the eradication of hookworm disease. Science 30, 635–636.

Anonymous, 2004. Thinking beyond deworming. Lancet 364, 1993–1994.

Anonymous, 2007. Is malaria eradication possible? Lancet 370, 1459.

Arunachalam, N., Tana, S., Espino, F., Kittayapong, P., Abeyewickreme, W., Thet, K., et al., 2010. Eco-bio-social determinants of dengue vector breeding: a multicountry study in urban and periurban Asia. Bull. World Health Organ. 88, 173–184.

Attwood, S.W., 2010. Studies on the parasitology, phylogeography and the evolution of host–parasite interactions, for the snail intermediate hosts of medically important trematode genera in Southeast Asia. Adv. Parasitol. 73, 405–440.

Attwood, S.W., Campbell, I., Upatham, E.S., Rollinson, D., 2004. Schistosomiasis in the Xe Kong river of Cambodia: the detection of *Schistosoma mekongi* in a natural population of snails and observations on intermediate host distribution. Ann. Trop. Med. Parasitol. 98, 221–230.

Attwood, S.W., Fatih, F.A., Campbell, I.C., Upatham, E.S., 2008. The distribution of Mekong schistosomiasis, past and future: preliminary indications from an analysis of genetic variation in the intermediate host. Parasitol. Int. 57, 256–270.

Bergquist, R., 2008. A century of schistosomiasis research. Acta Trop. 108, 65–68.

Bergquist, R., Lustigman, S., 2010. Control of important helminthic infections: vaccine development as part of the solution. Adv. Parasitol. 73, 297–326.

Bergquist, R., Rinaldi, L., 2010. Health research based on geospatial tools: a timely approach in a changing environment. J. Helminthol. 84, 1–11.

Bergquist, R., Tanner, M., 2010. Controlling schistosomiasis in Southeast Asia: a tale of two countries. Adv. Parasitol. 72, 109–144.

Bergquist, N.R., Leonardo, L.R., Mitchell, G.F., 2005. Vaccine-linked chemotherapy: can schistosomiasis control benefit from an integrated approach? Trends Parasitol. 21, 112–117.

Bergquist, R., Utzinger, J., McManus, D.P., 2008. Trick or treat: the role of vaccines in integrated schistosomiasis control. PLoS Negl. Trop. Dis. 2, e244.

Bergquist, R., Johansen, M.V., Utzinger, J., 2009. Diagnostic dilemmas in helminthology: what tools to use and when? Trends Parasitol. 25, 151–156.

Berriman, M., Haas, B.J., LoVerde, P.T., Wilson, R.A., Dillon, G.P., Cerqueira, G.C., et al., 2009. The genome of the blood fluke *Schistosoma mansoni*. Nature 460, 352–358.

Bethony, J., Brooker, S., Albonico, M., Geiger, S.M., Loukas, A., Diemert, D., et al., 2006. Soil-transmitted helminth infections: ascariasis, trichuriasis, and hookworm. Lancet 367, 1521–1532.

Brady, M.A., Hooper, P.J., Ottesen, E.A., 2006. Projected benefits from integrating NTD programs in sub-Saharan Africa. Trends Parasitol. 22, 285–291.

Brooker, S., Utzinger, J., 2007. Integrated disease mapping in a polyparasitic world. Geospat. Health 1, 141–146.

Brooker, S., Kabatereine, N.B., Gyapong, J.O., Stothard, J.R., Utzinger, J., 2009. Rapid assessment of schistosomiasis and other neglected tropical diseases in the context of integrated control programmes in Africa. Parasitology 136, 1707–1718.

Brown, E.R., 1976. Public health in imperialism: early Rockefeller programs at home and abroad. Am. J. Public Health 66, 897–903.

Budke, C.M., Qiu, J.M., Wang, Q., Torgerson, P.R., 2005. Economic effects of echinococcosis in a disease-endemic region of the Tibetan Plateau. Am. J. Trop. Med. Hyg. 73, 2–10.

Bundy, D.A.P., de Silva, N.R., 1998. Can we deworm this wormy world? Br. Med. Bull. 54, 421–432.

Caffrey, C.R., 2007. Chemotherapy of schistosomiasis: present and future. Curr. Opin. Chem. Biol. 11, 433–439.

Chan, M., 2007. The 2007 David E. Barmes Global Health Lecture "Climate change and health: preparing for unprecedented challenges" http://www.who.int/dg/speeches/2007/20071211_maryland/en/index.html. (accessed: 20 March 2010).

Cioli, D., 1998. Chemotherapy of schistosomiasis: an update. Parasitol. Today 14, 418–422.

Clements, A.C.A., Brooker, S., Nyandindi, U., Fenwick, A., Blair, L., 2008. Bayesian spatial analysis of a national urinary schistosomiasis questionnaire to assist geographic targeting of schistosomiasis control in Tanzania, East Africa. Int. J. Parasitol. 38, 401–415.

Conlan, J., Khounsy, S., Inthavong, P., Fenwick, S., Blacksell, S., Thompson, R.C.A., 2008. A review of taeniasis and cysticercosis in the Lao People's Democratic Republic. Parasitol. Int. 57, 252–255.

Crompton, D.W.T., 1999. How much human helminthiasis is there in the world? J. Parasitology 85, 397–403.

Da'dara, A.A., Li, Y.S., Xiong, T., Zhou, J., Williams, G.M., McManus, D.P., et al., 2008. DNA-based vaccines protect against zoonotic schistosomiasis in water buffalo. Vaccine 26, 3617–3625.

Daar, A.S., Berndtson, K., Persad, D.L., Singer, P.A., 2007. How can developing countries harness biotechnology to improve health? BMC Public Health 7, 346.

de Sherbinin, A., Balk, D., Yager, K., Jaiteh, M., Pozzi, F., Giri, C., et al., 2002. A CIESIN Thematic Guide to Social Science Applications of Remote Sensing. Center for International Earth Science Information Network (CIESIN). Columbia University, Palisades, NY, USA, pp. 68.

Ehrenberg, J.P., Ault, S.K., 2005. Neglected diseases of neglected populations: thinking to reshape the determinants of health in Latin America and the Caribbean. BMC Public Health 5, 119.

Erlanger, T.E., Sayasone, S., Krieger, G.R., Kaul, S., Sananikhom, P., Tanner, M., et al., 2008. Baseline health situation of communities affected by the Nam Theun 2 hydroelectric project in central Lao PDR and indicators for monitoring. Int. J. Environ. Health Res. 18, 223–242.

Ezeamama, A.E., Friedman, J.F., Olveda, R.M., Acosta, L.P., Kurtis, J.D., Mor, V., et al., 2005. Functional significance of low-intensity polyparasite helminth infections in anemia. J. Infect. Dis. 192, 2160–2170.

Fenwick, A., 2006. New initiatives against Africa's worms. Trans. R. Soc. Trop. Med. Hyg. 100, 200–207.

Fenwick, A., Webster, J.P., Bosque-Oliva, E., Blair, L., Fleming, F.M., Zhang, Y., et al., 2009. The Schistosomiasis Control Initiative (SCI): rationale, development and implementation from 2002–2008. Parasitology 136, 1719–1730.

Finkelstein, J.L., Schleinitz, M.D., Carabin, H., McGarvey, S.T., 2008. Decision-model estimation of the age-specific disability weight for schistosomiasis japonica: a systematic review of the literature. PLoS Negl. Trop. Dis. 2, e158.

Garjito, T.A., Sudomo, M., Abdullah, Dahlan, M., Nurwidayati, A., 2008. Schistosomiasis in Indonesia: past and present. Parasitol. Int. 57, 277–280.

Gray, D.J., Williams, G.M., Li, Y., Chen, H., Forsyth, S.J., Li, R.S., et al., 2009. A cluster-randomised intervention trial against *Schistosoma japonicum* in the People's Republic of China: bovine and human transmission. PLoS One 4, e5900.

Greenwood, B.M., Fidock, D.A., Kyle, D.E., Kappe, S.H., Alonso, P.L., Collins, F.H., et al., 2008. Malaria: progress, perils, and prospects for eradication. J. Clin. Invest. 118, 1266–1276.

Guo, J.G., Cao, C.L., Hu, G.H., Lin, H., Li, D., Zhu, R., et al., 2005. The role of 'passive chemotherapy' plus health education for schistosomiasis control in China during maintenance and consolidation phase. Acta Trop. 96, 177–183.

Hall, B.F., Fauci, A.S., 2009. Malaria control, elimination, and eradication: the role of the evolving biomedical research agenda. J. Infect. Dis. 200, 1639–1643.

Holveck, J.C., Ehrenberg, J.P., Ault, S.K., Rojas, R., Vasquez, J., Cerqueira, M.T., et al., 2007. Prevention, control, and elimination of neglected diseases in the Americas: pathways to integrated, inter-programmatic, inter-sectoral action for health and development. BMC Public Health 7, 6.

Hotez, P., 2008. Hookworm and poverty. Ann. N. Y. Acad. Sci. 1136, 38–44.

Hotez, P.J., Ehrenberg, J.P., 2010. Escalating the global fight against neglected tropical diseases through interventions in the Asia Pacific Region. Adv. Parasitol. 72, 31–53.

Hotez, P.J., Molyneux, D.H., Fenwick, A., Ottesen, E., Ehrlich Sachs, S., Sachs, J.D., 2006. Incorporating a rapid-impact package for neglected tropical diseases with programs for HIV/AIDS, tuberculosis, and malaria. PLoS Med. 3, e102.

Hotez, P.J., Molyneux, D.H., Fenwick, A., Kumaresan, J., Ehrlich Sachs, S., Sachs, J.D., et al., 2007. Control of neglected tropical diseases. N. Engl. J. Med. 357, 1018–1027.

Hotez, P.J., Brindley, P.J., Bethony, J.M., King, C.H., Pearce, E.J., Jacobson, J., 2008. Helminth infections: the great neglected tropical diseases. J. Clin. Invest. 118, 1311–1321.

Hotez, P.J., Fenwick, A., Savioli, L., Molyneux, D.H., 2009. Rescuing the bottom billion through control of neglected tropical diseases. Lancet 373, 1570–1575.

Huang, Y.X., Manderson, L., 2005. The social and economic context and determinants of schistosomiasis japonica. Acta Trop. 96, 223–231.

Jia, T.W., Zhou, X.N., Wang, X.H., Utzinger, J., Steinmann, P., Wu, X.H., 2007. Assessment of the age-specific disability weight of chronic schistosomiasis japonica. Bull. World Health Organ. 85, 458–465.

Johansen, M.V., Sithithaworn, P., Bergquist, R., Utzinger, J., 2010. Towards improved diagnosis of zoonotic trematode infections in Southeast Asia. Adv. Parasitol. 73, 171–195.

Ju, C., Zheng, F., Brindley, P.J., McManus, D.P., Han, Z.G., Wei, H., 2010. Our wormy world: genomics, proteomics and transcriptomics in East and Southeast Asia. Adv. Parasitol. 73, 327–371.

Keiser, J., Utzinger, J., 2005. Emerging foodborne trematodiasis. Emerg. Infect. Dis. 11, 1507–1514.

Keiser, J., Utzinger, J., 2007. Advances in the discovery and development of novel trematocidal drugs. Expert Opin. Drug Discov. 2 (Suppl. 1), S9–23.

Keiser, J., Utzinger, J., 2009. Food-borne trematodiases. Clin. Microbiol. Rev. 22, 466–483.

Keiser, J., Utzinger, J., 2010. The drugs we have and the drugs we need against major helminth infections. Adv. Parasitol. 73, 197–230.

Keiser, J., Utzinger, J., Singer, B.H., 2003. Gender composition of editorial boards of general medical journals. Lancet 362, 1336.

Keiser, J., Utzinger, J., Tanner, M., Singer, B.H., 2004. Representation of authors and editors from countries with different human development indexes in the leading literature on tropical medicine: survey of current evidence. BMJ 328, 1229–1232.

King, C.H., 2010a. Parasites and poverty: the case of schistosomiasis. Acta Trop. 113, 95–104.

King, C.H., 2010b. Health metrics for helminthic infections. Adv. Parasitol. 73, 51–69.

King, C.H., Bertino, A.M., 2008. Asymmetries of poverty: why global burden of disease valuations underestimate the burden of neglected tropical diseases. PLoS Negl. Trop. Dis. 2, e209.

King, C.H., Dickman, K., Tisch, D.J., 2005. Reassessment of the cost of chronic helmintic infection: a meta-analysis of disability-related outcomes in endemic schistosomiasis. Lancet 365, 1561–1569.

Kolaczinski, J.H., Kabatereine, N.B., Onapa, A.W., Ndyomugyenyi, R., Kakembo, A.S., Brooker, S., 2007. Neglected tropical diseases in Uganda: the prospect and challenge of integrated control. Trends Parasitol. 23, 485–493.

Lammie, P.J., Fenwick, A., Utzinger, J., 2006. A blueprint for success: integration of neglected tropical disease control programmes. Trends Parasitol. 22, 313–321.

Lammie, P., Milner, T., Houston, R., 2007. Unfulfilled potential: using diethylcarbamazine-fortified salt to eliminate lymphatic filariasis. Bull. World Health Organ. 85, 545–549.

Leonardo, L.R., Bergquist, R., 2002. Regional network on Asian schistosomiasis. Trends Parasitol. 18, 434–436.

Leonardo, L.R., Crisostomo, B.A., Solon, J.A., Rivera, P.T., Marcelo, A.B., Villasper, J.M., 2007. Geographical information systems in health research and services delivery in the Philippines. Geospat. Health 1, 147–155.

Leonardo, L.R., Rivera, P., Saniel, O., Villacorte, E., Crisostomo, B., Hernandez, L., et al., 2008. Prevalence survey of schistosomiasis in Mindanao and the Visayas, the Philippines. Parasitol. Int. 57, 246–251.

Liese, B., Rosenberg, M., Schratz, A., 2010. Programmes, partnerships, and governance for elimination and control of neglected tropical diseases. Lancet 375, 67–76.

Lightowlers, M.W., 2006. Cestode vaccines: origins, current status and future prospects. Parasitology 133 (Suppl.), S27–S42.

Lin, D.D., Liu, J.X., Liu, Y.M., Hu, F., Zhang, Y.Y., Xu, J.M., et al., 2008. Routine Kato-Katz technique underestimates the prevalence of *Schistosoma japonicum*: a case study in an endemic area of the People's Republic of China. Parasitol. Int. 57, 281–286.

Lun, Z.R., Gasser, R.B., Lai, D.H., Li, A.X., Zhu, X.Q., Yu, X.B., et al., 2005. Clonorchiasis: a key foodborne zoonosis in China. Lancet Infect. Dis. 5, 31–41.

Lv, S., Zhang, Y., Steinmann, P., Zhou, X.N., Utzinger, J., 2010. Helminth infections of the central nervous system occurring in Southeast Asia and the Far East. Adv. Parasitol. 72, 351–408.

Malone, J.B., Yang, G.J., Leonardo, L., Zhou, X.N., 2010. Implementing a geospatial health data infrastructure for control of Asian schistosomiasis in P.R. China and the Philippines. Adv. Parasitol. 73, 71–100.

Maudlin, I., Eisler, M.C., Welburn, S.C., 2009. Neglected and endemic zoonoses. Philos. Trans. R. Soc. Lond. B Biol. Sci. 364, 2777–2787.

May, R.M., 2007. Parasites, people and policy: infectious diseases and the millennium development goals. Trends Ecol. Evol. 22, 497–503.

McManus, D.P., 2010. Echinococcosis with particular reference to Southeast Asia. Adv. Parasitol. 72, 269–303.

McManus, D.P., Loukas, A., 2008. Current status of vaccines for schistosomiasis. Clin. Microbiol. Rev. 21, 225–242.

McManus, D.P., Li, Y.S., Gray, D.J., Ross, A.G., 2009. Conquering 'snail fever': schistosomiasis and its control in China. Expert Rev. Anti. Infect. Ther. 7, 473–485.

McManus, D.P., Gray, D.J., Li, Y., Feng, Z., Wiliams, G.M., Stewart, D., et al., 2010. Schistosomiasis in the People's Republic of China: the era of the Three Gorges Dam. Clin. Microbiol. Rev. 23, 442 –466.

Miguel, E., Kremer, M., 2004. Worms: identifying impacts on education and health in the presence of treatment externalities. Econometrica 72, 159–217.

Molyneux, D.H., 2006. Control of human parasitic diseases: context and overview. Adv. Parasitol. 61, 1–45.

Molyneux, D.H., 2008. Combating the "other diseases" of MDG 6: changing the paradigm to achieve equity and poverty reduction? Trans. R. Soc. Trop. Med. Hyg. 102, 509–519.

Molyneux, D.H., Hotez, P.J., Fenwick, A., 2005. ''Rapid-impact interventions'': how a policy of integrated control for Africa's neglected tropical diseases could benefit the poor. PLoS Med. 2, e336.

Moran, M., 2005. A breakthrough in R&D for neglected diseases: new ways to get the drugs we need. PLoS Med. 2, e302.

Moran, M., Guzman, J., Ropars, A.L., McDonald, A., Jameson, N., Omune, B., et al., 2009. Neglected disease research and development: how much are we really spending? PLoS Med. 6, e30.

Morel, C.M., Acharya, T., Broun, D., Dangi, A., Elias, C., Ganguly, N.K., et al., 2005. Health innovation networks to help developing countries address neglected diseases. Science 309, 401–404.

Morel, C.M., Serruya, S.J., Penna, G.O., Guimarães, R., 2009. Co-authorship network analysis: a powerful tool for strategic planning of research, development and capacity building programs on neglected diseases. PLoS Negl. Trop. Dis. 3, e501.

Murray, C.J.L., Lopez, A.D., 1996. The Global Burden of Disease: A Comprehensive Assessment of Mortality and Disability from Diseases, Injuries, and Risk Factors in 1990 and Projected to 2020. Harvard School of Public Health/World Bank, Cambridge, MA, USA.

Muth, S., Sayasone, S., Odermatt-Biays, S., Phompida, S., Duong, S., Odermatt, P., 2010. *Schistosoma mekongi* in Cambodia and Lao People's Democratic Republic. Adv. Parasitol. 72, 179–203.

Neumann, P.J., Greenberg, D., 2009. Is the United States ready for QALYs? Health Aff. (Millwood) 28, 1366–1371.

Odermatt, P., Lv, S., Sayasone, S., 2010. Less common parasitic infections in Southeast Asia that can produce outbreaks. Adv. Parasitol. 72, 409–435.

Olveda, R., Leonardo, L., Zheng, F., Sripa, B., Bergquist, R., Zhou, X.N., 2010. Coordinating research on neglected parasitic diseases in Southeast Asia through networking. Adv. Parasitol. 72, 55–77.

Peters, D.H., Phillips, T., 2004. Mectizan donation program: evaluation of a public–private partnership. Trop. Med. Int. Health 9, A4–A15.

Pullan, R., Brooker, S., 2008. The health impact of polyparasitism in humans: are we underestimating the burden of parasitic diseases? Parasitology 135, 783–794.

Reddy, M., Gill, S.S., Kalkar, S.R., Wu, W., Anderson, P.J., Rochon, P.A., 2007. Oral drug therapy for multiple neglected tropical diseases: a systematic review. JAMA 298, 1911–1924.

Rickard, M.D., Harrison, G.B., Heath, D.D., Lightowlers, M.W., 1995. *Taenia ovis* recombinant vaccine – 'quo vadit'. Parasitology 110 (Suppl.), S5–S9.

Savioli, L., Stansfield, S., Bundy, D.A.P., Mitchell, A., Bhatia, R., Engels, D., et al., 2002. Schistosomiasis and soil-transmitted helminth infections: forging control efforts. Trans. R. Soc. Trop. Med. Hyg. 96, 577–579.

Schistosoma japonicum Genome Sequencing and Functional Analysis Consortium, 2009. The *Schistosoma japonicum* genome reveals features of host–parasite interplay. Nature 460, 345–351.

Schratz, A., Fernanda Pineda, M., Reforma, L.G., Fox, N.M., Anh, T.L., Cavalli-Sforza, L.T., et al., 2010. Neglected diseases and ethnic minorities in the Western Pacific Region: exploring the links. Adv. Parasitol. 72, 79–107.

Sékétéli, A., Adeoye, G., Eyamba, A., Nnoruka, E., Drameh, P., Amazigo, U.V., et al., 2002. The achievements and challenges of the African Programme for Onchocerciasis Control (APOC). Ann. Trop. Med. Parasitol. 96 (Suppl. 1), S15–S28.

Simoonga, C., Utzinger, J., Brooker, S., Vounatsou, P., Appleton, C.C., Stensgaard, A.S., et al., 2009. Remote sensing, geographical information system and spatial analysis for schistosomiasis epidemiology and ecology in Africa. Parasitology 136, 1683–1693.

Singer, B.H., Castro, M.C., 2007. Bridges to sustainable tropical health. Proc. Natl. Acad. Sci. U.S.A. 104, 16038–16043.

Sinha, S., Sharma, B.S., 2009. Neurocysticercosis: a review of current status and management. J. Clin. Neurosci. 16, 867–876.

Smits, H.L., 2009. Prospects for the control of neglected tropical diseases by mass drug administration. Expert Rev. Anti. Infect. Ther. 7, 37–56.

Sripa, B., 2008. Concerted action is needed to tackle liver fluke infections in Asia. PLoS Negl. Trop. Dis. 2, e232.

Sripa, B., Kaewkes, S., Sithithaworn, P., Mairiang, E., Laha, T., Smout, M., et al., 2007. Liver fluke induces cholangiocarcinoma. PLoS Med. 4, e201.

Sripa, B., Kaewkes, S., Intapan, P.M., Maleewong, W., Brindley, P.J., 2010. Food-borne trematodiases in Southeast Asia: epidemiology, pathology, clinical manifestation and control. Adv. Parasitol. 72, 305–350.

Steinmann, P., Zhou, X.N., Matthys, B., Li, Y.L., Li, H.J., Chen, S.R., et al., 2007. Spatial risk profiling of *Schistosoma japonicum* in Eryuan county, Yunnan province, China. Geospat. Health 2, 59–73.

Steinmann, P., Du, Z.W., Wang, L.B., Wang, X.Z., Jiang, J.Y., Li, L.H., et al., 2008. Extensive multiparasitism in a village of Yunnan province, People's Republic of China, revealed by a suite of diagnostic methods. Am. J. Trop. Med. Hyg. 78, 760–769.

Steinmann, P., Utzinger, J., Du, Z.W., Zhou, X.N., 2010. Multiparasitism: a neglected reality on global, regional and local scale. Adv. Parasitol. 73, 21–50.

Stiles, C.W., 1939. Early history, in part esoteric, of the hookworm (uncinariasis) campaign in our southern United States. J. Parasitol. 25, 283–308.

Stoll, N.R., 1947. This wormy world. J. Parasitol. 33, 1–18.

Stothard, J.R., Chitsulo, L., Kristensen, T.K., Utzinger, J., 2009. Control of schistosomiasis in sub-Saharan Africa: progress made, new opportunities and remaining challenges. Parasitology 136, 1665–1675.

Sturrock, H.J., Picon, D., Sabasio, A., Oguttu, D., Robinson, E., Lado, M., et al., 2009. Integrated mapping of neglected tropical diseases: epidemiological findings and control implications for northern Bahr-el-Ghazal State, Southern Sudan. PLoS Negl. Trop. Dis. 3, e537.

Sudomo, M., Chayabejara, S., Socheat, D., Hernandez, L., Wu, W.P., Bergquist, R., 2010. Elimination of lymphatic filariasis in Southeast Asia. Adv. Parasitol. 72, 205–233.

Tendler, M., Simpson, A.J., 2008. The biotechnology-value chain: development of Sm14 as a schistosomiasis vaccine. Acta Trop. 108, 263–266.

The Global Fund to Fight AIDS, Tuberculosis and Malaria, 2010. The Global Fund 2010: Innovation and Impact. The Global Fund to Fight AIDS, Tuberculosis and Malaria, Geneva, pp. 125.

Utzinger, J., de Savigny, D., 2006. Control of neglected tropical diseases: integrated chemotherapy and beyond. PLoS Med. 3, e112.

Utzinger, J., Bergquist, R., Xiao, S.H., Singer, B.H., Tanner, M., 2003. Sustainable schistosomiasis control – the way forward. Lancet 362, 1932–1934.

Utzinger, J., Zhou, X.N., Chen, M.G., Bergquist, R., 2005. Conquering schistosomiasis in China: the long march. Acta Trop. 96, 69–96.

Utzinger, J., Xiao, S.H., Tanner, M., Keiser, J., 2007. Artemisinins for schistosomiasis and beyond. Curr. Opin. Investig. Drugs 8, 105–116.

Utzinger, J., Raso, G., Brooker, S., de Savigny, S., Tanner, M., Ørnbjerg, N., et al., 2009. Schistosomiasis and neglected tropical diseases: towards integrated and sustainable control and a word of caution. Parasitology 136, 1859–1874.

Vandemark, L.M., Jia, T.W., Zhou, X.N., 2010. Social science implications for control of helminth infections in Southeast Asia. Adv. Parasitol. 73, 137–170.

Wahlqvist, M.L., Kuo, K.N., 2009. Securing health through food systems: an initiative of the nutrition consortium of the National Health Research Institutes in Taiwan and Asia Pacific regional partners as a network. Asia Pac. J. Clin. Nutr. 18, 472–479.

Wang, T.P., Johansen, M.V., Zhang, S.Q., Wang, F.F., Wu, W.D., Zhang, G.H., et al., 2005. Transmission of *Schistosoma japonicum* by humans and domestic animals in the Yangtze River valley, Anhui province, China. Acta Trop. 96, 198–204.

Wang, Y.L., Utzinger, J., Xiao, S.H., Xue, J., Nicholson, J.K., Tanner, M., et al., 2006. System level metabolic effects of a *Schistosoma japonicum* infection in the Syrian hamster. Mol. Biochem. Parasitol. 146, 1–9.

Wang, L.D., Chen, H.G., Guo, J.G., Zeng, X.J., Hong, X.L., Xiong, J.J., et al., 2009a. A strategy to control transmission of *Schistosoma japonicum* in China. N. Engl. J. Med. 360, 121–128.

Wang, L.D., Guo, J.G., Wu, X.H., Chen, H.G., Wang, T.P., Zhu, S.P., et al., 2009b. China's new strategy to block *Schistosoma japonicum* transmission: experiences and impact beyond schistosomiasis. Trop. Med. Int. Health 14, 1475–1483.

Wang, Y.L., Xiao, S.H., Xue, J., Singer, B.H., Utzinger, J., Holmes, E., 2009c. Systems metabolic effects of a *Necator americanus* infection in Syrian hamster. J. Proteome Res. 8, 5442–5450.

Wang, Y.L., Li, J.V., Saric, J., Keiser, J., Wu, J.F., Utzinger, J., 2010. Advances in metabolic profiling of experimental nematode and trematode infections. Adv. Parasitol. 73, 373–404.

WHO, 2006a. Preventive Chemotherapy in Human Helminthiasis: Coordinated Use of Anthelminthic Drugs in Control Interventions: A Manual for Health Professionals and Programme Managers. World Health Organization, Geneva.

WHO, 2006b. Global programme to eliminate lymphatic filariasis. Wkly. Epidemiol. Rec. 81, 221–232.

WHO, 2009. Global programme to eliminate lymphatic filariasis. Wkly. Epidemiol. Rec. 84, 437–444.

WHO and UNICEF, 2010. Progress on Sanitation and Drinking-Water: 2010 Update. WHO/UNICEF Joint Monitoring Programme for Water Supply and Sanitation, Geneva.

Widdus, R., 2005. Public–private partnerships: an overview. Trans. R. Soc. Trop. Med. Hyg. 99 (Suppl. 1), S1–8.

Willingham 3rd, A.L., Engels, D., 2006. Control of *Taenia solium* cysticercosis/taeniosis. Adv. Parasitol. 61, 509–566.

Willingham III, A.L., Wu, H.W., Conlan, J., Satrija, F., 2010. Combating *Taenia solium* cysticercosis in Southeast Asia: an opportunity for improving human health and livestock production. Adv. Parasitol. 72, 235–266.

Wu, X.H., Wang, X.H., Utzinger, J., Yang, K., Kristensen, T.K., Berquist, R., et al., 2007. Spatio-temporal correlation between human and bovine schistosomiasis in China: insight from three national sampling surveys. Geospat. Health 2, 75–84.

Wu, X.H., Zhang, S.Q., Xu, X.J., Huang, Y.X., Steinmann, P., Utzinger, J., et al., 2008. Effect of floods on the transmission of schistosomiasis in the Yangtze River valley, People's Republic of China. Parasitol. Int. 57, 271–276.

Wu, J.F., Holmes, E., Xue, J., Xiao, S.H., Singer, B.H., Tang, H.R., et al., 2010. Metabolic alterations in the hamster coinfected with *Schistosoma japonicum* and *Necator americanus*. Int. J. Parastiol. 40, 695–703.

Xiao, S.H., Keiser, J., Chen, M.G., Tanner, T., Utzinger, J., 2010. Research and development of antischistosomal drugs in the People's Republic of China: a 60-year review. Adv. Parasitol. 73, 231–295.

Yaïch, M., 2009. Investing in vaccines for developing countries: how public-private partnerships can confront neglected diseases. Hum. Vaccin. 5, 368–369.

Yang, G.J., Vounatsou, P., Zhou, X.N., Utzinger, J., Tanner, M., 2005. A review of geographic information system and remote sensing with applications to the epidemiology and control of schistosomiasis in China. Acta Trop. 96, 117–129.

Yang, K., Zhou, X.N., Wu, X.H., Steinmann, P., Wang, X.H., Yang, G.J., et al., 2009. Landscape pattern analysis and Bayesian modeling for predicting *Oncomelania hupensis* distribution in Eryuan county, People's Republic of China. Am. J. Trop. Med. Hyg. 81, 416–423.

Yang, G.J., Utzinger, J., Lv, S., Qian, Y.J., Li, S.Z., Qiang, W., et al., 2010. Regional network for Asian Schistosomiasis and other Helminth Zoonoses ($RNAS^{+}$): target diseases in face of climate change. Adv. Parasitol. 73, 101–135.

Zhou, X.N., Acosta, L., Willingham 3rd, A.L., Leonardo, L.R., Chen, M.G., Aligui, G., et al., 2002. Regional network for research, surveillance and control of Asian schistosomiasis (RNAS). Acta Trop. 82, 305–311.

Zhou, X.N., Ohta, N., Utzinger, J., Bergquist, R., Olveda, R.M., 2008a. $RNAS^{+}$: a "win-win" collaboration to combat neglected tropical diseases in Southeast Asia. Parasitol. Int. 57, 243–245.

Zhou, X.N., Yang, G.J., Yang, K., Wang, X.H., Hong, Q.B., Sun, L.P., et al., 2008b. Potential impact of climate change on schistosomiasis transmission in China. Am. J. Trop. Med. Hyg. 78, 188–194.

Zhou, X.N., Lv, S., Yang, G.J., Kristensen, T.K., Bergquist, R., Utzinger, J., et al., 2009. Spatial epidemiology in zoonotic parasitic diseases: insights gained at the 1st International Symposium on Geospatial Health in Lijiang, China, 2007. Parasit. Vectors 2, 10.

Zhou, X.N., Bergquist, R., Leonardo, L., Yang, G.J., Yang, K., Sudomo, M., et al., 2010a. Schistosomiasis japonica: control and research needs. Adv. Parasitol. 72, 145–178.

Zhou, X.N., Wayling, S., Bergquist, R., 2010b. Concepts in research capabilities strengthening: positive experiences of network approaches by TDR in China and Eastern Asia. Adv. Parasitol. 73, 1–19.

CHAPTER 2

Escalating the Global Fight Against Neglected Tropical Diseases Through Interventions in the Asia Pacific Region

Peter J. Hotez[*,†] and **John P. Ehrenberg**[‡]

Contents

* Department of Microbiology, Immunology, and Tropical Medicine, George Washington University, Washington, District of Columbia, USA
† Sabin Vaccine Institute, Washington, District of Columbia, USA
‡ World Health Organization, Regional Office for the Western Pacific, Malaria, Vector-borne and other Parasitic Diseases, Manila, Philippines

Advances in Parasitology, Volume 72
ISSN 0065-308X, DOI: 10.1016/S0065-308X(10)72002-9

Abstract

As local, national and international control and elimination efforts for the neglected tropical diseases (NTDs) expand, there is increasing recognition that the 11 Southeast Asian countries together with the People's Republic of China (P.R. China) account for a significant burden of global poverty and disease. Indeed, approximately one-third of the world's intestinal helminthiases, most of the food-borne trematode infections, one-half of the active trachoma infections and a significant number of cases of lymphatic filariasis (LF), schistosomiasis and arboviral infections occur in this region. Among the Mekong countries, active programmes of mass drug administration are in place for the control and elimination of LF, as well as morbidity control aimed at school-aged children at risk of intestinal helminths. However, treatment coverage for intestinal helminth infections remains low in the largest Southeast Asian countries and in P.R. China's poorest provinces. The food-borne trematodiases, especially liver fluke infections, remain highly endemic in northern Thailand, Lao People's Democratic Republic and four provinces of P.R. China where they are an important risk factor for cholangiocarcinoma, while schistosomiasis continues to be an important zoonosis in P.R. China and the Philippines, although the former country has embarked on an ambitious elimination strategy. Through a global network for NTDs, an innovative finance mechanism Is being created to control the most common neglected diseases across Asia.

2.1. INTRODUCTION

The neglected tropical diseases (NTDs) are chronic and debilitating infections affecting the poorest people in low-income and middle-income countries. Together, the NTDs are the most common clinical conditions of the so-called 'bottom billion', referring to people living in the lowest economic tier, typically on less than US$ 1 per day (Hotez et al., 2009). In addition to their high prevalence and distribution, there is increasing awareness of the role that NTDs have as major global public health threats. Although they are not considered major causes of mortality, the NTDs are roughly equivalent to the 'big three' diseases, that is HIV/AIDS, malaria and tuberculosis in terms of their ability to cause chronic disability (often measured in disability-adjusted life years (DALYs) lost) (Hotez et al., 2007). Moreover, because these disabilities target disproportionately growing children, pregnant women and agricultural workers, the NTDs thwart economic development and these conditions are now recognised as stealth reasons why the bottom billion cannot escape the poverty trap (Hotez et al., 2009). As a result, global health policy makers have identified NTD control as a key element central to any strategy designed to achieve the United Nations millennium development goals (MDGs) for sustainable poverty reduction (Hotez, 2008). The seven most common NTDs, which include six helminth infections, that is, ascariasis, trichuriasis, hookworm disease, schistosomiasis, lymphatic filariasis (LF), onchocerciasis and trachoma, are being specifically targeted for mass drug administration (also sometimes referred to as preventive chemotherapy (WHO, 2006)) in recognition of their high prevalence, the observation that they account for at least 90% of the NTD global disease burden and because they frequently occur together in similar geographic areas where they are co-endemic (Hotez et al., 2006; Molyneux et al., 2005). These seven NTDs can be addressed with a 'rapid impact' package comprised of anti-infective agents, which are both donated by the major pharmaceutical companies and/or available as low-cost generic drugs (Hotez et al., 2006; Molyneux et al., 2005; WHO, 2006). Although not included in the group of NTDs due to helminths, a number of skin diseases caused by ectoparasites, fungi and bacteria have also been neglected despite the potential for elimination (e.g. yaws in selected countries of the Western Pacific Region). These neglected skin diseases can be the target of similar interventions utilising approaches such as school-based interventions.

As delivery of rapid impact packages has become attractive to some of the major donors as a low-cost and highly effective pro-poor strategy, beginning in 2007, both the United States and British Governments began providing up to US$ 400 million over a period of several years in order to finance the costs of procuring and delivering essential NTD drugs (Hotez et al., 2009). Most of the funding is being targeted for sub-Saharan Africa, because the highest NTD burden occurs in the World Health Organization's (WHO) African Region relative to any other WHO region (Hotez and Kamath, 2009; Molyneux et al., 2005). However, the reality is that the single largest number of cases of each of the seven NTDs (with the exception of schistosomiasis) is found in Asia (Hotez, 2009). Moreover, some investigators are contributing to raising the level of awareness regarding the high burden of food-borne trematode infections (Keiser and Utzinger, 2005, 2007, 2009; Sripa et al., 2007, 2010), most of which also occur in Asia. In response to the regional importance of NTDs both within and outside of Africa, the Bill & Melinda Gates Foundation recently provided US$ 34 million in seed funding to encourage the mobilisation of additional resources for treating over 200 million people through a system of self-sustaining resource mobilisation hubs in Africa, Latin America and the Caribbean and Asia (Hotez et al., 2009). An overview is hereby provided on the enormous NTD disease burden among the estimated 560 million people living in the 11 countries of Southeast Asia, that is, Brunei Darussalam, Cambodia, East Timor, Indonesia, Lao People's Democratic Republic (Lao PDR), Malaysia, Myanmar, the Philippines, Singapore, Thailand and Vietnam, as well as impoverished populations in the People's Republic of China (P.R. China), and the opportunities for large-scale NTD control in the region.

2.2. OVERVIEW OF THE NTDs IN THE ASIA PACIFIC REGION

Because of the extreme poverty that occurs in the 11 countries of Southeast Asia and some parts of P.R. China, there is a high prevalence of myriad NTDs in the region. With the possible exceptions of Brunei, Singapore and Malaysia, a significant number of the bottom billion live in Southeast Asia and also P.R. China (Table 2.1). Overall, 37% of the Southeast Asian population lives on less than US$ 1 per day, and only sub-Saharan Africa exceeds this region in terms of the percentage of people living in poverty (Szczepanski, 2009). Moreover, approximately two thirds of the population of Cambodia and Lao PDR lives on less than US$ 2 per day, and these two countries together with East Timor and Myanmar, rank near the bottom of all nations in terms of their development indicators (Szczepanski, 2009). Indigenous tribes and people in Southeast Asia are

TABLE 2.1 Poverty indicators in Southeast Asia and P.R. China[a,b]

Country	Percentage of population living below US$ 1 per day	Percentage of population living below US$ 2 per day	Year
Brunei	n.d.	n.d.	
Cambodia	18.5	61.7	2004
Indonesia	4.0	40.0	2005
Lao PDR	28.8	74.4	2003
Malaysia	0	9.8	2005
Myanmar	n.d.	n.d.	
Philippines	13.6	45.2	2006
Singapore	0	0	
Thailand	0	25.8	2002
Vietnam	8.4	43.2	2004
P.R. China	10.8	37.8	2004

n.d., not determined.
[a] From Asian Development Bank Key Indicators for Asia and the Pacific 2008.
[b] Sources: World Bank (2009), World Bank Group (2009).

also notable for their extreme poverty, as well as selected populations, which have been either previously or currently targeted for national government oppression, including those living in East Timor or Eastern Myanmar (Beyrer et al., 2007). As shown in Table 2.2, helminth infections represent the most common NTDs in the 11 countries of Southeast Asia, including the three major intestinal helminth infections (i.e. ascariasis, trichuriasis and hookworm disease), LF and the food-borne trematode infection, opisthorchiasis. Less common are trachoma, schistosomiasis and leprosy.

Approximately 11% of P.R. China's population of 1.3 billion people lives on less than US$ 1 per day (Table 2.1), thereby also accounting for a significant percentage of the world's bottom billion. Some of the highest rates of poverty and therefore the highest prevalence of NTDs occur in the southwestern provinces of Guangxi, Guizhou, Sichuan and Yunnan, which, compared to P.R. China's eastern provinces, have less benefited from P.R. China's boom in economic development over the last two decades (Hotez, 2002). The intestinal helminth infections are highly prevalent in P.R. China, as are two major food-borne trematode infections, namely clonorchiasis and paragonimiasis (Table 2.3). Trachoma is still highly prevalent in P.R. China and may represent the most common NTD behind the intestinal helminth infections. In addition to the food-borne trematode infections, other platyhelminth infections such as schistosomiasis, taeniasis and echinococcosis are also common, and leprosy still occurs (McManus, 2010; Muth et al., 2010; Zhou et al., 2010).

As shown in Table 2.4, there are also at least a dozen other NTDs in Southeast Asia and P.R. China for which prevalence data are insufficient or even non-existent. These include other helminth infections such as strongyloidiasis, echinococcosis and toxocariasis, which are most probably quite common. For example, Australian aboriginals have among the highest prevalence of echinococcosis in Australia and among ethnic minority populations (Schratz et al., 2010; WHO, 2008d), but also some important non-helminthic NTDs. These are discussed separately below.

2.3. INTESTINAL HELMINTH (SOIL-TRANSMITTED HELMINTH) INFECTIONS

The three major intestinal helminth infections are the most common NTDs in Southeast Asia. Approximately 40%, 36% and 26% of the 563 million people that live in the 11 countries are infected with *Ascaris lumbricoides*, *Trichuris trichiura* and the two major hookworms (with most of the cases caused by *Necator americanus*), respectively. Even though the populations living in the 11 Southeast Asian countries account for less than 10% of the global population, they account for up to one-third of the

TABLE 2.2 Ranking of NTDs in Southeast Asia by prevalence

Disease	Estimated number of cases (million)	Approximate prevalence in the region[a]	Approximate percentage of global disease burden	Reference(s)
Ascariasis	227	40%	28%	de Silva et al. (2003)
Trichuriasis	200	36%	33%	de Silva et al. (2003)
Hookworm infection	149	26%	26%	de Silva et al. (2003)
Lymphatic filariasis	<15, >64 (at risk)[b]	<3%	<14%	Michael et al. (1996); WHO (2008b)
Opisthorchiasis	9–10	2%	88%	Sithithaworn and Haswell-Elkins (2003); Keiser and Utzinger (2007); Andrews et al. (2008)
Trachoma	2	0.3%	3%	WHO Global Atlas (2009)[c]
Schistosomiasis	0.2	<0.1%	0.1%	Steinmann et al. (2006)
Leprosy	0.03	<0.1%	13%	WHO (2008c)

[a] Based on a population of 563 million: http://web.worldbank.org/WBSITE/EXTERNAL/DATASTATISTICS/0,contentMDK:20535285~menuPK:1192694~pagePK:64133150~piPK:64133175~theSitePK:239419,00.html.

[b] Includes 32 million in 'Mekong Plus' countries of Cambodia, Malaysia, Philippines and Vietnam, and approximately 32 million at risk in Indonesia, Myanmar, Thailand and East Timor.

[c] WHO Global Atlas for trachoma (http://apps.who.int/globalatlas/).

TABLE 2.3 Ranking of NTDs in P.R. China by prevalence

Disease	Estimated number of cases (million)	Approximate percentage of global disease burden	Reference(s)
Ascariasis	86	11%	Ministry of Health China (2005)
Trichuriasis	29	5%	Ministry of Health China (2005)
Hookworm infection	39	7%	Ministry of Health China (2005)
Trachoma	27	43%	WHO Global Atlas (2009)
Paragonimiasis	13.8[a]	66%[a]	Keiser and Utzinger (2005, 2007)
Clonorchiasis	12.5	<100%	Ministry of Health China (2005)
Schistosomiasis	0.8	0.4%	Steinmann et al. (2006)
Taeniais	0.5	ND	Ministry of Health China (2005)
Echinococcosis	0.4	ND	Ministry of Health China (2005)
Leprosy	0.003	1.4%	WHO (2008c)

[a] The 13.8 million number is an estimate based on the observation that 195 million of the 293 million at risk for paragonimiasis (66%) reside in P.R. China, multiplied by the total number of estimated cases (Keiser and Utzinger, 2005, 2007).

total number of cases (de Silva et al., 2003). This observation reflects the extreme poverty found in the region. Among the 11 countries, Indonesia has the greatest number of cases of ascariasis and trichuriasis (more than 90 million cases of each infection) as well as hookworm (60 million). Globally, Indonesia is exceeded only by India in terms of the total number of cases of intestinal helminth infections (de Silva et al., 2003). Behind Indonesia, the Philippines and Myanmar have the largest number of cases of intestinal helminth infections, followed by the Mekong countries (de Silva et al., 2003; Montresor et al., 2008; Rim et al., 2003; WHO, 2008d, 2009d,f). Based on limited surveys in the region and high rates of infection among Southeast Asian immigrants (Nutman et al., 1987), strongyloidiasis is believed to be highly endemic although there are only a few available prevalence estimates for this infection at a country or regional level (Olsen et al., 2009). High prevalence rates have recently been reported from Lao PDR (Sayasone et al., 2009).

TABLE 2.4 Major NTDs with no or minimal regional prevalence or incidence estimates in Southeast Asia and P.R. China

Helminth infections	Protozoan infections	Bacterial infections	Viral infections	Other conditions
Strongyloidiasis	Amoebiasis	Bovine tuberculosis	Dengue and other arboviral infections	Mycetoma
Toxocariasis	Balantidiasis	Cholera	Rabies	Paracoccidiomycosis
Taeniasis/cysticercosis	Leishmaniasis	Enteric pathogens		Scabies
Thelaziosis		Leptospirosis		
		Brucellosis		
		Melioidosis		

In P.R. China, there are an estimated 129 million infections with intestinal helminths based on the second nationwide survey that was completed prior to 2005, including 86 million cases of ascariasis, 29 million cases of trichuriasis and 39 million cases of hookworm infection (Ministry of Health China, 2005). The highest rates of intestinal helminth infection occur on the Chinese provincial island of Hainan, followed by the southwestern provinces of Guizhou, Sichuan and Guangxi (Ministry of Health China, 2005). High prevalence rates of strongyloidiasis and other intestinal helminthiases have also been reported from Yunnan province (Steinmann et al., 2007, 2010). These high prevalence rates reflect the high levels of rural poverty in these areas, with particularly high rates among farmers, fishermen and some indigenous populations living in remote and sometimes mountainous regions (Ministry of Health China, 2005). Among P.R. China's 31 provinces, autonomous regions and municipalities, Guizhou is the poorest, while the other provinces with high rates of intestinal helminth infections (e.g. Sichuan, Guangxi and Hainan) are in the bottom quartile (Ministry of Health China, 2005). Trichinellosis also occurs in Yunnan (and in Nei Mongolia) (Ministry of Health China, 2005). The high rates of intestinal nematode infections found in P.R. China's southwest were actually predicted during a period between the first nationwide survey (completed during the early 1990s) and the second, and were based on the observation that this area has not benefited from nearly the same levels of economic development that have taken place over the last two decades in P.R. China's eastern provinces and large eastern cities (Hotez, 2002). Previously, during the 1980s and early 1990s, high rates of infection were also found in east P.R. China where economic development had not yet occurred and living standards were poor (Hotez et al., 1997).

In 2001, the 54th World Health Assembly (WHA) adopted a resolution (i.e. WHA resolution 54.19) calling for periodic deworming of at least 75% of all school-aged children in highly endemic areas (Bethony et al., 2006; Colley et al., 2001; Savioli et al., 2002, 2009; WHO, 2002, 2008c,d, 2009d). Over the last 2 years, high coverage rates with anthelminthic drugs, typically either albendazole or mebendazole, have been achieved in some of the Mekong countries. For instance, since 2005, in Lao PDR, the government has organised a deworming campaign for approximately 1 million school-aged children that includes two rounds of annual treatments with 500 mg of mebendazole (Phommasack et al., 2008). Montresor et al. (2008) estimated that 9.6 million school-aged children received anthelminthic drugs in 2006, and beginning in 2007, national coverage reached 95% at a cost of only US$ 0.12 per child (Phommasack et al., 2008). Similar rates of high coverage for school-aged children have also been achieved in Cambodia (beginning in 2004) and Vietnam (beginning in 2008) at low cost (Montresor et al., 2007, 2008; Sinuon et al., 2005; WHO, 2008c). In Vietnam, women of reproductive age, including pregnant women, also receive anthelminthic drugs (Mihrshahi et al., 2009; Montresor et al., 2008). Outside of the Mekong countries, the coverage rates for deworming are not nearly as high. In Indonesia where the largest number of intestinal helminth infections occurs, only 3% of school-aged children and 2% of preschool-aged children receive deworming, with approximately 20% coverage for both age groups in Myanmar (Montresor et al., 2008; WHO, 2008c). In many of the larger Southeast Asian countries, deworming is linked almost exclusively to LF control, in which donated albendazole is added to diethylcarbamazine citrate (DEC) in children 2 years of age and older (Montresor et al., 2008). In the Philippines, an estimated 10 million children are dewormed annually as part of the Global Program to Eliminate Lymphatic Filariasis (GPELF), but approximately twice as many children would need to be treated to enable coverage to reach 75% as recommended by WHA resolution 54.19 (Montresor et al., 2008). WHO covers the Asian Pacific region out of its two regional offices, one for Southeast Asian countries and one for the Western Pacific regional countries. Few (3%) in the former region have achieved 75% of treatment coverage for deworming in comparison to almost half (44%) of the countries in the latter region (WHO, 2008c). In P.R. China, less than 1% of the at-risk population receives regular and periodic deworming (WHO, 2008c), although this number may represent an underestimate and does not reflect P.R. China's rapid economic gains especially in the rural areas, along with health promotion, and increasing use of chemical fertilisers in place of 'night soil' (Hotez, 2002; Montresor et al., 2008).

2.4. LYMPHATIC FILARIASIS

No recent estimates of the number of cases of LF in the 21 countries of the Asia Pacific Region are available (WHO, 2009e,f). In the mid-1990s, it was estimated that there were 15 million cases in Asia, excluding India and Pakistan (Michael et al., 1996). However, these estimates include the Pacific islands. The largest number of cases of LF is believed to occur in Indonesia and Myanmar, followed by the Philippines, Malaysia and Thailand (Michael et al., 1996), with most of the infections caused by *Wuchereria bancrofti*, except in Indonesia, the Philippines and Malaysia where infections caused by *Brugia malayi* are also endemic, and in East Timor *B. timori* infections are found. Among the major clinical differences between these filarial infections is the observation that genital involvement and disfigurement are much less common with *Brugia* infection. Typically, the endemic situation for LF is expressed in terms of the number of people at risk for infection. Approximately 32 million people are at risk for LF in the WHO South-East Asia Region (SEAR) countries of

Indonesia, Myanmar, Thailand and East Timor, while a similar number are at risk in the so-called 'Mekong Plus' countries of Cambodia, Malaysia, the Philippines and Vietnam (Montresor et al., 2008; WHO, 2008b, 2009d). In contrast, in 2006, P.R. China became the first country to certify verification of elimination of LF as a public health problem (Montresor et al., 2008). Since then, the Republic of Korea has also requested and obtained an official acknowledgement from WHO of having eliminated LF as a public health problem (WHO, 2009d).

In the 11 countries of Southeast Asia, DEC is provided through the GPELF either in salt or as an annual single dose together with albendazole for 5–6 consecutive years (Global Alliance to Eliminate Lymphatic Filariasis, 2009). According to the WHO SEAR office, both Indonesia and Myanmar have achieved high coverage exceeding 75%, as have Thailand and East Timor (WHO, 2008b). However, in the eastern frontiers of Myanmar, the ethnic minority groups have been engaged in civil military conflict for several decades and reportedly have been denied access to regular treatments for LF (Beyrer et al., 2007). Accordingly, the rates of LF infection Burmese immigrants coming across the border into Thailand remain high (Beyrer et al., 2007). In the Mekong Plus countries, approximately 64% of the 24 million people living in implementation units (out of a total of 32 million at risk) received DEC and albendazole in 2007 (WHO, 2008b). Among these implementing countries, Malaysia, and some parts of the Philippines and Vietnam, are expected to complete five rounds of annual treatments by the end of 2008 (WHO, 2008b, 2009d).

2.5. FOOD-BORNE TREMATODE INFECTIONS

Next to the nematode infections caused by intestinal helminths and filarial worms, trematode infections are the most common NTDs in Southeast Asia and P.R. China (WHO, 2008d, 2009d). The food-borne trematodiases opisthorchiasis, clonorchiasis and paragonimiasis are believed to be the most common, followed by schistosomiasis (Keiser and Utzinger, 2009).

Liver fluke infections (i.e. opisthorchiasis and clonorchiasis) are leading causes of both chronic disability and cholangiocarcinoma (cancer of the bile duct) (Sripa et al., 2010). Northern Thailand and Lao PDR represent hyperendemic areas for opisthorchiasis caused by *Opisthorchis viverrini*, as well as cholangiocarcinoma (Andrews et al., 2008; Sripa, 2008; Sripa et al., 2010). An estimated 10 million people are infected in these two countries (with most of the cases in north Thailand), with some additional cases in Cambodia. An estimated 67 million people are at risk for opisthorchiasis in Southeast Asia (Keiser and Utzinger, 2005). *Clonorchis sinensis* is the major liver fluke found in P.R. China, especially in the northeastern provinces of Heilongjiang and Jilin (Ministry of Health China, 2005), as well as in neighbouring regions of both North and South Korea (Hotez, 2003; Kim et al., 2009). A second major Chinese focus of *C. sinensis* infection occurs in the southern provinces of Guangdong and Guangxi (Ministry of Health China, 2005). In total, an estimated 12.5 million cases of clonorchiasis occur in P.R. China (Ministry of Health China, 2005), with approximately 570 million at risk of clonorchiasis in P.R. China and Taiwan (Keiser and Utzinger, 2005). Both *O. viverrini* and *C. sinensis* can cause chronic infections leading to long-standing bile duct inflammation and periductal fibrosis (sometimes leading to bile duct obstruction) (Sripa et al., 2009), which is accompanied by malnutrition and wasting. In the northern Thailand province of Khon Kaen, the prevalence of *O. viverrini* infection reaches 70%, with an incidence of almost 1 per 1000 (Andrews et al., 2008; Sripa, 2008).

Liver flukes are recognised as carcinogens and direct risk factors for cholangiocarcinoma (Andrews et al., 2008; Sripa, 2008), and over a period of 3–4 decades after initial infection, both species can produce cholangiocarcinoma in a subset of individuals. An estimated 5% of patients with chronic liver fluke infections develop cholangiocarcinoma. This translates to 5000 new cases of *O. viverrini*-induced cholangiocarcinoma that are diagnosed annually in Thailand, and several hundred additional cases in Lao PDR and elsewhere (Parkin, 2006). Approximately 1000 new cases of *C. sinensis*-induced cholangiocarcinoma also occur in P.R. China (Parkin, 2006), although these numbers may be underestimates (Parkin, 2006). Typically, death ensues within 3–6 months following a diagnosis of cholangiocarcinoma (Andrews et al., 2008), and so liver flukes are also a significant cause of mortality. It has been further determined that opisthorchiasis and cholangiocarcinoma exert a heavy socio-economic toll, particularly because of their disproportionate impact on male heads of households who are also family wage earners; Thailand loses an estimated US$ 120 million annually in lost wages and medical care costs (Andrews et al., 2008). There are also concerns about the emerging globalisation of liver fluke infections because of the expansion of aquaculture in Asia and increased exports of cultivated fish (Andrews et al., 2008). Although praziquantel is effective for treating opisthorchiasis and clonorchiasis, anthelminthic treatment does not always reverse periductal fibrosis and inflammation, and therefore may not prevent cholangiocarcinoma. Therefore, health education, especially for children, to reduce their consumption of infected fish, and for food preparers to cook their fish, are key elements for prevention. Since 1981, there has been a decline in the prevalence of opisthorchiasis in north Thailand as a result of control activities (Kaewpitoon et al., 2008), whereas the prevalence is believed to have actually increased in P.R. China (Lu et al., 2005; Ministry of Health China, 2005), possibly by as much as threefold (Keiser and Utzinger, 2007).

P.R. China accounts for approximately two-thirds of the people at risk for paragonimiasis (Keiser and Utzinger, 2005, 2007). *Paragonimus westermani* is the most common cause of lung fluke infection (pleuropulmonary infection) leading to chest pain and hemoptysis. Extrapulmonary infection caused by visceral and cutaneous larva migrans leading to cerebral and cutaneous paragonimiasis, respectively, is also common (WHO, 2008d, 2009d). *Paragonimus skrjabini* is a major cause of extrapulmonary disease in P.R. China. In P.R. China, paragonimiasis is reported most frequently in Shanghai and Chongqing, as well as among certain indigenous groups (Ministry of Health China, 2005), although the disease is believed to be highly underreported. In addition to paragonimiasis, there are up to 70 food-borne trematode species infecting the human gastrointestinal tract, with most of these infections caused by *Fasciolopsis buski*, heterophyid trematodes and echinostomes, occurring in Southeast Asia and P.R. China. At present, their prevalence and disease burden are unknown (Keiser and Utzinger, 2009).

2.6. SCHISTOSOMIASIS

Schistosoma japonicum is an important cause of intestinal schistosomiasis affecting up to 1 million people in P.R. China and the Philippines (Steinmann et al., 2006), with a small focus in Indonesia (Garjito et al., 2008), while *Schistosoma mekongi* cause intestinal schistosomiasis among thousands of people in Cambodia and Lao PDR (Muth et al., 2010).

Approximately 800,000 cases of intestinal schistosomiasis occur in the Chinese lake regions of the Yangtze River provinces of Anhui, Hubei, Hunan, Jiangsu and Jiangxi, as well as in the mountainous riverine areas of Sichuan and Yunnan provinces (Montresor et al., 2008; WHO, 2008d, 2009d; Zhou et al., 2007). These numbers represent a dramatic reduction from more than 10 million cases in 12 Chinese provinces that occurred during the middle part of the twentieth century (Wang et al., 2008), when intestinal schistosomiasis had a significant impact on P.R. China's geopolitics and socio-economic development (Hotez, 2008; Ross et al., 2001; Utzinger et al., 2003; Zhou et al., 2005, 2010). Despite P.R. China's enormous economic progress over the last two decades and its victories in reducing that country's schistosomiasis disease burden by more than 90%, eliminating the remaining cases has proven to be challenging. Schistosomiasis has been officially declared as a public health priority in P.R. China. A number of socio-economic, climatologic and economic factors have been cited for thwarting Chinese schistosomiasis elimination efforts, including the termination of an important World Bank loan project for schistosomiasis control in 2001 (Wang et al., 2008). Among the most compelling reasons for why schistosomiasis remains in P.R. China, however, are the observations that the intermediate *Oncomelania* snail hosts are amphibious and can proliferate in a diverse array of microhabitats, and that *S. japonicum* infection is a zoonosis transmitted from a diverse array of mammalian hosts but especially water buffaloes in the marshland region (Wang et al., 2008). In addition, the construction of the Three Gorges Dam on the Yangtze River and the resultant filling of an enormous reservoir have produced both positive and negative effects in terms of emerging schistosomiasis (Zhu et al., 2008). In 2004, the Ministry of Health of P.R. China launched a 10-year project for schistosomiasis control (Montresor et al., 2008; WHO, 2009d), and has set an elimination target for 2015 (Wang et al., 2009). The strategy has surprisingly little reliance on mass drug administration with praziquantel, possibly because of re-infection, and the anaemia associated with inflammation is often unaffected by treatment (Leenstra et al., 2006). Instead, schistosomiasis control and elimination in P.R. China focuses primarily on transmission from water buffaloes (responsible for up to 90% of the human transmission (Wang et al., 2005)) by replacing them with tractors, fencing them in restricted areas, and preventing them from pasturing in snail-infested marshland (Montresor et al., 2008), as well as by improving sanitation and providing mobile toilets for fishermen and other individuals with occupational commitments to the Yangtze River and its tributaries (Wang et al., 2008, 2009).

In the Philippines, an estimated 200,000 cases of intestinal schistosomiasis with *S. japonicum* occur and 6.7 million people are at risk in more than 1200 villages known as *barangays* in the islands of Leyte and Samar, and in the areas of Luzon and Mindanao (Tallo et al., 2008; WHO, 2009d). In contrast to P.R. China, control efforts rely heavily on mass drug administration with praziquantel to all residents 5 years of age and older in areas where the prevalence is $\geq$15% (Tallo et al., 2008). To date, however, treatment coverage is low, and it has been suggested that more behavioural and social science research is required to understand the basis for poor compliance among these populations (Tallo et al., 2008).

The largest number of cases of *S. mekongi* infection is believed to occur in Cambodia (WHO, 2009d) where mass drug administration with praziquantel is underway– according to one recent paper, no new cases have been reported since 2006 (Montresor et al., 2008).

2.7. CESTODE INFECTIONS

Based on the second nationwide survey, there are an estimated 550,000 cases of taeniasis in P.R. China, with the highest rates occurring in Tibet and among the Uyghur ethnic group (Ministry of Health China, 2005). Cysticercosis is also endemic throughout P.R. China. Cystic echinococcosis is endemic in northwestern P.R. China with an estimated 380,000 cases in Xinjiang and Inner Mongolia (Ministry of Health China, 2005; WHO,

2008d, 2009d). The highest rates of infection occur among farmers and herdsmen and in some ethnic minorities (Ministry of Health China, 2005). There are no available prevalence estimates of cestode infections in the 11 Southeast Asian countries.

2.8. NON-HELMINTHIC NTDs

2.8.1. Protozoan and bacterial infections

Unlike malaria, prevalence and disease burden estimates for protozoan and bacterial NTDs in Southeast Asia are especially poor, just as they are for sub-Saharan Africa (Hotez and Kamath, 2009). This absence of information may partly explain why there are no large-scale control efforts for these conditions. Among the protozoan infections, there are no available prevalence estimates for amoebiasis, while in P.R. China it has been noted that high rates of toxoplasmosis occur among some indigenous populations and kala-azar (visceral leishmaniasis) occurs in the western provinces of Xinjiang, Sichuan and Gansu (Ministry of Health China, 2005). Relatively high prevalence rates of kala-azar occur among Uighur indigenous populations in those regions (Ministry of Health China, 2005).

Among the bacterial NTDs, the most important is active trachoma. More than 40% of the global disease burden from trachoma occurs in P.R. China, where an estimated 27 million cases occur, while another 2 million cases occur in Indonesia, 1 million in Cambodia, and fewer than 500,000 in Vietnam (WHO, 2009c). Overall, approximately one-half of the world's active trachoma cases can be found in Southeast Asia and P.R. China. According to the Beijing Eye Study, a population-based, cross-sectional survey to determine the prevalence of trachoma among adult populations in P.R. China, up to 8% of Chinese adults in north P.R. China exhibited signs of active trachoma, with age, socio-economic status and rural habitats representing the major risk factors (Jie et al., 2008). Currently, Vietnam is the only asian country among the 18 countries where the International Trachoma Initiative applies its SAFE (i.e. surgery, antibiotics, facial cleanliness and environmental control) strategy (International Trachoma Initiative, 2009). There are very few published reports on efforts to scale-up trachoma control in either P.R. China or Cambodia.

Together Southeast Asia and P.R. China account for fewer than 15% of the world's leprosy cases (WHO, 2008a). Of the approximately 28,000 registered leprosy cases in Southeast Asia, 21,000 occur in Indonesia and 3000 each in P.R. China and Myanmar (WHO, 2008a). Melioidosis caused by *Burkholderia pseudomallei* is an important cause of septicemia in Southeast Asia, especially in parts of northern Thailand, Malaysia and Singapore (Currie et al., 2008), although no global estimates of disease burden are available.

2.8.2. Viral infections

The flaviruses that cause Japanese encephalitis (JE) and dengue are the most important arboviruses in the region. JE occurs in South and Southeast Asia and the Pacific, where there is an annual incidence of 30,000–50,000 cases, mostly transmitted to humans from infected water birds by *Culex* mosquitoes breeding in irrigated rice paddies (Erlanger et al., 2009). The number of cases is believed to be underreported because diagnostic surveillance centres have been established only in P.R. China and Thailand and not in less developed areas of Southeast Asia (Erlanger et al., 2009). Surveillance data from Myanmar are lacking, although JE is believed to be common there. Up to 15,000 deaths occur annually. Among the factors responsible for the emergence of JE in Southeast Asia are population growth and increases in irrigated rice farming required to support that growth, as well as the rearing of pigs, which are also an important animal reservoir (Erlanger et al., 2009).

Epidemic dengue as well as dengue hemorrhagic fever (DHF) and dengue shock syndrome (DSS) emerged out of Southeast Asia 50 years ago and the incidence has been steadily increasing (Kyle and Harris, 2008; WHO, 2009a,b,f). Globally, tens of millions of cases of dengue occur each year, along with approximately 0.5 million cases of DHF/DSS, which are major causes of paediatric hospitalisation in Southeast Asia (Kyle and Harris, 2008). For example, epidemics of DHF/DSS emerge out of Bangkok every 3 years and spread throughout the country at a rate of approximately 148 km per month (Kyle and Harris, 2008). *Aedes aegypti* is the major mosquito vector in urban areas, while the less efficient *Ae. albopictus* is a primary vector in rural areas. Global warming and urbanisation are major factors accounting for the emergence of dengue in Southeast Asia (Kyle and Harris, 2008). Although not the subject of the current chapter, other NTDs (caused by fungi, ecto-parasites, bacteria and viruses) are beginning to attract more attention within the public health community. Canine rabies is another important viral NTD, with more than one-half of the 55,000 annual deaths' cases occurring in Asia, principally in India followed by P.R. China (Knobel et al., 2005).

2.9. PRIORITIES FOR NTD CONTROL IN ASIA PACIFIC REGION

2.9.1. Integrated control of intestinal helminth infections and LF

The three major intestinal helminth infections and LF are by far and away the most common NTDs affecting the poorest people in Asia Pacific Region (Hotez, 2009). Most of the 300 million people who live in Southeast

Asia and P.R. China below the World Bank poverty level of US$ 1.25 per day suffer from one or more of these NTDs, as do many who live on less than US$ 2 per day. Moreover, based on selected disease burden calculations (Hotez et al., 2006, 2007), some investigators would rank these four infections among the most important health threats in the region. Therefore, an important priority for NTD control in the region is to reduce the morbidity of the intestinal helminths through mass drug administration with either albendazole or mebendazole as recommended by WHA resolution 54.19, as well as to target both adults and children at risk for LF by combining DEC and albendazole in mass drug administration, which will simultaneously target the intestinal helminth infections. These interventions are remarkably inexpensive, costing only around US$ 0.10 per person, so that the bottom 300 million living in Southeast Asia could receive annual mass treatments for only US$ 30 million annually. Through high treatment coverage, the Mekong countries have already made great strides in reducing the prevalence of intestinal helminth infections affecting school-aged children – for instance, Lao PDR has substantially reduced the prevalence of ascariasis and trichuriasis by reaching national coverage rates of 95%, with a virtual absence of high and moderate intensity infections (Phommasack et al., 2008). Similarly, several rounds of LF treatments have been achieved through the Mekong Plus programme (especially Malaysia, some parts of the Philippines and Vietnam) (WHO, 2008b, 2009d). It is critical that in instances where school-aged children receive albendazole for their intestinal helminth infections through Mekong Plus, these annual treatments continue even after LF is eliminated as a public health problem (Montresor et al., 2008). In contrast to the Mekong countries, among the largest Southeast Asian countries, both Indonesia and Myanmar have not achieved high coverage for their intestinal helminth infections despite the observation that globally they rank near the top in terms of prevalence for such infections. Escalating coverage in Indonesia and Myanmar is therefore a high priority, as well as intestinal helminth control in the four high prevalence Chinese provinces.

2.9.2. Integrated control of intestinal helminth and trematode infections

In selected areas of the Philippines, albendazole or mebendazole requires combination therapy with praziquantel to simultaneously target intestinal helminth infections and schistosomiasis; therefore coverage for these conditions remains a high priority (WHO, 2009d). Similarly in four Chinese provinces (mentioned earlier), as well as in northern Thailand and parts of Lao PDR, simultaneous coverage with albendazole/mebendazole and praziquantel for both intestinal helminth and liver fluke infections, respectively, must be considered. Possibly, there are regions in Cambodia, Lao PDR and the Philippines where the intestinal helminth infections overlap geographically with LF and either schistosomiasis or opisthorchiasis (WHO, 2009d). There are published safety data to support triple co-administration with albendazole, DEC and praziquantel, as there is for triple therapy with albendazole, ivermectin and praziquantel (Mohammed et al., 2008; Hotez, 2009).

2.9.3. Helminth elimination efforts and research needs

In addition to the integrated control efforts outlined earlier, over the next 5 years, LF could be eliminated as a public health problem in several Mekong countries, while, largely through interrupting transmission from water buffaloes, schistosomiasis could be eliminated as a public health problem in P.R. China (Wang et al., 2009). Such elimination efforts would leave the Philippines as having the largest population in the region at risk for both LF and schistosomiasis (Montresor et al., 2008). Considerable research opportunities exist for helminth control and elimination efforts, including operational research issues, to circumvent the biological and social barriers to helminth control in areas of low coverage, such as Indonesia, Myanmar and selected areas of the Philippines and P.R. China, as well as monitoring efforts to examine the sustainability of intestinal helminth and LF control in the high-coverage Mekong countries. In some cases, new control tools may be required, including improved diagnostics for food-borne trematode infections, (Keiser and Utzinger, 2008, 2010), and possibly vaccines to prevent hookworm infection, schistosomiasis and cysticercosis in high transmission areas either because of drug failure (especially mebendazole for hookworm) rapid re-infection (hookworm and schistosomiasis), or zoonotic transmission (schistosomiasis and cysticercosis) (Hotez and Ferris, 2006; McManus and Loukas, 2008). Finally, many important helminthic NTDs, including cysticercosis and the food-borne trematodiases, lack adequate disease prevalence and burden estimates, which are critical for advocacy and informed policy decisions. Many of the risk factors leading to NTDs lie outside the purview of the health sector. Socio-economic, environmental, cultural and other determinants of health need to be considered through interventions to sustain the gains of mass chemotherapy-based programmes (Ehrenberg and Ault, 2005; Schratz et al., 2010).

2.9.4. Non-helminthic NTD control and elimination efforts

SAFE strategy efforts need to be increased in areas highly endemic for trachoma in P.R. China and Cambodia, where the largest number of cases occurs, while leprosy elimination efforts with multi-drug therapy must continue, especially in Indonesia where the largest number of cases is registered. Vector control for JE and dengue remains a high priority in both urban and rural areas of Southeast Asia and P.R. China, along with ongoing operational research. New vaccines for JE and dengue are under development through both product development partnerships supported by the Bill & Melinda Gates Foundation and the vaccine manufacturer, Sanofi Pasteur (Hotez and Ferris, 2006).

2.10. CONCLUDING STATEMENT: INNOVATIVE FINANCING FOR NTD CONTROL AND ELIMINATION IN ASIA AND OTHER KEY ACTIONS

In addition to ongoing large-scale financial support for the Global Alliance to Eliminate LF, through initial support from the Bill & Melinda Gates Foundation, a regional hub for financing NTD control in Asia is also being established (Hotez et al., 2009). Currently, the funds are prioritised to emphasise helminth and trachoma control and elimination through mass drug administration, although in time vector control strategies would also be considered. Unfortunately, this pro-poor strategy is not balanced by a parallel research and development fund for new and priority NTD control tools, although as the global economy improves, perhaps such a fund may be considered in the future.

Regional plans of actions will need to be put in place for NTD prevention, control and/or elimination. These plans should be politically endorsed by the Ministers of Health of all affected countries during the annual WHO meetings (regional committee meetings). Such plans will provide the framework for the national plan and as a resource mobilisation tool to support regional fundraising efforts.

ACKNOWLEDGEMENTS

The authors wish to acknowledge the support of Dr. Jürg Utzinger from the Swiss Tropical and Public Health Institute for his helpful suggestions.

REFERENCES

Andrews, R.H., Sithithaworn, P., Petney, T.N., 2008. *Opisthorchis viverrini*: an underestimated parasite in world health. Trends Parasitol. 24, 497–501.

Bethony, J., Brooker, S., Albonico, M., Geiger, S.M., Loukas, A., Diemert, D., et al., 2006. Soil-transmitted helminth infections: ascariasis, trichuriasis, and hookworm. Lancet 367, 1521–1532.

Beyrer, C., Villar, J.C., Suwanvanichkij, V., Singh, S., Baral, S.D., Mills, E.J., 2007. Neglected diseases, civil conflicts, and the right to health. Lancet 370, 619–627.

Colley, D.G., LoVerde, P.T., Savioli, L., 2001. Medical helminthology in the 21st century. Science 293, 1437–1438.
Currie, B.J., Dance, D.A., Cheng, A.C., 2008. The global distribution of *Burkholderia pseudomallei* and melioidosis: an update. Trans. R. Soc. Trop. Med. Hyg. 102 (Suppl. 1), S1–S4.
de Silva, N.R., Brooker, S., Hotez, P.J., Montresor, A., Engels, D., Savioli, L., 2003. Soil-transmitted helminth infections: updating the global picture. Trends Parasitol. 19, 547–551.
Ehrenberg, J.P., Ault, S.K., 2005. Neglected diseases of neglected populations: thinking to reshape the determinants of health in Latin America and the Caribbean. BMC Public Health 5, 119.
Erlanger, T.E., Weiss, S., Keiser, J., Utzinger, J., Wiedenmayer, K., 2009. Past, present, and future of Japanese encephalitis. Emerg. Infect. Dis. 15, 1–7.
Garjito, T.A., Sudomo, M., Abdullah, Dahlan, M., Nurwidayati, A., 2008. Schistosomiasis in Indonesia: past and present. Parasitol. Int. 57, 277–280.
Global Alliance to Eliminate Lymphatic Filariasis, 2009. Global alliance to eliminate lymphatic filariasis. http://www.filariasis.org/.
Hotez, P.J., 2002. China's hookworms. China Q. 172, 1029–1041.
Hotez, P.J., 2003. The promise of medical science and biotechnology for North Korea and the relevance of U.S. "vaccine diplomacy." Korea Soc. Q. 3, 15–18.
Hotez, P.J., 2008. Forgotten People and Forgotten Diseases, the Neglected Tropical Diseases and their Impact on Global Health and Development. American Society of Microbiology.
Hotez, P.J., 2009. Mass drug administration and integrated control for the world's high-prevalence neglected tropical diseases. Clin. Pharmacol. Ther. 85, 659–664.
Hotez, P.J., Ferris, M.T., 2006. The antipoverty vaccines. Vaccine 24, 5787–5799.
Hotez, P.J., Kamath, A., 2009. Neglected tropical diseases is sub-Saharan Africa: review of their prevalence, distribution, and disease be den. PLoS Negl. Trop. Dis 3, e412.
Hotez, P.J., Feng, Z., Xu, L.Q., Chen, M.G., Xiao, S.H., Liu, S.X., et al., 1997. Emerging and reemerging helminthiases and the public health of China. Emerg. Infect. Dis. 3, 303–310.
Hotez, P.J., Molyneux, D.H., Fenwick, A., Ottesen, E., Ehrlich Sachs, S., Sachs, J.D., 2006. Incorporating a rapid-impact package for neglected tropical diseases with programs for HIV/AIDS, tuberculosis, and malaria. PLoS Med. 3, e102.
Hotez, P.J., Molyneux, D.H., Fenwick, A., Kumaresan, J., Ehrlich Sachs, S., Sachs, J.D., et al., 2007. Control of neglected tropical diseases. N. Engl. J. Med 357, 1018–1027.
Hotez, P.J., Fenwick, A., Savioli, L., Molyneux, D.H., 2009. Rescuing the bottom billion through control of neglected tropical diseases. Lancet 373, 1570–1575.
International Trachoma Initiative, 2009. Welcome to international trachoma initiative. http://www.trachoma.org/core/.
Jie, Y., Xu, L., Ma, K., Zhang, S., Zhu, J., Jonas, J.B., 2008. Prevalence of trachoma in the adult Chinese population. The Beijing eye study. Eye (Lond) 22, 790–791.
Kaewpitoon, N., Kaewpitoon, S.J., Pengsaa, P., Sripa, B., 2008. *Opisthorchis viverrini*: the carcinogenic human liver fluke. World J. Gastroenterol. 14, 666–674.
Keiser, J., Utzinger, J., 2005. Emerging foodborne trematodiasis. Emerg. Infect. Dis. 11, 1507–1514.
Keiser, J., Utzinger, J., 2007. Food-borne trematodiasis: current chemotherapy and advances with artemisinins and synthetic trioxolanes. Trends Parasitol. 23, 555–562.
Keiser, J., Utzinger, J., 2008. Efficacy of current drugs against soil-transmitted helminth infections: systematic review and meta-analysis. JAMA 299, 1937–1948.
Keiser, J., Utzinger, J., 2009. Food-borne trematodiases. Clin. Microbiol. Rev. 22, 466–483.
Keiser, J., Utzinger, J., 2010. The drugs we have and the drugs we need against major helminth infections. Adv. Parasitol. 73, 197–230.
Kim, H.G., Han, J., Kim, M.H., Cho, K.H., Shin, I.H., Kim, G.H., et al., 2009. Prevalence of clonorchiasis in patients with gastrointestinal disease: a Korean nationwide multicenter survey. World J. Gastroenterol. 15, 86–94.

Knobel, D.L., Cleaveland, S., Coleman, P.G., Fevre, E.M., Meltzer, M.I., Miranda, M.E., et al., 2005. Re-evaluating the burden of rabies in Africa and Asia. Bull. World Health Organ. 83, 360–368.

Kyle, J.L., Harris, E., 2008. Global spread and persistence of dengue. Annu. Rev. Microbiol. 62, 71–92.

Leenstra, T., Coutinho, H.M., Acosta, L.P., Langdon, G.C., Su, L., Olveda, R.M., et al., 2006. *Schistosoma japonicum* reinfection after praziquantel treatment causes anemia associated with inflammation. Infect. Immun. 74, 6398–6407.

Lu, Z.R., Gasser, R.B., Lai, D.H., Li, A.X., Zhu, X.Q., You, X.B., et al., 2005. Clonorchiasis: a key foodborne zoonosis in China. Lancet Infect. Dis. 5, 31–41.

McManus, D.P., 2010. Echinococcosis with particular reference to Southeast Asia. Adv. Parasitol. 72, 267–303.

McManus, D.P., Loukas, A., 2008. Current status of vaccines for schistosomiasis. Clin. Microbiol. Rev. 21, 225–242.

Michael, E., Bundy, D.A.P., Grenfell, B.T., 1996. Re-assessing the global prevalence and distribution of lymphatic filariasis. Parasitology 112, 409–428.

Mihrshahi, S., Casey, G.J., Montresor, A., Phuc, T.Q., Thach, D.T., Tien, N.T., et al., 2009. The effectiveness of 4 monthly albendazole treatment in the reduction of soil-transmitted helminth infections in women of reproductive age in Viet Nam. Int. J. Parasitol. 39, 1037–1043.

Ministry of Health China, 2005. Report on the national survey of current situation of major human parasite diseases in China. National Institute of Parasitic Diseases.

Mohammed, K.A., Haji, H.H., Gabrielli, A.F., Mubila, L., Biswas, G., Chitsulo, L., et al., 2008. Triple-co-administration of ivermectin, albendazole and praziquantel in Zanzibar: a safety study. PLoS Negl. Trop. Dis. 2, e171.

Molyneux, D.H., Hotez, P.J., Fenwick, A., 2005. ''Rapid-impact interventions'': how a policy of integrated control for Africa's neglected tropical diseases could benefit the poor. PLoS Med. 2, e336.

Montresor, A., Cong, D.T., Le Anh, T., Ehrhardt, A., Mondadori, E., Thi, T.D., et al., 2007. Cost containment in a school deworming programme targeting over 2.7 million children in Vietnam. Trans. R. Soc. Trop. Med. Hyg. 101, 461–464.

Montresor, A., Cong, D.T., Sinuon, M., Tsuyuoka, R., Chanthavisouk, C., Strandgaard, H., et al., 2008. Large-scale preventive chemotherapy for the control of helminth infection in Western Pacific countries: six years later. PLoS Negl. Trop. Dis. 2, e278.

Muth, S., Sayasone, S., Odermatt-Biays, S., Phompida, S., Duong, S., Odermatt, P., 2010. *Schistosoma mekongi* in Cambodia and Lao People's Democratic Republic. Adv. Parasitol. 72, 179–203.

Nutman, T.B., Ottesen, E.A., Ieng, S., Samuels, J., Kimball, E., Lutkoski, M., et al., 1987. Eosinophilia in Southeast Asian refugees: evaluation at a referral center. J. Infect. Dis. 155, 309–313.

Olsen, A., van Lieshout, L., Marti, H., Polderman, T., Polman, K., Steinmann, P., et al., 2009. Strongyloidiasis – the most neglected of the neglected tropical diseases? Trans. R. Soc. Trop. Med. Hyg. 103, 967–972.

Parkin, D.M., 2006. The global health burden of infection-associated cancers in the year 2002. Int. J. Cancer 118, 3030–3044.

Phommasack, B., Saklokham, K., Chanthavisouk, C., Nakhonesid-Fish, V., Strandgaard, H., Montresor, A., et al., 2008. Coverage and costs of a school deworming programme in 2007 targeting all primary schools in Lao PDR. Trans. R. Soc. Trop. Med. Hyg. 102, 1201–1206.

Rim, H.J., Chai, J.Y., Min, D.Y., Cho, S.Y., Eom, K.S., Hong, S.J., Sohn, W.M., et al., 2003. Prevalence of intestinal parasite infections on a national scale among primary schoolchildren in Laos. Parasitol. Res. 91, 267–272.

Ross, A.G.P., Sleigh, A.C., Li, Y., Davis, G.M., Williams, G.M., Jiang, Z., et al., 2001. Schistosomiasis in the People's Republic of China: prospects and challenges for the 21st century. Clin. Microbiol. Rev. 14, 270–295.

Savioli, L., Stansfield, S., Bundy, D.A.P., Mitchell, A., Bhatia, R., Engels, D., et al., 2002. Schistosomiasis and soil-transmitted helminth infections: forging control efforts. Trans. R. Soc. Trop. 96, 577–579.

Savioli, L., Gabrielli, A.F., Montresor, A., Chitsulo, L., Engels, D., 2009. Schistosomiasis control in Africa: 8 years after World Health Assembly Resolution 54.19. Parasitology 136, 1677–1681.

Sayasone, S., Vonghajack, Y., Vanmany, M., Rasphone, O., Tesana, S., Utzinger, J., et al., 2009. Diversity of human intestinal helminthiasis in Lao PDR. Trans. R. Soc. Trop. Med. Hyg. 103, 247–254.

Schratz, A., Fernanda Pineda, M., Reforma, L.G., Fox, N.M., Anh, T.L., Cavalli-Sforza, L.T., et al., 2010. Neglected diseases and ethnic minorities in the Western Pacific Region: exploring the links. Adv. Parasitol. 72, 79–107.

Sinuon, M., Tsuyuoka, R., Socheat, D., Montresor, A., Palmer, K., 2005. Financial costs of deworming children in all primary schools in Cambodia. Trans. R. Soc. Trop. Med. Hyg. 99, 664–668.

Sithithaworn, P., Haswell-Elkins, M., 2003. Epidemiology of *Opisthorchis viverrini*. Acta Trop. 88, 187–194.

Sripa, B., 2008. Concerted action is needed to tackle liver fluke infections in Asia. PLoS Negl. Trop. Dis. 2, e232.

Sripa, B., Kaewkes, S., Sithithaworn, P., Mairiang, E., Laha, T., Smout, M., et al., 2007. Liver fluke induces cholangiocarcinoma. PLoS Med. 4, e201.

Sripa, B., Mairian, E., Thinkhamrop, B., Laha, T., Kaewkes, S., Sithithaworn, P., et al., 2009. Advanced periductal fibrosis from infection with the carcinogenic human liver fluke *Opisthorchis viverrini* correlates with elevated levels of interleukin-6. Hepatology 50, 1273–1281.

Sripa, B., Kaewkes, S., Intapan, P.M., Maleewong, W., Brindley, P.J., 2010. Food-borne trematodiases: epidemiology, pathology, clinical manifestation and control. Adv. Parasitol. 72, 305–350.

Steinmann, P., Keiser, J., Bos, R., Tanner, M., Utzinger, J., 2006. Schistosomiasis and water resources development: systematic review, meta-analysis, and estimates of people at risk. Lancet Infect. Dis. 6, 411–425.

Steinmann, P., Zhou, X.N., Du, Z.W., Jiang, J.Y., Wang, L.B., Wang, X.Z., et al., 2007. Occurrence of *Strongyloides stercoralis* in Yunnan province, China, and comparison of diagnostic methods. PLoS Negl. Trop. Dis. 1, e75.

Steinmann, P., Utzinger, J., Du, Z.W., Zhou, X.N., 2010. Multiparasitism: a neglected reality on global, regional and local scale. Adv. Parasitol. 73, 21–50.

Szczepanski, K., 2009. Poverty in Southeast Asia. http://www.helium.com/items/998777-poverty-in-south-east-asia.

Tallo, V.L., Carabin, H., Alday, P.P., Balolong Jr, E., Olveda, R.M., McGarvey, S.T., 2008. Is mass treatment the appropriate schistosomiasis elimination strategy? Bull. World Health Organ. 86, 765–771.

Utzinger, J., Bergquist, R., Xiao, S.H., Singer, B.H., Tanner, M., 2003. Sustainable schistosomiasis control – the way forward. Lancet 362, 1932–1934.

Wang, T.P., Johansen, M.V., Zhang, S.Q., Wang, F.F., Wu, W.D., Zhang, G.H., et al., 2005. Transmission of *Schistosoma japonicum* by humans and domestic animals in the Yangtze River valley, Anhui province, China. Acta Trop. 96, 198–204.

Wang, L., Utzinger, J., Zhou, X.N., 2008. Schistosomiasis control: experiences and lessons from China. Lancet 372, 1793–1795.

Wang, L.D., Chen, H.G., Guo, J.G., Zeng, X.J., Hong, X.L., Xiong, J.J., et al., 2009. A strategy to control transmission of *Schistosoma japonicum* in China. N. Engl. J. Med. 360, 121–128.

WHO, 2002. Prevention and control of schistosomiasis and soil-transmitted helminthiasis: report of a WHO expert committee. WHO Tech. Rep. Ser. 912, 1–57.

WHO, 2006. Preventive chemotherapy in human helminthiasis: coordinated use of anthelminthic drugs in control interventions: a manual for health professionals and programme managers. http://whqlibdoc.who.int/publications/2006/9241547103_eng.pdf.
WHO, 2008a. Global leprosy situation, beginning of 2008. Wkly. Epidemiol. Rec. 83, 293–300.
WHO, 2008b. Global programme to eliminate lymphatic filariasis. Wkly. Epidemiol. Rec. 83, 333–348.
WHO, 2008c. Soil-transmitted helminthiasis. Wkly. Epidemiol. Rec. 83, 237–252.
WHO, 2008d. Review on the epidemiological profile of helminthiases and their control in the Western Pacific Region, 1997–2008. Manila: WHO/WPRO. http://www.wpro.who.int/internet/resources.ashx/MVP/Helminths+10+Year+Review+_reformatted+v2_.pdf.
WHO, 2009a. Asia-Pacific dengue programme managers meeting. Singapore, 5–9 May 2008. Manila: WHO/WPRO. http://www.wpro.who.int/sites/mvp/meetings/Asia-Pacific+Dengue+Programme+Managers+Meeting.htm.
WHO, 2009b. Dengue in the Western Pacific Region, 2009 Revision. Manila: WHO/WPRO. http://www.wpro.who.int/health_topics/dengue/.
WHO, 2009c. Global health atlas: global alliance for the elimination of blinding trachoma. http://apps.who.int/globalatlas/default.asp.
WHO, 2009d. First Mekong-Plus programme managers workshop on lymphatic filariasis and other helminthiasis. Phnom Penh, Cambodia, 23–26 March 2009. Manila: WHO/WPRO. http://www.wpro.who.int/internet/files/mvp/CambodiaLFNTD_report2.pdf.
WHO, 2009e. South-East Asia Regional Office, lymphatic filariasis, 2009 revision. New Delhi: WHO/SEARO. http://www.searo.who.int/EN/Section10/Section2096.htm.
WHO, 2009f. Western Pacific Regional Office, malaria, other vector-borne and parasitic diseases, 2009 revision. Manila: WHO/WPRO. http://www.wpro.who.int/sites/mvp.
World Bank, 2009. World bank poverty data, PovcalNet. http://iresearch.worldbank.org/PovcalNet/povcalSvy.html.
World Bank Group, 2009. Key development data and statistics. http://go.worldbank.org/1SF48T40L0.
Zhou, X.N., Wang, L.Y., Chen, M.G., Wu, X.H., Jiang, Q.W., Chen, X.Y., et al., 2005. The public health significance and control of schistosomiasis in China – then and now. Acta Trop. 96, 97–105.
Zhou, X.N., Guo, J.G., Wu, X.H., Jiang, Q.W., Zhen, J., Dang, H., et al., 2007. Epidemiology of schistosomiasis in the People's Republic of China, 2004. Emerg. Infect. Dis. 13, 1470–1476.
Zhou, X.N., Bergquist, R., Leonardo, L., Yang, G.J., Yang, K., Sudomo, M., et al., 2010. Schistosomiasis japonica: research and control. Adv. Parasitol. 72, 145–178.
Zhu, H.M., Xiang, S., Yang, K., Wu, X.H., Zhou, X.N., 2008. Three Gorges dam and its impact on the potential transmission of schistosomiasis in regions along the Yangtze River. Ecohealth 5, 137–148.

CHAPTER 3

Coordinating Research on Neglected Parasitic Diseases in Southeast Asia Through Networking

Remigio Olveda,* **Lydia Leonardo,**[†] **Feng Zheng,**[‡] **Banchob Sripa,**[§] **Robert Bergquist,**[¶] and **Xiao-Nong Zhou**[‡]

Contents

Abstract

The new dialogue between stakeholders, that is, scientists, research administrators and donors as well as the populations victimised by endemic infections, is initiating a virtuous circle leading to lower disease-burdens, improved public health and the mitigation of poverty. There is now general agreement that control activities need research collaboration to advance, while surveillance plays

* Department of Health, Research Institute of Tropical Medicine (RITM), Muntinlupa, Manila, Philippines
[†] Department of Parasitology, College of Public Health, University of the Philippines, Manila, Philippines
[‡] National Institute of Parasitic Diseases, Chinese Center for Disease Control and Prevention, Shanghai, People's Republic of China
[§] Tropical Disease Research Laboratory (TDR), Department of Pathology, Faculty of Medicine, Khon Kaen University, Thailand
[¶] Ingerod, Brastad, Sweden

Advances in Parasitology, Volume 72
ISSN 0065-308X, DOI: 10.1016/S0065-308X(10)72003-0

an increasingly important role in sustaining long-term relief. On the part of the Regional Network on Asian Schistosomiasis and Other Helminth Zoonoses (RNAS$^+$), this has led to a new vision not only focused on general strengthening of research capabilities but also on furthering efforts to close the gap between research and control and bridge different branches of science. From its original, exclusive focus on schistosomiasis, RNAS$^+$ has expanded to include food-borne and soil-transmitted helminth infections as well. Its current repository of data on the distribution, prevalence and severity of these diseases is increasingly utilised by decision makers charged with epidemiological control in the endemic countries. Thanks to a more rapid translation of research results into control applications and the dissemination of data and new technology through networking, the overall situation is improving. Working as a virtual organisation of researchers and control officers in the endemic countries of Southeast Asia, RNAS$^+$ is playing an important role in this conversion. Its responsibilities are divided along disease lines into five main areas, but no serious, endemic disease is considered to be outside the network's sphere of interest. This chapter recounts some of the more important RNAS$^+$ accomplishments, pinpoints potential directions for future operations and highlights areas where research is most needed.

3.1. ROLE OF NETWORKS IN PUBLIC HEALTH

Mechanisms for information-sharing play an increasingly important role with regards to the prompt accessing of information that is useful for the improvement of local technical standards. Networking can be defined as a process framework for empowering stakeholders not only to share and apply new knowledge but also to identify and prioritise problems systematically and to participate in the development of appropriate solutions. Geographical information systems (GIS) and satellite-based remote sensing (RS) are particularly interesting in this connection as these techniques generate databases that can be used for the distribution of continuously updated risk maps covering endemic areas for the various endemic diseases under study. When connected with national and regional databases, huge amounts of data can instantly be accessed, even in remote places, contributing to the perception of diseases in the wider social context. Stensgaard et al. (2009) discuss interactive map services based on satellite imagery as user-friendly tools that can make a difference with respect to presentation of the risk for different diseases in different places. Although public health-associated networks can act as clearing houses for this type of data, they are first and foremost interactive grids for the rapid dissemination of research news and progress of national control programmes, and for becoming acquainted with key technologies and evidence-based policies.

3.2. HISTORY AND OVERARCHING GOALS OF RNAS$^+$

The idea of establishing a regional network of scientists and control officers was initiated by the UNICEF/UNDP/World Bank/WHO Special Programme for Research and Training in Tropical Diseases (TDR) at the international workshop on "Research, Surveillance and Control of Schistosomiasis japonica", held in 1996 in Nanjing, People's Republic of China (P.R. China). The Regional Network on Asian Schistosomiasis (RNAS) started as a bid to coral stakeholders for research on schistosomiasis japonica in the region. A plan was presented at a later meeting in Wuxi, P.R. China, which attracted the interest of the 70+ researchers and representatives of control authorities. A status report (McGarvey et al., 1999) on schistosomiasis japonica produced after this meeting marked the informal beginning of the network based on intersectoral, interregional and international collaboration for work on schistosomiasis japonica. Further discussions at another TDR-supported project meeting entitled 'Establishment of a Regional Network for Research, Surveillance and Control of Asian Schistosomiasis', in 2000 in Tagaytay City, the Philippines, led to the formal establishment of RNAS (Zhou et al., 2002). The network consisted originally of a relatively small group of scientists, mainly from P.R. China and the Philippines, exclusively focused on oriental schistosomiasis. At this early stage, when activities were still exclusively focused on schistosomiasis, some important research priorities were identified which are still being pursued:

- improve sensitivity of stool examination and/or substitute it with serology;
- determine the contribution of animal reservoir hosts to transmission to humans;
- estimate production losses due to animal schistosomiasis and determine the effect of changing agricultural practices; and
- estimate the effect of climatic changes on transmission.

However, the interest in the network continued to grow and more diseases and member countries were added along the way (Zhou et al., 2004, 2008a,b). A strong reason underpinning the decision to formally establish RNAS was the need for a closer relation between research and control activities in the struggle against the endemic diseases in the region. RNAS has contributed to the strengthening of the dialogue between control programme managers and academic researchers and this task can now be regarded as essentially accomplished, as has been schematically illustrated in Fig. 3.1. Applied research continues to play a

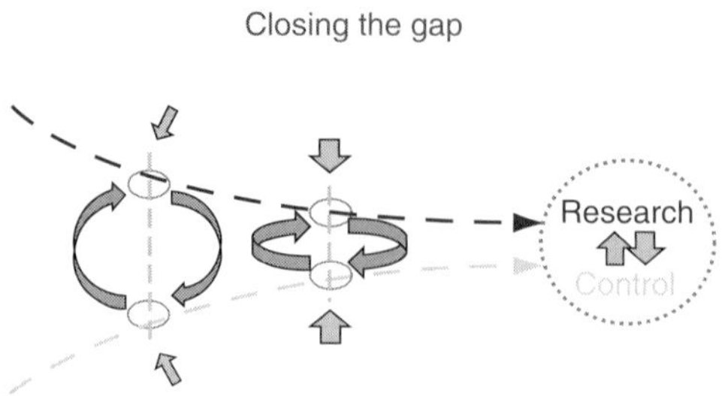

FIGURE 3.1 Closing the gap between research and control.

big role, but projects are always collaborative efforts initiated to solve specific problems in the control of one or more of the endemic diseases.

At its 5th annual meeting in 2005 in Bali, Indonesia, RNAS could look back on an impressive number of accomplishments and it was clear that the network had started to make an impact on problems related to schistosomiasis. The addition of cysticercosis/taeniasis, clonorchiasis, opisthorchiasis and fascioliasis and the change of the name to the 'RNAS^{+}' were agreed formally. Today, more than 90% of all research institutions and control authorities in the nine member countries working on the RNAS^{+} target diseases are represented in the network, which has become a force in multidisciplinary research and multisectoral collaboration among professionals, scientists and public health experts. The endemic diseases in Southeast Asia have been neglected, but there is now real hope that the situation is about to change, thanks to growing awareness of public health issues and also the economic impact of the diseases targeted for research and control by the network.

RNAS^{+} has passed through three stages of development during the last 10 years. In the establishment stage, from 1999 to 2001, regular scientific meetings were instituted and information-sharing and collaboration between the Chinese and Filipino scientists expanded noticeably. Between 2002 and 2006, in the second or strengthening stage, communications were further strengthened by the creation of the network's Internet homepage enabling continuous exchange on the diagnosis, surveillance and control of *Schistosoma japonicum*. Research and training benefited by efforts to survey the areas endemic for schistosomiasis in a standardised way. Research grants were awarded by TDR for three projects, that is, the application of immunodiagnostic kits, the standardisation of the ultrasonography protocol and the development of survey tools for animal schistosomiasis. These grants encouraged the expansion of the network—which was undertaken by the branches in Cambodia and Indonesia—to jointly study human and animal schistosomiasis prevalence in all four countries where oriental schistosomiasis (caused by *S. japonicum* or *S. mekongi*) is endemic. 'Ecology and transmission of schistosomiasis in Philippines (STEP)' is a good example of a well-managed project leading to another by another funding agency. In this case, the findings produced by the TDR projects resulted in 'add-on' funding from the National Institutes of Health (NIH), Bethesda, MD, USA. Similar funding has been awarded by NIH to research groups in P.R. China as well (Bergquist and Tanner, 2010).

The third stage, which can be called the expanding stage, started in 2005. In an example of technology-enhancing activities, data produced at a training course on GIS applications—offered during the RNAS$^+$ meeting—provided awareness of the utility of implementing GIS capability in each member country and created linkages with the Gnosis network (www.gnosisGIS.org). Alerted by this, several other funding agencies and research institutes took an interest in RNAS$^+$, providing input, collaboration and/or financial support. Examples include the Danish Centre for Experimental Parasitology (DCEP), Copenhagen, Denmark; the Danish International Development Agency (DANIDA), Copenhagen, Denmark; the Swedish International Development Cooperation Agency (SIDA), Stockholm, Sweden; the Wellcome Trust, London, UK; the Queensland Institute of Medical Research (QIMR), Brisbane, Australia; and the Swiss Tropical Institute (STI), Basel, Switzerland, as well as the WHO HQ and the WHO Western Pacific Regional Office (WPRO).

From only 20 participants and two member countries at the 2000 annual meeting, the network attracted increasing numbers of participants from universities, research institutes, control programmes, international organisations and industry, reaching 100 participants and nine member countries in 2008 (Fig. 3.2). The high number attending the 2007 annual meeting in Lijiang, P.R. China was due to the unusually high number of Chinese students who could find the financial means to participate when the meeting was held in their own country that year. Taking this into account, it seems that the core number of participants already reached a plateau of around 100 participants 3 years ago. On the other hand, if the RNAS$^+$ budget permitted the subsidising of students to allow them to attend its meetings (which is highly desirable), the regular number of attendees would probably be at least 50% higher.

Further strengthening of the RNAS$^+$ organisation in response to increased expectations from its members and partners led to the establishment of physical headquarters at the Research Institute of Tropical Medicine (RITM), Muntinlupa, the Philippines, where non-profit organisation legal status was obtained. Since 31 July 2007, RNAS$^+$ has been registered with the Securities and Exchange Commission (SEC), with its functions defined in by-laws and articles of incorporation approved by the SEC in the Philippines.

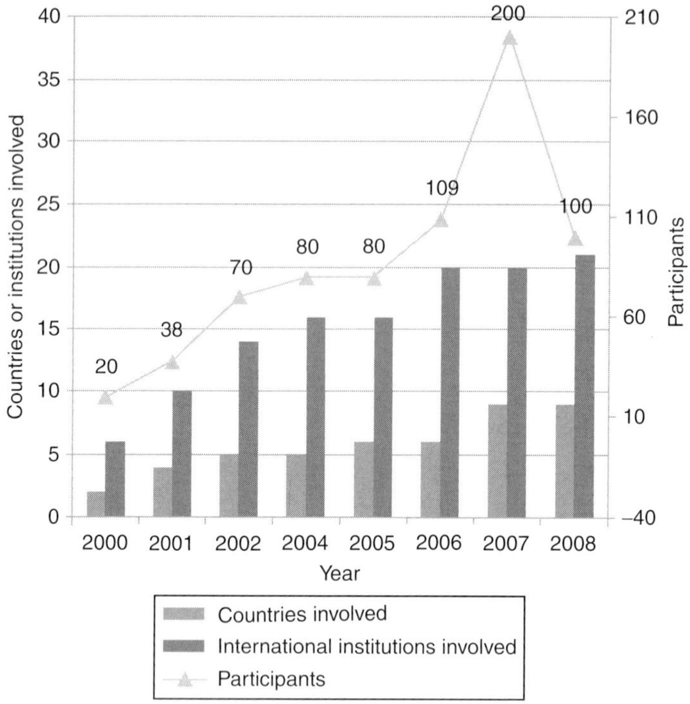

FIGURE 3.2 The number of participants, countries and international institutions involved in the RNAS+ annual meetings 2000–2008.

3.2.1. Organisational structure

Design and technical standardisation are important issues aiming at fostering research capacity, and fostering the development of the RNAS+ networking capacity and access to information databases. Figure 3.3 depicts a virtual organisation where the administrative body provides the platform connecting the RNAS+ members via the Internet; providing databases and administrative back-up. This design reflects the strategy to boost research on the target diseases by placing a strong emphasis on the ways and means to alleviate the spectre of the disease and poverty, as well as on the creation of interconnected, disease-specific groups capable of operating as 'nodes' on the RNAS+ website (http://www.rnas.org.cn). Although no serious, endemic disease is left outside the RNAS+ charter, the main disease 'nodes' are cysticercosis (CYS), food-borne trematode infections (FTI), schistosomiasis (SCH) and other helminth zoonoses (OHZ). Apart from these four main areas, there is also a crosscutting 'node' called trans-disease activities (TDA) that is concerned with the maintenance of databases, connectivity and other technical questions. The general work is concentrated on:

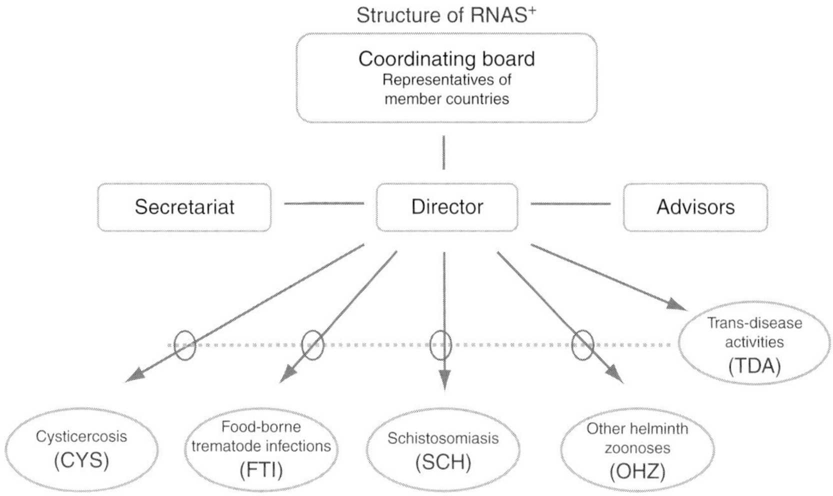

FIGURE 3.3 The RNAS$^+$ organisational chart.

- implementation of operational and control-associated research;
- retrieval of data of particular interest and identification of areas where RNAS$^+$ fills a need;
- identification of knowledge gaps and promotion of innovative synthesis of findings relevant to infectious diseases control in settings characterised by poverty; and
- acquainting researchers with the advantages of working via the RNAS$^+$ website as a knowledge management platform, encouraging active participation in the joint effort to continuously update information on the diseases of poverty.

The specific research priorities are to:

- support research on the impact of social determinants and economic issues on the epidemiology of helminth zoonotic infections in Southeast Asia;
- document, develop and apply health metrics in practice;
- promote GIS/RS techniques for the study of the impact of climate change on the RNAS$^+$ target diseases and other applications;
- improve and standardise diagnostic capabilities, including development of new products and techniques; and
- encourage the study of genetics and the immune responses against parasites to better understand the pathology caused and ultimately to apply the new knowledge to the development of new drugs and vaccines.

RNAS$^+$ aims to improve the research environment through the standardisation of technologies, procedures and protocols used in the prevention and control of endemic diseases and, in particular, to facilitate the dissemination of reliable and up-to-date information about helminth zoonotic infections. The vision is to become the recognised platform for evidence-based information and intersectoral communication bridging the gap between research scientists and control authorities for the prevention of neglected tropical diseases (NTDs) in Southeast Asia. Science is not easily regulated which contributes to increasing inequality at different levels. This is no different in the field of parasitic diseases, but the best way forward seems to be the establishment of a business model with 'accountables'. In contributing to reducing the burden and impact of NTDs in vulnerable populations, the immediate mission is to steer research progress onto specific targets and to harness new findings into easily accessible repositories with the aim to foster communication between scientists and control authorities. RNAS$^+$ also aims to be the primary centre in the region for specific research such as the assessment of health metrics, surveillance, diagnostics, GIS/RS, etc., introducing global standards and developing state-of-the-art technologies.

The internal connections and facilities within the overall structure of the RNAS$^+$ are described in Fig. 3.4. The platform represents the

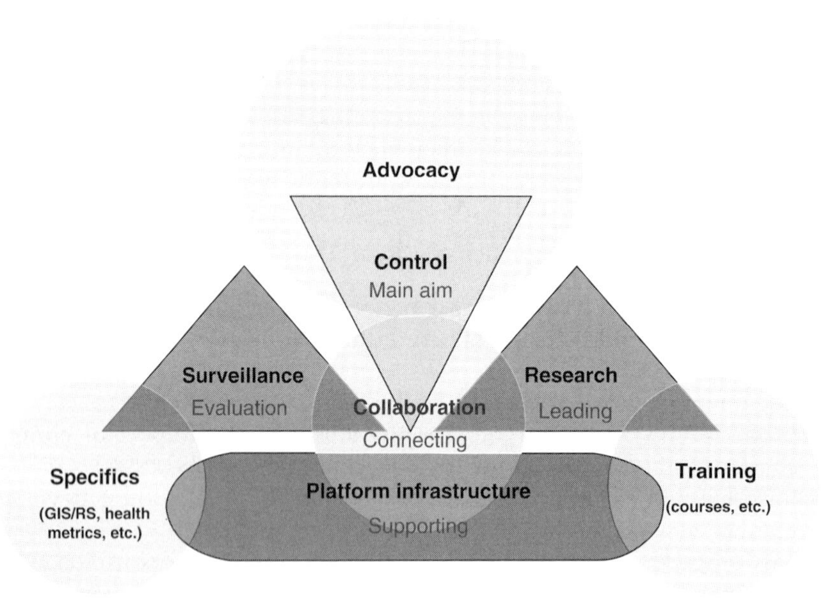

FIGURE 3.4 Schematic description of the internal functions and connections in RNAS$^+$.

supporting scaffolding of this virtual reality where collaboration is the connecting centrepiece. Research and surveillance, symbolised by the blue triangular shapes, are the bedrock activities that closely join with the main aim, that is, the progress of control activities. Advocacy, training and the short courses are peripheral to the central activities but the network could not work without them.

3.2.2. Achievements

The overall aim of RNAS$^+$ is to strengthen collaboration between researchers and control authorities in the endemic countries and the network has provided critical input in this respect for several parasitic diseases as highlighted in the following sections.

3.2.2.1. Diagnostics

Several problems plaguing control programmes are due to the insensitivity and variability of commonly used diagnostic assays as has been reported at several RNAS$^+$ meetings. For example, the Kato-Katz stool examination (Katz et al., 1972), generally used for the diagnosis of schistosomiasis, has become increasingly unreliable due to the lower parasite loads in controlled areas (Lin et al., 2008). In addition, the declining compliance rates commonly observed after repeated rounds of stool examinations and treatment (Guo et al., 2005a) have become a problem in the national control programmes, both in P.R. China and the Philippines. To overcome the aforementioned problems through the network, a diagnostic technique, developed at the Danish Bilharziasis Laboratory (DBL), used for the diagnosis of animal trematode infections, was shown to work well when tried in a survey (Anh et al., 2008). With respect to immunodiagnostic approaches, the DDIA kit for schistosomiasis, developed at the Jiangsu Institute of Parasitic Diseases (Zhu et al., 2002), was successfully transferred from P.R. China to Cambodia and Lao People's Democrabic Republic (Lao PDR) for the diagnosis of *S. mekongi* (Zhu et al., 2005).

3.2.2.2. Vaccine research

Owing to the role of domestic animals in the transmission of schistosomiasis japonica, vaccine research in P.R. China and the Philippines has focused on the possibility of transmission-blocking vaccines for livestock (Zhu et al., 2004, 2006). An experimental advantage with respect to *S. japonicum* vaccine research is the possibility to use full-size animal models thereby escaping the limitations of the mouse model (Johansen et al. 2000; Zhu et al., 2004). Based on the idea that reduced water buffalo infections would reduce transmission to humans, field trials of two *S. japonicum* antigens (Sj28-TPI, Sj23) are ongoing in P.R. China, (Da'dara et al., 2008; Dai et al., 2009). Results published so far show a greater than 50% protection of many animals, which could be further boosted by an integrated approach using praziquantel also.

In the Philippines, both RITM and the College of Public Health, University of the Philippines have had vaccine research groups for many years. More recently, RITM has analysed human immune responses to a panel of *S. japonicum* recombinant antigens in an effort to find out which antigens are the most promising (Acosta et al., 2002).

3.2.2.3. Drug development

Since it has now been convincingly shown that artemether and artesunate can kill schistosomula, they may be used as preventive drugs against schistosomiasis and also against food-borne trematodes (Xiao, 2005; Xiao et al., 2010). Indeed, impressive reductions in worm-burdens have been obtained with artemisinins and synthetic trioxolanes in rodents infected with either *S. japonicum*, *Clonorchis sinensis*, *Fasciola hepatica* or *Opisthorchis viverrini* (Keiser and Utzinger, 2007). A year after these reductions in worm-burdens were demonstrated, Hou et al. (2008) carried out and published the first randomised, double-blind, placebo-controlled trial evaluating combined artemether/praziquantel chemotherapy for the treatment of acute schistosomiasis japonica. Since these patients should harbour a comparatively high number of young parasite forms, an improved efficacy compared to praziquantel alone was expected. Surprisingly, however, apart from showing a good safety record, the results were negative. This could have various explanations. For example, acute schistosomiasis is a clinical diagnosis which, for obvious reasons, must leave out the determination of the number of schistosomula in the patients. One could speculate that the results might have been different if the drugs had been given earlier in the course of the infection. On the other hand, it would only be possible to test this occasionally. Possibly, a very large study in a very highly prevalent area could have shown a small difference between the different drug regimens. In spite of this difficulty, it would be useful to continue testing the effect of various combinations of various artemisinins together with praziquantel (Xiao et al., 2010).

3.2.2.4. Health metrics

The assessment of the personal impact of a disease is far from straightforward, in particular for chronic diseases with subtle pathologies. Already more than 50 years ago, Pesigan et al. (1958) noted the ravages caused by schistosomiasis and their paper marks the start of a long-lasting controversy about how to gauge the magnitude and duration of infection-related, chronic diseases. Stothard and Gabrielli (2007) argue that much of the morbidity caused by schistosomiasis appears one or two decades after the first incidence of infection in early childhood and that this fact was not sufficiently addressed in the original disability-adjusted life year (DALY) estimate by Murray and Lopez (1996). As pointed out by King et al. (2005) and King (2010a), the real impact of schistosomiasis can be 10 or even 15 times higher than current figures. Several courses have been given under the auspices of RNAS+ on the subject of health metrics and work along these lines has been initiated (Jia et al., 2007; King, 2010b; Li et al., 2005).

3.2.2.5. GIS/RS applications

It is now feasible to predict the distribution of the intermediate schistosomiasis host snail with the aid of remotely sensed environmental data (Guo et al., 2005b; Yang et al., 2005; Zhou et al., 2001). In addition, applied spatial analysis can be used to predict the distribution of the *Oncomelania hupensis* snail at the micro level (Zhang et al., 2005). While Guo et al. (2005b) only used the wetness feature in their approach, Zhang et al. (2005) also derived brightness and greenness. These two studies have enhanced our understanding of *S. japonicum* transmission at high resolution. As the research spectrum broadened, more applications, in particular with respect to climate change, were implemented and methodologies based on GIS/RS have led to a vastly improved knowledge base in the region (Chen et al., 2007; Leonardo et al., 2007; Li et al., 2009; Malone et al., 2010; Wu et al., 2007; Yang et al., 2006; Zhou et al., 2004, 2008c)

3.2.2.6. Control

An interesting report from Cambodia focuses on the cost of running the schistosomiasis control programme presenting an evaluation of its cost-effectiveness and cost-benefit (Croce et al., 2010). The drug cost amounted to about 17% of the implementation cost. The annual costs of keeping an individual free from infection was estimated at US$1, while that of restoring one severely infected adult to complete productivity, was estimated at US$114. It was calculated that the return in increased productivity was US$3.85 for each US$ invested.

The development of the schistosomiasis control programme in the Philippines can be followed in two papers (Leonardo et al., 2002, 2008). For example, instead of active case-finding, random sampling was implemented in a national prevalence survey, carried out between 2005 and 2008 (Leonardo et al., 2008). Although prevalence was found to have generally declined, places with high prevalence and high transmission were discovered in poor areas without proper sewage systems. The survey confirmed that more than 80% of all schistosomiasis in the Philippines is found in Mindanao and Visayas, the two big provinces in the south of the country.

Using diagnostic (stool examination + serology), demographic and environmental data obtained from a large area in P.R. China's Hunan province, Raso et al. (2009) found that demographic factors such as age, sex and occupation and the presence of reservoirs of infection (water buffaloes), rather than environmental factors, drive human transmission of schistosomiasis. The results, highly significant as they issue from a cross-sectional study comprising almost 50,000 participants from 47 villages, are practically useful for epidemiologic surveillance and future planning of interventions.

An advanced study on control strategy, looking towards the elimination of schistosomiasis, has been carried out in lake regions of P.R. China. This control strategy was implemented with an integrated approach which emphasised on elimination of the infectious sources or animal reservoir hosts in order to reduce the faecal contamination to oncomelanid snail intermediate host, since the previous approach of mass chemotherapy could not stop the transmission (Wang et al., 2009a,b). It encouraged us to put a greater effort into the elimination of schistosomiasis through long-term planning, intersectoral government coordination and commitment over a period of decades (King, 2009, 2010a).

3.2.2.7. Surveillance

Progress evolving from the links between monitoring activities and research has shown that surveillance represents more than just the collection of data. The situation has been reviewed with regard to efficiency of monitoring and the utility in relation to human diagnosis (Li et al., 2005; Wu et al., 2005). The questionnaire approach, developed by Lengeler et al. (2002) in Africa, was transferred and further developed for identification of high-risk individuals in areas prone to flooding (Tan et al., 2004).

The application of Bayesian multiple, logistic regression models helped Steinmann et al. (2007) identify associations between serologic results and environmental parameters in a county in Yunnan, P.R. China. Further use of serology has confirmed that infection in mobile populations, that is, fishermen and their families who move around the great lakes in central P.R. China, represent a so-called 'hot spot' of infection which cannot be easily eliminated (Zhu, 2005).

Naturally, this brief overview of a selection of recent research papers is far from exhaustive but it should suffice to make the point that research activities are numerous and that the projects with RNAS^{+} connections cover a broad range. It also goes to show that new knowledge is being generated and that projects have benefited the end-users (both at the policy and societal levels), contributed to capacity building (both at the individual and institutional level) and enhanced communication.

3.3. SEARCH FOR EVIDENCE

A large part of network-associated collaboration deals with the gathering of data and the presentation of this information in a reliable and understandable format which is easy to follow. Evidence-based medicine (EBM) and evidence-based practice (EBP) represent a rapidly growing area that includes information on Internet search engines for health care disciplines and ideas for handling the information (McKibbon, 1998). EBN and EBP are tools for knowledge dissemination that can support health care decisions by facilitating the identification of appropriate literature from various sources regarding therapy, diagnosis, etc. This approach, developed and applied to find the most efficacious interventions possible, was originally developed to improve individual patient care but could also be used for advising on control efforts in endemic countries. However, any external guidelines must be integrated with epidemiological expertise in order to decide whether and how it matches the endemic predicament and preferences and thus how it should be implemented. EBM is not restricted to randomised trials and meta-analyses but aspires to find the best external evidence with which to answer specific, clinical questions. Proper cross-sectional studies need to be identified in order to ensure the accuracy of diagnostic tests, while proper follow-up studies of infected subjects assembled at uniform points should be retrieved. With regard to therapy, non-experimental approaches should be avoided since these routinely lead to false-positive conclusions about efficacy. Because randomised trials, especially the systematic review of several such trials, are so much more likely to provide the information needed, it has become the "gold standard" for judging whether a treatment does more good than harm. Many different kinds of institutions (universities, donor agencies, non-profit organisations, or business-oriented companies) provide information for the assessment of health needs in the world. They differ in approach and scope as seen at the Lamar Soutter Library website of the University of Massachusetts Medical School (http://library.umassmed.edu/EBM/index.cfm). A few examples of the more well-known organisations involved with EBM and EBP are given as follows:

The Institute of Medicine (IOM) (http://www.iom.edu/) is an independent, not-for-profit organisation working outside of Government for the provision of unbiased and authoritative advice on matters of biomedical science, medicine and health. Established in 1970, the IOM is the health arm of the National Academy of Sciences, which has expanded into what is collectively known as the National Academies, comprising the National Academy of Sciences, the National Academy of Engineering and the National Research Council. The IOM's main mission is to serve as adviser to the United States in order to improve health in that country, but its resources are also open to outside users. It provides unbiased, evidence-based, authoritative information and advice concerning health and science policy to policy-makers, professionals, leaders in every secton of society and the public at large. Many of the studies undertaken begin as specific mandates from the US Congress, while others are requested by federal agencies and independent organisations. The IOM also convenes a series of forums, roundtables and standing committees, as well as other activities, to facilitate discussion, discovery and critical, cross-disciplinary thinking.

The Cochrane Collaboration (http://www.cochrane.org), founded in 1993, is another, not-for-profit, international, independent organisation that produces and disseminates systematic reviews of health care interventions. In particular, it promotes the search for evidence in the form of clinical trials. The Cochrane collaboration provides up-to-date, accurate information about the effects of health care worldwide. Its major product is the Cochrane Database of Systematic Reviews which is published quarterly as part of 'The Cochrane Library' which is accessible online through the Cochrane website. The reviewers are health care professionals who volunteer to work in one of the many 'Cochrane Review Groups', with editorial teams overseeing the preparation and maintenance of the reviews.

The Oxford Centre for Evidence-Based Medicine (http://www.cebm.net) was established in 1995 with the aim to develop, teach and promote evidence-based health care. EBM is the conscientious use of current best evidence in making decisions about the care of individual patients. The practice of EBM means integrating individual clinical expertise with the best available external clinical evidence from systematic research. It is based on clinical evidence and relevant research gleaned from the basic sciences of medicine but especially from patient-centred, clinical research into the accuracy and precision of diagnostic tests, the power of prognostic markers and the efficacy and safety of therapeutic, rehabilitative and preventive regimens.

3.4. THE FUTURE

New initiatives addressing NTDs are urgently needed and there is an increasing awareness of the role of polyparasitism (Hotez et al., 2007; Sayasone et al., 2009) and the role of the climate and the environment leading to changing epidemiological patterns (Spear et al., 2004; Yang et al., 2005, 2006; Zhou et al., 2004, 2008c). The rapid growth of key technologies (health metrics, GIS/RS, etc.) and the development of evidence-based policies are seen as important, although the latter is still controversial (Behague et al., 2009). To make progress towards these goals, it is necessary to foster research capacity and to develop networking capacities, as well as to provide easy access to information.

Faced with a situation where the means to control many of the different target diseases are available but the financial means to achieve this fully are lacking, RNAS+ is at an important juncture. Operating with nine member countries in Southeast Asia with the vision of becoming a recognised platform for evidence-based information and intersectoral communication, it has made progress in bridging the gap between research scientists and control authorities. RNAS+ also aims to be the forum for the exchange and dissemination of information about current research news and developments on prevention and control of NTDs in the area, through intersectoral collaboration and networking with scientists and control authorities. They intend to offer:

- expertise in diagnostics, GIS/RS and health metrics; drug/vaccine development; competence in developing training packages and short courses;
- mechanisms for sharing information through its website, databases, publications and meetings;
- the capacity to develop multidisciplinary approaches and multi-country proposals for disease control; and
- links with control programmes in member countries and collaborative activities with international organisations and research institutions.

The geospatial sciences have become a driving force in mapping diseases that are closely linked to the environment, ecology and climate. Current applications include a broad range of NTDs such as schistosomiasis, cysticercosis/taeniasis, echinococosis, hookworm disease, strongyloidiasis and food-borne diseases caused by helminth parasites as diverse as *Angiostrongylus*, *Clonorchis*, *Fasciola*, *Opisthorchis*, *Paragonimus*, *Haplorchis* and *Metorchis* (*Metagonimus*). The promotion of ethical issues, the establishment of guidelines for surveillance, the standardisation of diagnostic approaches and the production of training manuals for use in endemic areas are also priorities. To strengthen the research capacity through the network, a work plan has been drawn up in the form of 'business lines' corresponding to regional research needs:

Implementation research with focus on control strategies (Box 3.1);

Ecology and the environment: studies of the potential impact of climate change, large-scale, water resources development and environmental engineering projects;

Product development: the production of new drugs, vaccines, improved diagnostics and better molluscicides/pesticides;

Database development: the establishment of comprehensive databases containing epidemiological data on all the endemic diseases in the region and their vectors;

BOX 3.1 Regional research needs and priorities—implementation research with focus on control strategies:

(1) Identification of risk factors related to multi-helminth infections in different settings, including co-infections such as helminth/TB infections and helminth/HIV.
(2) Role of animal helminthiasis in different settings improving our understanding of the importance of animal infections for transmission to humans.
(3) Investigation of the factors leading to increased vulnerability for acute schistosomiasis.
(4) Assessment of treatment effectiveness after mass chemotherapy in large and diverse communities.
(5) Methods for the rapid evaluation of the community prevalence of *S. japonicum* infections, for example, by a combination of information from serological testing, stool examination and questionnaires used for research on both humans and livestock.
(6) Standardisation of morbidity assessment by ultrasonography for evaluation of the various disease-burdens.
(7) Investigation of the safety, efficacy, cost and effectiveness of drug treatment schedules and delivery mechanisms to assess the potential for novel chemotherapy strategies, for example, studies of the use of artemisinins, alone and in combination with praziquantel, are an integral part of this programme.
(8) Equity of control efforts—the study of the relationship between endemicity and control efforts in endemic areas should be encouraged to provide evidence for equitable allocation of resources.

Serum and specimen banks: the creation of a serum bank, a gene bank focused on *S. japonicum* and *O. hupensis* and a collection of parasite strains and their intermediate hosts;

Technical development and standardisation: the development and testing of diagnostic kits, GIS/RS implantation including expanded use of Bayesian statistics and modelling;

Surveillance (Box 3.2);

Parasite biology: molecular biology, bioinformatics, genome and proteome research, genetic basis for vector reinfection, genetic and the immunological background for human reinfection;

Vector/intermediate host biology and host/parasite relationship (Box 3.3);

Social determinants and human behaviour (Box 3.4);

Health metrics: to serve as a base for the planning and evaluation of efficacy and cost-effectiveness of control programmes;

BOX 3.2 Regional research needs and priorities—surveillance:

Determination of frequency and approach to monitoring, and criteria for changes therein; establishment of managerial tools and procedures for outbreak surveillance, classification and response to permit a timely and effective response; development and introduction of new tools for efficient surveillance of humans, animals and snail habitats after eradication and transmission interruption; and surveillance after interruption of transmission.

BOX 3.3 Regional research needs and priorities—vector/intermediate host biology and the host/parasite relationship:

(1) Development of simple methods for the detection of infected snails for surveillance and outbreak investigations.
(2) Host parasite interaction—acquaintance with systems biology to facilitate the understanding of the interaction between parasite and vector (intermediate host), including insights into their genetic coevolution.
(3) Intermediate host susceptibility to infection—the genetic basis and immunological mechanisms governing infection susceptibility of *O. hupensis* should be further studied.
(4) Genomic bases for infection resistance—genome and proteome studies should be employed to identify functional genes of *O. hupensis* conferring resistance against *S. japonicum* infection. Development of transmission models.

Modelling: employing environmental, demographic and socioeconomic variables to provide the theoretical basis for transmission estimates and the use of immunological and diagnostic variables for the evaluation of the efficacy of chemotherapy and vaccines.

In the latest annual RNAS$^+$ meeting, held in Vientiane, Lao PDR, in October 2009, the network aligned its activities with those of the WHO/WPRO Strategic Research Plan for NTDs, and formulated its vision and activities in terms of the Research Plan by conceptualising five research projects related to the control of NTDs. The projects were concerned with the following subjects:

BOX 3.4 Regional research needs and priorities—social determinants and human behavior:

(1) Socioeconomic context and impact on control approaches—the impact of the social and economic context should be studied in relation to control programmes with the aim to better respond to local conditions and requirements.
(2) Socioeconomic changes—the impact of socioeconomic factors should be studied, including rapid socioeconomic development, increased mobility and changes in agricultural and fisheries practices.

1. Integrated, multisectoral control of neglected tropical diseases.
2. Development of improved diagnostics, new drugs and trematode vaccines.
3. Impact of community-led total sanitation (CLTS) on helminth infections.
4. Risk-mapping of FTI using rapid epidemiological assessment.
5. Integration of large-scale distributions of praziquantel with control interventions against soil-transmitted helminth infections in an area with multiple helminth infections.

Over the coming years, RNAS$^+$ expects to spend most of its time on these projects, the concept and rationale of which can be summarised as follows:

(1) NTDs have common risk factors (socioeconomic, environmental, modes of transmission, etc.) and overlapping endemic areas. Hence, a multisectorial integrated control programme for NTDs would potentially be cost-effective and sustainable at the local level. Single vertical interventions, such as mass drug administration on its own, are challenging to maintain (primarily due to cost, compliance, reinfection rates and rebound morbidity).
(2) Diagnostic techniques need to become more sensitive. This is particularly well illustrated in the case of the national schistosomiasis control efforts in P.R. China, where intensity of infection is now often below the limit of detection by Kato-Katz stool examination, the traditionally used method, as has been unambiguously shown by Lin et al. (2008). New drugs are needed for many more diseases even after the introduction of artemisinin, used for the treatment of malaria as well as for the prevention of schistosomiasis (Xiao et al., 2010). Vaccines will increase in importance throughout the elimination phase for several

of the trematode infections (and also other helminths) when integrated with other control methods such as chemotherapy, targeted mollusciciding, sanitation and health education.

(3) It has been noted that poor sanitation is closely related to high prevalence of helminth infections in humans. The efficiency of preventive chemotherapy is thought to be low in poor sanitation scenarios because of high reinfection rates which rapidly engulf the positive effect. CLTS in conjunction with preventive chemotherapy (which would also affect protozoal and other diarrhoeal diseases) could bring added benefits (including cost savings) into facilitating the design of a control programme.

(4) Food-borne trematode infections and taeniasis/cysticercosis are prevalent in many parts of the region and together they constitute a major health problem in many countries of Southeast Asia. Infections occur in ethnic minorities who traditionally eat raw fish and pork (Sripa et al., 2010; Vandemark et al., 2010). High-risk areas should be targeted first and it is therefore imperative that a variety of rapid assessment tools be developed to cope with this situation.

(5) In Southeast Asia, many areas are endemic for multiple helminth infections, for example, lymphatic filariasis, schistosomiasis, opisthorchiasis, taeniasis/cysticercosis etc. Current interventions are limited to large-scale interventions with mebendazole (for soil-transmitted helminth infections) and albendazole/diethylcarbamazine (DEC) (for lymphatic filariasis) and focal distribution of praziquantel (for schistosomiasis). There is a need to expand the control of these diseases in an integrated manner, by piggybacking on existing control activities, for example, by expanding the target for praziquantel distribution to cover all individuals affected by at least two of the aforementioned infections.

3.5. CONCLUSIONS

RNAS$^+$'s aims are strongly supported as a result of long-term association with control programmes in its member countries and collaborative activities with international research institutions, but the network needs increased funding to grow. Its strengths can be summed up as consisting of experience in control strategies, coupled with available mechanisms for information-sharing and expertise in diagnostics, GIS/RS, health metrics and drug/vaccine development.

The network has provided critical research input with regard to several NTDs in Southeast Asia, and the ideas based on which RNAS$^+$ has been working over the last decade have shown that progress can be made with a relatively small network and limited funding. However, the current, larger vision demands the establishment of a permanent clearing house to support the continuous exchange of ideas and data and make it possible for national researchers and control managers to work together with international scientists on a daily basis.

REFERENCES

Acosta, L.P., Aligui, G.D., Tiu, W.U., McManus, D.P., Olveda, R.M., 2002. Immune correlate study on human *Schistosoma japonicum* in a well-defined population in Leyte, Philippines: I. Assessment of 'resistance' versus susceptibility to *Schistosoma japonicum* recombinant and native antigens. Acta Trop. 84, 127–136.

Anh, N.T., Phuong, N.T., Ha, G.H., Thu, L.T., Johansen, M.V., Murrell, D.K., et al., 2008. Evaluation of techniques for detection of small trematode eggs in faeces of domestic animals. Vet. Parasitol. 156, 346–349.

Behague, D., Tawiah, C., Rosato, M., Some, T., Morrison, J., 2009. Evidence-based policy-making: the implications of globally-applicable research for context-specific problem-solving in developing countries. Soc. Sci. Med. 69, 1539–1546.

Bergquist, R., Tanner, M., 2010. Controlling schistosomiasis in southeast Asia: a tale of two countries. Adv. Parasitol. 72, 109–144.

Chen, Z., Zhou, X.N., Yang, K., Wang, X.H., Yao, Z.Q., Wang, T.P., et al., 2007. Strategy formulation for schistosomiasis japonica control in different environmental settings supported by spatial analysis: a case study from China. Geospat. Health 1, 223–231.

Croce, D., Porazzi, E., Foglia, E., Restelli, U., Sinuon, M., Socheat, D., et al., 2010. Cost-effectiveness of a successful schistosomiasis control programme in Cambodia (1995-2006). Acta Trop. 113, 279–284.

Da'dara, A.A., Li, Y.S., Xiong, T., Zhou, J., Williams, G.M., McManus, D.P., et al., 2008. DNA-based vaccines protect against zoonotic schistosomiasis in water buffalo. Vaccine 26, 3617–3625.

Dai, Y., Zhu, Y., Harn, D.A., Wang, X., Tang, J., Zhao, S., et al., 2009. DNA vaccination by electroporation and boosting with recombinant proteins enhances the efficacy of DNA vaccines for schistosomiasis japonica. Clin. Vaccine Immunol. 16, 1796–1803.

Guo, J.G., Cao, C.L., Hu, G.H., Lin, H., Li, D., Zhu, R., et al., 2005a. The role of 'passive chemotherapy' plus health education for schistosomiasis control in China during maintenance and consolidation phase. Acta Trop. 96, 177–183.

Guo, J.G., Vounatsou, P., Cao, C.L., Utzinger, J., Zhu, H.Q., Anderegg, D., et al., 2005b. A geographic information and remote sensing based model for prediction of *Oncomelania hupensis* habitats in the Poyang Lake area, China. Acta Trop. 96, 213–222.

Hotez, P.J., Molyneux, D.H., Fenwick, A., Kumaresan, J., Ehrlich Sachs, S., Sachs, J.D., et al., 2007. Control of neglected tropical diseases. N. Engl. J. Med. 357, 1018–1027.

Hou, X.Y., McManus, D.P., Gray, D.J., Balen, J., Luo, X.S., He, Y.K., et al., 2008. A randomised, double-blind, placebo-controlled trial of safety and efficacy of combined praziquantel and artemether treatment for acute schistosomiasis japonica in China. Bull. World Health Organ. 86, 788–795.

Jia, T.W., Zhou, X.N., Wang, X.H., Utzinger, J., Steinmann, P., Wu, X.H., 2007. Assessment of the age-specific disability weight of chronic schistosomiasis japonica. Bull. World Health Organ. 85, 458–465.

Johansen, M.V., Bogh, H.O., Nansen, P., Christensen, N.O., 2000. *Schistosoma japonicum* infection in the pig as a model for human schistosomiasis japonica. Acta Trop. 76, 85–99.

Katz, N., Chaves, A., Pellegrino, J., 1972. A simple device for quantitative stool thick smear technique in schistosomiasis mansoni. Rev. Inst. Med.Trop. São Paulo 14, 397–400.

Keiser, J., Utzinger, J., 2007. Artemisinins and synthetic trioxolanes in the treatment of helminth infections. Curr. Opin. Infect. Dis. 20, 605–612.
King, C.H., 2009. Toward the elimination of schistosomiasis. New Engl. J. Med. 360, 106–109.
King, C.H., 2010a. Parasites and poverty: the case of schistosomiasis. Acta Trop. 113, 95–104.
King, C.H., 2010b. Health metrics for helminthic infections. Adv. Parasitol. 73, 51–69.
King, C.H., Dickman, K., Tisch, D.J., 2005. Reassessment of the cost of chronic helmintic infection: a meta-analysis of disability-related outcomes in endemic schistosomiasis. Lancet 365, 1561–1569.
Lengeler, C., Utzinger, J., Tanner, M., 2002. Questionnaires for rapid screening of schistosomiasis in sub-Saharan Africa and their contribution to control. Bull. World Health Organ. 80, 235–242.
Leonardo, L.R., Acosta, L.P., Olveda, R.M., Aligui, G.D., 2002. Difficulties and strategies in the control of schistosomiasis in the Philippines. Acta Trop. 82, 295–299.
Leonardo, L.R., Crisostomo, B.A., Solon, J.A.A., Rivera, P.T., Marcelo, A.B., Villasper, J.M., 2007. Geographical information systems in health research and services delivery in the Philippines. Geospat. Health 1, 147–155.
Leonardo, L.R., Rivera, P., Saniel, O., Villacorte, E., Crisostomo, B., Hernandez, L., et al., 2008. Prevalence survey of schistosomiasis in Mindanao and the Visayas, The Philippines. Parasitol. Int. 57, 246–251.
Li, Y.S., Zhao, Z.Y., Ellis, M., McManus, D.P., 2005. Applications and outcomes of periodic epidemiological surveys for schistosomiasis and related economic evaluation in the People's Republic of China. Acta Trop. 96, 266–275.
Li, S.Z., Wang, Y.X., Yang, K., Liu, Q., Wang, Q., Zhang, Y., et al., 2009. Landscape genetics: the correlation of spatial and genetic distances of *Oncomelania hupensis*, the intermediate host snail of *Schistosoma japonicum* in mainland China. Geospat. Health 3, 221–231.
Lin, D.D., Liu, J.X., Liu, Y.M., Hu, F., Zhang, Y.Y., Xu, J.M., et al., 2008. Routine Kato-Katz technique underestimates the prevalence of *Schistosoma japonicum*: a case study in an endemic area of the People's Republic of China. Parasitol. Int. 57, 281–286.
Malone, J.B., Yang, G.J., Leonardo, L., Zhou, X.N., 2010. Implementing a geospatial health data infrastructure for control of Asian schistosomiasis in P.R. China and the Philippines. Adv. Parasitol. 73, 71–100.
McGarvey, S.T., Zhou, X.N., Willingham 3rd, A.L., Feng, Z., Olveda, R., 1999. The epidemiology and host–parasite relationships of *Schistosoma japonicum* in definitive hosts. Parasitol. Today 15, 214–215.
McKibbon, K.A., 1998. Evidence-based practice. Bull. Med. Libr. Assoc. 86, 396–401.
Murray, C.J.L., Lopez, A.D., 1996. The Global Burden of Disease: A Comprehensive Assessment of Mortality and Disability from Diseases, Injuries, and Risk Factors in 1990 and Projected to 2020. Harvard School of Public Health/World Bank, Cambridge, MA.
Pesigan, T.P., Farooq, M., Hairston, N.G., Jauregui, J.J., Garcia, E.G., Santos, A.T., et al., 1958. Studies on *Schistosoma japonicum* infection in the Philippines. 1. General considerations and epidemiology. Bull. World Health Organ. 18, 345–455.
Raso, G., Li, Y., Zhao, Z., Balen, J., Williams, G.M., McManus, D.P., 2009. Spatial distribution of human *Schistosoma japonicum* infections in the Dongting Lake Region, China. PLoS One 4, e6947.
Sayasone, S., Vonghajack, Y., Vanmany, M., Rasphone, O., Tesana, S., Utzinger, J., et al., 2009. Diversity of human intestinal helminthiasis in Lao PDR. Trans. R. Soc. Trop. Med. Hyg. 103, 247–254.
Spear, R.C., Seto, E., Liang, S., Birkner, M., Hubbard, A., Qiu, D., et al., 2004. Factors influencing the transmission of *Schistosoma japonicum* in the mountains of Sichuan province of China. Am. J. Trop. Med. Hyg. 70, 48–56.

Sripa, B., Kaewkes, S., Intapan, P.M., Maleewong, W., Brindley, P.J., 2010. Food-borne trematodiases in Southeast Asia: epidemiology, pathology, clinical manifestation and control. Adv. Parasitol. 72, 305–350.

Steinmann, P., Zhou, X.N., Matthys, B., Li, Y.L., Li, H.J., Chen, S.R., et al., 2007. Spatial risk profiling of *Schistosoma japonicum* in Eryuan county, Yunnan province, China. Geospat. Health 2, 59–73.

Stensgaard, A.S., Saarnak, C.F.L., Utzinger, I., Vounatsou, P., Simoonga, C., Mushinge, G., et al., 2009. Virtual globes and geospatial health: The potentide of new tools in the management and control of vector-borne disease. Geospat. Health 3, 127–141.

Stothard, J.R., Gabrielli, A.F., 2007. Schistosomiasis in African infants and preschool children: to treat or not to treat? Trends Parasitol. 23, 83–86.

Tan, H.Z., Yang, M.X., Wu, Z.G., Zhou, J., Liu, A.Z., Li, S.Q., et al., 2004. Rapid screening method for *Schistosoma japonicum* infection using questionnaires in flood area of the People's Republic of China. Acta Trop. 90, 1–9.

Vandemark, L.M., Jia, T.W., Zhou, X.N., et al., 2010. Social science implications for control of helminth infections in Southeast Asia. Adv. Parasitol. 73, 137–170.

Wang, L.D., Chen, H.G., Guo, J.G., Zeng, X.J., Hong, X.L., Xiong, J.J., et al., 2009a. A strategy to control transmission of *Schistosoma japonicum* in China. N. Engl. J. Med. 360, 121–128.

Wang, L.D., Guo, J.G., Wu, X.H., Chen, H.G., Wang, T.P., et al., 2009b. China's new strategy to block transmission of schistosomiasis and beyond. Trop. Med. Int. Health 14, 1475–1483.

Wu, X.H., Chen, M.G., Zheng, J., 2005. Surveillance of schistosomiasis in five provinces of China which have reached the national criteria for elimination of the disease. Acta Trop. 96, 276–281.

Wu, X.H., Wang, X.H., Utzinger, J., Yang, J., Kristensen, T.K., Bergquist, R., 2007. Spatio-temporal correlation between human and bovine schistosomiasis in China: insight from three national sampling surveys. Geospat. Health 2, 75–84.

Xiao, S.H., 2005. Development of antischishosomal drugs in china, with particular consideration to praziquantel and the artemisimins. Acta Trop. 96, 153–167.

Xiao, S.H., Keises, J., Chen, M.G., Tanner, M., Utzinger, J., 2010. Research and development of antischishosomal drugs in the People's Republic of China: a 60-year review. Adv. Parasitol. 73, 231–295.

Yang, G.J., Vounatsou, P., Zhou, X.N., Utzinger, J., Tanner, M., 2005. A review of geographic information system and remote sensing with applications to the epidemiology and control of schistosomiasis in China. Acta Trop. 96, 117–129.

Yang, G.J., Vounatsou, P., Tanner, T., Zhou, X.N., Utzinger, J., 2006. Remote sensing for predicting potential habitats of *Oncomelania hupensis* in Hongze, Baima and Gaoyou lakes in Jiangsu province, China. Geospat. Health 1, 85–92.

Zhang, Z.Y., Xue, D.Z., Zhou, X.N., Zhou, Y., Liu, S.J., 2005. Remote sensing and spatial statistical analysis to predict the distribution of *Oncomelania hupensis* in the marshlands of China. Acta Trop. 96, 205–212.

Zhou, X.N., Malone, J.B., Kristensen, T.K., Bergquist, N.R., 2001. Application of geographic information systems and remote sensing to schistosomiasis control in China. Acta Trop. 79, 97–106.

Zhou, X., Acosta, L., Willingham 3rd, A.L., Leonardo, L.R., Minggang, C., Aligui, G., et al., 2002. Regional Network for Research, Surveillance and Control of Asian Schistosomiasis (RNAS). Acta Trop. 82, 305–311.

Zhou, X.N., Yang, K., Hong, Q.B., Sun, L.P., Yang, G.J., Liang, Y.S., et al., 2004. Prediction of the impact of climate warming on transmission of schistosomiasis in China. Zhongguo Ji Sheng Chong Xue Yu Ji Sheng Chong Bing Za Zhi 22, 262–265 (In Chinese with English abstract).

Zhou, X.N., Berquist, R., Leonardo, L., Olveda, R., 2008a. Important Helminth Infections in Southeast Asia: Regional Network for Asian Schistosomiasis and Other Helminth Zoonoses (RNAS$^+$). September, 2008.

Zhou, X.N., Ohta, N., Utzinger, J., Bergquist, R., Olveda, R.M., 2008b. RNAS$^+$: a win-win collaboration to combat neglected tropical diseases in Southeast Asia. Parasitol. Int. 57, 243–245.

Zhou, X.N., Yang, G.J., Yang, K., Wang, X.H., Hong, Q.B., Sun, L.P., et al., 2008c. Potential impact of climate change on schistosomiasis transmission in China. Am. J. Trop. Med. Hyg. 78, 188–194.

Zhu, Y.C., 2005. Immunodiagnosis and its role in schistosomiasis control in China: a review. Acta Trop. 96, 130–136.

Zhu, Y.C., He, W., Liang, Y.S., Xu, M., Yu, C.X., Hua, W.Q., et al., 2002. Development of a rapid, simple dipstick dye immunoassay for schistosomiasis diagnosis. J. Immunol. Methods 266, 1–5.

Zhu, Y., Ren, J., Da'dara, A., Harn, D., Xu, M., Si, J., et al., 2004. The protective effect of a *Schistosoma japonicum* Chinese strain 23 kDa plasmid DNA vaccine in pigs is enhanced with IL-12. Vaccine 23, 78–83.

Zhu, Y.C., Socheat, D., Bounlu, K., Liang, Y.S., Sinuon, M., Insisiengmay, S., et al., 2005. Application of dipstick dye immunoassay (DDIA) kit for the diagnosis of schistosomiasis mekongi. Acta Trop. 96, 137–141.

Zhu, Y., Si, J., Harn, D.A., Xu, M., Ren, J., Yu, C., et al., 2006. *Schistosoma japonicum* triose-phosphate isomerase plasmid DNA vaccine protects pigs against challenge infection. Parasitology 132, 67–71.

CHAPTER 4

Neglected Diseases and Ethnic Minorities in the Western Pacific Region: Exploring the Links

Alexander Schratz,* **Martha Fernanda Pineda,*** **Liberty G. Reforma,*** **Nicole M. Fox,*** **Tuan Le Anh,*** **L. Tommaso Cavalli-Sforza,*** **Mackenzie K. Henderson,*** **Raymond Mendoza,*** **Jürg Utzinger,**[†,‡] **John P. Ehrenberg,*** and **Ah Sian Tee***

Contents

* World Health Organization, Regional Office for the Western Pacific, Malaria, Vector-borne and other Parasitic Diseases, Manila, Philippines
† Department of Epidemiology and Public Health, Swiss Tropical and Public Health Institute, Basel, Switzerland
‡ University of Basel, Basel, Switzerland

Advances in Parasitology, Volume 72
ISSN 0065-308X, DOI: 10.1016/S0065-308X(10)72004-2

Abstract

Ethnic minority groups (EMGs) are often subject to exclusion, marginalisation and poverty. These characteristics render them particularly vulnerable to neglected diseases, a diverse group of diseases that comprise bacteria, ecto-parasites, fungi, helminths and viruses. Despite the health policy relevance, only little is known of the epidemiological profile of neglected diseases among EMGs. We reviewed country data from Australia, Cambodia, Lao People's Democratic Republic, Malaysia, the Philippines and Vietnam and found several overlaps between regions with high proportions of EMG population and high prevalence rates of neglected diseases (infections with soil-transmitted helminths, filarial worms, schistosomes, food-borne trematodes and cestodes). While the links are not always clearly evident and it is impossible to establish correlations among highly aggregated data without control variables—such as environmental factors—there appear indeed to be important linkages between EMGs, socio-economic status and prevalence of neglected diseases. Some determinants under consideration are lack of access to health care and general health status, poverty and social marginalisation, as well as education and literacy. Further research is needed to deepen the understanding of these linkages and to determine their public health and socio-economic significance. In particular, there is a need for more data from all countries in the Western Pacific Region that is disaggregated below the provincial level. Selected case studies that incorporate other control variables—such as risk factors from the physical environment—might be useful to inform policy makers about the feasibility of prevention and control interventions that are targeted at high-risk EMGs.

4.1. INTRODUCTION

Ethnic minority groups (EMGs) around the world are historically among the most vulnerable populations and often subject to exclusion, marginalisation and poverty (IWGIA, 2009; Roy, 2006). EMGs are usually isolated in remote geographical areas and often face seriously limited access to health care, education and other public services (ADB, 1998; Ehrenberg and Ault, 2005). This chapter explores the links between poverty, EMGs and a selected group of neglected diseases with a focus on the Western Pacific Region. Specifically, an attempt has been made to review socio-economic and demographic determinants that might explain why EMGs are at a higher risk of neglected diseases relative to the overall population of the Western Pacific Region. At present, little is known on the epidemiological profile of neglected diseases among EMGs. Yet, neglected diseases are regarded as diseases of poverty affecting marginalised groups where access to health care, adequate sanitation and clean water is limited (Hotez and Yamey, 2009; WHO/WPRO, 2008). Though scant, some studies suggest an unusually high burden due to neglected diseases among EMGs.

The low number of available publications and publicly available data on EMGs and neglected diseases reflects the neglect that both ethnic minorities and these diseases are subject to. The scope of this chapter is limited to six countries of the Western Pacific Region, for which data on EMGs and neglected diseases were available at the time of systematically reviewing the peer-reviewed literature and unpublished reports: Australia, Cambodia, Lao People's Democratic Republic (Lao PDR), Malaysia, the Philippines and Vietnam. To varying degrees, these countries have provided detailed data on both EMGs' socio-economic status and the epidemiology of neglected diseases. The authors hope that the current effort might encourage other countries and regions to collect and present their own data on EMGs and neglected diseases and explore the linkages so that setting-specific prevention, mitigation and control efforts can be enhanced.

4.2. EMGs AND NEGLECTED DISEASES

4.2.1. Working definitions

For the purpose of this chapter, the working definition of an EMG will be the one used by the Asian Development Bank (ADB). It refers to "those with a social or cultural identity distinct from the dominant or mainstream society, which makes them vulnerable to being disadvantaged in the process of development" (ADB, 1998). Some countries in the Western Pacific Region are comprised of a mosaic of ethnic groups, of which some may not be considered a minority, but may still be subject to socio-economic constraints that exceed those of the overall population (ADB, 1998). Further research should be conducted to determine the criteria required to differentiate or categorise these groups based on their population sizes. Recent immigrants and other non-indigenous migrant groups may eventually become a part of a country's EMG population. Studies suggest that they are also vulnerable to risk factors that may lead to high burdens of disease, particularly neglected diseases (de Silva et al., 2002; Einsiedel and Spelman, 2006). However, only indigenous groups were included in this chapter.

Unfortunately, inconsistent definitions of "EMG status" across the Western Pacific Regional Office's (WPRO) Member States impair comparability of data reported by different countries. Improved country-level reporting of official census figures on EMGs would therefore be helpful in order to provide a more comprehensive picture of the overall EMG distribution in the Western Pacific Region.

Notwithstanding these limitations, the proportion of EMGs relative to the total population ranges from 1.4% in Cambodia to as high as one third in Lao PDR (ABS and AIHW, 2008; IWGIA, 2009; PRB, 2008; Table 4.1). While these population groups do share common characteristics across the Region, specific characteristics of each EMG and the areas each lives in are crucial to understand the epidemiological pattern of neglected diseases.

Leading causes of morbidity and mortality vary from country to country, but more importantly between rural and urban settings as well as between EMG and non-EMG populations. EMGs' relatively poor standard of living translates into high susceptibility to infectious diseases, high infant mortality rates and low life expectancies. Given these poor health indicators, it is not surprising that they are also more vulnerable to neglected diseases, which tend to thrive in conditions of poverty and poor health (Hotez et al., 2006, 2007). Moreover, EMGs often have a large share of young people (children under the age of 15 years) and women in childbearing age, which represent the two major at-risk groups.

The limited political or social empowerment of EMGs greatly restricts their abilities to develop economically and negatively influences policies and programmes designed to serve their needs. Poverty fuels a cycle of poor access to quality health services and vulnerability to disease (communicable

TABLE 4.1 Percentages of total population belonging to an EMG in six selected countries of the Western Pacific Region

Country	Estimated population size (year)	% of population considered as belonging to an EMG	Estimated EMG population size	Sources
Lao PDR[a]		>30%		IWGIA (2009)
Vietnam	86.0 million (2008)	14%	12 million	IWGIA (2009)
Malaysia	28.6 million (2008)	12%	3.4 million	IWGIA (2009)
Philippines	90.4 million (2008)	10%	9 million	IWGIA (2009)
Australia	20.7 million (2006)	2.5%	520,000	ABS and AIHW (2008)
Cambodia	14.7 million (2008)	1.4%	190,000	PRB (2008) and IWGIA (2009)

[a] In Lao PDR, the concept of "indigenous peoples" is not officially recognised.

and non-communicable), presenting a challenge in achieving better health for EMGs and indeed overall developmental goals (e.g. achieving the United Nations (UN) millennium development goals (MDGs)).

As the list of the so-called neglected tropical diseases (NTDs)—over 35 worldwide, including bacteria, fungi, ecto-parasites, helminths and viruses—would far exceed the scope of this chapter, emphasis was placed on a group of selected neglected diseases, comprising infections with soil-transmitted helminths (*Ascaris lumbricoides*, hookworm, *Strongyloides stercoralis* and *Trichuris trichiura*), filarial worms (*Wuchereria bancrofti* and *Brugia malayi*), schistosomes (*Schistosoma japonicum* and *S. mekongi*), food-borne trematodes (*Clonorchis sinensis*, *Fasciola* spp., *Opisthorchis viverrini* and *Paragonimus* spp.) and cestodes (e.g. *Taenia solium*). For further details pertaining to the epidemiology, distribution, burden, prevention and control of these selected neglected diseases, the reader is referred to other chapters in this and an accompanying volume of the *Advances in Parasitology* (Hotez and Ehrenberg, 2010; Keiser and Utzinger, 2010; Muth et al., 2010; Sripa et al., 2010; Sudomo et al., 2010; Willingham et al., 2010; Zhou et al., 2010). Of note, although most of the neglected diseases discussed here will not cause death, they will often result in debilitating complications, contributing to malnutrition and severe disabilities.

4.2.2. Data sources

As indicated in Section 4.1, data on both EMGs and neglected diseases are scarce in the Western Pacific Region and elsewhere in the developing world. Hence, we made considerable efforts to obtain data from a multitude of different publicly available sources and focussed on the following countries: Australia, Cambodia, Lao PDR, Malaysia, the Philippines and Vietnam.

General epidemiological data on neglected diseases are based primarily on the World Health Organization's (WHO) recent review pertaining to the epidemiological profile of helminthiases and their control in the Western Pacific Region, completed in 2008 (WHO/WPRO, 2008). That report, for the first time, compiled and consolidated data provided by WPRO Member States, some of which have been published in peer-reviewed journals, in a comprehensive 10-year review. Where possible, we incorporated more recent data, such as the data presented during WHO's First Mekong-Plus Programme Managers Workshop on Lymphatic Filariasis and Other Helminthiases held in Phnom Penh, Cambodia, in March 2009 (WHO/WPRO, 2009).

EMG data are mostly based on official figures presented by the countries under review. We accessed these data either directly from government databases or from publications by international organisations like ADB and the United Nations Development Program (UNDP) and non-governmental organisations (NGOs), such as the International Working Group on Indigenous Affairs (IWGIA). Basic population data were verified with data provided by the Population Reference Bureau.

Additionally, we consulted individual articles published in the peer-reviewed literature that explored the links between EMGs and neglected diseases. For example, there is an existing body of research on soil-transmitted helminth infections in Australia and Malaysia. Moreover, we found one study from the Philippines that presents direct evidence for a higher susceptibility of an EMG to lymphatic filariasis. As the literature and research presented in this work may still not be exhaustive, we are grateful to additional pointers to published or unpublished data that we might have missed.

4.3. LINKAGES BETWEEN EMGs AND NEGLECTED DISEASES

4.3.1. Access to health care and general health status

In spite of the gradual improvements in health and general well-being worldwide and in such regions as the Greater Mekong Subregion, including Cambodia, Lao PDR, Myanmar, Thailand and Vietnam (ADB, 2001), data from Australia, Cambodia, the Philippines and Vietnam show that EMGs (and other poor groups) continue to live with marginal access to quality health care when compared to the general population. While those cases are well documented and underline these governments' awareness and appreciation of the challenges in providing equitable health care, one can only make informed guesses about EMGs' access to health care in other countries.

All helminth infections covered in this chapter can be readily treated in a cost-effective manner in their early stages (Hotez et al., 2007; WHO, 2006). Yet, limited health care access makes EMGs unlikely to receive timely diagnoses and adequate treatment that could prevent high morbidity rates due to neglected diseases. For example, Australian EMGs encounter limited availability of medical practitioners in remote areas and face long commuting distances to the nearest hospital (ABS and AIHW, 2008). Other challenges lie in the "transport availability, health insurance and health services affordability and in their English proficiency" (ABS and AIHW, 2008).

Moreover, EMGs have significantly different health-seeking behaviours than the general population. According to a Vietnam Living Standards Survey conducted in 1998, only 47% of ethnic minority mothers sought prenatal care, compared to 70% for mothers of the majority Kinh population. The survey also showed that 75% of ethnic minority parents consulted a health care provider when a young child (aged 5–60 months) was sick, compared to 88% for Kinh households (Baulch et al., 2002). This means that EMG children are at a higher risk of not receiving prompt diagnosis and treatment.

Health care access and coverage gaps remain in the Philippines—especially between rural and urban areas. Since most EMGs live in remote areas, their access to basic services is thus limited (UNDP, 2004). Particularly in the Cordillera Administrative Region (CAR), the number of health personnel such as nurses, midwives and village health workers was considered "barely adequate" by the ADB (2002b). The CAR is the region with the highest percentage of EMGs nationwide (NCIP, 2003; NSO, 2005).

For Cambodia, Fig. 4.1A illustrates that the regions with the highest proportion of EMGs have the lowest density of health care facilities (ADB, 2001; WHO, 2008a). In addition, there are intrinsic limitations to the Cambodian health system such as financial constraints and personnel available to cover remote areas (ADB, 2001). Interestingly, EMG-populated areas also tend to be very sparsely populated, which is usually linked to poor infrastructure overall, including transportation and communication (WHO, 2008b; Fig. 4.1B).

Regions where EMG populations live are also regions with high incidence rates of infectious diseases and related symptoms. Malaria, diarrhoea, acute respiratory infections, tuberculosis (TB) and intestinal parasites are all prevalent. Malaria is the most common cause of hospital admissions (ADB, 2001). While mortality and morbidity due to schistosomiasis have decreased due to interventions by health authorities (e.g. praziquantel-based morbidity control programmes; Sinuon et al., 2007), the remaining two endemic areas are situated in Kracheh and Stueng Traeng provinces (Muth et al., 2010; WHO/WPRO, 2008; Fig. 4.2A), which are two of the four provinces with the highest shares of EMGs (ADB, 2001). Lymphatic filariasis is also mainly endemic in provinces with a high share of ethnic minorities. While it is also prevalent in four provinces of Siem Reab and Preah Vihear, it is endemic in all of Stueng Traeng and Rotana Kiri's provinces (WHO/WPRO, 2009; Fig. 4.2B).

Given the limited access to health care, it would not be surprising if EMGs were not only more vulnerable to neglected diseases and other communicable diseases, but also to other non-communicable diseases. In the Western Pacific Region, EMG-specific health data are scant and only countries with relatively advanced health systems report disaggregated health data.

People's poor general nutritional and health status makes them even more susceptible to neglected diseases and leads to higher morbidity rates to one or more of these diseases. Multiple infections tend to be the rule rather than the exception (Steinmann et al., 2008, 2010; Utzinger and de Savigny, 2006). Infected individuals may not seek health care because symptoms of neglected diseases are often non-specific and sickness might be considered a "fact of life". Similarly, the Australian Bureau of Statistics reported indigenous life expectancy to be 59 years for males and 65 years for females. On average, that is 17–18 years less than the national life expectancy of 77 years for males and 82 years for females (ABS, 2008b). The National Agency for Health and Welfare Statistics and Information of Australia reported that "between 1999 and 2003, mortality rates for [EMG] infants were nearly three times higher than those for other Australian infants" (ABS, 2008a).

4.3.2. Poverty, social marginalisation and other risk factors

In terms of economic well-being, EMG indicators are often also below those of the non-EMG population. Even where the burden of low income and/or unemployment is high overall, it may be worse for EMGs. For example, Cambodia's EMGs live mainly in the four provinces in the north-east of

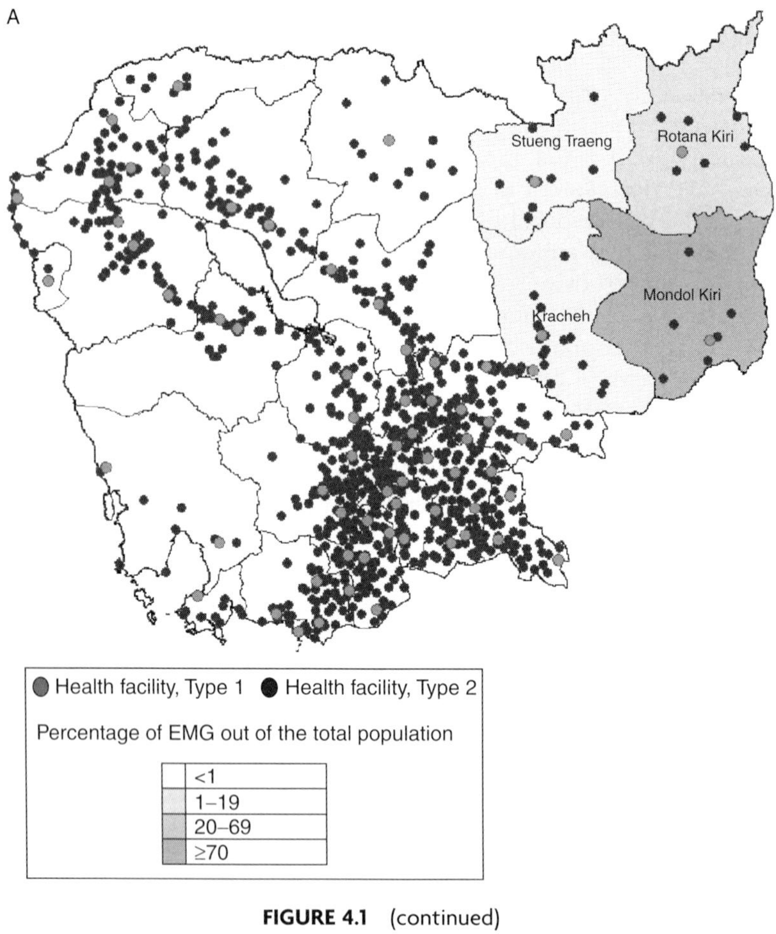

FIGURE 4.1 (continued)

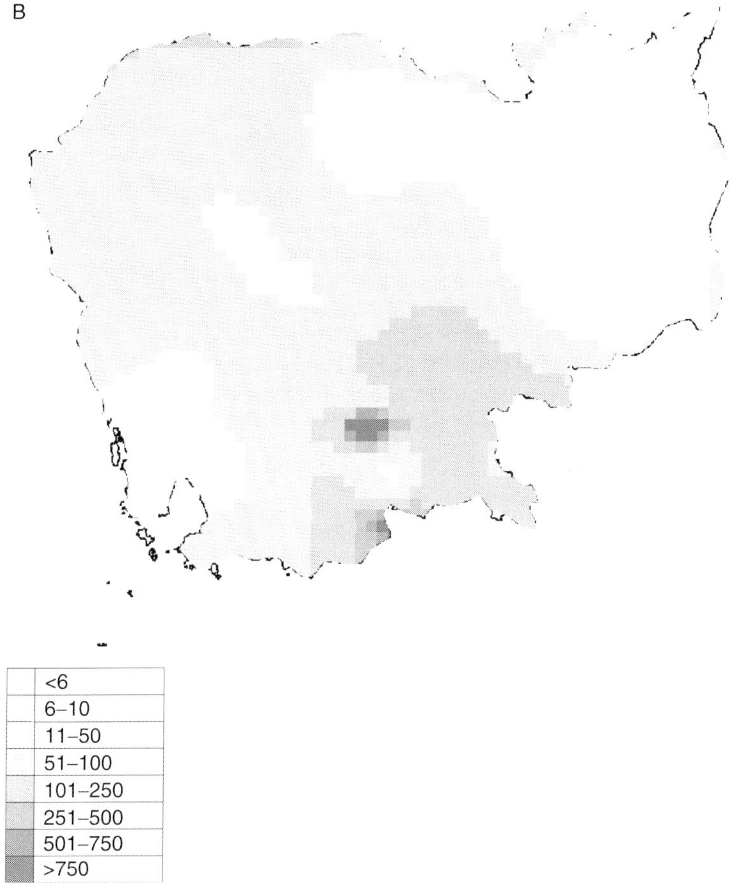

FIGURE 4.1 Maps of Cambodia as of 1997, showing the geographical distribution of EMGs and health facilities (A) and population density (B). Source: ADB (2001) and WHO (2008a,b).

Cambodia, which "are especially poor even by Cambodian standards" (MoP, 1999), where poverty affected up to 40% of the rural population country-wide in 1997 (ADB, 2002a). This is reflected in Fig. 4.3 (WFP, 2007).

Furthermore, poverty directly influences other determinants. Lack of financial resources may represent a barrier to health care and education, since it may lead to social exclusion. It may also result in precarious living conditions and low nutritional intake, strongly affecting the individual's general health status and susceptibility to disease. Neglected diseases disproportionately affect people living in poverty, including EMGs. Neglected diseases could be perceived as a human rights issue. Living in poverty increases the likelihood of contracting these diseases because access to

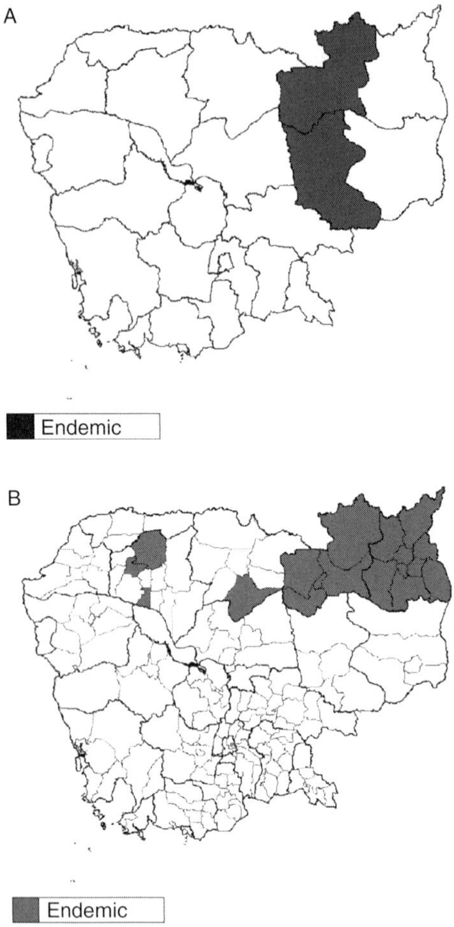

FIGURE 4.2 Maps of Cambodia showing the provinces where schistosomiasis mekongi as of 2006 (A) and lymphatic filariasis as of 2004 (B) were endemic. Source: WHO/WPRO (2008, 2009).

health care, education and housing cannot always be consistently assured (Hunt, 2007). Stigma is frequently associated with some of the sequelae of neglected diseases (e.g. elephantiasis and lymphatic filariasis). Stigma often leads to social exclusion and has been associated with treatment delays (Muela Ribera et al., 2009), an issue which would also fall within the human rights sphere (Weiss, 2008). Neglected diseases in EMGs need to be addressed from the perspective of equity in health care access and non-discrimination as an integral part of successfully preventing these diseases and their consequences among vulnerable populations (Hunt, 2007).

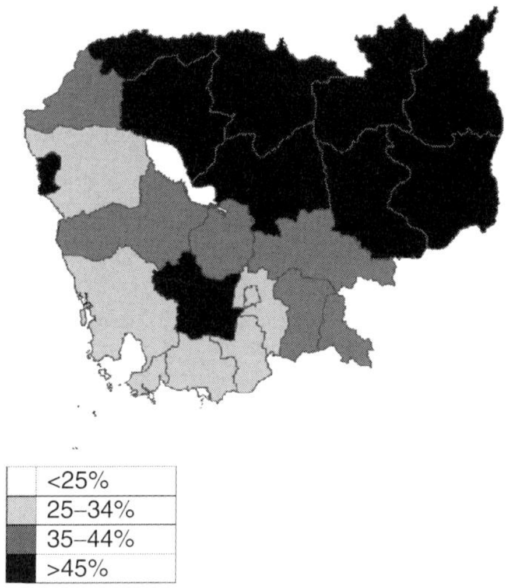

FIGURE 4.3 Poverty rates in Cambodia as of 2004. Source: WFP (2007)

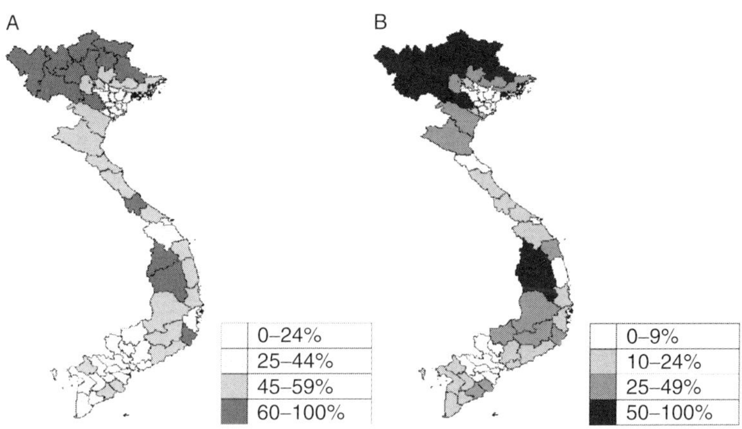

FIGURE 4.4 Linkage of rural poverty rates (A) and ethnic minorities (B) in Vietnam as of 2002. Sources: Henninger and Snel (2002) and WHO (2003).

An analysis of poverty rates in Lao PDR revealed that all EMGs showed substantially higher poverty rates than the majority Lao-Tai population (Engvall, 2007). Although rural EMGs make up less than a third of the population, rural ethnic minorities represent 47.4% of the poor (Engvall, 2007). This suggests that rural EMGs are almost two times more likely to be poor than the rural majority population and three times more than the urban population. Furthermore, Fig. 4.4A and B show a strong association between rural poverty and minority status in Vietnam, especially in the mountainous north-western provinces and in the Annamese highlands of the country's midsection (Henninger and Snel, 2002). EMGs represent the majority of the rural population in one central and almost all northern provinces.

Coincidentally, this northern region (Red River Delta, Northern Uplands) has a particularly high prevalence of soil-transmitted helminth infections (WHO/WPRO, 2008; Fig. 4.5A). Opisthorchiasis is mainly prevalent in the central part of Vietnam. No apparent overlap with EMG areas can be detected (WHO/WPRO, 2008; Fig. 4.5B). However, clonorchiasis and paragonimiasis do seem to be more prevalent in the northern areas with high EMG percentage (WHO/WPRO, 2008; Fig. 4.5B and C).

Social marginalisation is another determinant of neglected disease vulnerability in ethnic minorities. It can be due to various factors, such as culture, religion, poverty, certain stigmatised diseases, and, finally, ethnicity (Muela Ribera et al., 2009). EMGs often share several of these characteristics, which affect their health-seeking behaviour as well as access to health care to different extents. In Australia, for example, EMGs do not fully benefit from the socio-economic success of the general population: income rates for EMGs are lower than for the non-EMG population. Moreover, they have "poorer educational outcomes and lower rates of home ownership—all of which can impact upon a person's health and well-being" (ABS and AIHW, 2008). However, there is recent progress of Aboriginal groups in Australia both with regard to education and the labour market (ABS and AIHW, 2008).

In Vietnam, rapid economic growth has "provided young Vietnamese [with] new opportunities unheard of in previous generations" (Population Council, 2007). However, ethnic minority youths were less likely to benefit from these substantial improvements in living standards and positive

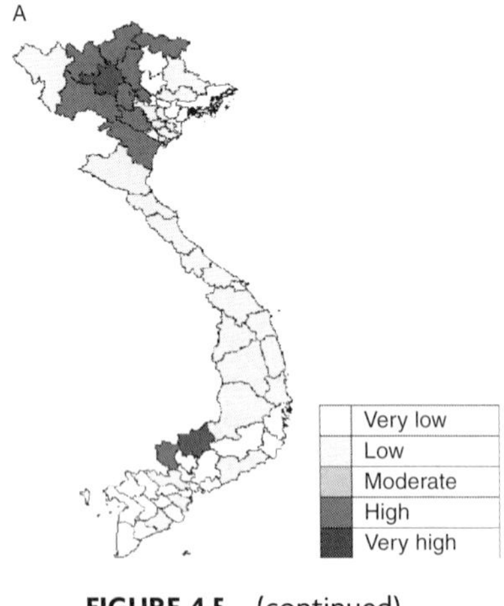

FIGURE 4.5 (continued)

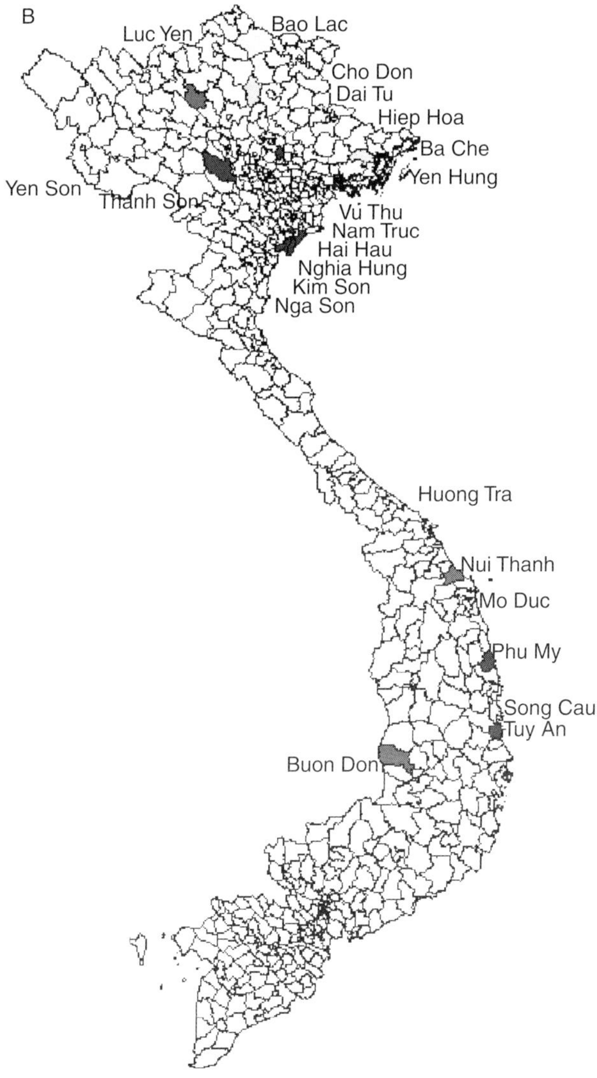

FIGURE 4.5 (continued)

economic changes, despite recent efforts by the Vietnamese government to reduce poverty in remote areas. "As these young people enter their working and reproductive years, they face an array of employment and health challenges" (Population Council, 2007). Many of them remain among the poorest, least healthy and least educated of Vietnam's population. The study concluded that social, economic and cultural factors such as family structures and lack of education all contribute to this (Population Council, 2007).

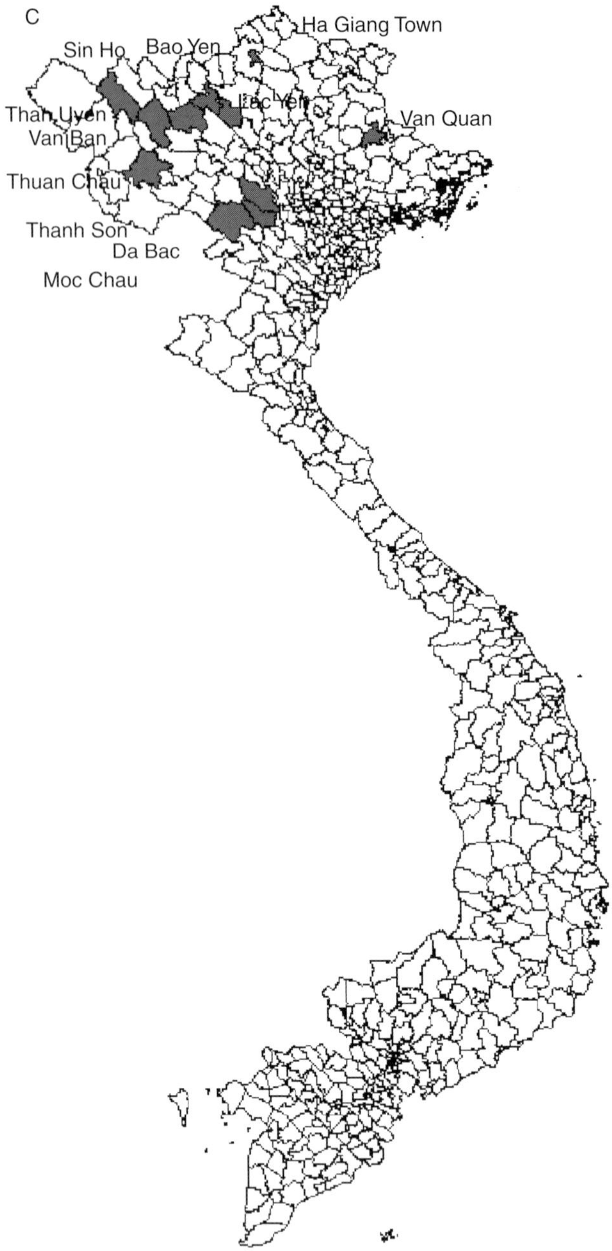

FIGURE 4.5 Maps of Vietnam showing the spatial distribution of soil-transmitted helminthiasis as of 2008 (A), clonorchiasis and opisthorchiasis as of 2006 (B), and paragonimiasis as of 2006 (C). Source: WHO/WPRO (2008).

Similarly, EMGs seem to benefit very little from the economic progress of the past decades in the Philippines. The ADB reports that "[o]n the whole, in the indigenous peoples' regions, the incidence of poor families and poor populations did not improve substantially between 1988 and 1997 despite the rise in average [national] income" (ADB, 2002b).

Epidemiological data from the Philippines do not show particularly high levels of neglected disease prevalence (e.g. soil-transmitted helminth infections (Fig. 4.6B), lymphatic filariasis (Fig. 4.6C) and schistosomiasis (Fig. 4.6D)) in diverse regions and provinces with a higher proportion of EMGs (NCIP, 2003; NSO, 2005; WHO/WPRO, 2009; Fig. 4.6A).

However, there might be links similar to the one that was identified for lymphatic filariasis in Mindoro Occidental. While prevalence rates in this province are not particularly high compared to the rest of the Philippines, a study in two neighbouring villages revealed significantly higher rates of lymphatic filariasis in the Mangyan EMG than the Tagalog majority, when considering and controlling for other risk factors (Ramirez et al., 2004). Carefully planned studies and data analysis below the province level should thus promote a better understanding of the epidemiological situation.

Information on EMGs' demographic profile is limited in most countries of the Western Pacific Region, including age distribution. Yet, the latter is a key in estimating figures for population at-risk of neglected diseases. At-risk estimates are critical in programme planning, a definite challenge when it comes to EMGs. However, it is well known that most developing countries have a higher population share of young people during early stages of the demographic and epidemiological transition. Evidence suggests that this is also true for EMGs within more developed countries. Table 4.2 presents data for the countries studied (PRB, 2008).

Preschool-aged children, school-aged children and women of child-bearing age are at highest risk of helminth infections. Even if EMG children were not more susceptible to neglected diseases than children in general, EMGs have a higher share of children and mothers than the general population. Therefore, EMGs overall would be expected to experience higher prevalence rates for neglected diseases.

In Australia, for example, EMGs had a median age of 21 years, compared to 37 years for the majority population, mainly due to "higher rates of fertility and deaths occurring at younger ages among the Indigenous population" (ABS and AIHW, 2008). This trend can also be illustrated in Australia's age pyramid, disaggregated by ethnicity (ABS and AIHW, 2008; Fig. 4.7). A similar age structure is found in New Zealand where 35% of the Māori population in New Zealand was under the age of 15 years compared to 21% for the general population (Māori Health, 2008).

In Malaysia, the Orang Asli population has a median age of 16.7 years, almost 6 years younger than the general population (22.4 years; Department of Statistics Malaysia, 2006). Moreover, 46% of the Orang

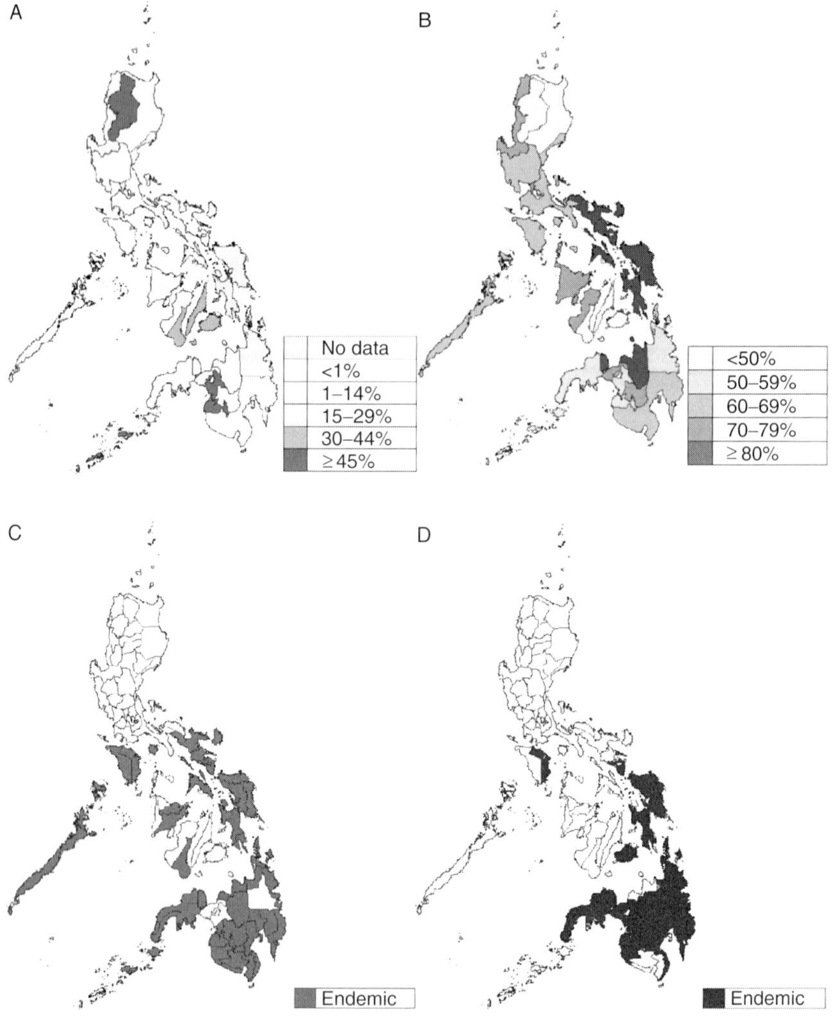

FIGURE 4.6 Maps of the Philippines showing the percentage of people belonging to EMGs as of 1996 (A) the spatial distribution of soil-transmitted helminthiasis as of 2008 (B), lymphatic filariasis as of 2008 (C) and schistosomiasis as of 2008 (D). Sources: NCIP (2003), NSO (2005) and WHO/WPRO (2009).

Asli population was below the age of 15 years compared to 32% for the total population in 2000 (Department of Statistics Malaysia, 2006). And lastly, the Orang Asli population in Malaysia has been growing at an annual rate of 3.3%, significantly higher than that of the total population (Department of Statistics Malaysia, 2006). These figures have implications

TABLE 4.2 Percentage of total population younger than 15 years in seven selected countries of the Western Pacific Region

Country	Estimated population		Population share younger than 15 years of age
	Total	Below age 15 years	
Lao PDR	5.9 million	2.6 million	44%
Cambodia	14.7 million	5.3 million	36%
Philippines	90.5 million	32 million	35%
Malaysia	27.7 million	8.9 million	32%
Vietnam	86.2 million	22 million	26%
New Zealand	4.3 million	0.9 million	21%
Australia	21.3 million	4 million	19%

Source: PRB (2008).

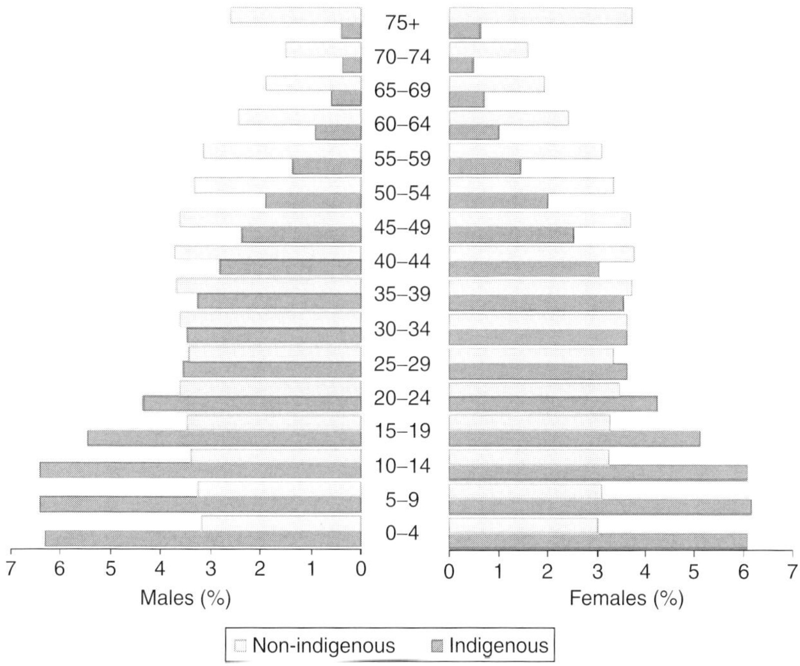

FIGURE 4.7 Age pyramid for Australia (in percent), disaggregated by ethnic status as of 2006. Source: ABS and AIHW (2008).

in terms of social care, including education, health and nutrition for certain population groups (Khor and Shariff, 2008) as well as macroeconomic repercussions due to a higher child dependency ratio, which implies reduced savings and investments.

Both Australia and Malaysia, which have no record of neglected disease endemicity in the general population, have pockets of very high prevalence rates of soil-transmitted helminth infections and other neglected diseases among their ethnic minorities. EMGs in Australia represent a small percentage of the total population. In 2006, the Australian Bureau of Statistics estimated that EMGs represented 2.5% of the total population (ABS and AIHW, 2008). Overall, 31% of EMGs live in urbanised areas, 45% in regional Australia and 24% in remote areas where general services and health-related infrastructure is likely to be weak (ABS and AIHW, 2008). Some studies investigating helminth infections among Australia's EMGs in the last 15 years suggest that these groups, mainly in the north-west and north of the country, bear a rather high burden of helminth infections (Meloni et al., 1993; Prociv and Luke, 1995; Reynoldson et al., 1997). For example, Prociv and Luke (1995) explain that presently hookworm infections are endemic only among EMGs of Northwest Australia and the Northern Territory, although they used to plague both European-descent (Caucasian) and Aboriginal communities (EMG) earlier in the last century. Meloni et al. (1993) studied five EMG communities in Western Australia and found that infections with intestinal parasites in children aged 1–5 years were very common. Another study found that hookworm infections (together with *Giardia intestinalis* and *Entamoeba coli*) were present in 30% of 180 fresh stools samples taken from Aboriginal communities in the Kimberley region (Reynoldson et al., 1997). *S. stercoralis*, another soil-transmitted helminth that is perhaps the most neglected nematode (Olsen et al., 2009), is also highly prevalent among EMG communities. It is indisputably more prevalent in rural and remote Aboriginal communities than in the mainstream Australian population (Adams et al., 2003). High-risk groups also include Aboriginal people living in remote communities of northern Australia (having prevalence rates above 25%) and immigrants from Southeast Asia, particularly Cambodia, Lao PDR and Vietnam. In one community, 41% of those tested were infected with *S. stercoralis* on a single stool specimen (Johnston et al., 2005). This strongly supports the need for more evidence-based research on the epidemiology of strongyloidiasis, especially among Aboriginal communities in Australia.

The most recent national prevalence data (1996) indicated that the prevalence of echinococcosis in Aboriginal EMGs was 12.2 times higher than that in other rural populations (WHO/WPRO, 2008). Updated research is needed on prevalence rates among the Aboriginal communities concerning cestode infections.

In Malaysia, EMGs represent approximately 12% of the total population (IWGIA, 2009). However, in peninsular Malaysia, EMGs account for only 3.5% of the population while they represent the majority in Malaysian Borneo (IWGIA, 2009). Several small-scale studies on the epidemiology of soil-transmitted helminth infections have been conducted in Malaysia in recent years. They revealed that soil-transmitted helminth infections are not

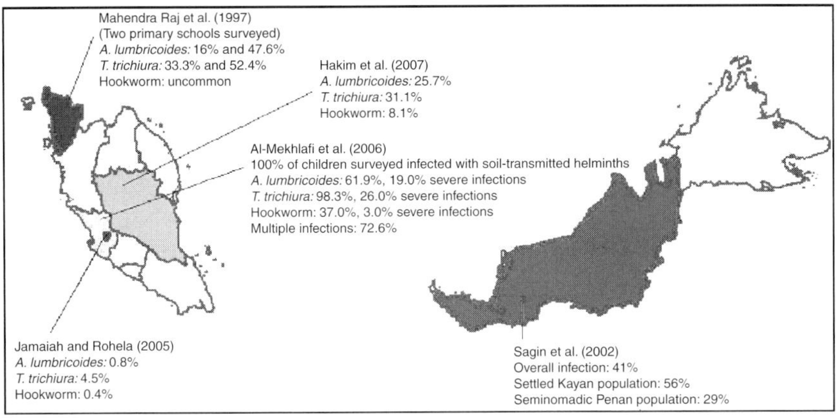

FIGURE 4.8 Location of selected study sites and prevalence of soil-transmitted helminth infections in Malaysia. Source: WHO/WPRO (2008).

a public health problem in this country (WHO/WPRO, 2008). Figure 4.8 shows varying rates of soil-transmitted helminth infection throughout Malaysia. The studies conducted by Al-Mekhlafi et al. (2006) and Hakim et al. (2007) focused specifically on Orang Asli communities in Cameron Highland and Selangor, respectively. In a survey of 74 stool samples taken from an Aboriginal settlement during a rotavirus outbreak, Hakim et al. (2007) found prevalence rates of *T. trichiura*, *A. lumbricoides* and hookworm of 31.1%, 25.7% and 8.1%, respectively. Al-Mekhlafi et al. (2006) diagnosed soil-transmitted helminth infections in all 281 children aged 12–15 years included in their survey. Three quarters of these subjects were infected with more than one helminth species concurrently. Another study by Sagin et al. (2002) showed that infection rates were higher among the settled Kayan population (56%) than among the semi-nomadic Penans (29%).

Singh and Cox-Singh (2001) summarised other small-scale studies pertaining to soil-transmitted helminth infections in selected communities (Table 4.3). Their review showed that soil-transmitted helminth infections were highly prevalent in rural communities where sanitation was inadequate. Aboriginal groups, inhabitants of islands and of forest fringe areas are among the most vulnerable groups. More large-scale studies are needed for a deeper understanding of prevalence rates of neglected diseases among EMGs in Malaysia.

4.3.3. Education and literacy

EMGs face a wide array of educational challenges in the Western Pacific Region, including limited access to, and funding for, schools, low pedagogical and infrastructure quality, conflicts between school and agricultural schedules (when families might need to rely on their children to help in the

TABLE 4.3 Prevalence of soil-transmitted helminth infections recorded in small-scale studies of selected communities in Malaysia

	A. lumbricoides	*T. trichiura*	Hookworm	Prevalence of all soil-transmitted helminth infections
		Peninsular Malaysia		
Dengkil *(aboriginal)*	62.9%	91.7%	28.8%	n.r.
Penang *(island)*	40.3%	33.3%	34.1%	n.r.
Post Brooke *(aboriginal)*	59.5%	41.7%	6.0%	79.8%
		Sarawak		
Serian (*forest*)	18.0%	34.3%	11.0%	47.5%

n.r., not reported.
Source: Singh and Cox-Singh (2001).

fields), gender issues, recruiting/retaining teachers in remote areas, isolation and poverty, lack of appropriate teaching/learning materials, language barriers and perceptions that returns from education are low (ADB, 2001, 2002a; IWGIA, 2009). A major issue of educational equity is the language of instruction in school systems: The language of instruction is often not the local language, and only few bilingual or alternative programmes are available throughout the Western Pacific Region. This pattern is also encountered in other regions of the world where it constitutes a barrier to education, including health education, for many EMGs.

Literacy rates are useful indicators for the problems EMGs face in the education sector and for their assimilation into the society as a whole (ADB, 2001). Disadvantaged EMGs often come from cultures with predominantly oral traditions such as the Aborigines in Australia. Most indigenous languages have no written scripts (Lyttleton, 2003). According to ADB, literacy rates for indigenous peoples are lower than the national literacy rates in Cambodia, Lao PDR and Vietnam. Moreover, women tend to have lower literacy rates than men, both in the general and the EMG population (ADB, 2001; Table 4.4).

Low educational attainment and literacy rates increase vulnerability to neglected diseases. Generally, this implies that EMGs have been exposed to less health education and are less accessible through written health information. Furthermore, a lack of education sustains poverty and promotes social marginalisation. Lastly, some health services such as large-scale de-worming campaigns are implemented through the school system (WHO/WPRO, 2008). If children of EMGs do not attend school, they will be missed out by these de-worming campaigns. More than a decade ago, it

TABLE 4.4 Literacy rates (%) for EMGs and the total population in three selected countries of the Western Pacific Region

	EMGs		Total	
Country	Female	Male	Female	Male
Cambodia	17	26	55	63
Lao PDR	17	33	48	60
Vietnam	n.d.	73	86	92

n.d., not determined.
Source: ADB (2001).

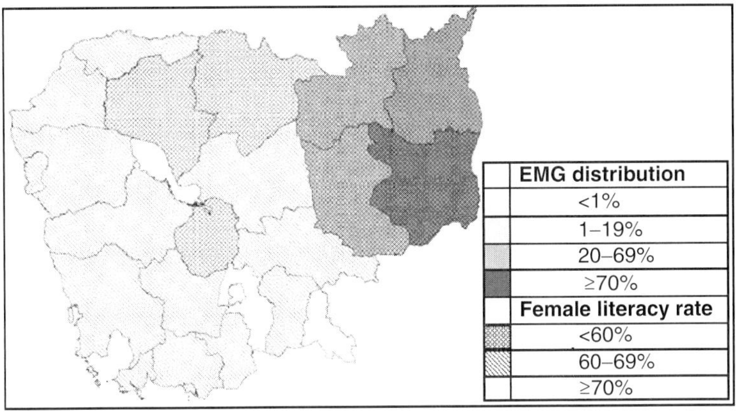

FIGURE 4.9 EMGs and female literacy rate in Cambodia, stratified by province as of 2004. Source: WFP (2007).

has been suggested that "school-based delivery may exacerbate existing inequalities in society" (Husein et al., 1996), a claim that warrants systematic inquiry.

Although EMGs, on average, achieve better educational levels in high-income countries like Australia, they face significant challenges in other settings. For example, 23% of EMG students in Australia completed secondary education in 2006, compared to 49% for non-EMG Australians (ABS and AIHW, 2008). However, Australia has succeeded in improving this rate by 3% between 2001 and 2006 (ABS and AIHW, 2008).

Figure 4.9 graphically shows the linkage between low female literacy rate in a high proportion of the EMG population of Cambodia, stratified by province (ADB, 2001; IWGIA, 2008).

Lao PDR has the most ethnically diverse population in mainland Southeast Asia and the largest share of EMGs among the six countries included in this chapter (IWGIA, 2009). The majority ethnic group in Lao

PDR, known as the Lao-Tai or ethnic Lao, accounts for 52% of the total country's population (ADB, 2001). The rest of the population is composed of several linguistically diverse EMGs (IWGIA, 2009). It should be noted that the link between EMG and high rates of neglected diseases is not always obvious. In the case of schistosomiasis, lymphatic filariasis and opisthorchiasis, there are no apparent links to areas with a higher concentration of EMGs at the provincial level in Lao PDR (Sayasone et al., 2007; WHO/WPRO, 2008). However, Fig. 4.10 clearly shows that high prevalence levels of *A. lumbricoides*, *T. trichiura* and hookworm in Lao PDR, in surveys carried out in 2000–2002, usually coincided with areas with high EMG population shares (Rim et al., 2003; WHO/WPRO, 2008).

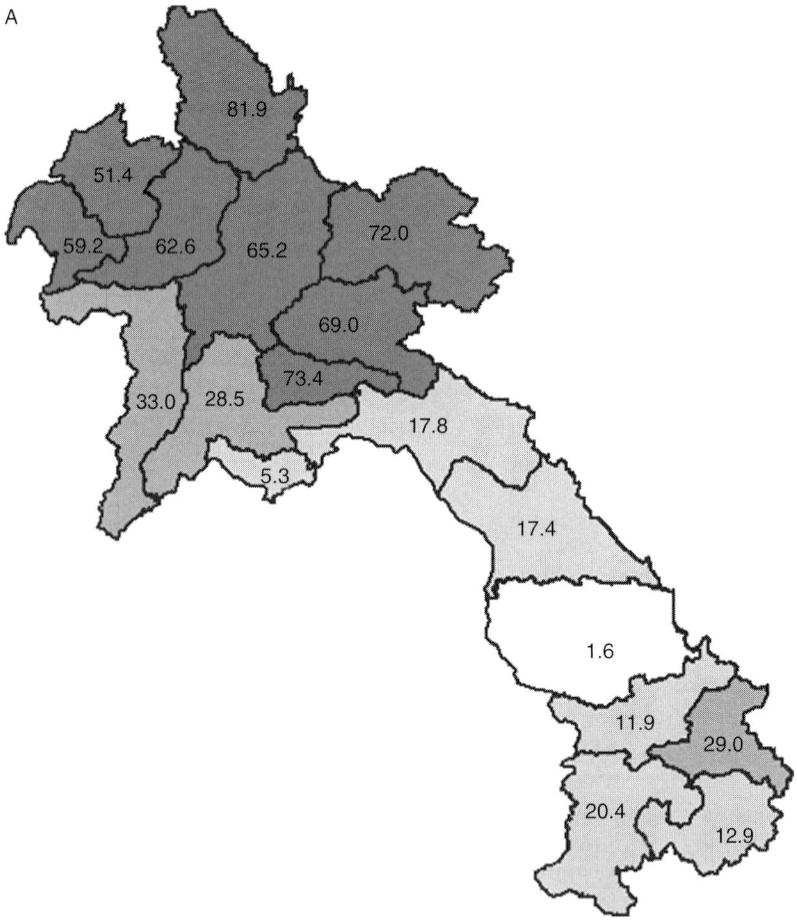

FIGURE 4.10 (continued)

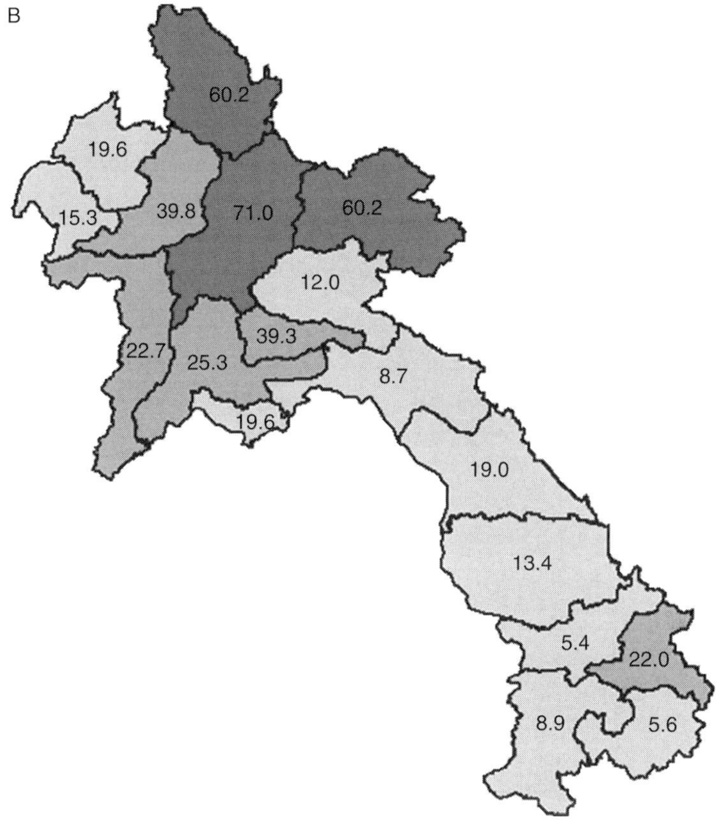

FIGURE 4.10 (continued)

4.4. CONCLUSION AND FUTURE RESEARCH NEEDS

This chapter provides a first systematic attempt in the Western Pacific Region to address the potential links between often marginalised EMG populations and the risk of acquiring and suffering the consequences of neglected diseases. Although limited in scope and depth, findings gathered primarily from public domain information sources for the purpose of this chapter show several overlaps between areas with high proportions of EMG population and high prevalence rates of neglected diseases across the region. These linkages may be attributed to a variety of determinants, most of which revolve around the poverty factor, such as lack of access to health care, clean water and sanitation, poor general health status, poor communication and social marginalisation, as well as deficient education and low literacy rates (Table 4.5).

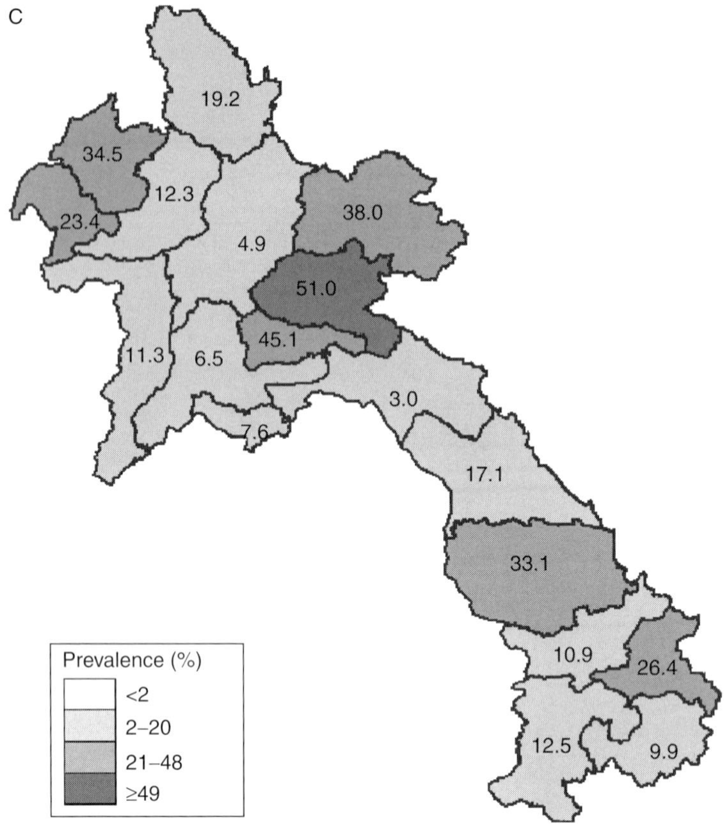

FIGURE 4.10 Prevalence of infections with *A. lumbricoides* (A), *T. trichiura* (B) and hookworm (C) in Lao PDR, 2000–2002. Source: WHO/WPRO (2008).

This pattern seems to be consistent with various degrees throughout the world in areas where there are EMGs. However, the linkages are not always clearly evident. It is difficult to establish correlations when only highly aggregated data are available. Neglected diseases are not subject to compulsory reporting, and hence their magnitude tends to be underestimated, probably even more so in EMGs. Concerted efforts need to take place at the national level to improve data collection and reporting on neglected diseases throughout the Western Pacific Region and elsewhere in the developing world. Further research should be conducted to determine the link between different risk factors (e.g. socio-economic and environmental, among others), EMGs and neglected diseases at national and sub-national levels. While more data will need to be collected, existing data should be refined and further disaggregated below the provincial level.

TABLE 4.5 Potential links between EMGs and neglected diseases

Determinants	Susceptibility to neglected diseases	Likelihood of treatment
Access to health care, clean water and sanitation as well as general health status	Poor underlying health conditions increase the risk of acquiring neglected diseases and higher morbidity rates	Weak health infrastructure reduces responsiveness of the health systems to the EMG health care needs General poor health may affect health-seeking behaviour
Poverty, social marginalisation and other risk factors	Precarious living conditions increase risk of infection Higher proportion of children means proportionally larger at-risk population	Limited financial means represent barrier to health care Social marginalisation may affect health-seeking behaviour
Education and literacy	Less health education may increase risk and affect health care-seeking behaviour	

Studies should also be conducted to establish new and cost-effective strategies potentially based on intersectoral synergies and articulating, where possible, with existing health systems.

Evidence-based strategies will help community health workers, volunteers and public health practitioners to implement effective surveillance, prevention and control measures of neglected diseases targeting specifically EMGs. Findings reported in the current review suggest that these diseases could be mainly clustered around EMGs and certainly around other economically marginalised population groups. Actions could be better targeted by the programmes to reach high-risk groups in resource-constrained environments, and hence optimising scarce financial and human resources. The authors hope that this chapter will help raise the profile of neglected diseases in the Western Pacific Region and in other parts of the world, particularly in the most vulnerable population groups such as EMGs. In doing so, it is further hoped that this will spur increased efforts to determine the magnitude of the problem more accurately and devote resources where they are needed most urgently.

ACKNOWLEDGEMENTS

The inclusion of the graphic materials is cited under the reference section. We would like to acknowledge the following for their contribution: Prof. Xiao-Nong Zhou, Mr. Norbert Henninger, the Western Pacific Regional Office and the Country Offices of the WHO, the General Statistics Office of Vietnam, the World Food Programme, the Australian Bureau of Statistics and the ADB. J. Utzinger acknowledges financial support from the Swiss National Science Foundation (project no. PPOOB-102883, PPOOB-119129).

Competing Interests: The authors (all, except J. Utzinger) declare that though they are employees or volunteers of the World Health Organization's Regional Office for the Western Pacific, the contents of this chapter are the sole responsibility of its authors and should not be construed as speaking for the policies of the World Health Organization's Regional Office for the Western Pacific. This chapter is a tool towards further scientific dialogue and discussion among public health professionals.

Disclaimer: The boundaries and names shown and the designations used on the maps in this document do not imply the expression of any opinion whatsoever on the part of the WHO concerning the legal status of any country, territory, city or area or of its authorities, or concerning the delimitation of its frontiers or boundaries. Dotted lines on maps represent approximate border lines for which there may not yet be full agreement.

REFERENCES

ABS, 2008a. Health of Children in Australia: A Snapshot, 2004–05. Australian Bureau of Statistics, Canberra.

ABS, 2008b. Year Book Australia, 2008. Australian Bureau of Statistics, Canberra.

ABS and AIHW, 2008. The Health and Welfare of Australia's Aboriginal and Torres Strait Islander Peoples, 2008. Australian Bureau of Statistics, Canberra.

Adams, M., Page, W., Speare, R., 2003. Strongyloidiasis: an issue in Aboriginal communities. Rural Remote Health 3, 152.

ADB, 1998. Policy on Indigenous People. Asian Development Bank, Manila.

ADB, 2001. Health and Education Needs of Ethnic Minorities in the Greater Mekong Subregion. Asian Development Bank, Manila.

ADB, 2002a. Indigenous Peoples/Ethnic Minorities and Poverty Reduction—Cambodia. Asian Development Bank, Manila.

ADB, 2002b. Indigenous Peoples/Ethnic Minorities and Poverty Reduction—Philippines. Asian Development Bank, Manila.

Al-Mekhlafi, M.S., Azlin, M., Nor Aini, U., Shaikh, A., Sa'iah, A., Fatmah, M.S., et al., 2006. Prevalence and distribution of soil-transmitted helminthiases among Orang Asli children living in peripheral Selangor, Malaysia. Southeast Asian J. Trop. Med. Public Health 37, 40–47.

Baulch, B., Haughton, D., Haughton, J.H., Chuyen, T.T.K., 2002. Ethnic Minority Development in Vietnam: A Socioeconomic Perspective. World Bank, Washington, DC (World Bank Policy Research Working Paper No. 2836).

Department of Statistics Malaysia, 2006. Profile of Orang Asli in Peninsular Malaysia. Department of Statistics Malaysia, Kuala Lumpur.

de Silva, S., Saykao, P., Kelly, H., MacIntyre, C.R., Ryan, N., Leydon, J., et al., 2002. Chronic *Strongyloides stercoralis* infection in Laotian immigrants and refugees 7–20 years after resettlement in Australia. Epidemiol. Infect. 128, 439–444.

Ehrenberg, J.P., Ault, S.K., 2005. Neglected diseases of neglected populations: thinking to reshape the determinants of health in Latin America and the Caribbean. BMC Public Health 5, 119.

Einsiedel, L., Spelman, D., 2006. *Strongyloides stercoralis*: risks posed to immigrant patients in an Australia tertiary referral centre. Intern. Med. J. 36, 632–637.

Engvall, A., 2007. Ethnic Minorities and Rural Poverty in Lao PDR. European Institute of Japanese Studies, Stockholm (European Institute of Japanese Studies Working Paper Series No. 232).

Hakim, S., Can, C.C., Malkit, K., Noor Azian, M., Chong, C.K., Shaari, N., et al., 2007. Parasitic infections among Orang Asli (Aborigine) in the Cameron Highland, Malaysia. Southeast Asian J. Trop. Med. Public Health 38, 415–419.

Henninger, N., Snel, M., 2002. Where are the Poor? Experiences with the Development and Use of Poverty Maps. World Resources Institute, Washington, DC.

Hotez, P.J., Ehrenberg, J.P., 2010. Escalating the global fight against neglected tropical diseases through interventions in the Asia Pacific Region. Adv. Parasitol. 72, 31–53.

Hotez, P.J., Yamey, G., 2009. The evolving scope of PLoS Neglected Tropical Diseases. PLoS Negl. Trop. Dis. 3, e379.

Hotez, P.J., Molyneux, D.H., Fenwick, A., Ottesen, E., Ehrlich Sachs, S., Sachs, J.D., 2006. Incorporating a rapid-impact package for neglected tropical diseases with programs for HIV/AIDS, tuberculosis, and malaria. PLoS Med. 3, e102.

Hotez, P.J., Molyneux, D.H., Fenwick, A., Kumaresan, J., Ehrlich Sachs, S., Sachs, J.D., et al., 2007. Control of neglected tropical diseases. N. Engl. J. Med. 357, 1018–1027.

Hunt, P., 2007. Neglected Diseases: A Human Rights Analysis. WHO/TDR, Geneva (Special Topics in Social, Economic and Behavioural Research, No. 6).

Husein, M.H., Talaat, M., El-Sayed, M.K., El-Badawi, A., Evans, D.B., 1996. Who misses out with school-based health programmes? A study of schistosomiasis control in Egypt. Trans. R. Soc. Trop. Med. Hyg. 90, 362–365.

IWGIA, 2008. The Indigenous World 2008. International Work Group for Indigenous Affairs, Copenhagen.

IWGIA, 2009. The Indigenous World 2009. International Work Group for Indigenous Affairs, Copenhagen.

Jamaiah, I., Rohela, M., 2005. Prevalence of intestinal parasites among members of the public in Kuala Lumpur, Malaysia. Southeast Asian J. Trop. Med. Public Health 36, 68–71.

Johnston, F.H., Morris, P.S., Speare, R., McCarthy, J., Currie, B., Ewald, D., et al., 2005. Strongyloidiasis: a review of the evidence for Australian practitioners. Aust. J. Rural Health 13, 247–254.

Keiser, J., Utzinger, J., 2010. The drugs we have and the drugs we need against major helminth infections. Adv. Parasitol. 73, 197–230.

Khor, G.K., Shariff, Z.M., 2008. The ecology of health and nutrition of "Orang Asli" (indigenous people) women and children in Peninsular Malaysia. Tribes and Tribals 2, 67–77. (Special volume).

Lyttleton, C., 2003. Prevention of HIV/AIDS among Ethnic Minorities of the Upper Mekong Region through Community-Based Non-Formal and Formal Education. UNESCO Asia Pacific Regional Bureau for Education, Bangkok.

Mahendra Raj, S., Sein, K.T., Khairul Anuar, A., Mustaffa, B.E., 1997. Effect of intestinal helminthiasis on school attendance by early primary schoolchildren. Trans. R. Soc. Trop. Med. Hyg. 91, 131–132.

Māori Health, 2008. Statistics, Demographics, Age Structure. http://www.maorihealth.govt.nz/moh.nsf/indexma/age-distribution (accessed: 18 February 2010).

Meloni, B.P., Thompson, R.C., Hopkins, R.M., Reynoldson, J.A., Gracey, M., 1993. The prevalence of *Giardia* and other intestinal parasites in children, dogs and cats from Aboriginal communities in the Kimberley. Med. J. Aust. 158, 157–159.

MoP, 1999. Cambodian Human Development Report, 1999: Village Economy and Development. Ministry of Planning, Phnom Penh.

Muela Ribera, J., Peeters Grietens, K., Toomer, E., Hausmann-Muela, S., 2009. A word of caution against the stigma trend in neglected tropical disease research and control. PLoS Negl. Trop. Dis. 3, e445.

Muth, S., Sayasone, S., Odermatt-Biays, S., Phompida, S., Odermatt, S., Duong, S., 2010. *Schistosoma mekongi* in Cambodia and Lao People's Democratic Republic. Adv. Parasitol. 72, 179–203.

NCIP, 2003. Ethnolinguistic Group Profiles. National Commission on Indigenous Peoples. http://www.ncip.gov.ph/ethno_region.php. (accessed: 18 February 2010).

NSO, 2005. 2000 Census of Population and Housing. National Statistics Office, Philippines. http://www.census.gov.ph/census2000/index.html (accessed: 18 February 2010).

Olsen, A., van Lieshout, L., Marti, H., Polderman, T., Polman, K., Steinmann, P., et al., 2009. Strongyloidiasis—the most neglected of the neglected tropical diseases? Trans. R. Soc. Trop. Med. Hyg. 103, 967–972.

Population Council, 2007. Changing Transitions to Adulthood in Vietnam's Remote Northern Uplands: A Focus on Ethnic Minority Youth and Their Families. Population Council, Hanoi.

PRB, 2008. 2008 World Population, Data Sheet. Population Reference Bureau, Washington, DC.

Prociv, P., Luke, R.A., 1995. The changing epidemiology of human hookworm infection in Australia. Med. J. Aust. 162, 150–154.

Ramirez, B.L., Hernandez, L., Alberto, F.F., Collins, M., Nfonsam, V., Punsalan, T., et al., 2004. Contrasting *Wucheria bancrofti* microfilaria rates in two Mangyan-populated Philippine villages. Am. J. Trop. Med. Hyg. 71, 17–23.

Reynoldson, J.A., Behnke, J.M., Pallant, L.J., Macnish, M.G., Gilbert, F., Giles, S., et al., 1997. Failure of pyrantel in treatment of human hookworm infections (*Ancylostoma duodenale*) in the Kimberley region of North West Australia. Acta Trop. 68, 301–312.

Rim, H.J., Chai, J.Y., Min, D.Y., Cho, S.Y., Eom, K.S., Hong, S.J., et al., 2003. Prevalence of intestinal parasite infections on a national scale among primary schoolchildren in Laos. Parasitol. Res. 91, 267–272.

Roy, P., 2006. Indigenous Peoples: Human Rights, Dignity and Development with Identity. Speech delivered at the International Day of the World's Indigenous Peoples, New York, 9 August 2006.

Sagin, D.D., Mohamed, M., Ismail, G., Jok, J.J., Lim, L.H., Pui, J.N.F., 2002. Intestinal parasitic infection among five interior communities at upper Rejang River, Sarawak, Malaysia. Southeast Asian J. Trop. Med. Public Health 33, 18–22.

Sayasone, S., Odermatt, P., Phoumindr, N., Vongsavarane, X., Sensombath, V., Phetsouvanh, X., et al., 2007. Epidemiology of *Opisthorchis viverrini* in a rural district of southern Lao PDR. Trans. R. Soc. Trop. Med. Hyg. 101, 40–47.

Singh, B., Cox-Singh, J., 2001. Parasites that cause problems in Malaysia: soil-transmitted helminths and malaria parasites. Trends Parasitol. 17, 597–600.

Sinuon, M., Tsuyuoka, R., Socheat, D., Odermatt, P., Ohmae, H., Matsuda, H., et al., 2007. Control of *Schistosoma mekongi* in Cambodia: results of eight years of control activities in the two endemic provinces. Trans. R. Soc. Trop. Med. Hyg. 101, 34–39.

Sripa, B., Kaewkes, S., Intapan, P.M., Maleewong, W., Brindley, P.J., 2010. Food-borne trematodiases in Southeast Asia: epidemiology, pathology, clinical manifestation and control. Adv. Parasitol. 72, 305–350.

Steinmann, P., Du, Z.W., Wang, L.B., Wang, X.Z., Jiang, J.Y., Li, L.H., et al., 2008. Extensive multiparasitism in a village of Yunnan province, People's Republic of China, revealed by a suite of diagnostic methods. Am. J. Trop. Med. Hyg. 78, 760–769.

Steinmann, P., Utzinger, J., Du, Z.W., Zhou, X.N., 2010. Multiparasitism: a neglected reality on global, regional and local scale. Adv. Parasitol. 73, 21–50.

Sudomo, M., Chayabejara, S., Socheat, D., Hernandez, L., Wu, W.P., Bergquist, R., 2010. Elimination of lymphatic filariasis in Southeast Asia. Adv. Parasitol. 72, 205–233.

UNDP, 2004. A Common View, a common Journey. A Common Country Assessment of the Philippines. United Nations Development Programme, Manila.

Utzinger, J., de Savigny, D., 2006. Control of neglected tropical diseases: integrated chemotherapy and beyond. PLoS Med. 3, e112.

Weiss, M., 2008. Stigma and the social burden of neglected tropical diseases. PLoS Negl. Trop. Dis. 2, e237.

WFP, 2007. Integrated Food Security and Humanitarian Phase Classification (IPC) Pilot in Cambodia. World Food Programme, Phnom Penh.

WHO, 2003. Health and Ethnic Minorities in Vietnam. World Health Organization, Hanoi. (Technical Series No. 1).

WHO, 2006. Preventive Chemotherapy in Human Helminthiasis: Coordinated Use of Anthelminthic Drugs in Control Interventions: A Manual for Health Professionals and Programme Managers. World Health Organization, Geneva.

WHO, 2008a. Cambodia—Health Facilities, 2004. In: WHO (Ed.), 2008a. The HealthMapper [database]. Version 4.3. World Health Organization, Geneva.

WHO, 2008b. Cambodia (Population Density), 1995. In: WHO (Ed.), 2008. The HealthMapper [database]. Version 4.3. World Health Organization, Geneva.

WHO/WPRO, 2008. Review on the Epidemiological Profile of Helminthiases and their Control in the Western Pacific Region, 1997–2008. World Health Organization/Western Pacific Regional Office, Manila.

WHO/WPRO, 2009. First Mekong-Plus Programme Managers Workshop on Lymphatic Filariasis and Other Helminthiasis. World Health Organization/Western Pacific Regional Office, Manila (Phnom Penh, Cambodia, 23–26 March 2009).

Willingham, A.L. III, Wu, H.W., Conlan, J., Satrija, F., 2010. Combating *Taenia solium* cysticercosis in Southeast Asia: an opportunity for improving human health and livestock production. Adv. Parasitol. 72, 235–266.

Zhou, X.N., Bergquist, R., Leonardo, L., Yang, G.J., Yang, K., Sudomo, M., et al., 2010. Schistosomiasis japonica: research and control. Adv. Parasitol. 72, 145–178.

CHAPTER 5

Controlling Schistosomiasis in Southeast Asia: A Tale of Two Countries

Robert Bergquist* and **Marcel Tanner**[†,‡]

Contents

Abstract

An overview of schistosomiasis control in the People's Republic of China and the Philippines is presented. Whilst the Chinese have managed to reduce the number of *Schistosoma japonicum* infections from an estimated 11.6 million to well below 1 million since 1950, the corresponding drop in the Philippines is less pronounced: from 700,000 in 1975 to currently 560,000. However, these figures should be seen in the context of the population growth, which approximately doubled the Chinese population over the past 60 years (from 557 million to 1.3 billion) whereas the number of

* Ingerod, Brastad, Sweden
† Department of Epidemiology and Public Health, Swiss Tropical and Public Health Institute, Basel, Switzerland
‡ University of Basel, Basel, Switzerland

Advances in Parasitology, Volume 72
ISSN 0065-308X, DOI: 10.1016/S0065-308X(10)72005-4

Filipinos during the same time more than quadrupled (from 21 to 93 million). The Philippine progress should also be judged against the backdrop of regional political instability combined with strong socio-ecological dynamics. Although substantial improvements have been achieved in both countries, compliance is waning in people repeatedly given praziquantel with or without prior diagnosis and this problem will not be reversed without sustained vigilance. In addition, the lower rates of excreted eggs per gram of stool in the new endemic situation characterised by widespread, low-intensity infections influence the accuracy of prevalence assessments negatively. Remaining pockets of high transmission further complicate the situation. Maintaining that advances in schistosomiasis control critically depend on technical progress, we discuss the problems currently facing control programmes from the viewpoint of what research can actually contribute at this stage of disease control. The need for flexible control approaches is emphasised and more sensitive diagnostics is highlighted. Above all, it is argued that strengthened, innovative surveillance approaches are called for if elimination of the disease is to succeed.

5.1. INTRODUCTION

With more than 12% of the world's population at risk with regard to schistosomiasis (Steinmann et al., 2006; WHO, 2009), the contention that this disease threatens the economy of many nations and that large numbers of people suffer is no exaggeration. Indeed, the full impact of schistosomiasis on a global level is no less than that caused by, for example, malaria and tuberculosis (King, 2010). Nevertheless, schistosomiasis remains a neglected tropical disease (NTD) and since transmission is only marginally affected by chemotherapy, rapid reinfection easily sustains prevalence, even in the face of well-run control programmes. Rebound morbidity, that is the aggressive pathology due to interference with the natural, immunological modulation noted in children in high-transmission areas after interrupted chemotherapy (Olveda et al., 1996; Reimert et al., 2008), can further complicate the situation. This is a good example of how previously unknown aspects of an infection require modified approaches to avoid unforeseen problems.

While academic research can develop and progress on its own as long as ideas and funding permit, control activities are demand-driven. Although progress has a strong foundation in academia, research and development (R&D) processes take the crucial middle position that drive control programmes. For example, without R&D, the serendipitous finding of a chemical compound with a broad anthelminthic activity (Gönnert and Andrews,

1977) would not have resulted in praziquantel (Andrews et al., 1980, 1983; Davis and Wegner, 1979), the cornerstone of current schistosomiasis control the world over. The importance of this point was brought home by the 10-year World Bank Loan Project (WBLP) to control schistosomiasis in the People's Republic of China (P.R. China) in the 1990s (Chen et al., 2005; Utzinger et al., 2005; Yuan et al., 2000a), which clearly showed that the outcome would have been handicapped without a well-designed, complementary research component. Although the utility of research was expected, it was a revelation that as little as 2.8% of the total WBLP budget was sufficient to usher in novel ideas which are still driving research in areas as diverse as diagnostics, risk-prediction, surveillance as well as vaccine and drug development (Utzinger et al., 2005; Xiao et al., 2010; Yuan et al., 2000a).

To illustrate the issue of controlling parasitic diseases in Southeast Asia, the activities in P.R. China and the Philippines were chosen as examples. In spite of good progress, both countries are still seriously affected by intestinal schistosomiasis due to *Schistosoma japonicum*. Both have devoted significant national funding and also received substantial outside financial help to control schistosomiasis, yet the results differ. Despite some incompleteness of the respective data sets, we have aimed at synthesizing available evidence on how these two countries adapted to the prevailing conditions, mobilized funding and developed their control strategies and activities accordingly.

5.2. TOWARDS THE 'TRUE' BURDEN OF SCHISTOSOMIASIS

To address the impact of human disease in a broad sense, Murray and Lopez (1996) introduced a new metric, the disability-adjusted life year (DALY) intended to gauge the gap between the prevailing health status and the ideal situation. In comparison to using mortality alone as a measure, their ideas represent a workable approach to gauge the impact of a particular disease or injury by giving weight also to morbidity and disability. However, as noted already by Pesigan et al. (1958), it is indeed a challenge to assess the impact on an individual, as well on the economy in general, of chronic diseases with subtle pathologies. Based on their research results, King et al. (2005) feel that the estimates for schistosomiasis require substantial revision. It has been argued that much of the morbidity caused by schistosomiasis appears one or two decades after the first incidence of infection in early childhood (Stothard and Gabrielli, 2007), which was not sufficiently addressed in the original DALY estimate. Moreover, as pointed out by King (2010), the removal of time-preference discounting of future events from the standard DALY calculation expands the present-day impact of schistosomiasis to between 24 and 29 million DALYs. These values are based on a conservative 2% average disability score, which increases to 49–56 million DALYs if a higher, still reasonable, 5% estimate of disability is used (King, 2010). Although these figures are many times higher than previous estimates, that is 1.7–4.5 million DALYs (WHO, 2002, 2004), it should be considered that they do not only reflect a more realistic assessment of infection-associated disability, but also account for the enduring effect of childhood infection throughout adult life. Although these recalculations strongly challenge the Global Burden of Disease (GBD) assessments by Murray and Lopez (1996) with regard to the influence of parasitic diseases on individual health, they make perfect sense in gauging the magnitude and duration of infection-related, chronic diseases on a global scale (Bustinduy and King, 2009).

5.3. CONTROL OF SCHISTOSOMIASIS

Although the global, human prevalence of schistosomiasis remains above 200 million with close to 800 million still at risk (Steinmann et al., 2006; WHO, 2009), durable progress has been made in many parts of the world. However, we need to look back to the mid-1980s to fully appreciate the advances made: praziquantel had just been introduced (Andrews et al., 1983; WHO, 1985) and there was hope that the cost of the drug would eventually be reduced. Conjecturing that chemotherapy could become the intervention of choice for large-scale control, the World Bank, the World health Organization (WHO) and the Edna McConnell Clark Foundation (EMCF) sponsored a workshop entitled 'Organization and Management of Schistosomiasis and other Tropical Disease Control Programmes' (Liese, 1986). The overarching issue of public health services was addressed by preparing the ground for the move from transmission control to morbidity control with regard to schistosomiasis. The subsequent WHO recommendation of morbidity control through chemotherapy (WHO, 1985, 1993) started an era of falling prices of praziquantel leading to an unprecedented, general investment in the endemic areas (Doenhoff et al., 2008; Fenwick et al., 2003). Indeed, in collaboration with WHO and international donors, national control programmes in P.R. China (Chen et al., 2005), Brazil (Katz, 1998), Egypt (El Khoby et al., 1998) and Morocco (Boelee and Laamrani, 2004) managed to reduce the number of infected people considerably and permanently.

Following the example of praziquantel, the Mectizan Donation Program (http://www.mectizan.org) was established in 1987 to oversee the donation by Merck & Co. (Whitehouse Station, NJ, USA), of Mectizan (ivermectin) for the control of onchocerciasis worldwide. The mandate was later expanded to include lymphatic filariasis (LF) elimination through co-administration of Mectizan and albendazole (donated by GlaxoSmithKline; GSK House, Brentford, London, UK) in African countries and Yemen where LF and onchocerciasis share the same geographic area. The partnership with Merck & Co., the Mectizan Donation Program, WHO and the African Programme for Onchocerciasis Control (APOC) is now considered a forerunner of the decentralized public–private partnerships that have sprung up in the last decade. Although it had originally been anticipated that the new drug-based approach should be administered by national control programmes, control of parasitic diseases is instead now moving in the direction of integrated approaches, spearheaded by support from international donor agencies working directly with pharmaceutical companies and private foundations such as the Bill and Melinda Gates Foundation (Seattle, WA, USA) (Hotez et al., 2007).

Ironically, the very model for this paradigm shift, praziquantel, still has to be paid for, while other drugs generally are donated and thus provided free. Schistosomiasis control continues to be based on a vertical approach in many countries, but has also been included in larger projects (Fenwick et al., 2009; Utzinger et al., 2009). As shown by work in Africa by the German Association for Technical Cooperation (GTZ) (http://www.gtz.de/en/) and the Schistosomiasis Control Initiative (SCI) (http://www.sci-ntds.org/), by their efforts to realize the Millennium Development Goals (MDGs) of sustainable poverty reduction (www.un.org/millenniumgoals/goals.html), activities are now becoming more integrated targeting several diseases concurrently in many countries (Fenwick, 2006; Fenwick et al., 2009; Lammie et al., 2006; Utzinger et al., 2009). For example, SCI has now added seven other NTDs to its original focus on schistosomiasis.

5.4. NATIONAL CONTROL PROGRAMMES

The trematode parasite *S. japonicum* (lifecycle at the back of this volume), one of the five main schistosome species that infect humans, exists mainly in P.R. China and the Philippines but can also be found in two restricted foci in the island of Sulawesi, Indonesia (Zhou et al., 2010). *S. mekongi* also belongs to the oriental schistosomes but this species is not discussed here as it is exclusively confined to a few limited areas in Cambodia and Lao People's Democratic Republic (Muth et al., 2010). In contrast to all other schistosome species adapted to humans, *S. japonicum* accepts a wide variety of vertebrate animals as its definitive host which can all act as reservoirs of infection, thus rendering control of this species a formidable challenge.

5.4.1. P.R. China

The magnitude of the schistosomiasis problem was not fully appreciated at the Government level until the founding of P.R. China. Almost immediately after the revolution in 1949, survey teams were dispatched to identify villages and areas affected. Their verdict was ready in the early 1950s: the number of infected people could exceed 11 million and more than 100 million were at risk (Chen and Feng, 1999; Mao and Shao, 1982). Once this alarm was sounded, offices at the various administrative levels were rapidly set up to implement countermeasures (Chen, 1989; Maegraith, 1958). The control activities were to be supervised by a network of provincial institutes led by the Institute for Parasitic Diseases (IPD) in Shanghai, which was also charged with coordination of control and research (Zhou et al., 2005a).

5.4.1.1. Control aspects

The shift to morbidity control, based on WHO's recommendation in the mid-1980s (WHO, 1985), was supported by research from Chinese scientists (Chen, 2005; Xiao, 2005) and initiated in the beginning of the 1990s under the guidance of the 10-year WBLP. The aim of this loan, awarded to P.R. China specifically for schistosomiasis control through large-scale, chemotherapy-based morbidity control, was to reduce the prevalence in both humans and bovines by at least 40% and to lower the snail infection prevalence by 50% (Chen et al., 2005). Central features of the approach implemented were standardised, large-scale chemotherapy accompanied with health education, sanitation and improved access to tap water. Importantly, snail control was not completely abandoned as in other parts of the world (Utzinger et al., 2005). Two years before the start of the WBLP in 1991, a national survey was carried out. The number of infected people, then estimated at 1.52–1.64 million (Chen and Feng, 1999; Zhen, 1993), should be compared to the 1995 national survey at the programme mid-term, which showed that the number of human infections had come down to an estimated 865,000. In addition, the prevalence in the endemic areas had fallen to 4.9% from 10.2% in 1989, while the average bovine infection rate had decreased from 13.3% to 9.1% (Ministry of Health, 1998; Zhou et al., 2005a).

Evaluations, based on stratified, randomised samples of at least 1% of the population living in endemic areas, were carried out three times during the WBLP; in 1989, 1995 and 2004 (Chen et al., 2005; Wu et al., 2007). The continuous, downward change of prevalence (green line) is illustrated in Fig. 5.1 together with the results of annual, less elaborate spot-checks (red line). The discrepancy between these two assessments is not great and depends probably on the lower ambition of the spot-checks but the seemingly sustained prevalence indicated by the spot-checks after 2000 is intriguing. Whether the results obtained after the end of the WBLP reflect a continued reduction of the prevalence, or whether a low-level stabilization has been attained, is currently unknown but will need to be established before long.

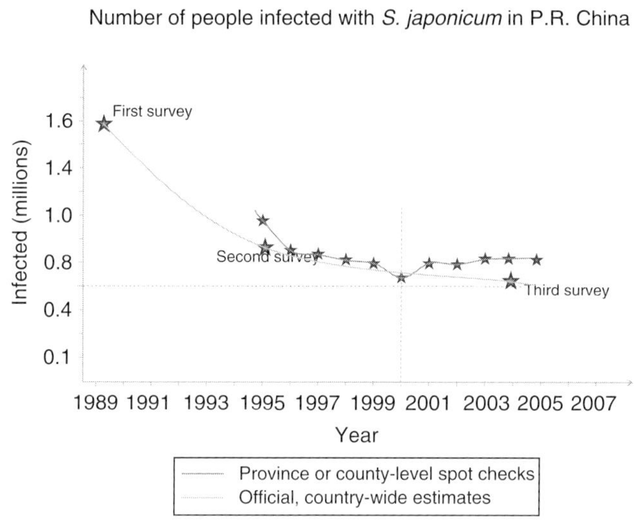

FIGURE 5.1 Estimated number of people infected with *S. japonicum* in P.R. China between 1989 and 2005.

In spite of the overall, unparalleled success of the Chinese control programme, schistosomiasis has in fact re-emerged in several counties where transmission control and interruption had been declared previously (Wu et al., 2007; Zhao et al., 2005; Zhou et al., 2005a). As a consequence, the initiative reflecting an understanding of the role of the water buffalo as infection reservoir is currently being launched in addition to the ongoing chemotherapy programme (Wang et al., 2009a). This revised strategy emphasizes transmission control by encouraging mechanized agriculture measures and fencing of water buffaloes in places where they cannot be replaced by tractors (Wang et al., 2009a, b).

Table 5.1 does not specify any data between 1950 and 1989 since no large-scale surveys were carried out during this time and existing province and/or county-based evaluations are difficult to come by. However, available data suggest that the strong focus on the snail during the second stage of the national control programme reduced the endemic areas by two-thirds and that the treatment of all infected humans and bovines that took place in conjunction with this concerted action must at least have halved the number of infected people in the country. Even if the snail-infested areas probably grew during the following 10 years, the situation was evidently quickly rectified. We also know that five provinces were declared free of the infection in the period 1985–1995 (Chen et al., 2005; Utzinger et al., 2005; Wu et al., 2005). It seems therefore safe to hypothesize that the biggest drop in prevalence took place in the five years prior to the first national survey in 1989.

TABLE 5.1 The evolving schistosomiasis situation in P.R. China since 1950

Year	Population[a] (billions)	At-risk population (millions)	Infected people (millions)	District prevalence (%)[b]	Bovines infected (millions)	References
1950	0.56	100	11.6	21.0	1.2	Mao and Shao (1982); Chen and Feng (1999)
1989	1.12		1.6	10.2	0.2 (13.3%)	Zhen (1993); Chen and Feng (1999)
1995	1.20		0.9	4.9	0.1 (9.1%)	Ministry of Health (1998)
2004	1.30	65	0.7	3.8	0.1 (5.7%)	Zhou et al. (2007); Wu et al. (2007)

[a] http://www.populstat.info/Asia/chinac.htm.
[b] highest value recorded.

To sum up the progress achieved and highlight future planning, the control programme can be shown as a project consisting of seven stages:

- 1950–1955: data collection and setting strategic goals;
- 1956–1965: environmental engineering plus treatment of humans and bovines;
- 1966–1976: intermission due to political upheaval;
- 1977–1980: reestablishment of the national control programme;
- 1980–1990: regaining lost momentum;
- 1991–2001: decade of the WBLP;
- 2002–2015: situation evaluation, planning for schistosomiasis elimination; and
- 2016–2120: elimination of schistosomiasis.

The large-scale administration of praziquantel provided good results initially, but there are growing concerns that a lasting effect might be unattainable with drugs alone. Still, in spite of the worrying tendency of stalling snail control, transmission seems to be receding which is supported by Fig. 5.2, which depicts the recent, strong decline in the number of acute cases of schistosomiasis in P.R. China (Li et al., 2009).

WBLP represents the largest effort of schistosomiasis control in the world by far. In addition, the Government provided financial support to the provinces (Table 5.1). The total cost of bringing down the number of

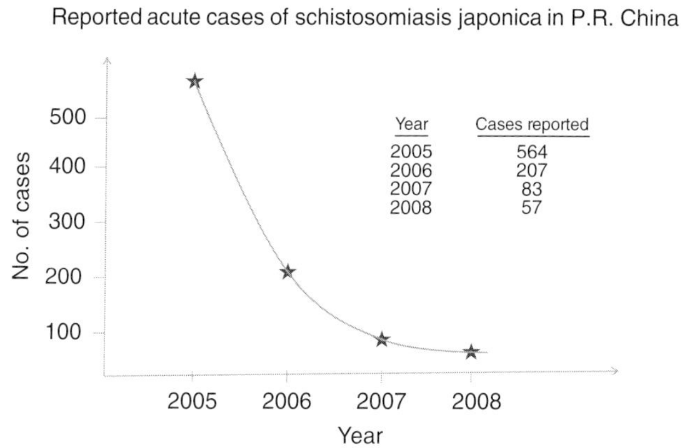

FIGURE 5.2 Reported acute cases of schistosomiasis japonica in P.R. China between 2005 and 2008.

infected people with more than 90% over 50 years must be considerable even if labour costs in P.R. China are traditionally low. It should in this connection be mentioned that an economic evaluation of the WBLP in six representative counties showed a benefit–cost ratio of 6.2, that is the project gained US$ 6.20 for every dollar spent (Zhou et al., 2005b). This suggests that further progress in schistosomiasis control will lead to growth of the local economy, particularly in areas where the disease had the highest impact previously.

5.4.1.2. The research component

Naturally, various research projects have been carried out in P.R. China over many years. However, these projects did not have a clear association with an overall plan for reduction and elimination of schistosomiasis (or any other disease). The first sign of a more planned approach came with a serology study, initiated and supported by the UNICEF/UNDP/World Bank/WHO Special Programme for Research and Training in Tropical Diseases (TDR), aimed at improving schistosomiasis diagnosis in the field. Based on two previous studies (Mott and Dixon, 1982; Mott et al., 1987), a collaborative study was set up to compare 12 serological assays in the different provincial parasitic institutes of the schistosome-endemic areas. Regretfully, due to a multitude of practical variations between the test systems, it was not possible to draw any firm conclusions from this study, which was therefore never published. The outcome was, however, not entirely in vain as a well-defined serum bank was collected and the study marked a start of Chinese collaborative research that was considered during the negotiations between the World Bank and the Government eventually leading to the WBLP. A decision was made to set aside a small part of the WBLP funds (2.8%) for research and training

(Table 5.1) and TDR was asked to support part of the Joint Research Management Committee (JRMC) that was established to watch over these activities (Yuan et al., 2000a). Supervised by the JRMC, training was intensified, resulting in improved applications and a better quality of the scientific level of the research carried out. After an overview of the internal organization and funding of the WBLP (Table 5.2), a brief inventory of current international collaborative research projects that directly issued from the training was provided by the JRMC (Table 5.3). The latest development in this connection is shown in Table 5.4, which depicts current and awarded grants for continued collaborative studies focused on risk factor analyses (Steinmann et al., 2007a,b), immunogenicity and vaccine-related research (Da'dara et al., 2008; Ellis and McManus, 2009) and morbidity control (Balen et al., 2007). These are just a few samples of finalized and ongoing collaborative projects in P.R. China, the number of which is currently growing exponentially.

5.4.1.2.1. Diagnostics The Kato-Katz stool examination (Katz et al., 1972), recommended by WHO for the diagnosis of intestinal schistosomiasis globally, is useful when the intensity of infection is generally high. However, it is less well suited for use in controlled areas when the parasite loads are lower and often result in eggs per gram (EPG) values below the limit of detection with this method, as was unambiguously shown by (Lin et al., 2008). Further support for a change in the diagnostics area was issued from the observation that compliance rates decline after repeated rounds of stool examinations (Guo et al., 2005a).

A number of new immunodiagnostics tests were developed in P.R. China, for example, the one-step enzyme immunoassay (Wang et al.,

TABLE 5.2 Research and control of *S. japonicum* in P.R. China: Spending under the WBLP

Title	Content	Duration	Funds (US$)	Sponsor
Schistosomiasis control in P.R. China	WBLP core funding	1991–2001	71,000,000	World Bank
Schistosomiasis control in P.R. China	Counterpart funding	1991–2001	82,000,000	Government of P.R. China
Control-oriented research (JRMC)	Research and training under the auspices of the WBLP	1992–2000	4,250,000	WBLP

TABLE 5.3 Research and control of *S. japonicum* in P.R. China: Outside funding for projects carried out by Chinese institutions

Title	Content	Duration	Funds (US$)	Sponsor
Emerging helminthiases in P.R. China I	Study on all aspects of schistosomiasis japonica, hookworm, clonorchiasis and paragonimiasis	1998–2002	2,500,000	TRMC grant from National Institutes of Health (NIH), Bethesda, MD, USA
Emerging helminthiases in P.R. China II	Continued studies concentrating on control aspects of schistosomiasis japonica and hookworm	2003–2008	3,000,000	TRMC grant from National Institutes of Health (NIH), Bethesda, MD, USA
Identification of vaccine molecules	Identification of *S. japonicum* target antigens by proteomic techniques	2004–2005	40,000	WHO/TDR
Bio-social risks of the schistosomiasis burden in the Yangtze River basin, P.R. China	Development and validation of new tools for assessment of risk factors for transmission and morbidity of *S. japonicum*; identification of key features of disease burdens in relation to social and economic status by gauging health inequities and DALYs	2004–2006	123,100	WHO
Schistosomiasis risks related to the construction of the Three Gorges Dam	Development of a model for the rapid determination of snail habitats in the Three Gorges reservoir based on remote sensing	2004–2006	15,000	WHO/TDR
Assessment of age-specific disability weight of chronic schistosomiasis japonica	Development of age-specific DALY estimates by assessing health outcomes and quality of life determinants exploring the link between environmental and socio-economic risk factors	2007–2008	9,900	WHO/WPRO/TDR

TABLE 5.4 Research and control of *S. japonicum* in P.R. China: international collaboration

Title	Content	Duration	Funds (US$)	Sponsor
Immune responses during *S. japonicum* infection	Immunogenetic studies in humans with *S. japonicum* infection around the Dongting Lake in Hunan province	2001–2003	235,775	Wellcome Trust; London, UK
Core grant allocation	General support for research on schistosomiasis in P.R. China	2004	275,000	National Health and Medical Research Council (NHMRC), Melbourne, Australia
Control of morbidity due to schistosomiasis	Progress towards sustainable morbidity control and prevention of schistosomiasis	2004–2009	2,450,000	Wellcome Trust, NHMRC and an International Collaborative Research Grant (ICRG)
Spatial distribution of *S. japonicum*	Risk factor analysis of *S. japonicum* (and other helminth infections) in Eryuan county, Yunnan province	2006–2007	30,000	Swiss National Science Foundation, Bern, Switzerland
Pathogenesis in schistosomiasis japonica	Study of the immunopathogenic mechanisms in human *S. japonicum* infection	2007–2009	440,000	DANA Foundation, New York, USA
S. japonicum in the Three Gorges Dam area	Impact of the Three Gorges Dam construction on control of human schistosomiasis with special reference to transmission	2010–2014	1,347,500	NHMRC

Determinants of schistosomiasis reemergence	Study of individual and village-level factors responsible for *S. japonicum* reemergence in Sichuan province and modelling the reemergence phenomenon	2007–2012	2,370,000	National Institute of Allergy and Infectious Diseases (NIAID), NIH
The influence of environmental change on parasite diffusion	Use of molecular genetic data for the quantification of parasite diffusion and its role in transmission in Sichuan province	2006–2011	1,964,000	National Science Foundation, NIH, Bethesda, MD, USA
Local strategies for schistosomiasis control	Model site-specific disease control strategies in Sichuan Province	2002–2007	1,584,000	NIAID, NIH, Bethesda, MD, USA
RS and GIS for schistosomiasis control	Determination of the feasibility of using remote sensing for large-scale surveillance of snail habitats for schistosomiasis control	1999–2002	907,000	NIAID, NIH, Bethesda, MD, USA

1999), the colloidal dye immunofiltration assay (Xiao et al., 2003, 2005), a dipstick dye immunoassay (Zhu et al., 2002; Zhu, 2005) and the dot immunogold filtration assay (Wen et al., 2005). This field of diagnostics flourished when technology advanced to the point that monoclonal antibodies could be produced which led to serology being integrated into the national schistosomiasis control programme in P.R. China at an early stage (Xiao et al., 2005; Zhao et al., 1993).

5.4.1.2.2. Demographic factors and health education The importance of health education was stressed from the beginning of the national schistosomiasis control programme (Maegraith, 1958). Research direct by the JRMC led to development and validation of new tools such as cartoons and video tapes (Hu et al., 2005; Yuan et al., 2000b). It was also found that health education does not only contribute to change in water contact behaviour, but can also be used to improve declining compliance due to numerous cycles of large-scale administration of praziquantel and community-based 'test-and-treat' campaigns (Guo et al., 2005a). Many communities have been repeatedly subjected to repeated rounds of praziquantel administration and some people have been treated with this drug up to 20 times (Wu et al., 2005). A two-year study compared routine mass chemotherapy with health education plus 'passive chemotherapy', an approach that involves medical teams treating individuals who request treatment based on symptoms or after recent water contact. With regard to treatment coverage among *S. japonicum*-infected people, 'passive chemotherapy' reached a level of 96.2–97.1% and the cost of 'passive chemotherapy' plus health education turned out to be only half that of mass chemotherapy (Guo et al., 2005a). Since 'passive chemotherapy' lends itself to integration into the primary health care system, it offers an attractive strategy for schistosomiasis control during the maintenance and consolidation phase.

Demographic factors and their associations with the risk of a schistosome infection have been investigated in different settings in many places. Huang and Manderson (2005) summarize a large body of mainly Chinese literature on the social and economic context of schistosomiasis japonica which, apart from purely social factors, covers environment policies (e.g. agricultural production systems), economic factors (e.g.occupation, wealth and income) and the domestic environment (e.g. safe water, sanitation and proximity to snail habitats). They also noted that the sustained growth of P.R. China's economy led to a significant urban immigration. This may indeed influence *S. japonicum* transmission negatively as increased population mobility enhances the risk of spreading the parasite to areas where transmission of the disease has previously been brought under control.

5.4.1.2.3. Drug experiences Chinese scientists have focussed on how praziquantel alters the adult worm metabolism in *S. japonicum* and also confirmed that the efficacy of praziquantel is antibody-dependent (Xiao, 2005; Xiao et al., 1987, 2010). The experience with large-scale morbidity control and case treatment with praziquantel (reviewed by Chen, 2005) has shown that the drug is not only a cornerstone for general treatment of schistosomiasis but is also highly efficacious against acute and chronic schistosomiasis japonica. A total dose of up to 120 mg/kg administered over 4–6 days is generally used in patients with acute schistosomiasis japonica. Chemotherapy is as much used for livestock as for humans to reduce transmission. Over 50 million doses of praziquantel have been administered to people infected with *S. japonicum* or to those at high risk of contracting the disease due to their occupation, for example fishermen and other people engaged in water-related occupations (Utzinger et al., 2005). So far, there are no indications of tolerance and/or resistance development in *S. japonicum* worms to praziquantel (Shi et al., 2004; Song et al., 2004).

The finding that the artemisinins (e.g. artemether and artesunate) have antischistosomal properties revived the interest in targeted drug research. After it had been demonstrated that the effect of the artemisinins is not general but directed against the young development stages (i.e. the schistosomula), it was shown by randomized, controlled trials that both artemether and artesunate could prevent the development of patent *S. japonicum* infections (for reviews see Utzinger et al., 2001a, 2001b, 2005, 2007; Xiao 2005; Xiao et al., 2000, 2002). The significance of developing both artemether and artesunate for use against schistosomiasis was emphasised early on (Yuan et al., 2000a) and the results have stimulated research also outside P.R. China, extending the scope from *S. japonicum* to *S. mansoni* (de Clercq et al., 2000; Utzinger et al., 2000), *S. haematobium* (de Clercq et al., 2002; N'Goran et al., 2003) and *S. mekongi* (Jiraungkoorskul et al., 2005).

Since it has now been convincingly shown that the artemisinins are capable of successfully preventing acute schistosomiasis japonica, there is no doubt that they have a place in the prophylactic and therapeutic arsenal. However, further applied research on the use of artemisinins alone and in combination with praziquantel is needed. In addition, the search for novel, orally active antischistosomal drugs with a broad spectrum of activity against the juvenile and adult stages of the parasite is being pursued (Xiao et al., 2007, 2010).

5.4.1.2.4. Mapping and prediction of snail habitats The advent of geographical information systems (GIS) and remote sensing (RS) techniques provides important advances to our understanding of key environmental factors. Traditionally, snail densities and infection rates are calculated after collection of the intermediate snail host *Oncomelania hupensis* on site. However, there is now ample evidence that it is feasible to predict the snail distribution with the aid of remotely sensed environmental data (Malone, 2005; Yang et al., 2005; Zhou et al., 2001). Based on satellite-derived data, Guo et al. (2005b) developed a useful model to predict snail habitats. The model holds promise for identifying high-risk areas with regard to infection and has revealed a gradient of high-to-low prevalence with increasing distance. This approach could play a role in schistosome-affected regions that lack accurate surveillance capabilities. Zhang et al. (2005) applied spatial analysis based on satellite imagery to predict the distribution of *O. hupensis* at the meso- and even at the micro-level. Although final proof of the presence of infected snails requires microscopy, this research group could confirm that snail densities in the marshlands relate to vegetation, wetness and temperature. In addition to more commonly used surrogate environmental measures, such as the normalized difference vegetation index (NDVI), features such as wetness, brightness and greenness were selected. These two studies have enhanced our understanding of the spatial distribution of *O. hupensis*, and hence *S. japonicum* transmission, at the meso-scale, that is the level generally used for the targeting of control interventions.

Agricultural and environmental factors associated with infection risk lend themselves to quantification by RS technology (Spear et al., 2004). Assessment of individual exposure to schistosomiasis is often part of such studies which are challenging even at the household level. However, the accuracy can be perfected with only a fraction of the normal workload if the study subjects are equipped with global positioning system (GPS) receivers to record their water-contact patterns. Seto et al. (2007) pioneered this approach creating time–activity maps which indicated that people are surprisingly mobile, averaging 1.4 ± 1.2 water-contacts per day. Their conclusion is that GPS units offer unique insights into the factors that influence schistosomiasis transmission.

5.4.1.2.5. Vaccine research In contrast to *S. mansoni* and *S. haematobium*, *S. japonicum* infection is zoonotic, which, from the vaccine development point of view, offers a shortcut by permitting the creation of a transmission-blocking vaccine for livestock. This has no doubt contributed to the increase of vaccine-related research on *S. japonicum* in the last few years (McManus and Dalton, 2006; McManus and Loukas, 2008; Zhu et al., 2004, 2006) which has now progressed to the level of field trials in P.R. China. These trials, based on the idea that reduced water buffalo infections would also reduce transmission of the disease to humans, have resulted in randomized double blind trials in water buffaloes using DNA vaccines encoding well-researched *S. japonicum* antigens (Sj28-TPI, Sj23) (Da'dara et al., 2008; Dai et al., 2009). The results showed protection of approximately 50% which could be further boosted by chemotherapy in an integrated approach that should have a significant impact on human risk in the future. The inclusion in an integrated control strategy of a vaccine approach targeting domestic animals would reinforce the effect of chemotherapy of humans, reduce the risk for transmission and enhance the possibilities of disease elimination.

5.4.1.2.6. Genome research Together with Brazil (DeMarco and Verjovski-Almeida, 2009; Verjovski-Almeida et al., 2004), P.R. China has taken the lead in mining the schistosome genome with the ultimate goal of identifying novel drug targets and vaccine candidates. The publication of the *S. japonicum* genome (*Schistosoma japonicum* Genome Sequencing and Functional Analysis Consortium et al., 2009) worked out through Chinese research collaboration represents a breakthrough in schistosomiasis research. Although products emanating from this project will not appear overnight, it is revolutionizing the search for new drug and vaccine targets. However, even if novel, superior antigens would be much welcome, progress in the field of vaccinology is now less a question of discovery and more one of industrial production and commercialization.

5.4.1.2.7. Surveillance The Government of P.R. China remains highly committed to consolidate the achievements made over the past 50 years in the control of schistosomiasis in the country and an important feature of the national control programme is rigorous surveillance. In the controlled areas, the emphasis is on monitoring active infections among local residents and domestic animals, as well as monitoring suspected snail infestations, while the situation is carefully followed at sentinel sites located in the known endemic areas (Zhao et al., 2005). Surveillance represents more than just the collection of data and can be regarded as an intervention in its own right. Its links with research activities are usefully illustrated by two innovative papers which analyse economic consideration and efficiency of epidemiological survey methods on the one hand (Li et al., 2005) and, on the other, the utility in relation to human diagnosis (Wu et al., 2005). Feedback and response mechanisms of this kind contribute to the evolution of the art of surveillance, while the development of mathematical transmission models will facilitate analysis of the indicators at play (Williams et al., 2002).

Based on extensive experience in Africa with other schistosome species, Lengeler et al. (2002a,b) developed a simple questionnaire that specifically aimed at schoolchildren for the rapid identification of high-risk areas. Transferring the questionnaire methodology to P.R. China demonstrated its efficiency to also identify *S. japonicum* infection in children, but it was also evident that the results depended critically on the questions selected (Zhou et al., 1998). Recently, the questionnaire approach was further developed for identification of high-risk individuals in areas prone to flooding (Tan et al., 2004) and in the mountainous areas of Yunnan province (Steinmann et al., 2007a).

Surveillance is of particular importance in the mountainous ecosystems which have so far resisted control activities. Research in the Yunnan and Sichuan provinces has shown that epidemiology in the mountainous areas is quite different from that in the plains. Steinmann et al. (2007b) used Bayesian multiple logistic regression models to identify associations between the local seroprevalence and various demographic and environmental parameters in a county in Yunnan. They found that *S. japonicum* seroprevalence was significantly associated with sex and age and that inhabitants of villages situated on steep slopes (inclination $\geq 20°$), or at higher altitudes (>2150 m), were at a comparatively lower risk. Working in the southwestern part of Sichuan, Spear et al. (2004) could show that the prevalence in domestic animals was relatively low, while the human prevalence, as well as intensity of disease, varied between wide margins. Infection intensity at the village level was found to be strongly associated with crop type, with low-intensity villages principally growing rice, in contrast to villages devoting more land to vegetables and tobacco.

Mobile populations represent a growing problem from the point of view of schistosomiasis control. Immunodiagnostic screening with positive results followed up by stool examination (Zhu, 2005) has confirmed that infection in this small, but increasingly important group of people (Liu et al., 1991; Tao and Li, 1999) cannot be easily eliminated. Although active infections are generally imported, they can also be due to residual habitats of infected *O. hupensis* found in areas where the transmission of *S. japonicum* has been officially interrupted (Wu et al., 2005). These observations show that chemotherapy on its own cannot contain the so-called 'endemic hot spots' (Jiang et al., 1996). A broad-based attack on the snail has historically been the key to schistosomiasis control in P.R. China and it is therefore a worry that snail habitats are now on the rise in quite a few places (Chen et al., 2003; Gao et al., 1998). To prevent further extension of habitats, snail surveillance would need to be carried out regularly, not only in the endemic areas, but also in well-controlled, non-endemic areas. Li et al. (2005b) note that an analysis of cost-effectiveness is necessary to identify the most financially feasible yet effective control options and stress the imperative need for periodic surveys using samples that are true representations of the population investigated.

The third national epidemiological sampling survey on schistosomiasis, carried out in 2004, incorporated improvements such as sampling of subjects for schistosome-induced fibrosis using ultrasonography and sampling of snails in a selection of sentinel sites in each of the seven provinces where *S. japonicum* remains endemic. The decline after the second survey in 1995 (Fig. 5.1) is not entirely convincing, as spot-checks suggest a low in 2000 after which prevalence seems to have increased again (Utzinger et al., 2005). On the other hand, the steep reduction of acute cases in the 2005–2008 period (Li et al., 2009; Fig. 5.2) corroborates the view of a continuing lowering of the risk for infection. This issue demands follow-up and a detailed analysis as the current control strategy will undoubtedly further improve the situation.

5.4.2. The Philippines

The scientific interest in the Philippines was originally focused on the biology of the parasite, but after the discovery of the local intermediate snail host, *Oncomelania quadrasi* (Tubangui, 1932), the focus shifted to a more control-oriented phase. This change first led to an initiative to map the endemic areas and then to increased research on clinical and pathological aspects of the disease. However, these activities declined at the beginning of World War II but intensified again as many allied soldiers were infected while based in the country (Garcia, 1976), in particular on the island of Leyte where the U.S. General McArthur first landed his forces. After the war, work to delineate the endemic areas continued and as the results accumulated, it became clear that schistosomiasis represented a potentially huge public health problem (McMullen et al., 1954; Pesigan et al., 1958). Further extensive research revealed the major foci located in the rice-growing areas of the islands Leyte, Samar and Mindanao (Santos, 1967). This line of research culminated with the first country-wide presentation of the endemic areas in 1975, indicating that an estimated 700,000 individuals were infected and that over 5 million were at risk (Santos, 1984). Foreign aid in the form of technical assistance, supplies, equipment and funds sustained many of the early epidemiological activities.

5.4.2.1. Control aspects

The first clear-cut reduction in national *S. japonicum* prevalence was accomplished in the first half of the 1980s (Santos, 1984), and this trend was accentuated by the implementation of the 5-year Philippine Health Development Project (PHDP) initiated in 1990. During this time, the National Schistosomiasis Control Programme (NSCP), with support from the World Bank, intensified case-finding and treatment in all endemic areas which resulted in further improvements.

In spite of difficulties encountered along the way, summarizing the schistosomiasis situation in the Philippines over the last 60 years gives a positive picture overall (Table 5.5). The figures in Table 5.5 are not

TABLE 5.5 Development of schistosomiasis control in the Philippines based on available data from the literature and the Department of Health (DOH)

Year	Population[a] (millions)	At risk (millions)	Infected (millions)	Endemic prevalence (%)[b]	References
1950	21	?	1.80[c]		
1953	23	?	Unknown but situation recognised as serious		McMullen et al. (1954)
1957	26	?	0.30–0.40	40–60	Pesigan et al. (1958)
1975	44	5?	0.70	34	Santos (1984)
1987	60			7	Zhou et al. (2010)
1994	70			5.4	DoH, unpublished
1997	75			4.7	DoH, unpublished
2005	88	6.7		1–2	Leonardo et al. (2008)
2008	93		0.56		WHO (2009)

[a] http://www.data360.org/dsg.aspx?Data_Set_Group_Id=216.
[b] highest value recorded
[c] 'guestestimate' based on McMullen et al. (1954) and Pesigan et al. (1958) and extent of the endemic areas known today

absolutely reliable, in the past due to resorting to case-finding rather than modern statistical approaches, and later due to probable underestimation of prevalence by the Kato-Katz technique. Nevertheless, the overall declining trend is evident even if its dynamics cannot be fixed exactly. Although elimination of the disease, as planned by the DoH, could theoretically be achieved in the next decades, the coherent implementation of an integrated, multisectoral approach with more sensitive diagnostics, well-designed treatment schedules and effective surveillance of the infection reservoirs represents a formidable challenge, where snail control in particular could form a major obstacle to success.

Following a national prevalence survey, carried out between 2005 and 2008, the DoH recommended chemotherapy in areas with prevalence of 2% or above. Instead of active case-finding, random sampling was implemented in this study to differentiate provinces with high and moderate prevalence from those with low prevalence and non-endemic locations. The first two phases of the survey, based on stratified, systematic cluster sampling and examining two Kato-Katz thick smears from each study participant, were completed in Mindanao in 2005 and in the Visayas in 2007. Although prevalence was found to have generally declined, 'hot spots' were discovered in areas characterised by poor environmental situations without proper sewage systems and where flooding is common. The survey confirmed that more than 60% of Mindanao and 45% of the Visayas are endemic, and that an estimated 80–90% of all schistosomiasis in the Philippines is concentrated to these two regions (Leonardo et al., 2008). Overall, the prevalence rate among males was higher than that of females, indicating the occupational hazard of farming and fishing, a fact borne out by the age distribution of the disease. Prevalence remained consistently high among the adults compared with the younger age groups (Leonardo et al., 2008).

Access to control has always been a problem in this region, especially in far-flung villages suffering from political unrest. In addition, the floods caused by recent typhoons are expected to have aggravated the exposure of residents in the whole area. Two new endemic provinces have been discovered in Mindanao in the last seven years.

5.4.2.2. Research projects

The Philippines has been able to attract substantial financial support for particular research projects (R. Olveda, personal communication) but has been less successful in finding funds for a large, backbone control project such as the WBLP in P.R. China.

5.4.2.2.1. Control-related research The multi-country collaboration on schistosomiasis control (Table 5.6), later expanded to cover also malaria, LF and leprosy in the form of a Tropical Medicine Research Center (TRMC) grant, comes close to what went on in P.R. China under the WBLP. It initiated collaboration between the Research Institute for Tropical Medicine (RITM) and the College of Public Health of the University of the Philippines (UP-CPH) and the Institute of Parasitic Diseases (IPD) in P.R. China, Brown University in the United States and the Walter and Eliza Hall Institute (WEHI) of Medical Research in Australia. In addition, scientists from the University of Queensland in Australia and the University of Cambridge in the United Kingdom participated in some of these studies. Together, these projects were funded for 10 years and provided insights useful for ongoing control activities. However, it differed from the WBLP in not being a control undertaking *per se* but rather represent a 'research-cum-action' project with a control component, more akin to that promoted by the JRMC, the research arm of the WBLP. In addition, the amount of funding was far lower.

Although this overview cannot provide an exhaustive examination of all schistosomiasis research in the Philippines, it aspires to give a flavour of what has been done there over the last few decades. The impetus for the

TABLE 5.6 Foreign research grants made available for schistosomiasis-related projects in the Philippines

Donor	Main objective	Time	Funds (US$)	Collaborators
World Bank	Schistosomiasis control			DoH
EMCF, USA	Community-based chemotherapy	1983–1985	90,000	RITM, the Philippines; Brown University, USA
TDR and Rockefeller Foundation's North-South Partnership	Collaborative project for control of schistosomiasis	1985–1990	180,000	RITM, the Philippines; UP-CPH, the Philippines; IPD, P.R. China; Brown University; WEHI, Australia
TRMC grant from National Institutes of Health (NIH), USA	Multidisciplinary control of malaria, leprosy, LF and schistosomiasis	1991–1995	250,000	RITM, the Philippines; UP-CPH, the Philippines; Brown University, USA
National Institutes of Health (NIH), USA	Ecology and the transmission of schistosomiasis	2000–2005	600,000	RITM, the Philippines; Brown University, USA
National Institutes of Health (NIH), USA	Puberty and resistance to schistosomiasis	2000–2005	600,000	RITM, the Philippines; Brown University, USA
National Institutes of Health (NIH), USA	Treatment of pregnant mothers with praziquantel	2006–2011	900,000	RITM, the Philippines; Brown University, USA

two projects discussed above came from a previous 3-year project on community-based control of schistosomiasis, funded by the EMCF, spearheading the then novel idea of chemotherapy-based morbidity control as the main approach. Much research was carried out within the framework of this control-oriented project, for example studies on the dynamics of transmission of infection including the association of *S. japonicum* infection in humans with that in animals and the relationship of prevalence of infection with morbidity (Olveda et al., 1983), as well as the long-term impact of chemotherapy with praziquantel on prevalence, transmission, intensity of disease and morbidity (Olveda et al., 1996).

5.4.2.2.2. Academic research The projects in the lower part of Table 5.6 are geared more at academic research than control-associated questions. However, important questions were approached and the results reported are of general interest for the schistosomiasis agenda. For example, studies conducted to measure the impact of *S. japonicum* infection on childhood growth and development in Filipino children showed that different intensities of infection with *S. japonicum* were associated with various degrees of growth reduction, which was most pronounced during adolescence (McGarvey et al., 1992). These effects were neither dependent on the presence of other intestinal parasites nor due to social and economic status. The authors also showed that the effects were greater in villages not yet receiving annual screening and treatment and that catch-up growth was modest compared to the magnitude of the defect. These results are of general interest to schistosomiasis research and have opened insights into the interplay between resistance to infection, reinfection and malnutrition induced by *S. japonicum* infection, showing that pro-inflammatory mediators have associations with schistosomiasis as well as with malnutrition (Coutinho et al., 2006). Another finding with potentially far-reaching consequences is that the hormone dehydroepiandrosterone sulphate (DHEA-S) seems to induce non-specific resistance against infection (Kurtis et al., 2006), suggesting that an intrinsic property of host puberty development mediates the resistance to infection observed in older individuals.

5.4.2.2.3. Vaccine research The DHEA-S finding mentioned above might be of interest for vaccine development, a research area intensely pursued through individual and national grants in the Philippines. Both UP-CPH and RITM established research groups for this purpose. The former institution not only pursued various proteases from egg and adult stages of the parasite as possible candidate vaccine molecules, but also specifically researched Sj26, a gluthione-*S*-transferase (GST) (Smith et al., 1986), a molecule which still remains on the vaccine agenda. In addition, though largely forgotten now, the demonstration of anti-embryonation immunity could still be revived as a vaccine against hepatosplenic disease (Mitchell et al., 1994). RITM focused on the identification of *S. japonicum* antigens recognised by specific antibody isotypes implicated in human immunity. Combining the tools of molecular biology and epidemiology, a cDNA library of adult worm antigens was screened for potential vaccine candidates using sera from infected humans. This strategy resulted in the identification of nine IgE clones and eight IgA clones reactive with soluble worm antigens (Santiago et al., 1998). Among the different candidate vaccine antigens analysed, paramyosin was shown to be significantly linked to resistance (Ramirez et al., 1996), while Sj22.6 was found to be associated with a specific IgE response (Santiago et al., 1998). In a TDR-supported study, RITM also analysed individual immune responses against a panel of *S. japonicum* recombinant antigens. Responses recorded from people who were identified as naturally resistant to *S. japonicum* infection were investigated to see if their immune reactions belonged to patterns of responses associated with protection against *S. japonicum* infection (Acosta et al., 2002a,b). This was found to be the case but there were also patterns associated with increased risk for infection, an approach described in more detail by Bergquist et al. (2002).

RITM has played an important role *vis-à-vis* industrial vaccine production by acquiring a modular, turnkey production facility for the production of a BCG vaccine for the domestic market. They are also interested in producing plasma-derived products and could add a research module for the scaling-up of experimental vaccines. TDR is a strong proponent of this idea and has successfully negotiated public–private and other types of partnerships for drug development both in industrialized and developing countries (Ridley, 2003) and might be open for a similar development in the vaccine field.

5.5. THE ROLE OF RESEARCH FOR CONTROL

International research collaboration catalyzes innovative approaches and contributes to the proliferation of know-how and novel methodology which is well illustrated by the aftermath of the WBLP activities in P.R. China. The legacy of WBLP is manifold but the ushering in of operational research under the guidance of its research arm JRMC might have been its most important accomplishment. This idea has been taken up and further developed by the Regional Network for Asian Schistosomiasis and other Helminth Zoonoses ($RNAS^+$) (http://www.rnas.org.cn), established through a small TDR grant in 2000. With an administrative base in P.R. China and the Philippines, $RNAS^+$ continues what was pioneered by the WBLP, that is providing a regional platform for research collaboration and strengthening communication among scientists and control authorities concerned with parasitic helminth diseases in Southeast Asia (Zhou et al., 2002, 2008a,b).

5.5.1. General observations

In P.R. China, the shift in focus from individual research projects to a structured research agenda was initiated by the JRMC. This body not only had full overview of the contemporary control activities but could also provide the funds needed for research on problems identified. The introduction of operational research marked a momentous change for control activities leading to the addition of a broad research agenda that involved collaborative, international studies with research groups in Australia, France, Switzerland and the United States to mention the most active ones. It also led to international training at the M.Sc. and Ph.D. levels for Chinese students abroad and, indeed, to such innovative arrangements as opening the possibility for postdoctoral studies in P.R. China for foreign scientists.

A large loan/grant comparable to the WBLP was not available in the Philippines and operations/interventions there were therefore not accompanied by management supervision, making a fair comparison of progress in the two countries difficult. The Philippines has several well-organized institutions such as UP-CPH and RITM, but control activities and the research agenda are fragmented. As a consequence, the many stakeholders involved lack the tools to effectively address perceived shortcomings in control approaches. In addition, the collaboration between the DoH and other Government departments as well as provincial Governments needs to find common ground when policies are developed. A Filipino WBLP should be contemplated as it would facilitate the development of a national umbrella organization that could prioritize and guide relevant operational research to supplement ongoing control activities.

A control programme needs to operationally respond to ecological and epidemiological challenges in a timely and cost-effective manner. Future progress in controlling schistosomiasis depends crucially on a surveillance system capable of accurately gauging and reporting ongoing activities in real time, with state-of-the-art GIS/RS technologies targeting interventions in a spatially explicit and cost-effective manner. It is thus important to move away from static, unguided data collection and engage a minimalist, more active search approach exclusively focusing on essential information. Given the vastly improved situation in many endemic areas, this would not only be feasible but also cost-effective. In particular, this approach entails designing the response to surveillance results, requiring rapid transfer of the information collected into risk-maps to be made accessible for public health action without delay. This is, in fact, already possible in P.R. China, as data are now continuously reported to the Chinese Ministry of Health over the Internet.

Research on the social sciences is important in reducing prevalence. Its broad agenda covers human behaviour from water-contact to compliance and political unrest. The latter is a particular problem for the Philippines, which is currently confronted with political upheaval in the South which destabilizes control activities in precisely those areas which harbour the great majority of all schistosomiasis in the country and where the need for control is the greatest. Finally, it must be emphasised that social science research that is not part of, or does not inspire or shape, modern surveillance approaches can be of great academic merit but is of little relevance for control and disease elimination in practice.

Intersectoral collaboration and community participation facilitated the creation of a working control strategy in P.R. China. The current examination shows that the various methods applied for the containment of schistosomiasis, primarily based on chemotherapy in concert with snail control, have been effective. The implementation of approaches flexible enough to change with the times and the adaptation of interventions suiting the local socio-economic and epidemiological settings facilitated the sustained, smooth reduction of prevalence in P.R. China. However, major ecological transformations such as the development of the country's water resources, intensification of agriculture and generation of electricity constitute examples of necessary activities that could impact schistosomiasis control negatively. Therefore, these activities must be addressed in order to develop and implement sound mitigation strategies in a timely and effective manner. Climate change, that seems now to have become an undeniable phenomenon, can only be addressed by global coordinated efforts, but its effects must also be included in any serious discussion of local, epidemiological developments (Zhou et al., 2008a).

5.5.2. Specifics

The establishment and operation of a surveillance system is a crucial feature of any developed, successful control programme. Research is needed to characterize and decide which specific measures are necessary to eliminate remaining or developing pockets of transmission or to establish contingency stations making 'ad hoc' treatment available when needed, for example for flood control workers. The growing mobile population living on their fleets of fishing boats is a particular challenge which has not found a solution. In addition, the resettlement of people from the now flooded upstream area of Three Gorges Dam to new homes in endemic areas has exposed well over a million people to the risk of *S. japonicum* infection. These examples all demand sound surveillance systems capable of consolidation and documentation of achievements, ready to address the situation at hand without undue loss of time. Both P.R. China and the Philippines would need to replace the often non-reactive monitoring and evaluation with a stronger focus on innovative surveillance.

Endemic countries need to take an active part in producing the products they need in order to contend with prevailing diseases. Both the Philippines and P.R. China have a clear interest in vaccine development and authorities should already now start thinking about industrial vaccine production. The capability to produce GMP-grade vaccines has already been demonstrated in the Philippines, and P.R. China is rapidly acquiring a strong industrial basis that would facilitate large-scale vaccine production. A transmission-blocking veterinary product will soon be ready for integrated control and a human schistosomiasis vaccine—even one with only partial efficacy—could play a decisive role in the final stages of elimination of this disease. With regard to drugs, praziquantel remains the drug of choice (Doenhoff et al., 2008; Fenwick et al., 2003; Xiao et al., 2010), but a combination with one of the artemisinins provides a distinct advantage as the former drug targets adult worms and the latter the immature larval forms. Although a praziquantel–artemisinin combination would increase the costs for chemotherapy, it could be useful for disease elimination in 'hot-spots', as prophylaxis for relief workers, and when the number of infected people is very low (Utzinger et al., 2003).

The move towards a market-oriented economy and the interrelated increase of private health care providers in P.R. China has stimulated readjustments of strategies and fostered the economic evaluation of strategies implemented to facilitate allocation of scarce resources in a cost-effective manner (Zhou et al., 2005b). It has also been demonstrated that selective chemotherapy significantly reduces the prevalence and infection intensity at a lower cost than large-scale administration (Tang et al., 2001). For example, the treatment costs can be halved by the 'passive chemotherapy' approach together with health education as shown by Guo et al. (2005a). Finally, it has been understood that innovations are needed to deal with the contamination of schistosome eggs in the environment (Huang and Zhang, 2007). The new 'countryside initiative for economic progress' that was launched in consequence is an interesting example of large, socio-economic projects which go hand in hand with measures improving the control of schistosomiasis (Wang et al., 2009a). The key of the new approach is a set of measures such as health education, access to tap water, adequate sanitation and, above all, the mechanization of agriculture. This initiative should not only contribute to the modernization of agricultural practices but in particular limit transmission through the replacement of water buffaloes by tractors. Importantly, such an integrated and intersectoral control approach has an impact beyond schistosomiasis, as witnessed by significant drops in the prevalence of common soil-transmitted helminth infections (Wang et al., 2009b).

Diminishing prevalence and intensity of *S. japonicum* infection in controlled areas has highlighted the shortcomings of current diagnostic approaches. There is an increasing need for new tests which are sufficiently sensitive to gauge and ascertain the achievements of control programmes with high accuracy (Bergquist et al., 2009; Johansen et al., 2010). However, the generally lower infection levels and insensitivity of currently applied diagnostic techniques conspire to produce increasingly inaccurate estimates of disease. In this situation, serology is an alternative as it can be adopted for inexpensive, large-scale screening with the particular aim to capture recent exposures and 'hot spots'. The integration of serology into national control programmes is a natural development but to work well good collaboration between research laboratories, health service laboratories and epidemiologists is required. A major advantage is that the use of standardized assays would permit comparisons between different socio-geographical areas providing a sound basis for decisions regarding national policies and strategies.

During the last 30 years, P.R. China's economy has been developing as fast as that of Japan in the 1950s. Ironically, this has harmed the control programme as it finds itself in conflict with ongoing water resources developments, a situation that might become aggravated due to climate change. Population movements from non-endemic to endemic areas have already caused new infections (Xu et al., 2000) and, in a warmer climate, the Three Gorges Dam and the South-to-North water transfer (SNWT) project will undoubtedly create new *O. hupensis* habitats (Yang et al., 2005, 2006; Zhou et al., 2008a,b). Another looming problem is the concept of post-transmission schistosomiasis (Giboda and Bergquist, 2000), which will require medical care and attention long after transmission has been interrupted.

5.6. CONCLUDING REMARKS

Awareness of the magnitude of the schistosomiasis problem was the signal, both in P.R. China and the Philippines, for the political leadership to initiate and strongly guide control activities. The concept of control based on different interventions operating in an integrated manner is a flexible approach that evolves with time. International collaboration supports this process by facilitating and encouraging the training of the next generations of researchers, control cadres and public health specialists.

Sustained control requires an innovative surveillance system that makes use of modern technologies capturing the current, rapid dynamics of population movements, including environmental as well as social changes. Surveillance systems designed to capture the foci of transmission and to launch swift responses are part of the new, integrated intervention packages which are replacing classical monitoring and evaluation approaches in the endemic areas.

The outlook for schistosomiasis control is bright and current activities demonstrate that it is possible, not only to control the disease but also to move towards its elimination. As there is no clear boundary indicating when to change from control to elimination, the situation is best judged in relation to the prevailing socio-ecological and the geographical situations. However, evaluations should go beyond schistosomiasis-specific outcome measures to include appraisal of general well-being and equity. Since assessment and control is accomplished by the same or similar epidemiological approaches and surveillance systems, the progress achieved opens the door to the future amalgamation of the separate strategies developed for diverse NTDs such as food-borne trematodiases, soil-transmitted helminthiases and other zoonoses. The analysis of schistosomiasis epidemiology and control in the two countries discussed here can thus provide practical insight into the challenges of modern public health, leading to highly cost-effective tactics and favourable cost-benefit ratios for all concerned.

ACKNOWLEDGEMENTS

The authors thank Dr. Lydia Leonardo, Professor Donald P. McManus, Professor Remigio Olveda, Dr. Edmund Seto, Professor Robert Spear and Professor Xiao-Nong Zhou for providing some of the data this article is based on.

REFERENCES

Acosta, L.P., Aligui, G.D., Tiu, W.U., McManus, D.P., Olveda, R.M., 2002a. Immune correlate study on human *Schistosoma japonicum* in a well-defined population in Leyte, Philippines: I. Assessment of 'resistance' versus susceptibility to *Schistosoma japonicum* recombinant and native antigens. Acta Trop. 84, 127–136.

Acosta, L.P., Waine, G., Aligui, G.D., Tiu, W.U., Olveda, R.M., McManus, D.P., 2002b. Immune correlate study on human *Schistosoma japonicum* in a well-defined population in Leyte Philippines: II. Cellular immune responses to S. japonicum recombinant and native antigens. Acta Trop. 84, 137–149.

Andrews, P., Dycka, J., Frank, G., 1980. Effect of praziquantel on clinical-chemical parameters in healthy and schistosome-infected mice. Ann. Trop. Med. Parasitol. 74, 167–177.

Andrews, P., Thomas, H., Pohlke, R., Seubert, J., 1983. Praziquantel. Med. Res. Rev. 3, 147–200.

Balen, J., Zhao, Z.Y., Williams, G.M., McManus, D.P., Raso, G., Utzinger, J., et al., 2007. Prevalence, intensity and associated morbidity of *Schistosoma japonicum* infection in the Dongting Lake region, China. Bull. World Health Organ. 85, 519–526.

Bergquist, R., Al-Sherbiny, M., Barakat, R., Olds, R., 2002. Blueprint for schistosomiasis vaccine development. Acta Trop. 82, 183–192.

Bergquist, R., Johansen, M.V., Utzinger, J., 2009. Diagnostic dilemmas in helminthology: what tools to use and when? Trends Parasitol. 25, 151–156.

Boelee, E., Laamrani, H., 2004. Environmental control of schistosomiasis through community participation in a Moroccan oasis. Trop. Med. Int. Health 9, 997–1004.
Bustinduy, A.L., King, C.H., 2009. Parasitic helminths. In: Fratamico, Smith, Brogden (Eds.), Post-infectious sequelae and long-term consequences of infectious diseases. American Society for Microbiology Press, Washington, pp. 291–329.
Chen, M.G., 1989. Schistosomiasis control program in the People's Republic of China: a review. Southeast Asian J. Trop. Med. Public Health 20, 511–517.
Chen, M.G., 2005. Use of praziquantel for clinical treatment and morbidity control of schistosomiasis japonica in China: a review of 30 years' experience. Acta Trop. 96, 168–176.
Chen, M.G., Feng, Z., 1999. Schistosomiasis control in China. Parasitol. Int. 48, 11–19.
Chen, X.Y., Wu, X.H., Wang, L.Y., Dang, H., Wang, Q., Zheng, J., et al., 2003. Schistosomiasis situation in the People's Republic of China in 2002. Chin. J. Schisto. Control 15, 241–243.
Chen, X.Y., Wang, L.Y., Cai, J.M., Zhou, X.N., Zheng, J., Guo, J.G., et al., 2005. Schistosomiasis control in China: the impact of a 10-year World Bank loan project (1992–2001). Bull. World Health Organ. 83, 43–48.
Coutinho, H.M., Leenstra, T., Acosta, L.P., Su, L., Jarilla, B., Jiz, M.A., et al., 2006. Pro-inflammatory cytokines and C-reactive protein are associated with undernutrition in the context of *Schistosoma japonicum* infection. Am. J. Trop. Med. Hyg. 75, 720–726.
Da'dara, A.A., Li, Y.S., Xiong, T., Zhou, J., Williams, G.M., McManus, D.P., Feng, Z., Yu, X.L., Gray, D.J., Harn, D.A., 2008. DNA-based vaccines protect against zoonotic schistosomiasis in water buffalo. Vaccine 26, 3617–3625.
Dai, Y., Zhu, Y., Harn, D.A., Wang, X., Tang, J., Zhao, S., Lu, F., Guan, X., 2009. DNA vaccination by electroporation and boosting with recombinant proteins enhances the efficacy of DNA vaccines for Schistosomiasis japonica. Clin. Vaccine Immunol. 16, 1796–1803.
Davis, A., Wegner, D.H., 1979. Multicentre trials of praziquantel in human schistosomiasis: design and techniques. Bull. World Health Organ. 57, 767–771.
de Clercq, D., Vercruysse, J., Verlé, P., Niasse, F., Kongs, A., Diop, M., 2000. Efficacy of artesunate against *Schistosoma mansoni* infections in Richard Toll, Senegal. Trans. R. Soc. Trop. Med. Hyg. 94, 90–91.
de Clercq, D., Vercruysse, J., Kongs, A., Verlé, P., Dompnier, J.P., Faye, P.C., 2002. Efficacy of artesunate and praziquantel in *Schistosoma haematobium* infected schoolchildren. Acta Trop. 82, 61–66.
DeMarco, R., Verjovski-Almeida, S., 2009. Schistosomes–proteomics studies for potential novel vaccines and drug targets. Drug Discov. Today 14, 472–478.
Doenhoff, M.J., Cioli, D., Utzinger, J., 2008. Praziquantel: mechanisms of action, resistance and new derivatives for schistosomiasis. Curr. Opin. Infect. Dis. 21, 659–667.
El Khoby, T., Galal, N., Fenwick, A., 1998. The USAID/Government of Egypt's Schistosomiasis Research Project (SRP). Parasitol. Today 14, 92–96.
Ellis, M.K., McManus, D.P., 2009. Familial aggregation of human helminth infection in the Poyang lake area of China with a focus on genetic susceptibility to schistosomiasis japonica and associated markers of disease. Parasitology. 136, 699–712.
Fenwick, A., 2006. New initiatives against Africa's worms. Trans. R. Soc. Trop. Med. Hyg. 100, 200–207.
Fenwick, A., Savioli, L., Engels, D., Bergquist, N.R., Todd, M.H., 2003. Drugs for the control of parasitic diseases: current status and development in schistosomiasis. Trends Parasitol. 19, 509–515.
Fenwick, A., Webster, J.P., Bosque-Oliva, E., Blair, L., Fleming, F.M., Zhang, Y., et al., 2009. The Schistosomiasis Control Initiative (SCI): rationale, development and implementation from 2002–2008. Parasitology 136, 1719–1730.

Gao, Z.Q., Jiang, X.J., Cai, Z.R., Wang, L.X., Zheng, Z.G., Huang, D.S., 1998. Surveillance report on schistosomiasis ten years after reaching the criteria for elimination in Shanghai Municipality. Chin. J. Schisto. Control 10, 159–161.

Garcia, E.G., 1976. Clinical studies on schistosomiasis japonica in the Philippines: a review. Southeast Asian J. Trop. Med. Public Health 7, 247–256.

Giboda, M., Bergquist, N.R., 2000. Post-transmission schistosomiasis: a new agenda. Acta Trop. 77, 3–7.

Gönnert, R., Andrews, P., 1977. Praziquantel, a new board-spectrum antischistosomal agent. Z. Parasitenkd. 52, 129–150.

Guo, J.G., Cao, C.L., Hu, G.H., Lin, H., Li, D., Zhu, R., et al., 2005a. The role of 'passive chemotherapy' plus health education for schistosomiasis control in China during maintenance and consolidation phase. Acta Trop. 96, 177–183.

Guo, J.G., Vounatsou, P., Cao, C.L., Utzinger, J., Zhu, H.Q., Anderegg, D., et al., 2005b. A geographic information and remote sensing based model for prediction of *Oncomelania hupensis* habitats in the Poyang Lake area, China. Acta Trop. 96, 213–222.

Hotez, P.J., Molyneux, D.H., Fenwick, A., Kumaresan, J., Ehrlich Sachs, S., Sachs, J.D., et al., 2007. Control of neglected tropical diseases. N. Engl. J. Med. 357, 1018–1027.

Hu, G.H., Hu, J., Song, K.Y., Lin, D.D., Zhang, J., Cao, C.L., et al., 2005. The role of health education and health promotion in the control of schistosomiasis: experiences from a 12-year intervention study in Poyang Lake area. Acta Trop. 96, 232–241.

Huang, Y.X., Manderson, L., 2005. The social and economic determinants of schistosomiasis japonica. Acta Trop. 96, 223–231.

Huang, S.Q., Zhang, M.L., 2007. The medical and health service system in building socialist new countryside. Chin. Health Serv. Manage. 230, 535–536.

Jiang, Q.W., Zhang, S.J., Yuan, H.C., Liu, Z., Zhao, G.M., Brinkmann, U., 1996. The effect of a combined approach to schistosomiasis control on the transmission of *Schistosoma japonicum* in Xingzi of Poyang Lake area, China. Southeast Asian J. Trop. Med. Public Health 27, 535–541.

Jiraungkoorskul, W., Sahaphong, S., Sobhon, P., Riengrojpitak, S., Kangwanrangsan, N., 2005. Effects of praziquantel and artesunate on the tegument of adult *Schistosoma mekongi* harboured in mice. Parasitol. Int. 54, 177–183.

Johansen, M.V., Sithithaworn, P., Bergquist, R., Utzinger, J., 2010. Towards improved diagnosis of zoonotic trematodes in Asia. Adv. Parasitol. 73, 171–195.

Katz, N., 1998. Control in Brazil. Mem. Inst. Oswaldo Cruz 93 (Suppl. 1), 33–35.

Katz, N., Chaves, A., Pellegrino, J., 1972. A simple device for quantitative stool thick smear technique in schistosomiasis mansoni. Rev. Inst. Med.Trop. São Paulo 14, 397–400.

King, C.H., 2010. Parasites and poverty: the case of schistosomiasis. Acta Trop. 113, 95–104.

King, C.H., Dickman, K., Tisch, D.J., 2005. Reassessment of the cost of chronic helmintic infection: a meta-analysis of disability-related outcomes in endemic schistosomiasis. Lancet 365, 1561–1569.

Kurtis, J.D., Friedman, J.F., Leenstra, T., Langdon, G.C., Wu, H.W., Manalo, D.L., et al., 2006. Pubertal development predicts resistance to infection and reinfection with *Schistosoma japonicum*. Clin. Infect. Dis. 42, 1692–1698.

Lammie, P.J., Fenwick, A., Utzinger, J., 2006. A blueprint for success: integration of neglected tropical disease control programmes. Trends Parasitol. 22, 313–321.

Lengeler, C., Utzinger, J., Tanner, M., 2002a. Questionnaires for rapid screening of schistosomiasis in sub-Saharan Africa and their contribution to control. Bull. World Health Organ. 80, 235–242.

Lengeler, C., Utzinger, J., Tanner, M., 2002b. Screening for schistosomiasis in sub-Saharan Africa. Trends Parasitol. 18, 375–377.

Leonardo, L.R., Rivera, P., Saniel, O., Villacorte, E., Crisostomo, B., Hernandez, L., et al., 2008. Prevalence survey of schistosomiasis in Mindanao and the Visayas, the Philippines. Parasitol. Int. 57, 246–251.

Li, Y.S., Zhao, Z.Y., Ellis, M., McManus, D.P., 2005. Applications and outcomes of periodic epidemiological surveys for schistosomiasis and related economic evaluation in the People's Republic of China. Acta Trop. 96, 266–275.

Li, S.Z., Luz, A., Wang, X.H., Xu, L.L., Wang, Q., Qian, Y.J., et al., 2009. Schistosomiasis in China: acute infections during 2005–2008. Chin. Med. J. (Engl). 122, 1009–1014.

Liese, B., 1986. The organization of schistosomiasis control programmes. Parasitol. Today. 2, 339–345.

Lin, D.D., Liu, J.X., Liu, Y.M., Hu, F., Zhang, Y.Y., Xu, J.M., et al., 2008. Routine Kato-Katz technique underestimates the prevalence of *Schistosoma japonicum*: a case study in an endemic area of the People's Republic of China. Parasitol. Int. 57, 281–286.

Liu, X.Y., Li, D.J., Lin, P.C., Lin, J.X., 1991. Analysis on schistosomiasis surveillance for four years in Fujian province. Chin. J. Schisto. Control 3, 229–230.

Maegraith, B., 1958. Schistosomiasis in China. Lancet 271, 208–214.

Malone, J.B., 2005. Biology-based mapping of vector-borne parasites by geographic information systems and remote sensing. Parassitologia 47, 27–50.

Mao, S.P., Shao, B.R., 1982. Schistosomiasis control in the People's Republic of China. Am. J. Trop. Med. Hyg. 31, 92–99.

McGarvey, S.T., Aligui, G., Daniel, B.L., Peters, P., Olveda, R., Olds, G.R., 1992. Child growth and schistosomiasis japonica in northeastern Leyte, the Philippines: cross-sectional results. Am. J. Trop. Med. Hyg. 46, 571–581.

McManus, D.P., Dalton, J.P., 2006. Vaccines against the zoonotic trematodes *Schistosoma japonicum, Fasciola hepatica* and *Fasciola gigantica*. Parasitology 133, (Suppl.), S43-61.

McManus, D.P., Loukas, A., 2008. The current status of vaccines for schistosomiasis. Clin. Microbiol. Rev. 21, 225–242.

McMullen, D.B., Hubendick, B., Pesigan, T.P., Bierstein, P., 1954. Observations made by the World Health Organization schistosomiasis team in the Philippines. J. Philipp. Med. Assoc. 30, 615–627.

Ministry of Health, 1998. Epidemic Status of Schistosomiasis in China: A Nation Wide Sampling Survey in 1995. Nanjing University Press, Nanjing, China.

Mitchell, G.F., Garcia, E.G., Rivera, P.T., Tiu, W.U., Davern, K.M., 1994. Evidence for and implications of anti-embryonation immunity in schistosomiasis. Exp. Parasitol. 79, 546–549.

Mott, K.E., Dixon, H., 1982. Collaborative study on antigens for immunodiagnosis of schistosomiasis. Bull. World Health Organ. 60, 729–753.

Mott, K.E., Dixon, H., Carter, C.E., Garcia, E., Ishii, A., Matsuda, H., et al., 1987. Collaborative study on antigens for immunodiagnosis of *Schistosoma japonicum* infection. Bull. World Health Organ. 65, 233–244.

Murray, C.J.L., Lopez, A.D., 1996. The Global Burden of Disease: A comprehensive assessment of mortality and disability from diseases, injuries, and risk factors in 1990 and projected to 2020. Harvard School of Public Health/World Bank, Cambridge, MA, USA.

Muth, S., Sayasone, S., Odermatt-Biays, S., Phompida, S., Duong, S., Odermatt, P., et al., 2010. Schistosoma mekongi in Cambodia and Lao People's Democratic Republic. Adv. Parasitol. 72, 179–203.

N'Goran, E.K., Utzinger, J., Gnaka, H.N., Yapi, A., N'Guessan, N.A., Kigbafori, S.D., et al., 2003. Randomized, double-blind, placebo-controlled trial of oral artemether for the prevention of patent *Schistosoma haematobium* infections. Am. J. Trop. Med. Hyg. 68, 24–32.

Olveda, R.M., Tiu, E., Fevidal, P., Jr., De Veyra, F., Jr., Icatlo, F., Jr., Domingo, E.O., 1983. The relationship of prevalence and intensity of infection with morbidity in schistosomiasis japonica: a study of three communities in Leyte, Philippines. Am. J. Trop. Med. Hyg. 32, 1312–1321.

Olveda, R.M., Daniel, B.L., Ramirez, B.D., Aligui, G.L., Acosta, L.P., Fevidal, P., et al., 1996. Schistosomiasis japonica in the Philippines: the long-term impact of population-based chemotherapy on infection, transmission and morbidity. J. Infect. Dis. 174, 163–172.

Pesigan, T.P., Farooq, M., Hairston, N.G., Jauregui, J.J., Garcia, E.G., Santos, A.T., et al., 1958. Studies on Schistosoma japonicum infection in the Philippines. 1. General considerations and epidemiology. Bull. World Health Organ. 18, 345–455.

Ramirez, B.L., Kurtis, J.D., Wiest, P.M., Arias, P., Aligui, F., Acosta, L., et al., 1996. Paramyosin: a candidate vaccine antigen against *Schistosoma japonicum*. Parasite Immunol. 18, 49–52.

Reimert, C.M., Tukahebwa, E.M., Kabatereine, N.B., Dunne, D.W., Vennervald, B.J., 2008. Assessment of *Schistosoma mansoni* induced intestinal inflammation by means of eosinophil cationic protein eosinophil protein X and myeloperoxidase before and after treatment with praziquantel. Acta Trop. 105, 253–259.

Ridley, R.G., 2003. Product R&D for neglected diseases. Twenty-seven years of WHO/TDR experiences with public-private partnerships. EMBO Rep. 4, S43–S46.

Santiago, M.L.O., Hafalla, J.C.R., Kurtis, J.D., Aligui, G.L., Wiest, P.M., Olveda, R.M., et al., 1998. Identification of *Schistosoma japonicum* 22.6-kDa: a major target of human IgE response: similarity of IgE binding epitopes to allergen peptides. Int. Arch. Allergy Immunol. 117, 94–104.

Santos, A.T., 1967. The schistosomiasis control program in the Philippines. World Med. J. 14, 23–24.

Santos, A.T., 1984. The present status of schistosomiasis in the Philippines. Southeast Asian J. Trop. Med. Public Health 15, 439–445.

Schistosoma japonicum Genome Sequencing and Functional Analysis Consortium, Zhou, Y., Zheng, F., Liu, F., Hu, W., Wang, Z.Q., Gang, L., Ren, S., 2009. The *Schistosoma japonicum* genome reveals features of host–parasite interplay. Nature 460, 345–351.

Seto, E.Y.W., Knapp, F., Zhong, B., Yang, C., 2007. The use of a vest equipped with a global positioning system to assess water-contact patterns associated with schistosomiasis. Geospat. Health 2, 233–241.

Shi, M.Z., Yu, D.B., Wei, W.Y., Zhang, C.S., He, H.B., Yang, G.F., et al., 2004. Experimental study on susceptibility of praziquantel against *Schistosoma japonicum* in repeated chemotherapy areas in Dongting Lake region. Chin. J. Schisto. Control 16, 171–173.

Smith, D.B., Davern, K.M., Board, P.G., Tiu, W.U., Garcia, E.G., Mitchell, G.F., 1986. Mr 26,000 antigen of *Schistosoma japonicum* recognized by resistant WEHI 129/J mice is a parasite glutathione S-transferase. Proc. Natl Acad. Sci. USA 83, 8703–8707.

Song, H.T., Liang, Y.S., Dai, J.R., Li, L.G., Shen, X.H., Tian, Q.A., et al., 2004. Studies on sensitivity of *Schistosoma japonicum* to praziquantel - situation in low endemic areas. Chin. J. Schisto. Control 16, 58–59.

Spear, R.C., Seto, E., Liang, S., Birkner, M., Hubbard, A., Qiu, D., et al., 2004. Factors influencing the transmission of *Schistosoma japonicum* in the mountains of Sichuan province of China. Am. J. Trop. Med. Hyg. 70, 48–56.

Steinmann, P., Keiser, J., Bos, R., Tanner, M., Utzinger, J., 2006. Schistosomiasis and water resources development: systematic review, meta-analysis, and estimates of people at risk. Lancet Infect. Dis. 6, 411–425.

Steinmann, P., Zhou, X.N., Li, Y.L., Li, H.J., Chen, S.R., Yang, Z., et al., 2007a. Helminth infections and risk factor analysis among residents in Eryuan county, Yunnan province, China. Acta Trop. 104, 38–51.

Steinmann, P., Zhou, X.N., Matthys, B., Li, Y.L., Li, H.J., Chen, S.R., et al., 2007b. Spatial risk profiling of *Schistosoma japonicum* in Eryuan county, Yunnan province, China. Geospat. Health 2, 59–73.

Stothard, J.R., Gabrielli, A.F., 2007. Schistosomiasis in African infants and preschool children: to treat or not to treat? Trends Parasitol. 23, 83–86.

Tan, H.Z., Yang, M.X., Wu, Z.G., Zhou, J., Liu, A.Z., Li, S.Q., et al., 2004. Rapid screening method for *Schistosoma japonicum* infection using questionnaires in flood area of the People's Republic of China. Acta Trop. 90, 1–9.

Tang, D.L., Yu, D.B., Li, Y.Y., Xie, M.S., Wen, H.M., Cai, W.B., et al., 2001. Analysis of cost-effectiveness on two chemotherapy schemes to schistosomiasis in hyperendemic villages of Hunan province. Prac. Prev. Med. 8, 165–168.

Tao, H.Q., Li, S.W., 1999. Consolidation and surveillance situation and suggestion for schistosomiasis control in Zhejiang province. Chin. J. Schisto. Control 11, 226–227.

Tubangui, M.A., 1932. The molluscan intermediate host in the Philippines of the oriental blood fluke *Schistosoma japonicum* Kutsurada. Philipp. J. Sci. 49, 295–304.

Utzinger, J., N'Goran, E.K., N'Dri, A., Lengeler, C., Xiao, S.H., Tanner, M., 2000. Oral artemether for prevention of *Schistosoma mansoni* infection: randomised controlled trial. Lancet 355, 1320–1325.

Utzinger, J., Booth, M., N'Goran, E.K., Müller, I., Tanner, M., Lengeler, C., 2001a. Relative contribution of day-to-day and intra-specimen variation in faecal egg counts of *Schistosoma mansoni* before and after treatment with praziquantel. Parasitology 122, 537–544.

Utzinger, J., Xiao, S.H., N'Goran, E.K., Bergquist, R., Tanner, M., 2001b. The potential of artemether for the control of schistosomiasis. Int. J. Parasitol. 31, 1549–1562.

Utzinger, J., Keiser, J., Xiao, S.H., Tanner, M., Singer, B.H., 2003. Combination chemotherapy of schistosomiasis in laboratory studies and clinical trials. Antimicrob. Agents Chemother. 47, 1487–1495.

Utzinger, J., Zhou, X.N., Chen, M.G., Bergquist, R., 2005. Conquering schistosomiasis in China: the long march. Acta Trop. 96, 69–96.

Utzinger, J., Xiao, S.H., Tanner, M., Keiser, J., 2007. Artemisinins for schistosomiasis and beyond. Curr. Opin. Investig. Drugs 8, 105–116.

Utzinger, J., Raso, G., Brooker, S., de Savigny, D., Tanner, M., Ørnbjerg, N., et al., 2009. Schistosomiasis and neglected tropical diseases: towards integrated and sustainable control and a word of caution. Parasitology 136, 1859–1874.

Verjovski-Almeida, S., Leite, L.C.C., Dias-Neto, E., Menck, C.F.M., Wilson, R.A., 2004. Schistosome transcriptome: insights and perspectives for functional genomics. Trends Parasitol. 20, 304–308.

Wang, X.Z., Li, S.T., Zhou, Z.X., 1999. A rapid one-step method of EIA for detection of circulating antigen of *Schistosoma japonicum*. Chin. Med. J. 112, 124–128.

Wang, L.D., Chen, H.G., Guo, J.G., Zeng, X.J., Hong, X.L., Xiong, J.J., et al., 2009a. A strategy to control transmission of *Schistosoma japonicum* in China. N. Engl. J. Med. 360, 121–128.

Wang, L.D., Guo, J.G., Wu, X.H., Chen, H.G., Wang, T.P., Zhu, S.P., et al., 2009b. China's new strategy to block *Schistosoma japonicum* transmission: experiences and impact beyond schistosomiasis. Trop. Med. Int. Health 14, 1475–1483.

Wen, L.Y., Chen, J.H., Ding, J.Z., Zhang, J.F., Lu, S.H., Yu, L.L., et al., 2005. Evaluation on the applied value of the dot immunogold filtration assay (DIGFA) for rapid detection of anti-*Schistosoma japonicum* antibody. Acta Trop. 96, 142–147.

WHO, 1985. The control of schistosomiasis. Report of a WHO expert committee. WHO Tech. Rep. Ser. 728, 1–113.

WHO, 1993. The control of schistosomiasis. Second report of the WHO expert committee. WHO Tech. Rep. Ser. 830, 1–86.

WHO, 2002. Prevention and control of schistosomiasis and soil-transmitted helminthiasis: report of a WHO expert committee. WHO Tech. Rep. Ser. 912, 1–57.

WHO, 2004. The World Health Report 2004 – Changing History. World Health Organization, Geneva.

WHO, 2009. Preventive chemotherapy (PCT) databank.http://www.who.int/neglected_diseases/preventive_chemotherapy/databank/en/index.html (Accessed: 15 December 2009).

Williams, G.M., Sleigh, A.C., Li, Y.S., Feng, Z., Davis, G.M., Chen, H., et al., 2002. Mathematical modelling of schistosomiasis japonica: comparison of control strategies in the People's Republic of China. Acta Trop. 82, 253–262.

Wu, X.H., Chen, M.G., Zheng, J., 2005. Surveillance of schistosomiasis in five provinces of China which have reached the national criteria for elimination of the disease. Acta Trop. 96, 276–281.

Wu, X.H., Wang, X.H., Utzinger, J., Yang, K., Kristensen, T.K., Bergquist, R., et al., 2007. Spatio-temporal correlation between human and bovine schistosomiasis in China: insight from three national sampling surveys. Geospat. Health 2, 75–84.

Xiao, S.H., 2005. Development of antischistosomal drugs in China, with particular consideration to praziquantel and the artemisinins. Acta Trop. 96, 153–167.

Xiao, S.H., Yue, W.J., Yang, Y.Q., You, J.Q., 1987. Susceptibility of *Schistosoma japonicum* to different developmental stages to praziquantel. Chin. Med. J. 100, 759–768.

Xiao, S.H., Booth, M., Tanner, M., 2000. The prophylactic effects of artemether against *Schistosoma japonicum* infections. Parasitol. Today 16, 122–126.

Xiao, S.H., Tanner, M., N'Goran, E.K., Utzinger, J., Chollet, J., Bergquist, R., et al., 2002. Recent investigations of artemether, a novel agent for the prevention of schistosomiasis japonica, mansoni and haematobia. Acta Trop. 82, 175–181.

Xiao, X., Wang, T.P., Tian, Z.G., 2003. Development of a rapid, sensitive, dye immunoassay for schistosomiasis diagnosis: a colloidal dye immunofiltration assay. J. Immunol. Methods 280, 49–57.

Xiao, X., Wang, T.P., Ye, H.Z., Qiang, G.X., Wei, H.M., Tian, Z.G., 2005. Field evaluation of a rapid, visually-read colloidal dye immunofiltration assay for *Schistosoma japonicum* for screening in areas of low transmission. Bull. World Health Organ. 83, 526–533.

Xiao, S.H., Keiser, J., Chollet, J., Utzinger, J., Dong, Y., Endriss, Y., et al., 2007. *In vitro* and *in vivo* activities of synthetic trioxolanes against major human schistosome species. Antimicrob. Agents Chemother. 51, 1440–1445.

Xiao, S.H., Keiser, J., Chen, M.G., Tanner, M., Utzinger, J., 2010. Research and development of antischistosomal drugs in the People's Republic of China: a 60-year review. Adv. Parasitol. 73, 231–295.

Xu, X.J., Wei, F.H., Yang, X.X., Dai, Y.H., Yu, G.Y., Chen, L.Y., et al., 2000. Possible effects of the Three Gorges dam on the transmission of *Schistosoma japonicum* on the Jiang Han plain China. Ann. Trop. Med. Parasitol. 94, 333–341.

Yang, G.J., Vounatsou, P., Zhou, X.N., Utzinger, J., Tanner, M., 2005. A review of geographic information system and remote sensing with applications to the epidemiology and control of schistosomiasis in China. Acta Trop. 96, 117–129.

Yang, G.J., Vounatsou, P., Tanner, M., Zhou, X.N., Utzinger, J., 2006. Remote sensing for predicting potential habitats of *Oncomelania hupensis* in Hongze, Baima and Gaoyou lakes in Jiangsu province, China. Geospat. Health 1, 85–92.

Yuan, H., Jiagang, G., Bergquist, R., Tanner, M., Xianyi, C., Huanzeng, W., 2000a. The 1992–1999 World Bank Schistosomiasis Research Initiative in China: outcome and perspectives. Parasitol. Int. 49, 195–207.

Yuan, L.P., Manderson, L., Tempongko, M.S.B., Wei, W.Y., Aiguo, P., 2000b. The impact of educational videotapes on water contact behaviour of primary school students in the Dongting Lakes region, China. Trop. Med. Int. Health 5, 538–544.

Zhang, Z.Y., Xue, D.Z., Zhou, X.N., Zhou, Y., Liu, S.J., 2005. Remote sensing and spatial statistical analysis to predict the distribution of Oncomelania hupensis in the marshlands of China. Acta Trop. 96, 205–212.

Zhao, W.X., Wu, G.L., Guan, X.H., 1993. Immunodiagnosis of *Schistosoma japonicum* infection in China. Chin. Med. J. 106, 623–627.

Zhao, G.M., Zhao, Q., Jiang, Q.W., Chen, X.Y., Wang, L.Y., Yuan, H.C., 2005. Surveillance for schistosomiasis japonica in China from 2000 to 2003. Acta Trop. 96, 288–295.

Zhen, J., 1993. A brief introduction to a nation-wide sampling survey on schistosomiasis. Chin. Med. J. 106, 569–575.

Zhou, H., Ross, A.G.P., Hartel, G.F., Sleigh, A.C., Williams, G.M., McManus, D.P., et al., 1998. Diagnosis of schistosomiasis japonica in Chinese schoolchildren by administration of a questionnaire. Trans. R. Soc. Trop. Med. Hyg. 92, 245–250.

Zhou, X.N., Malone, J.B., Kristensen, T.K., Bergquist, N.R., 2001. Application of geographic information systems and remote sensing to schistosomiasis control in China. Acta Trop. 79, 97–106.

Zhou, X.N., Acosta, L., Willingham, A.L., 3rd, Leonardo, L.R., Chen, M.G., Aligui, G., et al., 2002. Regional Network for Research, Surveillance and Control of Asian Schistosomiasis (RNAS). Acta Trop. 82, 305–311.

Zhou, X.N., Wang, L.Y., Chen, M.G., Wang, T.P., Guo, J.G., Wu, X.H., et al., 2005a. An economic evaluation of the national schistosomiasis control programme in China from 1992 to 2000. Acta Trop. 96, 255–265.

Zhou, X.N., Wang, L.Y., Chen, M.G., Wu, X.H., Jiang, Q.W., Chen, X.Y., et al., 2005b. The public health significance and control of schistosomiasis in China – then and now. Acta Trop. 96, 97–105.

Zhou, X.N., Guo, J.G., Wu, X.H., Jiang, Q.W., Zheng, J., Dang, H., et al., 2007. Epidemiology of schistosomiasis in the People's Republic of China, 2004. Emerg. Infect. Dis. 13, 1470–1476.

Zhou, X.N., Ohta, N., Utzinger, J., Bergquist, R., Olveda, R.M., 2008a. $RNAS^+$: a win-win collaboration to combat neglected tropical diseases in Southeast Asia. Parasitol. Int. 57, 243–245.

Zhou, X.N., Yang, G.J., Yang, K., Wang, X.H., Hong, Q.B., Sun, L.P., et al., 2008b. Potential impact of climate change on schistosomiasis transmission in China. Am. J. Trop. Med. Hyg. 78, 188–194.

Zhou, X.N., Bergquist, R., Leonardo, L., Yang, G.J., Yang, K., Sudomo, M., et al., 2010. Schistosomiasis japonica: research and control. Adv. Parasitol. 72, 145–178.

Zhu, Y.C., 2005. Immunodiagnosis and its role in schistosomiasis control in China: a review. Acta Trop. 96, 130–136.

Zhu, Y.C., He, W., Liang, Y.S., Xu, M., Yu, C.X., Hua, W.Q., et al., 2002. Development of a rapid, simple dipstick dye immunoassay for schistosomiasis diagnosis. J. Immunol. Methods 266, 1–5.

Zhu, Y., Ren, J., Da'dara, A., Harn, D., Xu, M., Si, J., et al., 2004. The protective effect of a *Schistosoma japonicum* Chinese strain 23 kDa plasmid DNA vaccine in pigs is enhanced with IL-12. Vaccine 23, 78–83.

Zhu, Y., Si, J., Harn, D.A., Xu, M., Ren, J., Yu, C., et al., 2006. *Schistosoma japonicum* triose-phosphate isomerase plasmid DNA vaccine protects pigs against challenge infection. Parasitology 132, 67–71.

CHAPTER 6

Schistosomiasis Japonica: Control and Research Needs

Xiao-Nong Zhou,*[*] Robert Bergquist,[†] Lydia Leonardo,[‡] Guo-Jing Yang,[§] Kun Yang,[§] Mohammad Sudomo,[¶] and Remigio Olveda[#]

Contents

Abstract

Schistosomiasis japonica, a chronic and debilitating disease caused by the blood fluke *Schistosoma japonicum*, is still of considerable economic and public health concern in the People's Republic of

[*] National Institute of Parasitic Diseases, Chinese Center for Disease Control and Prevention, Shanghai, People's Republic of China
[†] Ingerod, Brastad, Sweden
[‡] Department of Parasitology, College of Public Health, University of the Philippines, Manila, Philippines
[§] Jiangsu Institute of Parasitic Diseases, Wuxi, People's Republic of China
[¶] Ecology and Health Status Research and Development Centre, National Institute of Health Research and Development, Ministry of Health, Jakarta, Indonesia
[#] Department of Health, Research Institute for Tropical Medicine (RITM), Muntinlupa, Manila, Philippines

Advances in Parasitology, Volume 72
ISSN 0065-308X, DOI: 10.1016/S0065-308X(10)72006-6

China, the Philippines, and Indonesia. Despite major progress made over the past several decades with the control of schistosomiasis japonica in the aforementioned countries, the disease is emerging in some areas. We review the epidemiological status and transmission patterns of schistosomiasis japonica, placing it into a historical context, and discuss experiences and lessons with national control efforts. Our analyses reveal that an integrated control approach, implemented through intersectoral collaboration, is essential to bring down the prevalence and intensity of *Schistosoma japonicum* infections and disease-related morbidity, and to sustain these parameters at low levels. The need for innovation and a sufficiently flexible control approach to adapt interventions in response to the changing nature and challenges of schistosomiasis control from the initial phase of morbidity control to the final state of elimination is emphasised. The aim of the presentation and the analyses is to inspire researchers and disease control managers elsewhere in Asia, Africa, and the Americas to harness the experiences gained and the lessons presented here to improve the control and eventual elimination of schistosomiasis and parasitic diseases.

6.1. INTRODUCTION

Approximately, 12% of all people on Earth are at risk for schistosomiasis, a disease widely spread access the tropical belt where a third of the global population lives. More than 200 million people are infected by schistosomiasis and close to 800 million are daily at risk (Steinmann et al., 2006). There is a great variation in prevalence estimates, which results from the focal character of this disease (Brooker et al., 2009; Engels et al., 2002; Utzinger et al., 2009). The distribution is not easy to pin down in detail and most overviews therefore express countries as either endemic or not. However, this is a spurious way of viewing the situation, as the endemic areas in most cases, including Africa, are limited to particular places suitable for transmission such as natural water bodies (ponds, lakes, and rivers) and man-made constructions such as multi-purpose small dams, large dams for hydropower production, feeding irrigation systems, and large-scale irrigation schemes (Steinmann et al., 2006). Thus, most countries are characterised by large stretches of safe land punctuated by numerous small areas of high transmission. Schistosomiasis can be controlled where the public health importance of the disease has been recognised, political will and commitment prevail, and financial and technical resources exist (Engels et al., 2002; Wang et al., 2008a). However, elimination has proved difficult in many places, particularly in sub-Saharan Africa (Stothard et al., 2009).

6.1.1. Life cycle of *Schistosoma japonicum*

Schistosomes are parasitic, trematode worms with a complicated life cycle (Gryseels et al., 2006; Ross et al., 2002). Mammals act as the definitive host in which large amounts of eggs, the cause of almost all symptoms, are produced by the adult female worm. Humans have been implicated in the transmission of five species of *Schistosoma*, but more than 90% of all infections are caused by just three: *S. mansoni* (mainly in Africa and South America) and *S. japonicum* (predominantly in the People's Republic of China (P.R. China), the Philippines, and Indonesia) produce intestinal disease, while *Schistosoma haematobium* (common in Africa and some countries in the Middle East) causes urinary schistosomiasis. The two less common species with human involvement are *S. intercalatum* in Western and Central Africa, and *S. mekongi* in Cambodia and Lao People's Democratic Republic (Lao PDR). *S. malyayensis*, a species only reported in Malaysia, is known to cause natural infections in humans, but sustained transmission through human populations has not been confirmed.

In most cases (in four of the five species involved in human transmission), the adult worms live in the capillary network around the intestines where they release hundreds or thousands of eggs daily, many of which end up in the liver, and remaining eggs move to the membrane layer of intestine, thereby causing intestinal schistosomiasis. *S. haematobium*, being the exception, causes the urinary form of the disease due to its location around the bladder, where the inflammatory reaction to the eggs not only affects the bladder but also the urethra, ureters, and kidneys. Up to 50% of all eggs become sequestered in the final host, but the life cycle requires that at least some eggs work themselves through the tissues to eventually become excreted with the faeces or, in the case of *S. haematobium* infection, the urine. Those eggs that are deposited in water hatch and release the miracidium, an intermediate form capable of infecting snail intermediate hosts in which several generations of asexual sporocyst stages develop. The life cycle is completed when cercariae from the snails return to the final host, penetrate the skin and rapidly develop into schistosomula upon skin penetration, which finally mature into millimeter-long adult worms as shown in Fig. 6.1.

6.1.2. Morbidity of schistosomiasis japonica

The human symptoms caused by schistosomiasis vary from hardly detectable to very serious. The majority of all infected people might not even know that they are infected, far from all develop clinical symptoms and only a minority become seriously affected. In principle, three clinical stages of schistosomiasis are recognised, the first or acute phase, the second or "silent" phase, and the third or chronic phase. These clinical

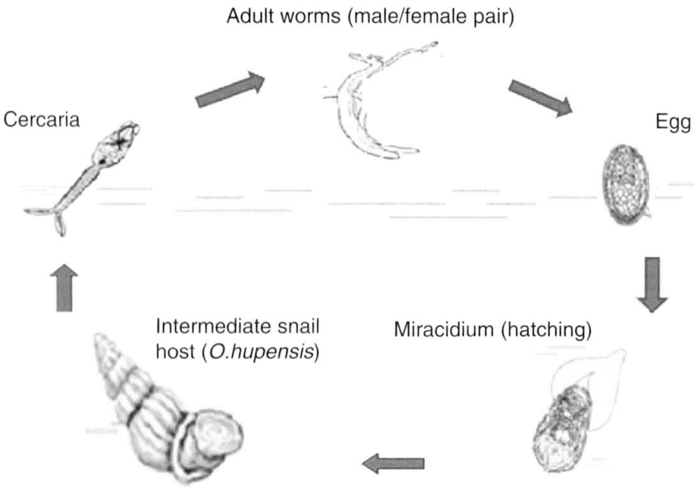

FIGURE 6.1 Simplified *Schistosoma japonicum* life cycle.

stages are similar in all forms of the disease with some exceptions, that is, the *S. haematobium* infection presents differently due it its focus in the bladder and the acute form seems to be more pronounced in schistosomiasis japonica compared to the other forms of intestinal schistosomiasis.

Mortality due to schistosomiasis is comparatively low, but the chronic character of the disease causes widespread human suffering. The social impact resulting from the fact that most people in the endemic areas are more or less continuously infected has yet to be fully appreciated. In our opinion, and that of others (King, 2010; King et al., 2005; Li et al., 2005), the full impact of schistosomiasis on a global level is not far less than that caused by malaria and tuberculosis. This may appear counterintuitive considering the success of praziquantel, the safe and effective treatment, which has contributed to the remarkable reduction of morbidity due to schistosomiasis worldwide (Chen, 2005; Doenhoff et al., 2008; Fenwick et al., 2003; Xiao et al., 2010).

In spite of the major public health impact of schistosomiasis in endemic countries, research on this parasite has not received the levels of funding required to make sustained progress. The current situation in Southeast Asia is summarised in Table 6.1. Even if vigilance is high in some countries, for example, P.R. China and in private initiatives such as the Schistosomiasis Control Initiative (SCI) in Africa (Fenwick et al., 2009), the overall problem caused by this disease remains large. However, since transmission is only marginally affected by treatment of the human host, rapid reinfection limits the success of drug-based control due to the need for indefinitely continued treatment (Utzinger et al., 2009). This disease

TABLE 6.1 Current status of schistosomiasis in Southeast Asia

Country	Prevalence (%)	No. of cases[a]	No. at risk[a]	Disease distribution	Risk and problems	Country goals
P.R. China	2.5	720	56,000	In seven provinces. New endemic foci found in the lake region	Three Gorges Dam, water-development projects, animal reservoirs, global warming	Infection rate <5% by 2008, <1% by 2015
Indonesia	0.17–1.7	0.269	30.5	Two foci (the Lindu and Napu valleys). New endemic area found in Bada valley	Mobile populations, domestic and wild animal reservoirs	Elimination by the year 2010
Philippines	3	100	1900	Three regions (Luzon, Visayas, Mindanao). New endemic foci found in the northern part and central parts of the country	Environmental changes, changes of land cover, animal reservoirs	Lowered to <1% by 2010
Total		820.3	57,930	Three countries in Asia	Natural, social, and economic factors	

[a] × 1000.

thus remains a hurdle for economic development, posing a threat that can be kept at bay only by regular re-treatment; therefore only a strong research initiative resulting in new approaches can make a decisive impact (Utzinger et al., 2005).

Regardless of the angle from which morbidity due to schistosomiasis is viewed, it is beyond doubt that the widespread use of praziquantel is the main reason for the global, dramatic drop of morbidity due to this disease. Prevalence, on the other hand, is more difficult to pin down. Stool examination, using the Kato-Katz thick smear technique (Katz et al., 1972), recommended by the World Health Organization (WHO) for the diagnosis of intestinal schistosomiasis, is useful when the intensity of disease is generally high. However, it is less well suited for application in controlled areas since many low-level infections are missed when the number of parasites in the host falls below the threshold needed to produce above 100 eggs per gram (EPG) of stool (Bergquist et al., 2009; de Vlas and Gryseels, 1992; de Vlas et al., 1997; Utzinger et al., 2001). *S. japonicum* may also be more difficult to diagnose due to the pronounced propensity of the eggs of this species to aggregate (Pesigan et al., 1958; Yu et al., 1998). Indeed, based on three Kato-Katz thick smears from two separate stool samples as the diagnostic "gold" standard, Lin et al. (2008a, b) found the rate of underestimation in a well-controlled area in P.R. China to be as high as 36% when compared to records based on two Kato-Katz thick smear readings.

6.2. SCHISTOSOMIASIS JAPONICA IN ASIA

6.2.1. Regional status of schistosomiasis japonica

6.2.1.1. Historical records

S. japonicum was first discovered in Japan (Katsurada, 1904) and its life cycle was established by Fujinami and Nakamura (1909). At the beginning of the 1900s, *S. japonicum* was also found in P.R. China (Logan, 1905) and in the Philippines (Wooley, 1906). The eggs of this parasite have been found in ancient corpses (Mao and Shao, 1982), which serves as a reminder that the parasite has been a human companion for millennia and probably much longer than that. In 1906, human infections were found in the Philippines and later (in 1937) also in Indonesia (Tanaka and Tsuji, 1997). Schistosomiasis was thus established in four countries of the region. Transmission of *S. japonicum* has been interrupted in Japan and, although animal reservoirs still remain, no more new human cases have been discovered there since 1978 (Tanaka and Tsuji, 1997; WHO, 2001). Therefore at present, *S. japonicum* only exists in three Asian countries, namely P.R. China, the Philippines, and Indonesia.

6.2.1.2. Current status

Although transmission intensity has been reduced significantly during the past 50 years, a total of 820,300 human cases are currently reported from P.R. China, Indonesia, and the Philippines (Coutinho et al., 2005; Garjito et al., 2008; Zhou et al., 2007). However, there are great differences in the distribution and impact of schistosomiasis as it affects large areas and large numbers of people in some areas, while it is limited to a few foci in other places. Table 6.1 gives an overview of the situation based on estimates from 2005.

6.2.2. Schistosomiasis in P.R. China

6.2.2.1. Historical background and geographical distribution

P.R. China has been spectacularly successful in managing to reduce the extent of the endemic areas. The hard work aimed at elimination of schistosomiasis in all feasible and eradicable areas bore fruit relatively early on, but the lower reaches of the Yangtze River valley and some high-altitude areas in the Sichuan and Yunnan provinces remain severely affected to this day. The endemic areas were traditionally stratified into three types, that is, (i) "plains and waterways", (ii) "marshlands and lakes", and (iii) "mountainous regions", an ecosystem stratification which is still in use. The main thrust was snail control through environmental engineering (Mao and Shao, 1982), but the strategy also offered free diagnosis and treatment, including health education to everyone living in an area at risk (Maegraith, 1958). Irrigation ditches were reconstructed by turning over the soil in a scheme to destroy the snail intermediate host using an environmental approach that also involved lowering of the water level of canals and the building of dykes along the lake shores (Mao and Shao, 1982). This course of action was effective and rapidly reduced the endemic areas by more than two-thirds, leading to disappearance of the disease; first in Shanghai and Guangdong (1985) and later in Fujian (1987), Guangxi (1989), and Zhejiang (1995) (Wu et al., 2005; Zhou et al., 2005). After these achievements, the pace slowed as the problems in the seven remaining endemic provinces were more difficult to deal with (Utzinger et al., 2005; Zhou et al., 2005). Nevertheless, national prevalence has continued its downward trend. The most severely affected areas were, and still are, the Yangtze River valley, the marshlands around the Dongting and Poyang lakes, and certain mountainous areas in the West (Fig. 6.2) (Hao et al., 2007).

6.2.2.2. Control programme

Compared with the 1989 baseline data, the final 2002 evaluation of the impact of the World Bank Loan Project (WBLP) revealed that most of the objectives had been met, that is, the total number of infected people had

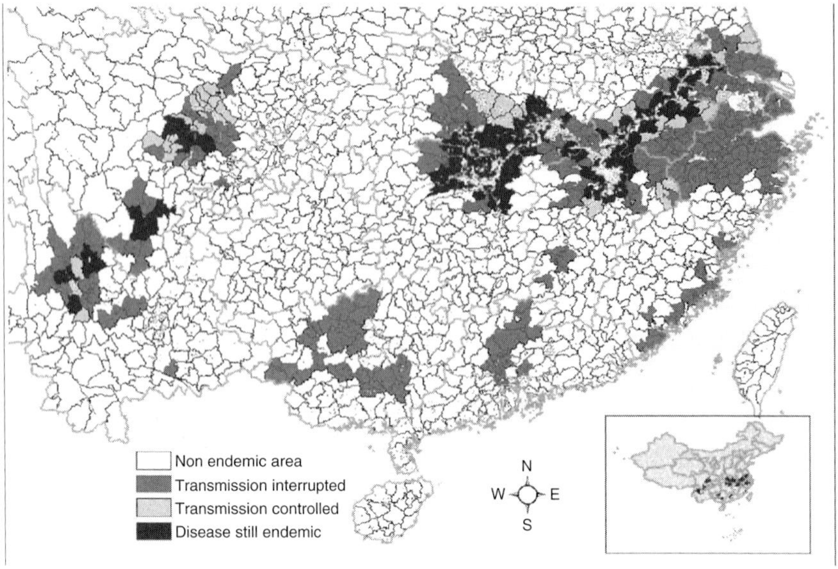

FIGURE 6.2 The epidemiological status of schistosomiasis in P.R. China in 2006.

dropped to somewhere between 700,000 and 800,000, the prevalence in the remaining endemic areas had been halved in both humans and bovines, and the snail-infested areas had been reduced by three-quarters (Chen et al., 2005). However, there were also problems, for example, the diminishing trend of snail infection had stalled with rates fluctuating at a low level rather than disappearing completely (Chen et al., 2005). Indeed, although the infection rate and density of infected snails had decreased by 69% and 45%, respectively, the areas affected had again increased by the end of the project (Zhang and Wong, 2003). The control of schistosomiasis japonica became a priority after a survey carried out in the 1950s. The national control programme was initiated soon after that and has now continued uninterrupted for more than 50 years (Utzinger et al., 2005; Zhou et al., 2005). By employing vast resources and diverse approaches, the national control programme led to the elimination of the disease from a large area involving 260 counties and transmission has been controlled in another 63 counties. Substantial progress has also been made in most of the remaining endemic areas and, as can be seen in Fig. 6.3 (Wu et al., 2006), the total number of infected people has been reduced by over 90% since 1950 (Wang et al., 2008a). A recent nationwide sampling survey provided a detailed picture of the contemporary epidemiological situation (Fig. 6.3). According to this survey, the number of infected people in 2005 was estimated at 725,000 (Zhou et al., 2007).

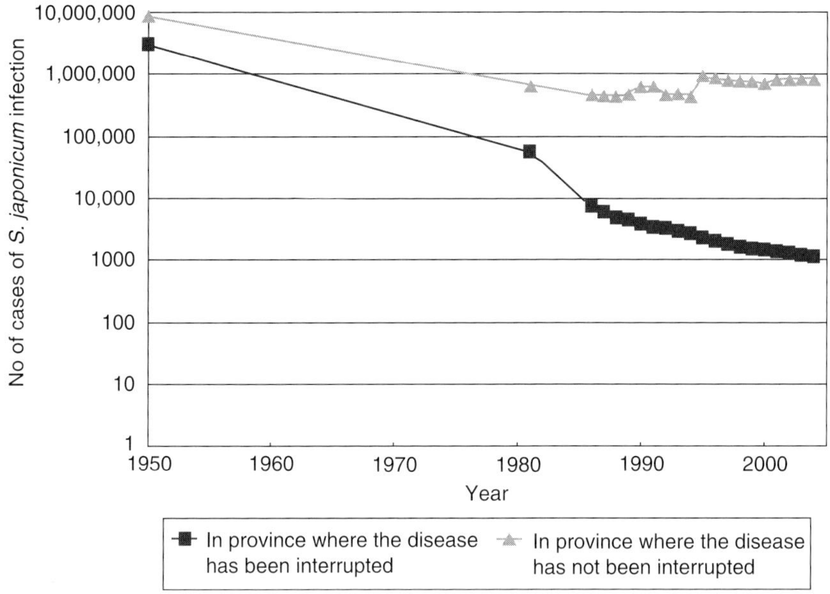

FIGURE 6.3 Reduction of schistosomiasis cases in P.R. China in the period 1950–2000.

6.2.2.3. Experience and lessons from the control programme

Although the fact that the overall epidemiological situation has much improved since the national control programme was initiated in the early 1950s, recent survey results confirm that progress is now less vigorous. In fact, there has been only little progress since the end of the 10-year WBLP that lasted from 1992 to 2001 (Chen et al., 2005; Utzinger et al., 2005). Schistosomiasis japonica even re-emerged in at least 38 counties where transmission control and interruption had been declared previously (Liang et al., 2006). There has also been a resurgence of schistosomiasis in terms of the total number of infected cases, also following the termination of the WBLP (Fig. 6.4) (Utzinger et al., 2005). In addition, foci of intensive transmission and high prevalence rates in humans and cattle are still found in the areas mentioned earlier. The ongoing transmission in other endemic areas, albeit at a lower level, is also of considerable concern, as the situation is likely to deteriorate as soon as control efforts are scaled down (Utzinger et al., 2005; Wang et al., 2008a). It is therefore crucial for continued success to maintain and sustain the current efforts to further reduce transmission.

As a consequence, the Government of P.R. China has renewed its commitment by assigning equal priority to schistosomiasis, tuberculosis, HIV/AIDS, and hepatitis B (Engels et al., 2005). New and ambitious targets for control have been set: infection control (prevalence $<5\%$) for

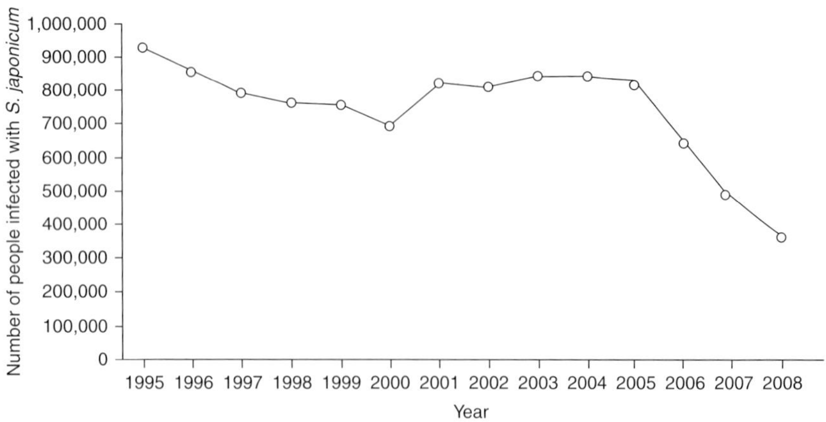

FIGURE 6.4 People infected with *S. japonicum* in P.R. China between 1995 and 2008.

the whole country by 2008 and transmission control (prevalence $<1\%$) by 2015 (Wang et al., 2008a, 2009a).

6.2.2.4. Contribution of research to the control programme

The main research achievements related to schistosomiasis in P.R. China during the last five decades have contributed to the improvement of the national control programme; these improvements are reflected in three main fields. Firstly, new tools of diagnostics and intervention have been developed, secondly, epidemiological knowledge has been gained from field settings and, thirdly, new control approaches have been developed and field-tested (Liu et al., 2008).

The discovery and development of antischistosomal drugs and diagnostic assays related to schistosomiasis has provided good tools for the detection and treatment of infected cases, and has reduced the disease burden through preventive chemotherapy. For example, the local production of praziquantel, in collaboration with several Chinese institutions since 1982, facilitated widespread use of the drug at low cost for individual treatment and large-scale community-based morbidity control. Numerous reports on the clinical use of praziquantel in P.R. China have been published since the late 1970s (Chen, 2005; Chen et al., 2007; Wu, 2002; Xiao, 2005a,b; Xiao et al., 2000; Yang et al., 2009b; Zhu, 2005).

More than 50 million treatment courses have been administered in P.R. China, and several studies on the optimisation of praziquantel at the individual patient level and within community-based control programmes have been described (Chen, 2005; Song et al., 1998; Wu, 2002; Xiao, 2005a,b; Xiao et al., 2000; Zhu, 2005). Large-scale use of praziquantel was particularly widespread during WBLP, with a significant reduction in morbidity due to *S. japonicum* by more than 30% (Chen et al., 2005).

In 1980, Chinese scientists discovered that artemisinin and its derivatives (e.g. artemether and artesunate) could kill the early developmental stages of *S. japonicum*, which makes it possible to prevent the development of egg-laying adult worms, and hence prevent morbidity associated with the immunological reactions to schistosome eggs trapped in the host tissue (Xiao, 2005a,b; Xiao et al., 2000, 2002, 2010).

Based on the finding that the artemisinins exhibited highest activity against juvenile *S. japonicum* worms, these drugs have been used as a "chemoprophylactic" agent against schistosomiasis. Nowadays, artemisinin is used to prevent patent infections in high-risk populations, for example, flood relief workers, who are exposed to schistosome-infested water for a short period of time (Song et al., 1998).

With regard to diagnostic assays, in P.R. China, more than 20 serologic assays have been developed during the last 30 years in different institutions (Wu, 2002). These immunodiagnostic kits, often in combination with stool examination among those individuals who showed a positive immunodiagnostic test result, have improved the screening of cases, especially in communities with low prevalence and low intensity infection, resulting in more cost-effective control programmes (Zhu, 2005).

Epidemiological studies on schistosomiasis have improved the understanding of schistosomiasis transmission in natural field settings, leading to the classification of endemic areas into specific ecosystem types (Wang et al., 2008a; Zhou et al., 2005). Classification based on ecological characteristics helped greatly in the development of both short-term and long-term goals and monitoring and evaluation (M&E) indicators in the national control programme. Model-based epidemiological findings have also improved control strategy adaptation at the base-level or community-level in different environmental settings (Chen et al., 2007; Yang et al., 2009b).

In terms of control approaches, numerous investigations focused on environmental management for enhancing the national schistosomiasis control programme. In particular, approaches that integrated with other sectors improved the efficiency of the control programme significantly (Wang et al., 2009a). In the last 30 years, control was integrated with (i) agricultural activities, for example, alteration of crops planted, reclamation of land and plantations to eliminate snail habitats (Gao, 2002); (ii) water resources development projects, for example, cement lining of irrigation canals, installation of sinks to obstruct snail dispersal, and construction of flood gates in the connection areas of main irrigation canals or rivers(Li et al., 2007; Wang et al., 2002); (iii) forestry projects, for example, planting trees in the marshlands to change the ecology of snail habitats and to discourage buffaloes from grazing on the marshland, and establishing new forests in the mountainous areas (Zhang et al., 2003; Zuo et al., 1999); and (iv) agricultural projects, for example, construction of fish ponds, rearrangement of irrigation systems and establishment of drainage systems (Zhang et al., 2003). These approaches have contributed to the gradual elimination of transmission of *S. japonicum* in vast endemic areas of P.R. China (Zhou et al., 2005).

6.2.3. Schistosomiasis in the Philippines

6.2.3.1. Historical background

As elsewhere, snail control dominated schistosomiasis-related activities in the Philippines before the 1980s (Pesigan and Hairston, 1961). Drainage, stream canalization and pond management were tried in combination with molluscicides, but the Chinese success could not be duplicated due to ecological differences (Blas, 1976). Health education and environmental hygiene were essential components of the control programme, but efforts to enforce sanitation were not successful as only a third of the population had satisfactory latrines. In the end, it was not possible to mount an initiative capable of reducing the national prevalence of *S. japonicum* infection until chemotherapy was introduced as the main control approach (Santos et al., 1979).

The first case, a Filipino male who had never been out of the country, was reported in 1906 (Crowell and Hammack, 1913). Subsequently, schistosome ova were found in several cases among 500 autopsies reported in 1908 and in the faeces of some prisoners admitted to the Bilibid Prison, City of Manila in 1914 (Ramos, 1928). Several years later, in 1928, a case of Katayama disease presenting as chronic appendicitis was reported (Tubangui, 1932). However, in spite of all these human cases, attempts to identify the intermediate host of the parasite were not successful until the discovery of the small, amphibious *Oncomelania hupensis quadrasi* freshwater snail in Palo, Leyte in 1932 (Garcia, 1976). The life cycle and the multi-host characteristics of the parasite were confirmed when the infection could be transferred to mice, rabbits, and monkeys by cercariae obtained from the *Oncomelania* snails. Since then, the distribution of *O. h. quadrasi* has been well characterised and shown to correspond to the major endemic areas for human schistosomiasis.

6.2.3.2. Epidemiology and distribution

Following the identification of the intermediate host snail, *Onchomelania quadrasi*, research on the basic biology of the parasite was overtaken by field surveys delineating the schistosomiasis-endemic areas and by studies on the clinical and pathological aspects of schistosomiasis japonica. Research activities were disrupted in the 1940s during World War II but revived when an outbreak of schistosomiasis occurred in the Americans and Allied Armed Forces landing on the island of Leyte in 1945 (Santos, 1984). In 1953, schistosomiasis was recognised as a public health problem in the Philippines and from the early 1960s to the latter part of the 1970s, extensive research activities were conducted, ranging from parasite biology and transmission and control to clinical and pathological aspects of the disease. By 1975, the endemic areas of *S. japonicum* infection in the Philippines had been delineated (Hernandez, 2003) and indicated that approximately 5 million people lived in schistosomiasis-endemic areas. It was estimated that over 700,000 individuals were infected. The major foci of schistosomiasis japonica were, and still are, the islands of Leyte, Samar, and Mindanao covering 24 provinces of eight regions of the country as shown in Fig. 6.5.

These regions are predominantly rice-growing areas as there are no distinct dry seasons, a fact which maximizes contact between humans and freshwater snails. In 2006, it was estimated that the population in the endemic areas had grown to 12 million. However, thanks to the implementation of extensive preventive chemotherapy programmes, the number of individuals with active infection had been reduced from the mid-1970s estimate to around 150,000 in the new millennium (Olveda, 2006). The current endemic areas in the Philippines cover 11 regions and 28

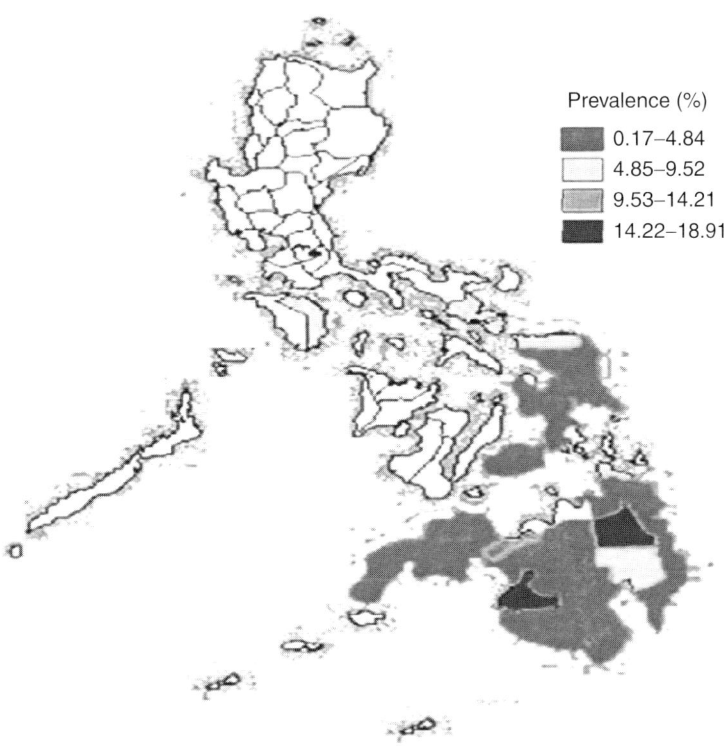

FIGURE 6.5 Provinces endemic for schistosomiasis in the Philippines in 1997.

provinces, affecting 189 municipalities, and 2222 barangays (villages). The total population at risk is 12 million people, 2.5 million of which are directly exposed to the disease. The 3391 positive snail colonies in the endemic barangays cover approximately 11,250 ha.

In the period 1981–1985, prevalence in the endemic areas first declined to an average 10%, in 1987, it reached 7%, and then stabilised at a level thereabouts until eventually dropping to near 4% in 1992 (Blas et al., 2004). In 1997, a report from the Department of Health (DoH) put the prevalence of schistosomiasis at 4.7% (DoH, unpublished). The same report classified three provinces as endemic with a prevalence rate of 18.9%, two provinces as moderately affected and 19 provinces with low endemicity, that is, less than 2% prevalence. This progress first gave the impression that the schistosomiasis problem was manageable and that it should be possible to eliminate the disease by community-based mass treatment. However, prevalence increased to 5.4% in 1994 as the looming termination of the PHDP led to less regular prevalence surveys, which had to be concentrated on highly endemic areas with sampling limited to 10–20% of the population (Bergquist and Tanner, 2010). Indeed, with 10 out of 16 regions in the country affected by schistosomiasis japonica in 2002 (Leonardo et al., 2002), the disease remained a public health problem.

6.2.3.3. Research activities

The early 1980s saw the beginning of a multi-disciplinary approach in the study of the disease. This was made possible with inputs from WHO, the UNICEF/UNDP/World Bank/WHO Special Programme for Research and Training in Tropical Diseases (TDR) and the Rockefeller Foundation, followed by a Tropical Medicine Research Center (TMRC) grant from U.S. National Institutes of Health (NIH) in the United States.

In addition to direct control approaches, the University of the Philippines, College of Public Health (UP-CPH) Schistosomiasis Research Group (UP-CPH SRG) focused on vaccine development as a long-term solution. That work led to the identification of several candidate vaccine molecules such as Sj 26, glutathione-*S*-transferase (GST), Sj 23, and several promising proteases from egg and adult stages of the parasite (Olveda, 2006). A strong supporting factor for pursuing vaccine development was that vaccines would also be effective against transmission by reducing the excretion of mature eggs in the faeces of infected humans and animals (Santiago et al., 1998).

Based on its immunological expertise, the Research Institute for Tropical Medicine (RITM) Schistosomiasis Study Group (RITM SSG), which also contributed greatly to the vaccine approach through the WHO/TDR vaccine initiative programme, also carried out a study of human immune responses as correlates of protection to specific *S. japonicum* recombinant antigens. Immune responses of individuals identified as resistant or susceptible to *S. japonicum* infection to the different antigens were analysed (Acosta et al., 2002). Studies were also conducted to measure the impact of *S. japonicum* infection on childhood growth and development of Filipino children (McGarvey et al., 1992).

6.2.3.4. Control efforts

Before the advent of effective chemotherapy, the Government focused on health education, limiting human exposure to the infective form of the parasite, and efforts to break the parasite life cycle through control of the intermediate host snail using agro-engineering methods and environmental modification. Then, as now, the constraint was mainly financial, that is, the prohibitive cost of agro-engineering methods and the protracted effect of environmental sanitation and health education. Hence, pilot projects were conducted with assistance from WHO and UNICEF and other foreign agencies. Control programmes evolved from these projects became integrated with existing health structures or functioned as independent bodies solely aimed at disease control. Foreign aid in the form of technical assistance, supplies and equipment, and funds sustained many of the components of the early control programme activities. There were significant achievements but none sufficiently effective to significantly reduce the national prevalence of *S. japonicum* infection. For example, environmental manipulations such as drainage, stream canalization, and pond management in combination with molluscicides were used but found to be too expensive. In addition, pilot studies have shown that this approach does not have a significant impact on transmission. Improved environmental hygiene was an essential component of the control programme but was difficult to sustain in a population no more than one-third of which had satisfactory latrines. The successful snail control approach used in P.R. China was not implemented due to differences in ecology and habitat of the snails found in the Philippines, while chemotherapy was not possible because the drugs available at the time showed unsatisfactory safety profiles and had significant side effects (Antimony potassium tartrate trihydrate).

A dramatic decrease in national prevalence of *S. japonicum* infection was noted after the introduction in 1978 of praziquantel in the Philippines. The most impressive effect was in the first half of the 1990s and was attributed to the implementation of the Philippine Health Development Plan. With support from the World Bank, the National Schistosomiasis Control Service of the DoH was able to intensify case finding and treatment in all endemic areas in the country and managed to reduce national prevalence from more than 10% before 1990 to less than 5% after 1995. The significant drop in the national prevalence of *S. japonicum*, which was sustained at less than 5% from 1996 to 2006, gave the impression that schistosomiasis was in retreat and that elimination could be achieved with the next few years. However, longitudinal studies, carried out by the RITM SSG showed that chemotherapy alone would only lower morbidity and prevalence but not eliminate schistosomiasis due to continuous transmission supported by animal reservoirs. In addition, interruption of treatment for more than 2 years was shown to produce rebound morbidity and increased intensity of *S. japonicum* infection (Leonardo et al., 2002; Olveda et al., 1983, 1996). These findings, and the decreasing compliance encountered by the control programme, strongly suggest that chemotherapy-based control programmes must be sustained with high compliance and in combination with other control measures until a more effective alternative approach has been developed (e.g. vaccination).

It is, in this connection, important to realize that the national prevalence data in the Philippines for the last 5 years may be significantly underestimated because only around 10–20% of all individuals in the endemic areas were examined. In addition, it is known that examination of a single stool sample from each individual using the Kato-Katz technique considerably underestimates the prevalence of infection (Lin et al., 2008a; Zhang et al., 2009; Zhou et al., 2008a,c).

The discovery of praziquantel brought about a shift of focus from the highly expensive snail control approach to a more manageable strategy involving case detection and treatment. This significant development renewed hopes of eventually gaining control of the disease with the limited resources available. From a four-pronged approach that included treatment of cases, environmental sanitation, snail control, and health education intended to control transmission or eliminate schistosomiasis, the government adopted the more feasible objective of morbidity control through praziquantel-based chemotherapy supplemented by environmental sanitation, health education, and mollusciciding.

Figure 6.6 shows the dramatic drop in disease prevalence in the 1980s. This trend continued up to the early 1990s. This period marks the intensification of the control programme, which was sustained for several years by influx of external funds, particularly by loans from the World Bank. In 1990, the Philippine Health Development Project (PHDP) provided the push to expand the target to 95% case detection and 100% treatment coverage. However, in 1994, prevalence increased to 5.4% from a low of 4.0%, coinciding with the end of PHDP support (Fig. 6.6). Thereafter, prevalence surveys became irregular and limited mostly to the highly endemic areas and in those provinces where research was being undertaken.

RITM contributed greatly in terms of policy formulation, which brought about a significant drop in prevalence and morbidity in many areas. In some municipalities, prevalence was sharply reduced in just 3 years, that is, from a high of 42–50% prevalence to a plateau level of 10%, a level that has been maintained for 6 years, but the fear of resurgence is still there. A 1997 report from the DoH puts the overall prevalence of

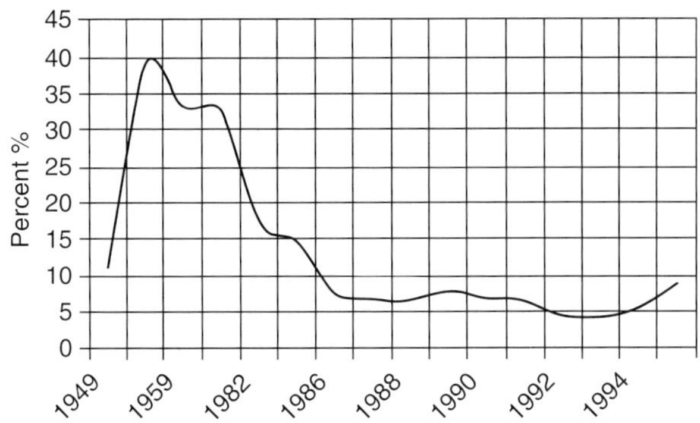

FIGURE 6.6 Mean schistosomiasis prevalence in the Philippines from 1953 to 1997.

schistosomiasis in the country at 4.7%. The same report classified three provinces as endemic with a prevalence rate of 18.9%, two provinces as moderately endemic and 19 provinces with low endemicity. One province is reported to have reached the point of elimination as the prevalence rate had reached a very low value (0.17%). In the National Objectives for Health, which is a statement of the national goals for health of the Philippine Government, schistosomiasis was targeted for elimination as a public health problem in endemic areas over the next 4 years (Fig. 6.7).

Although problems in the control of schistosomiasis have recently been aggravated by the diminishing attention given to it as a result of the growing problems posed by other diseases such as tuberculosis, malaria, and HIV/AIDS, the government hopes to achieve the goal of elimination of the disease by embarking on a multi-sectoral and more vigorous approach; this approach will continue to involve interventions in treatment, environmental sanitation, snail control, and other preventive actions (Leonardo et al., 2008).

A WHO-assisted project, initiated in order to determine the baseline prevalence of schistosomiasis in the country from 2005 to 2007, marked the first time that a stratified two-step systematic cluster design was used for sampling in a prevalence study. Of the three largest islands, Luzon, Visayas, and Mindanao, the latter showed the widest coverage of the disease at 60% compared with 45% in the Visayas and 37.5% in Luzon. Figure 6.8 shows the distribution and intensity of schistosomiasis in the three island groups. The highest prevalence is along the southeastern part of the Visayas and Mindanao. The lower coverage in Luzon and the Visayas could be due to the geographical separation of the regions into islands deterring easy transport of the disease into other regions. Considering the situation by region: Region 13 or Caraga in Mindanao, which includes the provinces of Surigao del Norte, Agusan del Norte, Surigao del Sur, and Agusan del Sur, ranked first in prevalence at 1.6%, followed

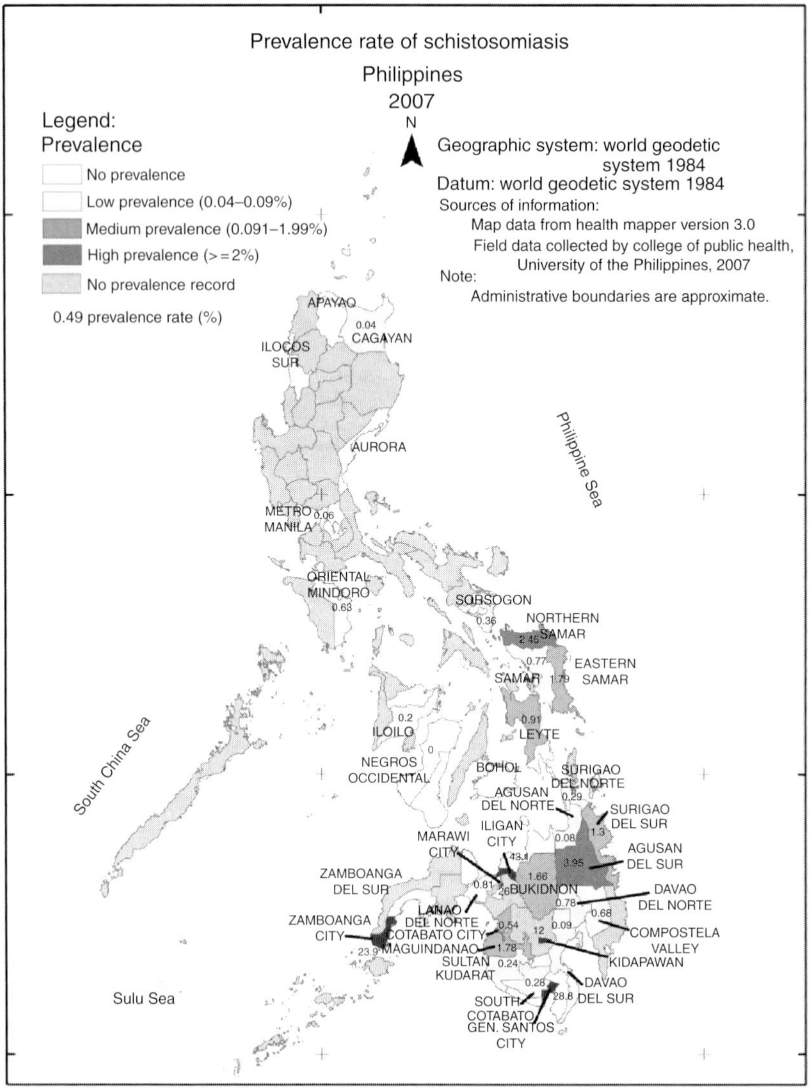

FIGURE 6.7 The distribution and intensity of *S. japonicum* infection in the Luzon, Visayas, and Mindanao regions.

by Region 8 in Visayas, which is composed of Northern Samar, Eastern Samar, Leyte, Southern Leyte, and Biliran at 1.5%. By province, Agusan del Sur, as in previous records, showed the highest prevalence at 4.0%, followed by Northern Samar at 2.5% and Eastern Samar at 1.8%. Overall, the prevalence rate among males was higher than that of females suggesting occupational hazards related to farming and fishing. The higher

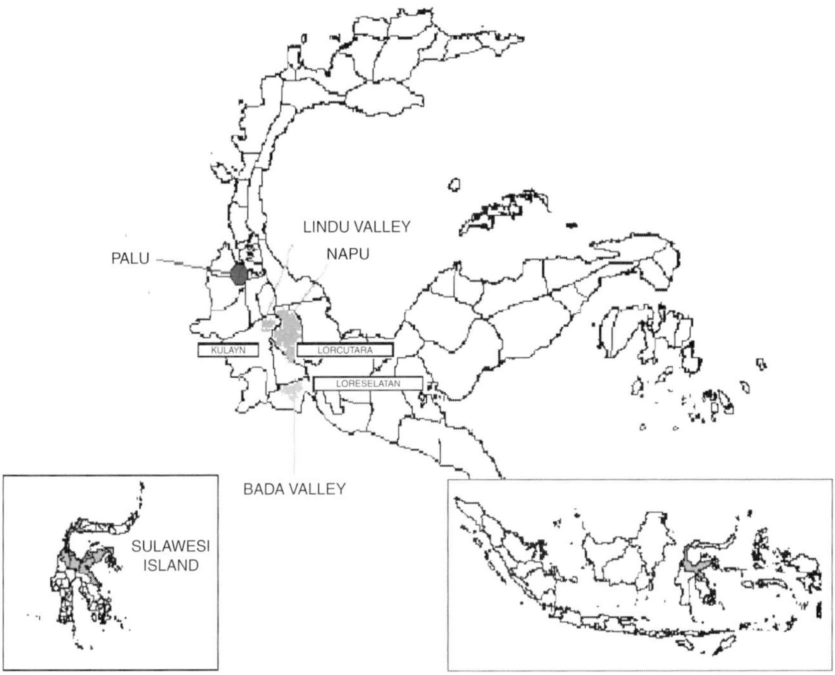

FIGURE 6.8 Schistosomiasis prevalence in humans between 1984 and 2006 in Napu and Lindu Valleys, Central Sulawesi Province, Indonesia.

occupational exposure is also borne out by the age distribution, which showed the prevalence to be consistently high among the adults compared with the younger age groups in all the regions.

New endemic foci have been discovered in the last 7 years. These new endemic areas are found in Gonzaga, a municipality in Cagayan Valley located in the northernmost part of Luzon and in the municipality of Calatrava in Negros Occidental in the Visayas region. WHO-funded research showed the presence of indigenous cases, infected snails and infected animals in several villages in the new endemic municipalities. It is proposed that *Oncomelania* snails must have been there even before the discovery of the disease and that population movement due to job opportunities must have brought cases into the new endemic sites.

The national survey showed that schistosomiasis occurs together with other helminthic infections, most importantly, soil-transmitted helminthiasis and also heterophyidiasis, taeniasis, and echinostomiasis, demonstrating that inadequate environmental sanitation facilitates transmission of schistosomiasis, soil-transmitted helminthiasis, and other coinfections. The wisdom of an integrated approach to helminth control that could effectively target as many helminths as possible is supported by the survey results and underscores recent recommendations for integrated control of helminths and other neglected diseases (Steinmann et al., 2010; Utzinger et al., 2009; Wang et al., 2009b).

6.2.4. Schistosomiasis in Indonesia

6.2.4.1. Historical background and geographical distribution

The unusually limited distribution of schistosomiasis to only two very isolated regions of central Sulawesi, that is, the marshes around Lake Lindu and an area in the Napu Valley, illustrates the strong focal character of human schistosomiasis (Fig. 6.8). As in P.R. China and the Philippines, the disease is caused by *S. japonicum*, with the first case in Indonesia discovered in 1937 by Müller and Tesch in a male patient who later died in a hospital (Garjito et al., 2008; Hadidjaja, 1985; Hadidjaja and Sudomo, 1976). Later, in the same year, Brug and Tesch traced the infection to the patient's home village, which was recognised as a schistosomiasis-endemic area (Garjito et al., 2008; Leonardo et al., 2008). A large-scale study of schistosomiasis in the area was initiated in 1940 when the prevalence of infection was reported to be 56% in this village (Leonardo et al., 2008). The reservoir of infection seemed to be important, comprising mammals other than humans, notably deer and dogs. However, the intermediate host snail was not identified until 1971 when an oncomelanid snail was found under the grass of abandoned rice fields in the Paku subvillage of Anca in Lindu valley. It was named *O. hupensis lindoensis* Davis & Carney 1973 (Hadidjaja and Sudomo, 1976).

Napu valley is located about 30 km southeast from Lindu and was recognised as an endemic area in 1972 and first reported by Carney et al. (1974). As a pilot to a comprehensive control programme, a study in the Napu area was conducted in 1974, which reported an extraordinarily high prevalence among the local population, which numbered about 4000 people, for example, as high as 72% in Winowanga village. Data for the same year also reported that *S. japonicum* was infecting 13 mammalian species, nine of them wild animals, in the region (Carney et al., 1974). Schistosomiasis surveillance and control are a public health priority of the province of central Sulawesi. The Directorate General of Communicable Diseases Control of Indonesia estimated that more than 10,000 people were at risk of infection in both areas. Further coordinated surveys focused on Lindu valley in 1975 and found schistosomiasis in seven villages in the upper valley of Lindu where the highest prevalences observed were 70.6%, 56.3%, and 56.0% in Anca, Langko, and Tomado, respectively. The intermediate host snails were also found to be focally distributed around Lindu Lake.

6.2.4.2. The control programme

Over the past six decades, schistosomiasis has been successfully controlled through five phases, and the average infection rate is currently much lower than prior to initiation of the control programme. The average prevalence was 0.49% in seven villages in Lindu valley during 2005 and 2006. In Napu valley, the average prevalence among 17 villages was 0.79% (2005) and 1.08% (2006). In the same period, the infection rate among snails ranged from 0% to 13.4% and 0–9.1% in Napu and Lindu valleys, respectively. The prevalence in the main reservoir host (*Rattus* spp.) ranged from 0% to 20%. The highest prevalences in both humans and reservoir hosts were found in Dodolo village.

Even though the endemic areas are very limited, schistosomiasis control in Indonesia has faced many difficulties. Diminishing funding after the termination of the Central Sulawesi Integrated Area Development Project (CSIADC-P), funded by the Asian Development Bank (ADB) in 2005, resulted in staff reductions in schistosomiasis control stations in both endemic regions, and in inconsistent surveillance and control. A relatively stable level of very low prevalence has been achieved, but additional efforts are needed to eliminate the disease. The full participation of the health sector and intersectoral collaboration has been identified as key factors in the struggle to eliminate schistosomiasis in Indonesia. Unfortunately, a lack of coordination and collaboration between the Ministry of Health and other departments repeatedly occurred, which possibly led to increased reinfection rates and control failures. Increasing awareness among the local community is essential to support the environmental management programme, as this approach has proved to be the best one in Napu and Lindu valleys.

6.3. REGIONAL RESEARCH NEEDS

Basic research on schistosomiasis has a long tradition and operational research has always been an important component of the national control programmes in Southeast Asia (Liu et al., 2008; Utzinger et al., 2005). Both have contributed much to the past successes in control, now paving the road towards elimination. For instance, research was an integral part of the WBLP on schistosomiasis control in P.R. China; about 2% of the total loan was used for this purpose (Bergquist and Tanner, 2010; Chen et al., 2005).

The identification of research needs and determination of priorities are always important to a control programme, particularly in the initial stages of a new control initiative, so as to ensure the quality and progress of the control activities in coordination with new technological developments (Hotez and Ehrenberg, 2010; WHO, 1993). Therefore, considering the current status of schistosomiasis in Asia, it is important to define weak points in current control programmes and thereby identify areas that would benefit from further research. This goal has already been approached through the annual workshops organised by the Regional Network of Asian Schistosomiasis and Other Helminth Zoonoses (RNAS^{+}) that have taken place during the last 10 years. These meetings have proved to be a good basis for setting research priorities (McGarvey et al., 1990; Zhou et al., 2005, 2008a).

6.3.1. Research needs orientated by control goal

Based on an overview of all the national schistosomiasis control programmes in all endemic countries in the region, a general goal seems to be to reduce the prevalence to a sustainable, low level. As prevalence approaches levels as low as around 1%, it becomes increasingly difficult to find the remaining cases (Leonardo et al., 2008; Li et al., 2009a). At this stage, it is also essential to know how to maintain the control efforts and to move decidedly forward on several fronts, such as the control of snail intermediate hosts and animal infection reservoirs (WHO, 2007).

6.3.1.1. Tackling the challenges faced by the control programme

Evaluation of the present epidemiological situation and development of the new control strategy have revealed that some critical tools for completing the task of national schistosomiasis control and elimination are lacking (King, 2009). Shortcomings in presently available knowledge and control approaches are among the reasons for the persistence of pockets of uncontrolled snail propagation, parasite transmission, and faecal contamination of the environment by the many species of infected definitive hosts. The problem of re-emergence has also made it obvious that not all measures employed thus far are sustainable in the long term. The envisaged intersectoral collaboration is also considered crucial for the success of the control programme, yet there are many unsolved questions with reference to this issue (Zhou et al., 2008a).

Research should be done proactively and planned with a consideration of future challenges, for example, the effects of global warming and large-scale water resource development projects (Yang et al., 2007, 2010; Zhou et al., 2008b). Finally, the profound socio-economic changes taking place in all realms of society require constant readaptation of control programmes. Therefore, new efforts in operational as well as institutional and basic research are needed to develop improved tools and strategies for schistosomiasis control and to make them available to the control programme (Utzinger et al., 2005; Wang et al., 2009b).

6.3.1.2. Improvement of the quality of the control programme and surveillance

6.3.1.2.1. Development of improved tools and strategies The current set of control tools and guiding strategies is not sufficient to cope with the challenges in hyper-endemic areas and in places where endemicity is low, but stable. Detailed study of the local conditions is required to guide the development of new strategies to overcome the deadlock of the control programmes. Some of the issues which have to be investigated are the failure of traditional methods to permanently reduce endemicity in hyper-endemic areas, the decreased compliance rates for stool sample collection in residents after massive morbidity reductions by repeated rounds of praziquantel administered to at-risk populations, and the low sensitivity of the Kato-Katz method that results in failure to detect light infections (Lin et al., 2008b). Another factor compromising further progress in schistosomiasis control is the high cost and environmental toxicity of niclosamide, the only commercially available molluscicide.

The multitude of serological diagnostic tests for case detection and surveillance has made it difficult to come up with reliable national data and to analyse trends (Bergquist et al., 2009; Lin et al., 2008b). Standardisation of serological tests and rapid diagnostic reagents is therefore of utmost importance. In P.R. China, the adaptation of the control programme to the rapid changes in socio-economic and environmental conditions triggered by the ongoing market reforms and the major ecological transformations brought along with these changes in society and economy are further crucial areas which must be investigated. Finally, the development of a vaccine and a strategy for its use in areas with persisting high prevalence levels could be the much-needed additional tool to achieve sustained control by breaking the transmission cycle even in areas that have proved resistant to control attempts so far (Da'dara et al., 2008; McManus and Loukas, 2008).

6.3.1.2.2. Efficient management structures The transformation from a planned to a market-oriented economy system and the process of decentralisation in P.R. China has made it increasingly difficult to maintain the old system of administration in schistosomiasis control. Collaboration with other sectors such as agriculture, water resources, forestry, and infrastructure development becomes ever more important (Utzinger et al., 2005; Zhou et al., 2005). The present system of reporting cases and surveillance data for central evaluation and epidemiological trend analysis has to be improved, and there are pressing needs to design control strategies which are adapted to the local eco-epidemiological conditions and versatile enough to respond to changing needs while maintaining comparability for evaluation (Chen et al., 2007; Wang et al., 2008b, 2009a).

6.3.1.3. Requirements for locally tailored control strategies

The rapid pace at which enormous water resources development projects such as the Three Gorges dam, anti-flood measures, and the South–North water transfer project are implemented in P.R. China makes it imperative to closely evaluate their effects in all endemic or at-risk areas and to develop predictive models allowing a more reliable evaluation of the potential effects of future projects (Yang et al., 2006; Zhu et al., 2008). The effects of flooding events on snail dispersal into previously snail-free areas and especially of climate change are further topics where research is urgently needed into the possible impact on the epidemiology of schistosomiasis (Yang et al., 2007, 2009a; Zhou et al., 2008b).

The mobilisation of people has become more difficult for research and control efforts, the increased mobility of the population, especially of migrant workers, has made surveillance less comprehensive, and there is an increased risk of schistosomiasis cases moving to non-endemic areas where they are not recognised (Leonardo et al., 2002). Such migrations could also spread the parasite to new locations, establishing new foci of transmission. Economic development can mean that more people have access to safe infrastructure such as running water but this is not always reflected in the individual risk behaviour. Economic hardship can also force people to take greater risks and it is conceivable that high infection risks are increasingly concentrated in a fraction of the society, possibly leading to a dilution effect which makes it more difficult to identify them. Last but not least, the livestock numbers have vastly increased, partly without adaptation to the production system and thus enlarging the pool of definitive hosts (Zhou et al., 2007a,b).

6.3.2. Areas in need of further research

Further progress in schistosomiasis control critically depends on the diversification of the tools and strategies available to the national control programme. More research is needed in a wide range of fields, covering operational, institutional, and basic biological aspects. Emphasis should be laid on operational research and capacity building and on the close collaboration between research and control; and priority should be assigned to those areas to be able to directly improve the control activities.

6.3.2.1. Operational research relevant to control

The emphasis of operational research should be on new strategies and tools, technical standardization, investigation of eco-epidemiological determinants, and social justice. The ultimate goal is to further focus the control programme on crucial issues so as to make it more sustainable and cost-effective.

6.3.2.1.1. New technologies The effectiveness of the national control programme could be boosted by the development of new tools and techniques to broaden the available selection and to better respond to local as well as future requirements. New tools should be developed in the following fields: (i) assessment of treatment effectiveness, (ii) rapid epidemiological assessment of community prevalence, (iii) detection of infected snails, and (iv) surveillance of existing and suspected snail habitats.

6.3.2.1.2. Eco-epidemiological determinants The epidemiology of schistosomiasis japonica is not yet fully understood in all settings and current rapid socio-economic development as well as shifts in environmental conditions make it imperative to study further the contextual determinants of schistosomiasis japonica, the optimal allocation of health-care resources, and to evaluate the true morbidity associated with different infection intensities (Jia et al., 2007). The following priorities are proposed: (i) interaction between ecosystem and schistosomiasis transmission, (ii) burden of disease estimates, (iii) animal schistosomiasis in different settings, (iv) new animal management strategies, (v) environmental changes and their epidemiological impact, and (vi) socio-economic context and impact on control approaches, including the impact of climate changes and socio-economic changes.

6.3.2.1.3. Technical standardization The technical standardization of policies and procedures, which can nevertheless be readily adapted to changing local socio-economic and eco-epidemiological conditions, is of utmost importance to ensure that data can be compared across endemic areas, and thereby to facilitate quality assurance and communication between all parties (Steinmann et al., 2006; Wu et al., 2008). Uniform standards are required in strategy adjustment, surveillance, and responses to outbreaks.

6.3.2.1.4. Novel products The development of new, standardized products to be used in the control programme is important as this will allow a certain technical harmonization of the programme, thereby broadening its range of activities and enhancing its ability to respond to specific requirements. New products are required as drugs and treatment procedures, diagnostic kits, molluscicides, and vaccines.

6.3.2.2. Innovative approaches to control

Sustained research on basic questions of the biology of *S. japonicum* and its epidemiology will produce new insights into this complex parasite, its life cycle, and the determining factors for transmission and infection (Zhou et al., 2009). This could result in new concepts and innovative methods for control, most welcome additions to the current arsenal of tools and approaches. Research should focus on the following domains:

6.3.2.2.1. Biology of S. japonicum Reinfections in different settings cause resurgence of the diseases. The genetic and immunological background for human reinfection with *S. japonicum* should be elucidated to better understand human reinfection in hyper-endemic areas. At the same time, bioinformatics, genome and proteome research is suitable for application to *S. japonicum* and their reservoir hosts in an effort to find specific molecular and immunological markers characteristic of different stages and to elucidate the molecular interplay between the parasite and its host (Liu et al., 2009). This information could inform the development of novel diagnostic tools, drugs, and vaccines to improve the control programme.

6.3.2.2.2. Biology of snail intermediate hosts Studies of the biological interactions between *S. japonicum* and *O. hupensis* could help improve our understanding of the genetic co-evolution among *S. japonicum* and its snail intermediate host. The genetic basis and immunological mechanisms governing the infection susceptibility of *O. hupensis* and variations therein should be further studied. Genome and proteome studies are, in principle, able to identify the functional genes of *O. hupensis* conferring resistance against *S. japonicum* infection (Li et al., 2009b).

6.3.2.2.3. Epidemiology and immunology of schistosomiasis Transmission models employing environmental, demographic, and socio-economic variables should be developed in order to provide the theoretical basis for transmission estimations and forecasting, a valuable tool for the management of the control programme (Spear et al., 2004; Wang et al., 2006).

The immunological events following an infection in end hosts should be further investigated to provide detailed information for the development and field evaluation of diagnostic kits and vaccines (Da'dara et al., 2008; Hotez et al., 2007). Defining the immunological factors causing this type of morbidity and study of the factors leading to the increased vulnerability should be investigated. This would allow the creation of specific control programmes focusing on acute infections in hyper-endemic areas (Bergquist et al., 2009; Hafalla et al., 1999; Planas, 2008).

6.3.2.3. Capacity building and construction of a research platform

Closer collaboration between all involved scientists and institutions will considerably strengthen research by sharing limited resources, information, and experience (Zhou et al., 2008a). It will also facilitate the development of standardized products and foster the education of the next generation of scientists. The following steps and structures are proposed:

6.3.2.3.1. Networking between laboratories in the region Networks connecting laboratories and institutions could combine their respective potential and special experiences, resulting in superior performance of research and control. Networking is also crucial to standardize the quality of control approaches and diagnostic products and to unify reporting. The following networks should be set up: (i) a network of laboratories working on the development of diagnostic kits to standardize existing ones and develop a generally accepted standard kit which is available to the whole control programme; (ii) a network of laboratories involved in drug screening will enable them to share the work and to engage in large-scale projects (allocation of specific tasks to the most suitable laboratory will also be much easier); and (iii) a similarly designated network for the development of novel vaccine candidates.

Easy access to standardized reference samples of *S. japonicum*, *O. hupensis*, and human serum will improve and facilitate research in many fields. Therefore, it is proposed to set up a serum bank containing blood samples from well-characterised infected humans, a gene bank of *S. japonicum* and *O. hupensis*, and a collection of standardized strains of the parasite and its intermediate host.

6.3.2.3.2. Information databases The establishment of comprehensive computerized databases containing epidemiological and snail distribution data, and of a geographical information system (GIS) database on schistosomiasis and intermediate host snail distribution will grant rapid access to information and facilitate the exchange between all involved parties. Easy and fast access to information is crucial for the management of the control programme, for surveillance and outbreak response and the ready detection of epidemiological trends (Chen et al., 2007; Leonardo et al. 2005; Yang et al., 2006, 2009b; Zhou et al., 2008a,b,c). A specific research database could improve the exchange and knowledge sharing among the scientific community.

6.4. CONCLUSIONS

It is essential to attract more funds for the neglected areas. Support of local government units, non-government organizations, other government organizations, and the community is expected to sustain regular control activities, for example, clearing of vegetation, drainage, provision of safe source of water supply and water-sealed toilets, construction of footbridges, and agro-engineering measures that will cut disease transmission. In addition to these, research activities, for example, basic research, implementation research, and product development, also have a role to play in reaching the goal of eliminating schistosomiasis in Asia as a public health problem, and to save lives among those vulnerable populations, for example, children, women, and workers in affected water-bodies.

More attention has recently been focused on research activities related to the elimination of schistosomiasis japonica in Asia, after the prevalence is reduced to the 1% level. However, global research activities related to elimination of the disease are still neglected with respect to tools for the assessment of progress towards elimination, with respect to the scheme of surveillance to consolidate the achievement of low prevalence, and with respect to the alerting system to detect and combat resurgence of the disease. Therefore, the schistosomiasis control programmes in Asia are facing the problem of sustainability. There is a great need to approach the declining transmission intensity and scale with an integrated strategy that would include agricultural development programmes, modernization programmes in water/irrigation projects, and local socio-economic development programmes.

Both research and control will benefit from international collaboration. Such cooperation will enhance the exchange of information and expertise in research, surveillance and control, and encourage the training of the next generation of researchers and control staff. The existing RNAS$^+$ is an excellent platform for this purpose and should be further strengthened in the fields of training, risk mapping, and advocacy of integrated control to broaden the focus from schistosomiasis to other parasitic diseases such as food-borne trematodiases and soil-transmitted helminthiases. It should also encourage information exchange in spite of language barriers and the publication of research findings in internationally accessible journals.

ACKNOWLEDGEMENTS

X.N. Zhou received financial support from the National Natural Science Foundation of China (grant no. 30590373), the National S & T Mayor Project (grant no. 2008ZX10004-011), and UNICEF/UNDP/World Bank/WHO Special Programme on Research and Training in Tropical Diseases (grant no. 200020548). Thanks to Dr. Peter Steinmann for his help on manuscript improvement.

REFERENCES

Acosta, L.P., Waine, G., Aligui, G.D., Tiu, W.U., Olveda, R.M., McManus, D.P., 2002. Immune correlate study on human *Schistosoma japonicum* in a well-defined population in Leyte, Philippines: II. Cellular immune responses to *S. japonicum* recombinant and native antigens. Acta Trop. 84, 137–149.

Bergquist, R., Tanner, M., 2010. Controlling schistosomiasis in Southeast Asia: a tale of two countries Adv. Parasitol. 72, 109–144.

Bergquist, R., Johansen, M.V., Utzinger, J., 2009. Diagnostic dilemmas in helminthology: what tools to use and when? Trends Parasitol. 25, 151–156.

Blas, B.L., 1976. Agro-engineering and sanitation improvement in the control of schistosomiasis japonica in the Philippines: a review. Southeast Asian J. Trop. Med. Public Health 7, 341–345.

Blas, B.L., Rosales, M.I., Lipayon, I.L., Yasuraoka, K., Matsuda, H., Hayashi, M., 2004. The schistosomiasis problem in the Philippines: a review. Parasitol. Int. 53, 127–134.

Brooker, S., Kabatereine, N.B., Gyapong, J.O., Stothard, J.R., Utzinger, J., 2009. Rapid assessment of schistosomiasis and other neglected tropical diseases in the context of integrated control programmes in Africa. Parasitology 136, 1707–1718.

Carney, W.P., Masri, S., Salludin, Putrali J., 1974. The Napu Valley, a new schistosomiasis area in Sulawesi, Indonesia. Southeast Asian J. Trop. Med. Pub. Health 5, 246–251.

Chen, M.G., 2005. Use of praziquantel for clinical treatment and morbidity control of schistosomiasis japonica in China: a review of 30 years' experience. Acta Trop. 96, 168–176.

Chen, X.Y., Wang, L.Y., Cai, J.M., Zhou, X.N., Zheng, J., Guo, J.G., et al., 2005. Schistosomiasis control in China: the impact of a 10-year World Bank Loan Project (1992–2001). Bull. World Health Organ. 83, 43–48.

Chen, Z., Zhou, X.N., Yang, K., Wang, X.H., Yao, Z.Q., Wang, T.P., et al., 2007. Strategy formulation for schistosomiasis japonica control in different environmental settings supported by spatial analysis: a case study from China. Geospat. Health 2, 223–231.

Coutinho, H.M., McGarvey, S.T., Acosta, L.P., Manalo, D.L., Langdon, G.C., Leenstra, T., et al., 2005. Nutritional status and serum cytokine profiles in children, adolescents, and young adults with *Schistosoma japonicum*-associated hepatic fibrosis, in Leyte, Philippines. J. Infect. Dis. 192, 528–536.

Crowell, B., Hammack, R., 1913. Intestinal parasites encountered in five hundred autopsies, with reports of cases. Philip. J. Sci. B 8, 157.

Da'dara, A.A., Li, Y.S., Xiong, T., Zhou, J., Williams, G.M., McManus, D.P., et al., 2008. DNA-based vaccines protect against zoonotic schistosomiasis in water buffalo. Vaccine 26, 3617–3625.

de Vlas, S.J., Gryseels, B., 1992. Underestimation of *Schistosoma mansoni* prevalences. Parasitol. Today 8, 274–277.

de Vlas, S.J., Engels, D., Rabello, A.L., Oostburg, B.F., Van Lieshout, L., Polderman, A.M., et al., 1997. Validation of a chart to estimate true *Schistosoma mansoni* prevalences from simple egg counts. Parasitology 114, 113–121.

Doenhoff, M.J., Cioli, D., Utzinger, J., 2008. Praziquantel: mechanisms of action, resistance and new derivatives for schistosomiasis. Curr. Opin. Infect. Dis. 21, 659–667.

Engels, D., Chitsulo, L., Montresor, A., Savioli, L., 2002. The global epidemiological situation of schistosomiasis and new approaches to control and research. Acta Trop. 82, 139–146.

Engels, D., Wang, L.Y., Palmer, K.L., 2005. Control of schistosomiasis in China. Acta Trop. 96, 67–68.

Fenwick, A., Savioli, L., Engels, D., Bergquist, N.R., Todd, M.H., 2003. Drugs for the control of parasitic diseases: current status and development in schistosomiasis. Trends Parasitol. 19, 509–515.

Fenwick, A., Webster, J.P., Bosque-Oliva, E., Blair, L., Fleming, F.M., Zhang, Y., et al., 2009. The Schistosomiasis Control Initiative (SCI): rationale, development and implementation from 2002–2008. Parasitology 136, 1719–1730.

Fujinami, A., Nakamura, H., 1909. The route of infection, the development of the parasite of Katayama disease and its infection in animals. Kyoto Med. J. 6, 224–252.

Gao, L.L., 2002. Considerations on snail control by environmental modification in Zhejiang province. Chin. J. Schisto. Cont. 14, 299–302.

Garcia, E.G., 1976. Clinical studies on schistosomiasis japonica in the Philippines: a review. Southeast Asian J. Trop. Med. Pub. Health 7, 247–256.

Garjito, T.A., Sudomo, M., Dahlan, M., Nurwidayati, A., 2008. Schistosomiasis in Indonesia: past and present. Parasitol. Int. 57, 277–280.

Gryseels, B., Polman, K., Clerinx, J., Kestens, L., 2006. Human schistosomiasis. Lancet 368, 1106–1118.

Hadidjaja, P., 1985. Schistosomiasis in central Sulawesi. Faculty of Medicine, University of Indonesia, Indonesia.

Hadidjaja, P., Sudomo, M., 1976. Some aspects on the ecology and biology of *Oncomelania hupensis lindoensis*. Southeast Asian J. Trop. Med. Pub. Health 7, 227.

Hafalla, J.C., Alamares 2nd, J.G., Acosta, L.P., Dunne, D.W., Ramirez, B.L., Santiago, M.L., 1999. Molecular identification of a 21.7 kDa *Schistosoma japonicum* antigen as a target of the human IgE response. Mol. Biochem. Parasitol. 98, 157–161.

Hao, Y., Wu, X.H., Zhen, H., Wang, L.Y., Guo, J.G., Xia, G., et al., 2007. Schistosomiasis situation in People's Republic of China in 2006. Chin. J. Schisto. Cont. 19, 401–406.

Hernandez, L.M., 2003. International Symposium on Schistosomiasis. September 11–12, Alabang, Muntinlupa City, the Philippines.

Hotez, P.J., Ehrenberg, J.P., 2010. Escalating the global fight against neglected tropical diseases through interventions in the Asia Pacific Region. Adv. Parasitol. 72, 31–53.

Hotez, P.J., Molyneux, D.H., Fenwick, A., Kumaresan, J., Sachs Ehrlich, S., Sachs, J.D., et al., 2007. Control of neglected tropical diseases. N. Engl. J. Med. 357, 1018–1027.

Jia, T.W., Zhou, X.N., Wang, X.H., Utzinger, J., Steinmann, P., Wu, X.H., 2007. Assessment of the age-specific disability weight of chronic schistosomiasis japonica. Bull. World Health Organ. 85, 458–465.

Katsurada, F., 1904. Determination of the cause of a new parasite disease seen in Yamanashi and other prefectures. Tokyo Iji Shinshi 1371, 13–32.

Katz, N., Chaves, A., Pellegrino, J., 1972. A simple device for quantitative stool thick smear technique in schistosomiasis mansoni. Rev. Inst. Med. Trop. São Paulo 14, 397–400.

King, C.H., 2009. Toward the elimination of schistosomiasis. N. Engl. J. Med. 360, 106–109.

King, C.H., 2010. Parasites and poverty: the case of schistosomiasis. Acta Trop. 113, 95–104.

King, C.H., Dickman, K., Tisch, D.J., 2005. Reassessment of the cost of chronic helmintic infection: a meta-analysis of disability-related outcomes in endemic schistosomiasis. Lancet 365, 1561–1569.

Leonardo, L.R., Acosta, L.P., Olveda, R.M., Aligui, G.D., 2002. Difficulties and strategies in the control of schistosomiasis in the Philippines. Acta Trop. 82, 295–299.

Leonardo, L.R., Rivera, P.T., Crisostomo, B.A., Sarol, J.N., Bantayan, N.C., Tiu, W.U., et al., 2005. A study of the environmental determinants of malaria and schistosomiasis in the Philippines using Remote Sensing and Geographic Information Systems. Parassitologia 47, 105–114.

Leonardo, L.R., Rivera, P., Saniel, O., Villacorte, E., Crisostomo, B., Hernandez, L., et al., 2008. Prevalence survey of schistosomiasis in Mindanao and the Visayas, The Philippines. Parasitol. Int. 57, 246–251.

Li, Y.S., Zhao, Z.Y., Ellis, M., McManus, D.P., 2005. Applications and outcomes of periodic epidemiological surveys for schistosomiasis and related economic evaluation in the People's Republic of China. Acta Trop. 96, 266–275.

Li, Y.S., Raso, G., Zhao, Z.Y., He, Y.K., Ellis, M.K., McManus, D.P., 2007. Large water management projects and schistosomiasis control, Dongting Lake region, China. Emerg. Infect. Dis. 13, 973–979.

Li, S.Z., Luz, A., Wang, X.H., Xu, L.L., Wang, Q., Qian, Y.J., et al., 2009a. Schistosomiasis in China: acute infections during 2005–2008. Chin. Med. J. (Engl.) 122, 1009–1014.

Li, S.Z., Wang, Y.X., Yang, K., Liu, Q., Wang, Q., Zhang, Y., et al., 2009b. Landscape genetics: the correlation of special and genetic distances of Oncomelania hupensis, the intermediate host snail of *Schistosoma japonicum* in mainland China. Geospat. Health 3, 221–231.

Liang, S., Yang, C., Zhong, B., Qiu, D., 2006. Re-emerging schistosomiasis in hilly and mountainous areas of Sichuan, China. Bull. World Health Organ. 84, 139–144.

Lin, D.D., Liu, J.X., Liu, Y.M., Hu, F., Zhang, Y.Y., Xu, J.M., et al., 2008a. Routine Kato-Katz technique underestimates the prevalence of *Schistosoma japonicum*: a case study in an endemic area of the People's Republic of China. Parasitol. Int. 57, 281–286.

Lin, D.D., Xu, J.M., Zhang, Y.Y., Liu, Y.M., Hu, F., Xu, X.L., et al., 2008b. Evaluation of IgG-ELISA for the diagnosis of *Schistosoma japonicum* in a high prevalence, low intensity endemic area of China. Acta Trop. 107, 128–133.

Liu, Q., Tian, L.G., Xiao, S.H., Qi, Z., Steinmann, P., Mak, T.K., et al., 2008. Harnessing the wealth of Chinese scientific literature: schistosomiasis research and control in China. Emerg. Themes Epidemiol. 5, 19.

Liu, F., Zhou, Y., Wang, Z.Q., Lu, G., Zheng, H., Brindley, P.J., et al., 2009. The *Schistosoma japonicum* genome reveals features of host–parasite interplay. Nature 460, 345–351.

Logan, O., 1905. A case of dysentery in Hunan province caused by the trematode *Schistosoma japonicum*. Chin. Med. J. 19, 243–245.

Maegraith, B., 1958. Schistosomiasis in China. Lancet 271, 208–214.

Mao, S.P., Shao, B.R., 1982. Schistosomiasis control in the People's Republic of China. Am. J. Trop. Med. Hyg. 31, 92–99.

McGarvey, S.T., Aligui, G., Daniel, B.L., Peters, P., Olveda, R., Olds, G.R., 1992. Child growth, and Schistosomiasis japonica in Northeastern Leyte, The Philippines: cross-sectional results. Am. J. Trop. Med. Hyg. 46, 571–581.

McManus, D.P., Loukas, A., 2008. Current status of vaccines for schistosomiasis. Clin. Microbiol. Rev. 21, 225–242.

Olveda, R.M., 2006. Schistosomiasis in the Philippines: accomplishments over the last 100 years. In: Presented at the International Symposium on Schistosomiasis, September 11–12 Alabang, Muntinlupa City, the Philippines.

Olveda, R.M., Tiu, E., Fevidal, Jr., P., De Veyra, Jr., F., Icatlo, Jr., F., Domingo, E.O., 1983. The relationship of prevalence and intensity of infection with morbidity in schistosomiasis japonica: a study of three communities in Leyte, Philippines. Am. J. Trop. Med. Hyg. 32, 1312–1321.

Olveda, R.M., Daniel, B.L., Ramirez, B.D., Aligui, G.L., Acosta, L.P., Fevidal, P., et al., 1996. Schistosomiasis japonica in the Philippines: the long-term impact of population-based chemotherapy on infection, transmission and morbidity. J. Infect. Dis. 174, 163–172.

Pesigan, T.P., Hairston, N., 1961. The effect of snail control on the prevalence of *Schistosoma japonicum* infection in the Philippines. Bull. World Health Organ. 25, 479–482.

Pesigan, T.P., Farooq, M., Hairston, N.G., Jauregui, J.J., Garcia, E.G., Santos, A.T., et al., 1958. Studies on *Schistosoma japonicum* infection in the Philippines. 1. General considerations and epidemiology. Bull. World Health Organ. 18, 345–455.

Planas, L.G., 2008. Intervention design, implementation, and evaluation. Am. J. Health Syst. Pharm. 65, 1854–1863.

Ramos, V., 1928. Estudio de un caso de enfermedad de Katayam que se ha manifesto como una appendecitis cronica. Bull. San Juan de Dios Hosp. 2, 127–136.

Ross, A.G.P., Bartley, P.B., Sleigh, A.C., Olds, G.R., Li, Y., Williams, G.M., et al., 2002. Schistosomiasis. N. Engl. J. Med. 346, 1212–1220.

Santiago, M.L., Hafalla, J.C., Kurtis, J.D., Aligui, G.L., Wiest, P.M., Olveda, R.M., et al., 1998. Identification of the *Schistosoma japonicum* 22.6-kDa antigen as a major target of the human IgE response: similarity of IgE-binding epitopes to allergen peptides. Int. Arch. Allergy Immunol. 117, 94–104.

Santos, A.T., 1984. The present status of schistosomiasis in the Philippines. Southeast Asian J. Trop. Med. Pub. Health 15, 439–445.

Santos, A.T., Blas, B.L., Noseñas, J.S., Portillo, G.P., Ortega, O.M., Hayashi, M., et al., 1979. Preliminary clinical trials with praziquantel in *Schistosoma japonicum* infections in the Philippines. Bull. World Health Organ. 57, 793–799.

Song, Y., Xiao, S., Wu, W., Zhang, S., Xie, H., Xu, X., et al., 1998. Preventive effect of artemether on schistosome infection. Chin. Med. J. (Engl.) 111, 123–127.

Spear, R.C., Seto, E., Liang, S., Birkner, M., Hubbard, A., Qiu, D., et al., 2004. Factors influencing the transmission of *Schistosoma japonicum* in the mountains of Sichuan province of China. Am. J. Trop. Med. Hyg. 70, 48–56.

Steinmann, P., Keiser, J., Bos, R., Tanner, M., Utzinger, J., 2006. Schistosomiasis and water resources development: systematic review, meta-analysis, and estimates of people at risk. Lancet Infect. Dis. 6, 411–425.
Steinmann, P., Utzinger, J., Du, Z.W., Zhou, X.N., et al., 2010. Multiparasitism: a neglected reality on global, regional and local scale. Adv. Parasitol. 73, 21–50.
Stothard, J.R., Chitsulo, L., Kristensen, T.K., Utzinger, J., 2009. Control of schistosomiasis in sub-Saharan Africa: progress made, new opportunities and remaining challenges. Parasitology 136, 1665–1675.
Tanaka, H., Tsuji, M., 1997. Discovery to eradication of schistosomiasis in Japan 1847–1996. Int. J. Parasitol. 27, 1465–1480.
Tubangui, M., 1932. The molluscan intermediate host in the Philippines of the oriental blood fluke *Schistosoma japonicum* Katsurada. Philipp. J. Sci. 49, 295.
Utzinger, J., Xiao, S.H., N'Goran, E.K., Bergquist, R., Tanner, M., 2001. The potential of artemether for the control of schistosomiasis. Int. J. Parasitol. 31, 1549–1562.
Utzinger, J., Zhou, X.N., Chen, M.G., Bergquist, R., 2005. Conquering schistosomiasis in China: the long march. Acta Trop. 96, 69–96.
Utzinger, J., Raso, G., Brooker, S., de Savigny, D., Tanner, M., Ørnbjerg, N., et al., 2009. Schistosomiasis and neglected tropical diseases: towards integrated and sustainable control and a word of caution. Parasitology 136, 1859–1874.
Wang, J.G., Liao, H.Y., Zhong, G.T., Yu, B.G., Huang, S.S., 2002. Observation on the effect on schistosomiasis through snail control by environmental modification. Chin. J. Schisto. Cont. 14, 200–202.
Wang, X.H., Wu, X.H., Zhou, X.N., 2006. Bayesian estimation of community prevalences of Schistosoma japonicum infection in China. Int. J. Parasitol. 36, 895–902.
Wang, L., Utzinger, J., Zhou, X.N., 2008a. Schistosomiasis control: experiences and lessons from China. Lancet 372, 1793–1795.
Wang, X.H., Zhou, X.N., Vounatsou, P., Chen, Z., Utzinger, J., Yang, K., et al., 2008b. Bayesian spatio-temporal modeling of *Schistosoma japonicum* prevalence data in the absence of a diagnostic 'gold' standard. PLoS Negl. Trop. Dis. 2, e250.
Wang, L.D., Chen, H.G., Guo, J.G., Zeng, X.J., Hong, X.L., Xiong, J.J., et al., 2009a. A strategy to control transmission of *Schistosoma japonicum* in China. N. Engl. J. Med. 360, 121–128.
Wang, L.D., Guo, J.G., Wu, X.H., Chen, H.G., Wang, T.P., Zhu, S.P., et al., 2009b. China's new strategy to block transmission of schistosomiasis and beyond. Trop. Med. Int. Health 14, 1475–1583.
WHO, 1993. The Control of Schistosomiasis: Second Report of the WHO Expert Committee. World Health Organization, Geneva pp. 1–61.
WHO, 2001. Report of the WHO Informal Consultation on Schistosomiasis in Low Transmission Areas: Control Strategies and Criteria for Elimination. WHO/CDS/CPE/SIP/2001.1.
WHO, 2007. Schistosomiasis and Soil Transmitted Helminths Country Profile Laos PDR. World Health Organization, Geneva.
Wooley, P.G., 1906. The occurrence of *Schistoma japonicum* Vel Cattol in the Philippines. Philipp. J. Sci. 1, 83–90.
Wu, G.L., 2002. A historical perspective on the immunodiagnosis of schistosomiasis in China. Acta Trop. 82, 193–198.
Wu, X.H., Chen, M.G., Zheng, J., 2005. Surveillance of schistosomiasis in five provinces of China which have reached the national criteria for elimination of the disease. Acta Trop. 96, 276–281.
Wu, X.H., Wang, L.P., Li, S.Z., Wang, X.H., Tao, H.Q., Pan, H.D., et al., 2006. The process and strategy in elimination of schistosomiasis in Guangdong, Shanghai, Fujian, Guangxi, Zhejiang provinces. In: Wang, L.D. (Ed.), The Course and Perspectives in Schistosomiasis Control in China. People's Health Press, Beijing, p. 401.

Wu, X.H., Zhang, S.Q., Xu, X.J., Huang, Y.X., Steinmann, P., Utzinger, J., et al., 2008. Effect of floods on the transmission of schistosomiasis in the Yangtze River valley, People's Republic of China. Parasitol. Int. 57, 271–276.

Xiao, S.H., 2005a. Development of antischistosomal drugs in China, with particular consideration to praziquantel and the artemisinins. Acta Trop. 96, 153–167.

Xiao, S.H., 2005b. Study on the prevention and cure efficacy of artemether against schistosomiasis. Chin. J. Schisto. Cont. 17, 310–320.

Xiao, S.H., Booth, M., Tanner, M., 2000. The prophylactic effects of artemether against *Schistosoma japonicum* infections. Parasitol. Today 16, 122–126.

Xiao, S.H., Tanner, M., N'Goran, E.K., Utzinger, J., Chollet, J., Bergquist, R., et al., 2002. Recent investigations of artemether, a novel agent for the prevention of schistosomiasis japonica, mansoni and haematobia. Acta Trop. 82, 175–181.

Xiao, S.H., Keiser, J., Chen, M.G., Tanner, M., Utzinger, J., 2010. Research and development of antischistosomal drugs in The People's Republic of China: a 60-year review. Adv. Parasitol. 73, 231–295.

Yang, G.J., Vounatsou, P., Tanner, M., Zhou, X.N., Utzinger, J., 2006. Remote sensing for predicting potential habitats of *Oncomelania hupensis* in Hongze, Baima and Gaoyou lakes in Jiangsu province, China. Geospat. Health 1, 85–92.

Yang, G.J., Utzinger, J., Sun, L.P., Hong, Q.B., Vounatsou, P., Tanner, M., et al., 2007. Effect of temperature on the development of *Schistosoma japonicum* within *Oncomelania hupensis*, and hibernation of *O. hupensis*. Parasitol. Res. 100, 695–700.

Yang, K., Li, H.J., Yang, W.C., Shi, X.W., Qi, Y.L., 2009a. Effect of comprehensive schistosomiasis control measures with emphasis on infetious source control in dam areas of mountainous region, Yunnan Province. Chin. J. Schisto. Cont. 21, 272–275.

Yang, K., Zhou, X.N., Wu, X.H., Steinmann, P., Wang, X.H., Yang, G.J., et al., 2009b. Landscape pattern analysis and Bayesian modeling for predicting *Oncomelania hupensis* distribution in Eryuan County, People's Republic of China. Am. J. Trop. Med. Hyg. 81, 416–423.

Yang, G.J., Utzinger, J., Lv, S., Qian, Y.J., Li, S.Z., Wang, Q., et al., 2010. The Regional Network of Asian Schistosomiasis and other Helminth Zoonoses ($RNAS^+$): target diseases in face of climatic change. Adv. Parasitol 73, 101–135.

Yu, J.M., de Vlas, S.J., Yuan, H.C., Gryseels, B., 1998. Variations in fecal *Schistosoma japonicum* egg counts. Am. J. Trop. Med. Hyg. 59, 370–375.

Zhang, W., Wong, C.M., 2003. Evaluation of the 1992–1999 World Bank Schistosomiasis Control Project in China. Acta Trop. 85, 303–313.

Zhang, Y.Q., Zhang, J., Shu, R.R., He, Q.X., Qi, L.J., Zhang, R., et al., 2003. Effect of schistosomiasis control by environment alteration and chemotherapy in lake regions. Chin. J. Schisto. Cont. 15, 304–305.

Zhang, Y.Y., Luo, J.P., Liu, Y.M., Wang, Q.Z., Chen, J.H., Xu, M.X., et al., 2009. Evaluation of Kato-Katz examination method in three areas with low-level endemicity of schistosomiasis japonica in China: a Bayesian modeling approach. Acta Trop. 112, 16–22.

Zhou, X.N., Wang, L.Y., Chen, M.G., Wu, X.H., Jiang, Q.W., Chen, X.Y., et al., 2005. The public health significance and control of schistosomiasis in China—then and now. Acta Trop. 96, 97–105.

Zhou, X.N., Guo, J.G., Wu, X.H., Jiang, Q.W., Zheng, J., Dang, H., et al., 2007. Epidemiology of schistosomiasis in the People's Republic of China, 2004. Emerg. Infect. Dis. 13, 1470–1476.

Zhou, X.N., Ohta, N., Utzinger, J., Bergquist, R., Olveda, R.M., 2008a. $RNAS^+$: a win–win collaboration to combat neglected tropical diseases in Southeast Asia. Parasitol. Int. 57, 243–245.

Zhou, X.N., Yang, G.J., Yang, K., Wang, X.H., Hong, Q.B., Sun, L.P., et al., 2008b. Potential impact of climate change on schistosomiasis transmission in China. Am. J. Trop. Med. Hyg. 78, 188–194.

Zhou, Y.B., Yang, M.X., Tao, P., Jiang, Q.L., Zhao, G.M., Wei, J.G., et al., 2008c. A longitudinal study of comparison of the Kato-Katz technique and indirect hemagglutination assay (IHA) for the detection of schistosomiasis japonica in China, 2001–2006. Acta Trop. 107, 251–254.

Zhou, X.N., Lv, S., Yang, G.J., Kristensen, T.K., Bergquist, N.R., Utzinger, J., et al., 2009. Spatial epidemiology in zoonotic parasitic diseases: insights gained at the 1st International Symposium on Geospatial Health in Lijiang, China, 2007. Parasit. Vectors 2, 10.

Zhu, Y.C., 2005. Immunodiagnosis and its role in schistosomiasis control in China: a review. Acta Trop. 96, 130–136.

Zhu, H.M., Xiang, S., Yang, K., Wu, X.H., Zhou, X.N., 2008. Three Gorges Dam and its impact on the potential transmission of schistosomiasis in regions along the Yangtze River. Ecohealth 5, 137–148.

Zuo, J., Ren, M.Y., He, H.B., Gao, J.X., Huang, C.L., Lin, B., et al., 1999. Control of schistosomiasis in lake regions through snail control and environmental measures. Chin. J. Schisto. Cont. 11, 146–148.

CHAPTER 7

Schistosoma mekongi in Cambodia and Lao People's Democratic Republic

Sinuon Muth,* **Somphou Sayasone,**[†,‡,§] **Sophie Odermatt-Biays,**[‡,§] **Samlane Phompida,**[¶] **Socheat Duong,*** and **Peter Odermatt**[‡,§]

Contents

Abstract

Schistosomiasis found in communities along the Mekong River in Cambodia and Lao People's Democratic Republic (Lao PDR) is caused by the blood fluke *Schistosoma mekongi*. Early observations on patients in 1957 revealed severe intestinal and hepatosplenic

* National Centre for Parasitology, Entomology and Malaria Control, Phnom Penh, Cambodia
† National Institute of Public Health, Ministry of Health, Vientiane, Lao People's Democratic Republic
‡ Department of Epidemiology and Public Health, Swiss Tropical and Public Health Institute, Basel, Switzerland
§ University of Basel, Basel, Switzerland
¶ Centre for Malariology, Parasitology and Entomology, Vientiane, Lao People's Democratic Republic

Advances in Parasitology, Volume 72
ISSN 0065-308X, DOI: 10.1016/S0065-308X(10)72007-8

disease. High mortality rates and widespread disease were reported from the provinces of northern Cambodia (Stung Treng and Kratié) and southern Lao PDR (Champasack) in the early 1970s and 1990s. Control programmes built around mass drug administration, with praziquantel, and combined with information and education campaigns, were carried out. In Cambodia, such programmes were started in 1995 in the endemic provinces and sustained until today; these efforts resolved the public health problem of schistosomiasis mekongi and led to a significant reduction in transmission. In Lao PDR, the interventions started in the late 1980s, but suffered several interruptions which permitted transmission to resume. Today, a number of small foci continue to show substantial prevalence rates. The snail intermediate host, *Neotricula aperta*, is present in the Mekong River and some of its tributaries. There is evidence that the snail might not yet have reached its full geographical distribution emphasising the need to sustain vigilance. New infections with *S. mekongi* occur in the endemic population and travellers alike. Comprehensive guidelines for the elimination of *S. mekongi* and bilateral efforts between Cambodia and Lao PDR are required.

7.1. INTRODUCTION

Schistosomiasis mekongi is endemic along the Mekong River and its certain tributaries in the lower Mekong basin. The blood fluke *Schistosoma mekongi* is the causative agent. It is a close relative of *Schistosoma japonicum* (McManus et al., 2009; Zhou et al., 2010), both species potentially lead to severe disease outcomes if left untreated. Foci of *S. mekongi* were described along the Mekong River and its tributaries in two northern provinces in Cambodia, namely Kratié and Stung Treng, and in two districts (Khong and Mounlapamok) of Champasack province, the most southern province of Lao People's Democratic Republic (Lao PDR). As shown in Fig. 7.1, *S. mekongi* infection is also known from eastern Thailand (Harinasuta, 1984). Approximately 140,000 people are at risk for *S. mekongi* infection: 80,000 people in Cambodia and 60,000 in Lao PDR (Urbani et al., 2002).

The intermediate host snail, *Neotricula aperta*, is particularly frequent in the Mekong main river but it can also be found in tributaries (Attwood et al., 2008a). The transmission period, March–April, coincides with the dry season when the water level is low and the observed snail populations reach their maximum. Most human communities depend on fishing and use the river water for recreational activities (e.g. bathing and swimming) and occupational activities (e.g. washing clothes and dishes and performing other daily household activities).

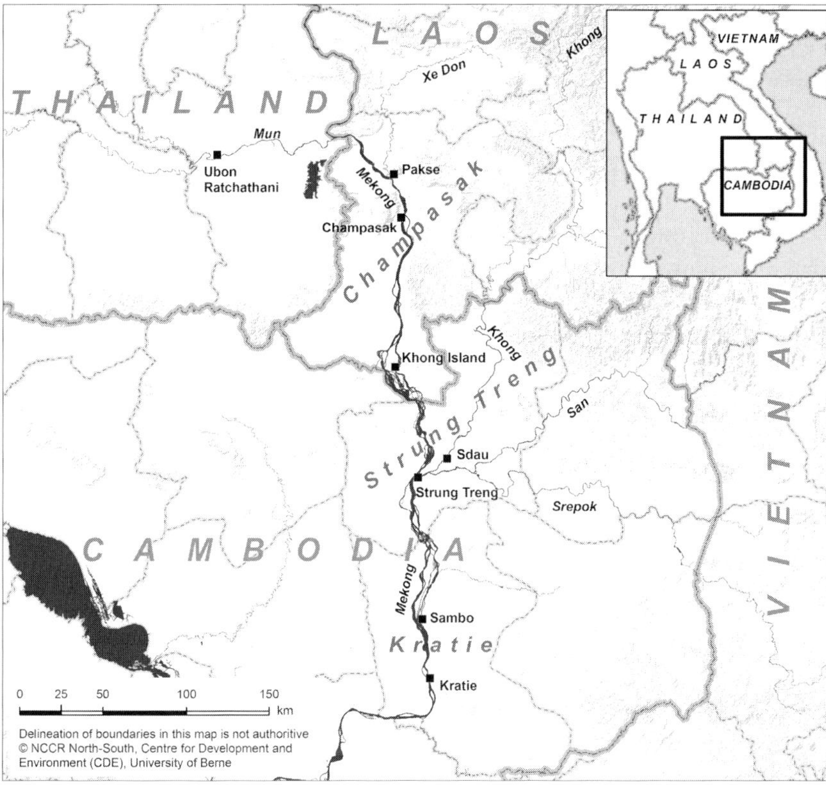

FIGURE 7.1 Map of Lao PDR, Cambodia and Thailand with endemic area of *Schistosoma mekongi*.

The purpose of this chapter is to review the public health importance of schistosomiasis mekongi, its epidemiology and control of the disease and infection, and to provide a historical background of this *Schistosoma* species. The chapter concludes on current challenges of control.

7.2. DISCOVERY AND RE-DISCOVERY

7.2.1. First reports in Cambodia and Lao PDR

Early reports of schistosomiasis in Southeast Asia date back to 1957 when Vic-Dupont and colleagues described a case of hepatosplenic schistosomiasis in Saint Joseph hospital in Paris (Vic-Dupont et al., 1957). An 18-year-old male Laotian patient was hospitalised in a state of shock following an episode of severe haematemesis. In the course of treatment, the patient underwent a splenectomy. The patient spent his first 9 years of life on Khong Island, located in Champasack province in south Lao PDR, where he most probably acquired the infection. Due to the similar clinical presentation and the similar shape and size of eggs, the patient was initially classified as suffering from a *S. japonicum*-like infection. Subsequent cases of Laotian patients referred to and reported in hospitals in Paris led to the hypothesis that a significant transmission focus must be present in southern Lao PDR (Barbier, 1966, 1967). In 1967, the presence of such a focus was confirmed by a mission convened by the World Health Organization (WHO) to the area (Iijima and Garcia, 1967).

In the same year, Audebaud and Tournier-Lasserve and their colleagues (Audebaud et al., 1968; Tournier-Lasserve et al., 1970) reported cases of severe schistosomiasis in Phnom Penh hospitals. All the patients originated from Kratié town (Kratié province). An epidemiological study was carried out in schoolchildren of Kratié town and neighbouring villages (Jolly et al., 1970a,b). The investigators looked in particular at the population of the floating villages that were attached to the Mekong shores. High infection rates were diagnosed, for example, in 70 examined children in a floating village close to Kratié, 46 (65.7%) were found with *Schistosoma* eggs in their stool. Virtually all children were in a deprived general and nutritional status, and most of them had marked hepatomegaly. The stools were stained with blood and mucus, and mostly decolourized and liquid. In order to further determine the zone of transmission, an extended survey was undertaken mainly in primary schools from villages along the Mekong River from northern Cambodia in Strung Treng province downstream to Kratié province, through Khamphong Cham province to the border of Vietnam (Iijima, 1970). Intradermal sensitivity tests using *S. japonicum* antigens were performed in 3767 children. Highest positivity rates of 35.6% were found in villages of the province of Kratié. Again, particularly affected were the inhabitants of the floating villages (59.6%). Lower positivity rates were observed in Stung Treng province (13.6%), and in the provinces further downstream, rates below 10% were observed. The findings were consistent with the parasitological stool examination. Only in stool samples from children originating from Kratié (33.6%) and Strung Treng (3.6%) were *Schistosoma* eggs detected.

In the 1970s, in southern Lao PDR, particularly on Khong Island, further studies revealed the parasitological and epidemiological features of *Schistosoma* foci in this area. During extensive malacological surveys, potential snail intermediate hosts were collected and brought to the laboratory at Mahidol University, Bangkok, for analysis. Furthermore, *Schistosoma*-infected dogs from the Mekong Island were found and examined (Sornmani et al., 1973a). Although initially recognised as *S. japonicum*, Sornmani et al. (1973b), Kitikoon et al. (1971) soon began to note differences in the size and shape of the eggs of the Mekong strain and argued that it may be a new species, distinct from *S. japonicum*. Analysis showed that *Lithoglyphopsis aperta* was the most likely intermediate host (Kitikoon, 1984; Kitikoon and Schneider, 1976). Later, this snail species was renamed as *N. aperta* (Davis et al., 1976). The discovery that the intermediate host of the Mekong strain was a triculine snail added support to the case that this was a new species (*S. japonicum* is only transmitted by species of *Oncomelania*—a pomatiopsine snail). The Mekong parasite was able to develop successfully in dogs and eggs were shed after 6–7 weeks post-infection. In addition, stool samples from 104 water buffaloes were collected and analyzed. None of them were found to be positive with *Schistosoma eggs* (Schneider et al., 1975), a marked contrast with the high infection among buffaloes in *S. japonicum*-endemic areas. It was in 1978 that the parasite was confirmed to be a separate species: *S. mekongi* (Voge et al., 1978).

Observations on Khong Island concerning the clinical manifestation documented the severity of the infection (Sornmani et al., 1976). In 1976, among 90 persons examined, several patients were seen with signs of portal hypertension such as dilated superficial abdominal veins or advanced ascites. Hepatomegaly and splenomegaly were also diagnosed at high frequencies. Among the surveyed population, adolescents and young adults were most heavily affected. Stool examinations revealed *Schistosoma* eggs in 62.5% of the subjects. Other parasites were also documented, most notably, *Opisthorchis viverrini* (63.9%) and hookworm (44.4%). Although, severe cases were described, Sornmani et al. (1976) did not report on mortality, that is, in the course of an episode of haemoptysis.

7.2.2. Re-discovery of Mekong schistosomiasis

During the dramatic historical events of war and civil unrest that Lao PDR but more so Cambodia suffered in the 1970s and 1980s, interventions and follow-up studies on the first cases of schistosomiasis could not be pursued.

In 1986, the Lao Ministry of Health (MoH) requested the assistance of the WHO to evaluate the endemicity level of schistosomiasis in the districts of Khong and Mounlapamok (Mott, 1991). In a subsequent survey conducted in primary schools of four villages on Khong Island, *S. mekongi* infection rates between 25% and 50% were documented. The high rates were confirmed in an examination of 869 children aged between 7 and 14 years of which 30% were found to be infected (Mott, 1991). Based on this information, the WHO recommended the launch of a community-based intervention programme where treatment was the main pillar.

In Cambodia, the importance of schistosomiasis was recognised later. It was only in 1992 that the non-governmental organization *Action Internationale Contre la Faim* (AICF) "re-discovered" schistosomiasis in

Kratié province. Rapidly, the public health dimension became clear. Half of 120 schoolchildren examined in Ampil Tuk village were diagnosed with a marked hepato-splenomegaly (Biays, 1995). Subsequently, an additional 1021 persons from various villages north of Kratié town were examined. The overall infection rate was 27.3%. The rates varied considerably between villages from 1.1% to 68.3% (A.W.J. Van der Velden, personal communication). Interestingly, the infection was significantly correlated with the river bed substratum at the water-contact sites. Study participants who reported bathing regularly in Mekong River sites with rocky substrata had a 9.1-times higher risk (95% confidence interval (CI): 4.9–16.8) of infection than those who reported bathing on sandy shores only. Those who reported clay and rock underground in their sites had a 7.9-times (95% CI: 4.2–14.8) higher risk for infection. These observations are consistent with the ecological requirement of the intermediate snail host, *N. aperta*. Indeed, the snails' preferred habitats are river stretches with fast flowing and well-oxygenated waters, which are mostly locations with rocky and stony substrata (Attwood, 2001).

Based on the initial epidemiological observations, the Cambodian MoH, the health authorities in the province of Kratié in collaboration with *Médecins sans Frontières* (MSF) initiated a rehabilitation programme at the provincial hospital of Kratié and the district hospital of Sambo, into which community-based and hospital-based schistosomiasis control was integrated. The district of Sambo in the north of Kratié town was recognised as the "epicenter" of the Cambodian schistosomiasis foci.

7.3. INFECTION, MORBIDITY AND PUBLIC HEALTH IMPORTANCE

7.3.1. Morbidity assessments

That the public health importance of schistosomiasis focused around Kratié town and Sambo district became clear during the course of the implementation of the rehabilitation programme. In the first months of 1994, in Sambo hospital, more than 120 patients per month were diagnosed with schistosomiasis, which corresponded to about 40% of all outpatients of the newly established district hospital (Biays et al., 1999). Between two and 11 patients with severe schistosomiasis were hospitalised every month.

The clinical picture of *S. mekongi* infection resembled in manifestation and severity the picture of *S. japonicum*. The most severe disease manifestation were observed among patients aged between 7 and 54 years (Biays et al., 1999). Poor general health status, stunted growth, cachexia, anaemia, and signs of portal hypertension such as collateral venous circulation, organomegaly (specifically of the left liver lobe and spleen), and ascites were commonly observed. Diarrhoea with blood in stool was often reported. Social consequences of infection resulted from high rates of school absenteeism, impaired cognitive function and the inability to work due to physical disability. In addition, delayed puberty in heavily infected individuals adversely affected their ability to find marriage partners. Death most frequently occurred after an episode of gastrointestinal bleeding as a result of ruptured oesophageal varices. Katayama syndrome, typical for *S. japonicum* (Ross et al., 2007), was never recorded for *S. mekongi*. However, a few cases of ectopic Mekong schistosomiasis were diagnosed and reported (Carmody et al., 2008; Houston et al., 2004).

The public health importance of the disease was underlined by the fact that villagers have seen and reported typical severe chronic signs and given names according to their interpretations, for example, widely reported were ''falling turtle'' and ''hornets' nest'' in the belly, which referred to the enlargement of the spleen and the left liver lobe, respectively (Biays et al., 1999). ''Pregnant men'' referred to organomegaly or ascites in men. The traditional treatment for these signs consisted of burning the turtle hidden in the belly, with hot stones or smouldering wooden sticks applied to the skin to combat the hidden turtle and hornets. In addition, in numerous communities, villagers reported sudden death of individuals following episodes of ''vomiting blood'' (hematemesis) or after falling (probably due to rupture of spleen) and liquid flowing from the umbilicus (probably due to ascites and subsequent infection) (Biays et al., 1999).

A large-scale community survey in primary schools of 20 accessible villages of the northern Kratié province was performed in 1995, with 2391 individuals aged 6–16 years examined parasitologically (Stich et al., 1999). It showed an overall infection rate of 40.0%, ranging from 7.7% to 72.9%. As the Kato-Katz technique used has only a low sensitivity, and as only one stool sample per individual was examined, the true infection rates were certainly higher than noted (Lin et al., 2008; Utzinger et al., 2001; Yu et al., 2007; Zhang et al., 2009). In Sambok village, the sensitivity of examination of several stool samples was assessed. A total of 118 children provided stool samples over three consecutive days, which were examined for *S. mekongi* and other intestinal parasite infection, using a single Kato-Katz thick smear per stool sample (Katz et al., 1972). The cumulative prevalence of infection with *S. mekongi* increased from 68% after the first day to 89% after triplicate Kato-Katz thick smears were obtained from consecutive days (Biays, 1995). Co-infection with other intestinal helminths was common; 82% of the children were infected with hookworm, and 15% and 8% were infected with *Ascaris lumbricoides* and *Trichuris trichiura*, respectively. *O. viverrini* eggs were diagnosed in only a few children (<10 children). Eating raw or insufficiently cooked fish was rarely reported and occurred mainly in individuals with a travel history to southern Lao PDR. There was also an infection with *Capillariasis philippinensis*, a severe nematode infection often confused with *T. trichiura* (Soukhathammavong et al., 2008).

Further epidemiological investigations showed that *S. mekongi* prevalence rates were similar in males and females (Stich et al., 1999). The age distribution in infection rate and intensity peaked in the school-aged children and adolescents (age range: 5–20 years). Substantial clinical morbidity was diagnosed in children, for example, 55.2% suffered from a marked hepatomegaly, and a quarter of the children reported blood (26.7%) and mucus (24.3%) in their stool. In 4.1% of the children, abdominal collateral circulation was seen, and 12 children (0.5%) were diagnosed with ascites. Based on these results, mass drug administration (MDA) with praziquantel (orally administered at the standard dose of 40 mg/kg body weight in a single dose) was clearly warranted and was instituted at the community level.

7.3.2. Geographical distribution of infection and morbidity

The only known intermediate host of *S. mekongi* is the aquatic snail *N. aperta*. It is most commonly found in cracks of partially submerged rocks along the Mekong River (Attwood, 2001). For example, in a malacological in-depth study on the Mekong shores in Kratie town in 1995, on average, 3000 snails were found per m^2 (Mouchet, 1995). Of the three snail strains (α-, β- and γ-strain), the α-strain was found only in the Mekong River of Ubon Ratchanthane. *N. γ-aperta* is found in the lower Mekong River and several of its tributaries. In contrast, the β-strain is found in the Mun River (Ubon Ratchathane). As far as is known, *N. γ-aperta* is the only snail transmitting *S. mekongi* in nature. Furthermore, evidence suggests that the Cambodian population of *N. aperta* γ-strain is more susceptible than *N. aperta* γ-strain from southern Lao PDR (Shimada et al., 2007). In addition to the Mekong River, *N. aperta* is found in tributaries such as the Xe Khong River in northern Cambodia (Attwood et al., 2004, 2008a).

Reservoir animals such as dogs (Matsumoto et al., 2002) and pigs (Strandgaard et al., 2001) have been reported. Buffaloes were suspected as potential hosts but their involvement has yet to be proven; this is in contrast to *S. japonicum* where buffaloes play a key role in the transmission of the disease (Gray et al., 2009; Wang et al., 2005, 2008, 2009a). The specific contribution of various reservoir hosts for the transmission and distribution of *S. mekongi* remains to be fully elucidated.

During the period of political instability, the stool examinations of refugees in the 1970s and 1980s suggested transmission of schistosomiasis mekongi in new areas such as Battambang province in Cambodia

(Keittivuti et al., 1982) or northern Lao PDR (Wittes et al., 1984). These areas, however, could not be confirmed when larger studies were conducted later. For example, in a large survey carried out around the Cambodian Tonle Sap Lake, no evidence of schistosomiasis transmission was obtained (Chhakda et al., 2006).

The Mekong River basin is a fascinating ecologically and socio-culturally rich area. In recent years, the number of travellers has increased markedly. Eco-tourism and leisure activities in the Mekong River and its tributaries put travellers at risk of infection. A Canadian traveller became infected in 2000 and suffered neurological complications (Houston et al., 2004). Recently, Leshem et al. (2009) reported on a group of 12 travellers who swam in the Mekong River in Lao PDR. Seven of them subsequently suffered from acute schistosomiasis. In one patient, eggs of *S. mekongi* were found in stool, whilst all seven were seropositive for *S. japonicum*. Surprisingly, four of the travellers did not visit any of the known schistosomiasis-endemic areas in southern Lao PDR, but bathed in the Mekong River in Vang Vieng, which is located in northern Lao PDR between the capital of Vientiane and Luang Prabang. No schistosomiasis cases had previously been reported from this part of Lao PDR. Although other factors might explain these findings, for example, cross-reactions of serological tests, in-depth follow-up studies are warranted.

7.4. CONTROL OF SCHISTOSOMIASIS IN CAMBODIA

Integration of control activities into the health system was a main concern and considered a prerequisite to sustain interventions and guarantee a durable impact. At the outset of the programme in the province of Kratié, intervention activities were planned and carried out by MSF in close collaboration with the provincial and district health authorities. Although, the funding of the programme exclusively originated from MSF, responsibility for implementation activities was largely held by the local authorities. When the programme commenced, the dimensions of the *S. mekongi* foci were unclear and difficult to assess as political conditions hampered the free movement of communities along the Mekong River. Human populations in at least two provinces, Kratié and Strung Treng, were thought to be at risk. As a consequence, MSF advised the MoH to appoint a national centre for the coordination of the schistosomiasis-related intervention. In 1995, the National Centre for Parasitology, Entomology and Malaria Control was officially assigned by the MoH.

The control programme at the hospital and community level started in the first months of 1994. The various control measures led to the present-day virtual disappearance of schistosomiasis mekongi cases. In sentinel schools of four villages in Kratié province (i.e. Achen, Chatnaol,

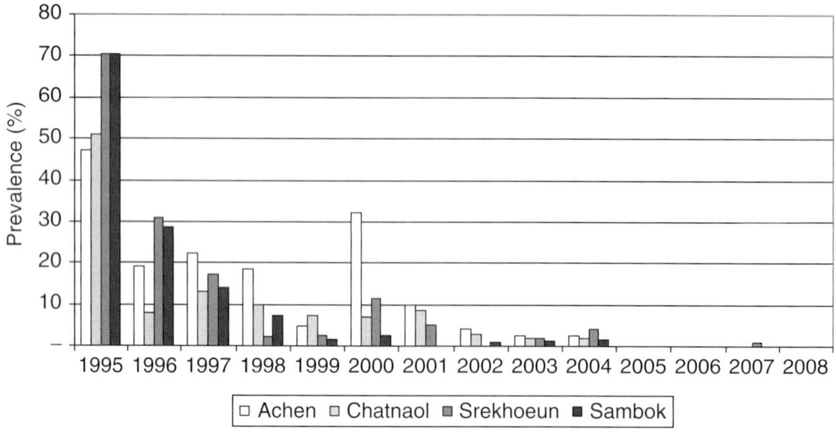

FIGURE 7.2 Evolution of *S. mekongi* prevalence in all four sentinel primary schools in the province of Kratie from 1995 to 2003 after implementing a control programme consisting of praziquantel mass drug administration and health education (data source: National Centre for Parasitology, Entomology and Malaria Control, Phnom Penh, Cambodia).

Srekhoeurn and Sambok), the impact of control was monitored by annual stool examinations using the Kato-Katz technique (Katz et al., 1972) for a random sample of 120–150 children per village (Fig. 7.2). From the baseline infection prevalence of more than 70% (Stich et al., 1999), the prevalences dropped to below 5% in 2002 (Ohmae et al., 2004) and to zero in 2004 (Sinuon et al., 2007). Similar achievements were observed in Stung Treng province. From infection rates of 6–88% in 1997, a reduction to 0.7–3.5% in 2005 was achieved (Sinuon et al., 2007). The central feature of interventions was MDA using praziquantel against schistosomiasis (single 40 mg/kg oral dose) and mebendazole against soil-transmitted helminth infections (single 500 mg oral dose) for all individuals except children under the age of 2 years and pregnant women. Health education was an integral part in all community intervention activities.

In early 1994, control activities started in the district hospital of Sambo. In the first months, a large proportion of the outpatients were schistosomiasis mekongi cases (60% in March 1994, Fig. 7.3). This percentage dropped to below 10% after January 1995 when MDA commenced in the communities. Large-scale treatments led to rapid improvements in health of the general population. A cohort of 118 primary schoolchildren of Sambok village was followed. At baseline in December 1994, only 18% of the subjects had a normal-sized liver; one and a half years later, most children improved and 70% of them had a normal-sized liver (Fig. 7.4). The transmission of *S. mekongi* was only marginally affected by a single round of MDA and health education. In the Sambok cohort, the infection

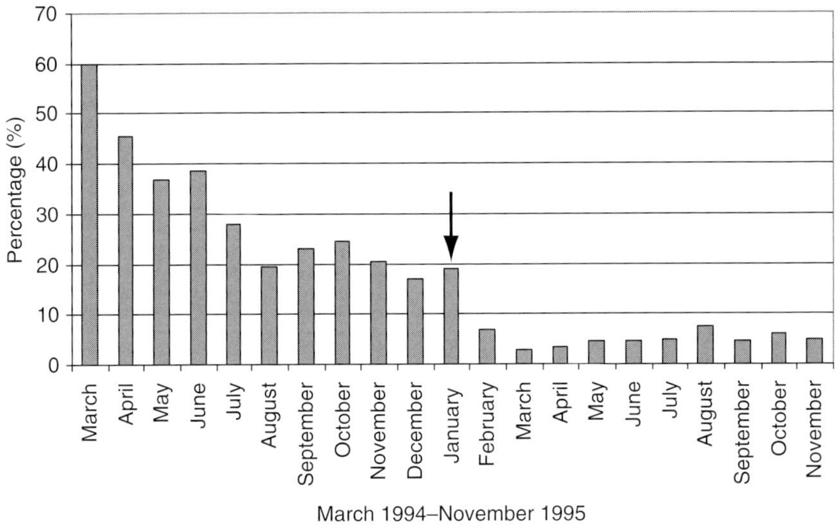

FIGURE 7.3 District hospital of Sambo: proportion of schistosomiasis patients among all outpatients from March 1994 to November 1995 (arrow: start of first mass drug administration with praziquantel in the communities).

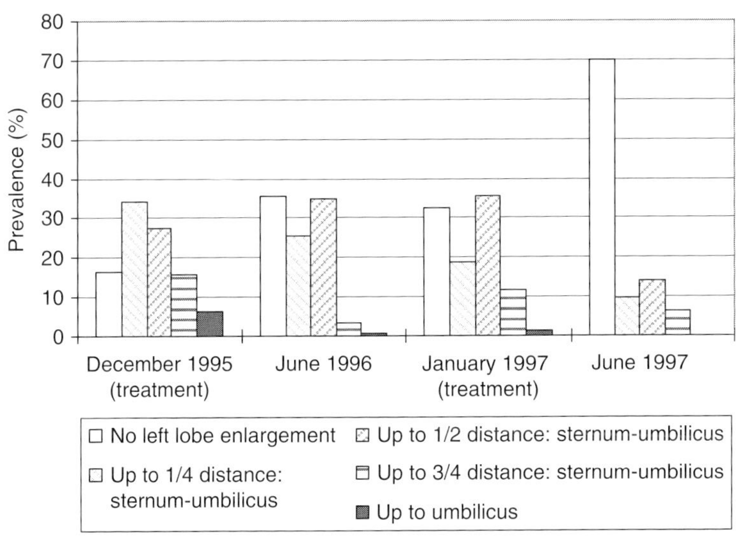

FIGURE 7.4 Cohort of schoolchildren in Sambok ($n = 118$): cumulative prevalence and intensity of infection with *S. mekongi* of five stool examination at baseline (December 1995), and 6 months (June 1996) and 12 months (January 1997) with praziquantel treatment (single 40 mg/kg oral dose) at baseline and 12 months.

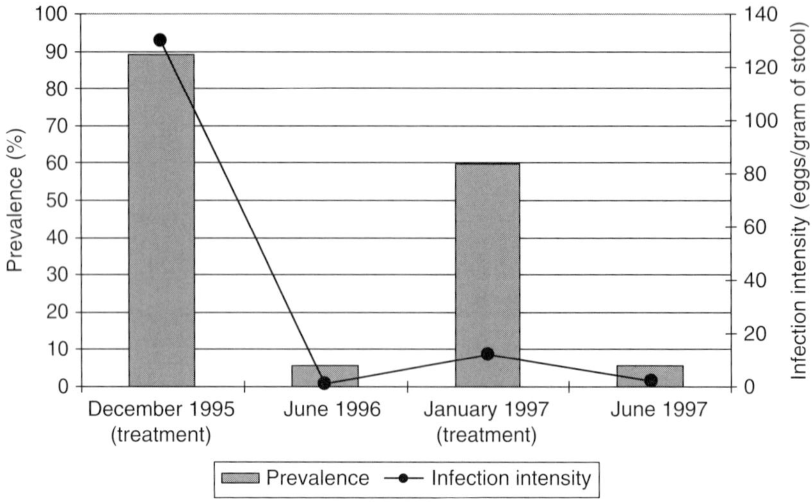

FIGURE 7.5 Cohort of schoolchildren in Sambok ($n = 118$): left liver lobe enlargement (classification used in Biays et al., 1999) at baseline (December 1995), and 6 months (June 1996), 12 months (January 1997), and 18 months (June 1997) with praziquantel treatment (single 40 mg/kg oral dose) at baseline and 12 months.

rates of 90% in December 1994 dropped after treatment to below 5% in June 1996 but returned to 60% when evaluated 12 months after treatment (Fig. 7.5). However, intensity of infection remained very low.

Although after 1997, hepatomegaly in the communities became relatively rare, subclinical pathology in the community was still of concern. The difficult political situation at the start of the programme did not allow a proper baseline survey to be conducted on the presence of subclinical liver pathology associated with *S. mekongi* infection. Only in the village of Sdau in Stung Treng province was a pre-intervention ultrasound assessment carried out and this revealed a high rate of liver pathology (Urbani et al., 2002). However, later studies assessed liver pathology in the schistosomiasis-endemic Kratie provinces with ultrasonography and linked it to the control measures. In 2001 and 2002, Chigusa et al. (2006) examined more than 300 individuals from 10 villages. The researchers chose the presence of thickening of the portal vein wall and formation of meandering collateral circulation of the splenic vein as the main parameters examined, as they can be assessed with little inter-observer variations. The study showed that thickening of the portal vein wall diameter had the potential to improve with successive rounds of treatment. However, other parameters such as established hard splenomegaly and meandering collateral circulation of the splenic vein remained unchanged. In 2002, after the seventh round of MDA, Keang et al. (2007) compared subclinical liver morbidity of adult villagers living in areas endemic for schistosomiasis with non-endemic areas of Kratié province. There was a clear difference between the two areas. While in the non-endemic control district of Chhlong, subclinical liver morbidity was absent, substantial morbidity was diagnosed in the schistosomiasis-endemic district, for example, in 45.5% of 342 study participants in the endemic setting, advanced periportal fibrosis with portal hypertension was detected *versus* none in the non-endemic district. Although other causes such as hepatitis cannot be entirely excluded, it was concluded that a large extent of the observed morbidity was residual morbidity due to *S. mekongi* infection. Hence, these two in-depth investigations showed that partial resolution of subclinical liver morbidity following praziquantel administration was possible. However, a complete resolution of *S. mekongi* was certainly not possible. These findings were in line with observations on liver morbidity induced by the closely related species of *S. japonicum* (Li et al., 2000, 2002).

At the individual case level, remarkable success was achieved in the treatment of some patients who recovered. This is exemplified by the following two cases: First, a 14-year-old boy was initially seen in November 1994 in poor general status (Fig. 7.6A), weighed only 14 kg and had a height of only 115 cm, which corresponded to severe stunting with a height for age *z*-score of −5 standard deviations (Biays et al., 1999). The boy suffered for several years from chronic, bloody diarrhoea. Hepato- and splenomegaly were diagnosed. Four months after treatment with praziquantel (25 mg/kg body weight for 3 days), he had gained 8 kg in weight (Fig. 7.6B). Two years after the initial treatment (January 1997,

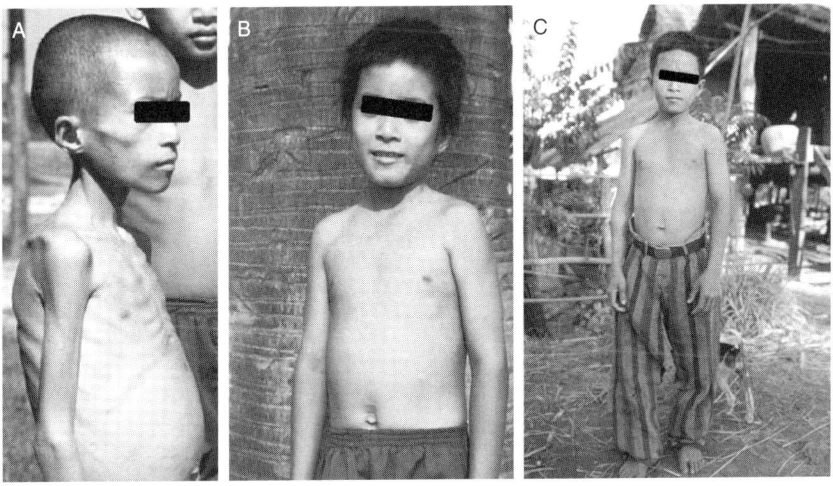

FIGURE 7.6 Fourteen-year-old boy from Sre-Khoeurn infected with *S. mekongi* in November 1994 (A), and 4 months (March 1995; B) and 2 years (January 1997; C) after praziquantel treatment.

Fig. 7.6C), he recovered completely and resumed fishing activities but remained small for his age. Second, a severely affected 7-year-old girl developed into a healthy adolescent over a 10-year period following treatment with praziquantel (Fig. 7.7A–C).

Those patients with severe schistosomiasis and complications linked to portal hypertension were mostly found hospitalised at the district hospital of Sambo. Very few patients who had been hospitalised, treated and discharged in 1994 and 1995 were found alive during a follow-up visit in 1999 (unpublished data).

In 1998, a considerable number of patients with signs of portal vein hypertension remained. In district and provincial hospitals, patients with severe gastrointestinal bleeding due to rupture of oesophageal varices were regularly seen. Mortality in the course of these events was high. In consideration of a potential surgical intervention, 106 patients with signs of portal hypertension were identified and further evaluated (Dumurgier et al., 2006). Eleven patients were identified with favourable general health status such that a surgical intervention was proposed (four mesenterico-cave shunt with an interposition of a graft, one operation of ''Hassap'' after splenectomy and six proximal spleno-renal diversions after splenectomy). Surgeries were carried out at Calmette hospital in Phnom Penh. One patient died 10 days after operation due to hepatic insufficiency. The remaining patients were followed up for a mean duration of 42 months and all of them resumed work. None of the patients suffered from subsequent episodes of bleeding. A liver biopsy taken during

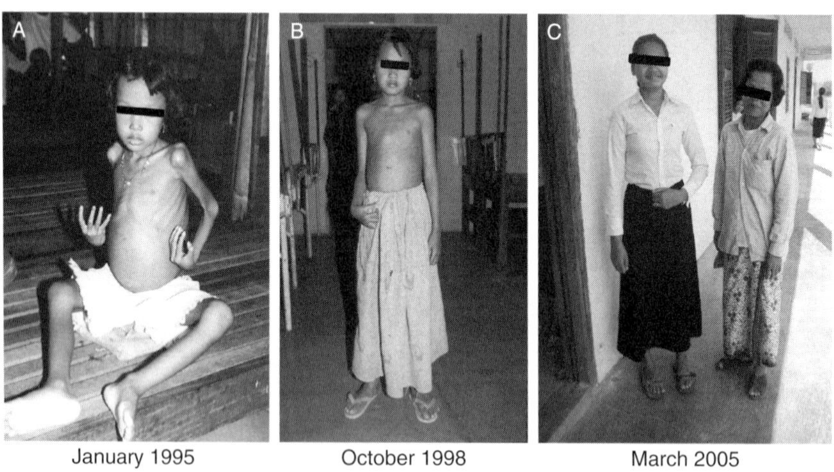

FIGURE 7.7 Seven-year-old girl at Sambo district hospital infected with *S. mekongi* in January 1995 (A), and 3.5 years (October 1998; B) and 10 years after praziquantel treatment (March 2005; C).

surgical intervention in these patients showed a high degree of liver pathology, including a severe degree of fibrosis, normally not seen in schistosomiasis (Monchy et al., 2006).

Annual universal MDA was carried out in Kratie from 1994/1995 and in Stung Treng from 1997 with an exception in 1998 when insufficient funds were available for the intervention. Under universal MDA, everybody other than children under the age of 2 years and women who were pregnant or breastfeeding, was offered a single 40 mg/kg oral dose of praziquantel. Coverage was between 62% and 67% until 2004, subsequently coverage increased to 83% (data from CNM). In 2003, targeted rather than universal MDA was carried out. In 2004, a few newly infected individuals were detected at several localities (Sinuon et al., 2007), thus indicating that the danger of re-emergence of transmission was real. Reservoir animal hosts such as dogs and pigs are believed to have contributed to the persistence, suggesting that sustained control, in concert with rigorous surveillance, is an indispensable element of control in the future. Currently, coverage remains high (84.8% in Kratie in 2008) due to the efforts of provincial and local health staff. The education campaign included local radio spots and poster messages (CNM report 2008). When interviewed, local people also reported that they received information from teachers, village volunteers and community leaders. This local support and ownership of the project is encouraging.

With the use of mathematical modelling, Hisakane et al. (2008) studied the impact of different interventions on the prevalence of *S. mekongi* (Ishikawa and Ohmae, 2009). In particular, they compared the effects of universal treatment *versus* targeted treatment (drugs administered to infected individuals only). Their simulations indicated that both strategies reduce high infection rates, such as those observed in Cambodia (70%), to prevalences below 5%. However, it is essential that the interventions are conducted for at least 8 years. Therefore, it is the commitment to long-lasting interventions (8 consecutive years at least), which is a key factor for success.

Consequently, the funding of successful control of Mekong schistosomiasis is a central issue. Although the Cambodian experience must be considered as cost-effective, for example, to treat an individual amounted to US$ 1.02 per year and the cost of averting severe infection was estimated at US$ 61.50; the overall cost of the intervention was too high to be covered by the Cambodian MoH (Croce et al., 2010). Hence, partners for control with a long-term commitment are essential. In Cambodia, MSF's initiatives have been taken up successfully by the MoH and WHO, with the support of the Sasakawa Memorial Health Foundation. In addition, at all stages, international organizations were involved with an interest in operational research. This led to significant scientific support of Cambodian national staff, to improved quality of routine data on the intervention and to the examination of pertinent operational questions, for example, the dipstick dye immunoassay (DDIA) developed in the People's Republic of China (P.R. China) for the detection of *S. japonicum* infection was validated to diagnose *S. mekongi* infection in Cambodia. This rapid and cheap test proved to be highly sensitive. Unfortunately, the DDIA showed substantial cross-reactivity with *O. viverrini* infection (Zhu et al., 2005). Importantly though, in *S. mekongi*-endemic provinces of Cambodia, *O. viverrini* infection does not play a major role, and hence the DDIA will be useful for immunodiagnosis of *S. mekongi*, although results have to be interpreted with caution. However, in southern Lao PDR where *S. mekongi* and *O. viverrini* co-infections are common, the DDIA will not be applicable.

7.5. CONTROL OF SCHISTOSOMIASIS IN LAO PDR

In view of the documented severe cases and community investigations carried out in the 1970s, together with the epidemiological surveys conducted in the late 1980s, it was concluded that the control of schistosomiasis was of pressing necessity (Mott, 1991). Furthermore, observations on Khong Island showed that risk factors for *S. mekongi* transmission were highly prevalent; almost all households were using exclusively the Mekong River for bathing and household-related activities. Most of the river shores were suitable habitats for the *N. aperta* snails, and almost half of the population did not use any type of latrine (Thamkeo and Pholsena, 2003).

With technical support from the WHO, the MoH of Lao PDR designed a community-based intervention, which was launched in 1989. By 1995, five rounds of MDA with praziquantel (40 mg/kg body weight) were implemented in Khong and Mounlapamok districts in Champasack province (Kimura, 1994; Thamkeo and Pholsena, 2003). The treatment strategy depended on the prevalence of *S. mekongi* infection. In villages with an infection prevalence of more than 50%, the entire population received treatment. All children (2–14 years) and infected children only received treatment in villages with an infection prevalence between 25% and 50% and below 25%, respectively. The exact number of people who benefited from the intervention varies according to authors, but it is clear that tremendous efforts were undertaken to reach a large fraction of the at-risk population with preventive chemotherapy. For example, Thamkeo and Pholsena (2003) reported that in the first year, 37,689 persons in 129 villages received the intervention, corresponding to 88% of the targeted population. In the fifth year, almost 20,000 people in 108 villages were treated, with a somewhat lower coverage of 46% (Thamkeo and Pholsena, 2003). As the strategy employed required parallel stool examination, substantial effort was made to develop human resources to deliver the interventions and to monitor the progress made. In order to support these efforts, a workshop on schistosomiasis was held in October 1990 (Mott, 1991).

In the selective treatment of children aged between 4 and 16 years at the initial round of treatment, some 3000 individuals received praziquantel (Swillen, 1990). The efficacy of the intervention (praziquantel, single 40 mg/kg oral dose) was assessed, which revealed an overall cure rate of 88% in 53 individuals subjected to pre- and post-treatment evaluation. This efficacy was regarded as sufficiently high to continue with this treatment regimen, given the advantage that praziquantel could be administered in a single dose. For subsequent treatment rounds, all individuals aged 4–69 years were eligible, except pregnant and lactating women. The frequency of side effects after praziquantel treatment was of concern. Complaints were very frequent. In 102 schoolchildren followed up after treatment, headache, diarrhoea and abdominal pain were reported in 52.9%, 42.1% and 19.6%, respectively (Thamkeo and Pholsena, 2003). Vomiting (16.6%) was also frequent. It was thought that these adverse events might also contribute to lower compliance in re-treatment efforts.

In 1998, a further treatment round was performed targeting 424 villages (8 communes) in the Champasack province bordering the Mekong; 129,585 persons were reached, resulting in an overall coverage of 52.2% (Thamkeo and Pholsena, 2003).

After completion of treatment, in a thorough evaluation of infection status in the targeted communities, it was found that the prevalence of infection had been reduced dramatically. In 1994, only 0.4% of schoolchildren were diagnosed with a *S. mekongi* infection, as compared to an estimated baseline prevalence of 30%. The sharp decline in both prevalence and intensity of infection was also confirmed in other community members (Kimura, 1994). In 1999, *S. mekongi* infections occurred only in 5 out of 21 villages surveyed; all rates observed were below 8% (Thamkeo and Pholsena, 2003). In this context, it is interesting to note that while *S. mekongi* infection prevalences were dramatically reduced, the prevalence of *O. viverrini* infection in the same villages remained unchanged (Thamkeo and Pholsena, 2003).

Over the intervention period, a clear reduction in the overall coverage rate was observed. While at the start, in some villages, 70% of the eligible population were given praziquantel (Swillen, 1993a,b), coverage rates dropped to 40% in subsequent years (Kimura, 1994). The disappearance, in endemic villages, of recognised gastrointestinal symptoms such as blood in stool and abdominal pain reduced the perceived importance of infection in the community, and hence the perceived need for re-treatment. Furthermore, on several occasions, the treatment was provided during the months with the highest precipitation (July and August), and hence it was difficult to reach community members, as many farmers and their families were working in the rice fields and were therefore not available to receive free treatment.

In 1991, as a further preventive measure, control of *N. aperta* intermediate host snail was attempted. Niclosamide, wrapped into small bags, was introduced into water, and before and after the snail population was monitored. The trial, however, proved disappointing. While *N. aperta* could not be found 1 day after the niclosamide application, snail densities were back to pre-trial levels 5–9 days after the application (Thamkeo and Pholsena, 2003).

The altogether encouraging results of the MDA activities were also attributed to the additional health education and water and sanitation interventions, which took place alongside preventive chemotherapy. In 1989, for example, in Khong district, the *Adventist Development Relief Agency* (ADRA) installed over 100 water pumps and more than 460 latrines (Swillen, 1993a). Emphasis was also put on health education; that is, informing the communities and in particular schoolchildren, on how schistosomiasis is transmitted, and how the disease can be recognised, prevented and treated. In the final examination before leaving school, a question pertaining to schistosomiasis was systematically included (Swillen, 1993a). Research carried out in P.R. China and elsewhere clearly documented that a package of interventions is necessary to produce a lasting effect on schistosomiasis and that such efforts can also have an impact beyond the target diseases, most notably on soil-transmitted helminth infections (Utzinger et al., 2009; Wang et al., 2009b).

The final evaluation in 1994 stated that schistosomiasis had been successfully controlled. At the same time, it was emphasised that transmission was not interrupted, and therefore, that the infection prevalence and intensity will almost certainly increase if water contact along the Mekong River does not cease.

Indeed, the fears that *S. mekongi* infections might re-emerge proved correct. In 2000, during a community-based cross-sectional survey in the province of Champasack, infection rates between 3% and 10% were found in several villages. In one village, the infection rate reached 26.8% (H. Strandgaarts, personal communication). In 2006, a quarter of 225 habitants of Don Long Island in Khong district tested positive for *S. mekongi* (unpublished data).

In recent follow-up studies of earlier patients, several patients with severe complications of schistosomiasis were detected (Phonephasong Soukhathammavong, personal communication). On Don Long Island, nine patients were diagnosed and followed up after treatment. Most importantly, in addition to patients aged 30 years and above, infection and morbidity were also diagnosed in young children aged only 5 or 7 years. This observation is of particular concern as infections in younger individuals point to recent and ongoing transmission at a level that is sufficiently high as to lead to the development of severe schistosomiasis.

In 2008, annual MDA has resumed, targeting the entire population in schistosomiasis-endemic districts in southern Lao PDR (Dr. Keoka, Provincial Malaria Station, Pakse, personal communication). Detailed reports on the activity of the newly started control efforts are not available yet.

7.6. REMAINING CHALLENGES AND A WAY FORWARD

During the past 20+ years, our understanding of the epidemiology and control of schistosomiasis mekongi has deepened and the burden of disease in the affected populations in Cambodia and Lao PDR has been substantially reduced. In parallel, individual and institutional capacity to conduct research and control has been built up and strengthened. The main challenge now is to organize, implement and sustain control activities consistent with the specific needs of the two countries involved. In Cambodia, the population in the schistosomiasis-endemic provinces has benefited from 15+ years of intensive control efforts. The programme has led to a virtual elimination of schistosomiasis as a public health problem (Montresor et al., 2008). Some authors argue that elimination could be envisaged in this setting even with the ongoing presence of *N. aperta* (Ohmae et al., 2004). Given the fact that in the southern part of Lao PDR substantial transmission is still ongoing, elimination in neighbouring Cambodia might be a too optimistic goal, as the introduction of the parasite into the downstream area is very likely. In our view, vigilant follow up and further consolidation of the achievements made to date is a viable option for the near future.

Before setting a more ambitious goal such as elimination of the parasite from the region, substantial and long-term investment must re-enforce the control in Lao PDR. In recent years, with the renewed interest in the control of neglected tropical diseases, schistosomiasis control resumed in the country. However, long-term commitment from Lao PDR and regional and international communities is required to reduce infection and transmission to a close to zero level.

At the same time, it must be stressed that schistosomiasis-endemic areas are known to be endemic for several other helminthic diseases and tropical diseases that are often neglected. Indeed, multiple parasitic infections are the norm rather than the exception across large parts of Southeast Asia (Steinmann et al., 2010). Control initiatives in schistosomiasis-endemic areas need to take into account this fact and enhance synergies within and between programmes and initiatives (Hotez and Ehrenberg, 2010).

The distribution of the snail intermediate host of *S. mekongi* is closely linked to the transmission of the disease. It has been assumed that the snail invaded Southeast Asia from southern P.R. China and that the presently observed state of distribution was the final pattern the snail species could reach due to its ecological requirements for microhabitats. However, recent work has shed new light on the distribution patterns of *N. aperta* and *S. mekongi* from an entirely different angle. Attwood and colleagues analysed genetic variation and delineated clades of *N. aperta* from locations throughout Southeast Asia—from Lao PDR, Cambodia and Thailand with a view to better explain the current distribution pattern (Attwood et al., 2008a,b). Based on their analyses, it appears that the distribution of *S. mekongi* shows a historical expansion that is lagging behind that of the snail intermediate host. According to these authors, *N. aperta* is in the process of invading Lao PDR (where many *N. aperta* populations occur in the absence of *S. mekongi*) from the South; therefore, the potential maximum distribution of *S. mekongi* has yet to be reached. These predictions are of considerable public health importance. For example, the absence of snails in lakes, small ponds and other freshwater habitats, which has been explained by the unsuitability of these sites for the snail due to their ecological conditions, may be due to the fact that the snail has not yet had the chance to reach these environments. Hence, there is no likely ecological barrier to a wider distribution of *N. aperta* in the future, which would invaluably result in wider and more intense transmission potential of the parasite. Recent observations in *Schistosoma*-infected Israeli travellers to Lao PDR provide some evidence that transmission might occur in places where it has not been reported earlier, for example, north of Vientiane (Leshem et al., 2009).

Clearly, these findings warrant careful follow up, and must trigger prudence when large-scale demographic, environmental and social transformations occur within the framework of major water resource developments (Steinmann et al., 2006). While a recent health impact assessment pertaining to a large hydroelectric project in central Lao PDR concluded that schistosomiasis does not currently represent a major health threat, the risk profile might change in the years to come (Erlanger et al., 2008). In this context, it is of considerable interest that in Lao PDR, more than 70 hydroelectric projects at various scales are in the planning stage, several of which include substantial water body development.

As infection prevalence and intensity will be lower in the future, the choice of diagnostic techniques will become a critical issue. The Kato-Katz method has a low sensitivity for diagnosing *S. mekongi* and other schistosome species, particularly when infection intensities are low (Bergquist et al., 2009). Besides repeated stool examination, the development and validation of new techniques must be considered and given due attention.

The other significant challenge is the lack of available guidelines on schistosomiasis elimination and specifically experience about *S. mekongi* elimination. There is considerable support from the local people as many have been personally affected by schistosomiasis. It is a serious disease in the endemic areas with many deaths and distinctive symptoms. It is due to this support that the MDA programme has been so successful. However, this means that any attempt to reduce the frequency of MDA is met with criticism and resentment. Rates of schistosomiasis are now very low, but when there are no specific guidelines, little research on re-infection, and (from the Lao PDR's experience) rapid re-infection when control efforts are lowered, it is tempting to continue indefinitely. Cambodia, however, has limited resources and so must use what it has to maximum cost-effectiveness. Continuing programmes unnecessarily divert funds from other projects that could have more impact on the overall community health status.

ACKNOWLEDGEMENTS

We thank the guest editors for inviting us to prepare this manuscript, two external referees for a series of helpful comments and Mr. Kaspar Hurni for the preparation of Fig. 7.1.

REFERENCES

Attwood, S.W., 2001. Schistosomiasis in the Mekong region: epidemiology and phylogeography. Adv. Parasitol. 50, 87–152.

Attwood, S.W., Campbell, I., Upatham, E.S., Rollinson, D., 2004. Schistosomes in the Xe Kong River of Cambodia: the detection of *Schistosoma mekongi* in a natural population of snails and observations on the intermediate host's distribution. Ann. Trop. Med. Parasitol. 98, 221–230.

Attwood, S.W., Fatih, F.A., Campbell, I., Upatham, E.S., 2008a. The distribution of Mekong schistosomiasis, past and future: preliminary indications from an analysis of genetic variation in the intermediate host. Parasitol. Int. 57, 256–270.

Attwood, S.W., Fatih, F.A., Upatham, E.S., 2008b. DNA-sequence variation among *Schistosoma mekongi* populations and related taxa; phylogeography and the current distribution of Asian schistosomiasis. PLoS Negl. Trop. Dis. 2, e200.

Audebaud, G., Tournier-Lasserve, C., Brumpt, V., Jolly, M., Mazaud, R., Imbert, X., et al., 1968. Premier cas de bilharziose humane observé au Cambodge (région de Kratie). Bull. Soc. Pathol. Exot. Filiales 61, 778–784.

Barbier, M., 1966. Détermination d'un foyer de bilharziose artério-veigneuse au Sud-Laos. Bull. Soc. Pathol. Exot. Filiales 59, 974–983.

Barbier, M., 1967. Determination d'un foyer limite de bilharziose arterio-veineuse dan la province de Sithadone (sud Laos). Organisation Mondiale de la santé WHO/BILH/67.61.

Bergquist, R., Johansen, M.V., Utzinger, J., 2009. Diagnostic dilemmas in helminthology: what tools to use and when? Trends Parasitol. 25, 151–156.

Biays, S., 1995. La bilharziose à *Schistosoma mekongi*: aspects cliniques et données epidémiologiques dans la province de Kratie, Cambodge. Mémoire de DEA. Institut Santé et Développement, Paris V.

Biays, S., Stich, A.H., Odermatt, P., Long, C., Yersin, C., Men, C., et al., 1999. Foyer de bilharziose à *Schistosoma mekongi* redécouvert au Nord du Cambodge: I. Perception culturelle de la maladie; description et suivi de 20 cas cliniques graves. Trop. Med. Int. Health 4, 662–673.

Carmody, D., Nolan, C., Allcutt, D., 2008. Intracranial *Schistosoma mekongi* infection. Ir. Med. J. 101, 315.

Chhakda, T., Muth, S., Socheat, D., Odermatt, P., 2006. Intestinal parasites in school-aged children in villages bordering Tonle Sap Lake, Cambodia. Southeast Asian J. Trop. Med. Public Health 37, 859–864.

Chigusa, Y., Ohmae, H., Otake, H., Keang, H., Sinuon, M., Saem, C., et al., 2006. Effects of repeated praziquantel treatment on schistosomiasis mekongi morbidity as detected by ultrasonography. Parasitol. Int. 55, 261–265.

Croce, D., Porazzi, E., Foglia, E., Restelli, U., Sinuon, M., Socheat, D., et al., 2010. Cost-effectiveness of a successful schistosomiasis control programme in Cambodia (1995–2006). Acta Trop. 113, 279–284.

Davis, G.M., Kitikoon, V., Temcharoen, P., 1976. Monograph on ''Lithoglyphopsis'' aperta, the snail host of Mekong River schistosomiasis. Malacologia 15, 241–287.

Dumurgier, C., Tay, K.H., Surith, T.N., Rathat, C., Buisson, Y., Monchy, D., et al., 2006. Place de la chirurgie dans la prévention des récidives d'hémorragies digestives chez les sujets présentant une hypertension portale due à *Schistosoma mekongi*. Bull. Soc. Pathol. Exot. 99, 365–371.

Erlanger, T.E., Sayasone, S., Krieger, G.R., Kaul, S., Sananikhom, P., Tanner, M., et al., 2008. Baseline health situation of communities affected by the Nam Theun 2 hydroelectric project in central Lao PDR and indicators for monitoring. Int. J. Environ. Health Res. 18, 223–242.

Gray, D.J., Williams, G.M., Li, Y., Chen, H., Forsyth, S.J., Li, R.S., et al., 2009. A cluster-randomised intervention trial against *Schistosoma japonicum* in the People's Republic of China: bovine and human transmission. PLoS One 4, e5900.

Harinasuta, C., 1984. Epidemiology and control of schistosomiasis in Southeast Asia. Southeast Asian J. Trop. Med. Public Health 15, 431–438.

Hisakane, N., Kirinoki, M., Chigusa, Y., Sinuon, M., Socheat, D., Matsuda, H., et al., 2008. The evaluation of control measures against *Schistosoma mekongi* in Cambodia by a mathematical model. Parasitol. Int. 57, 379–385.

Hotez, P.J., Ehrenberg, J.P., 2010. Escalating the global fight against neglected tropical diseases through interventions in the Asia Pacific Region. Adv. Parasitol. 72, 31–53.

Houston, S., Kowalewska-Grochowska, K., Naik, S., McKean, J., Johnson, E.S., Warren, K., 2004. First report of *Schistosoma mekongi* infection with brain involvement. Clin. Infect. Dis. 38, e1–e6.

Iijima, T., 1970. Enquête épidémiologique sur la bilharziose. Rapport de mission: 13 novembre 1968 - 8 mai 1969. -WPR/059-70.

Iijima, T., Garcia, R.G., 1967. Rapport d'affectation (enquête préliminaire sur la bilharziose au Laos Méridional). O.M.S. Bureau Rég. Pacif. Occid. Doc. WPRO-80, 23 mai 1967 (11 pages, 3 cartes).

Ishikawa, H., Ohmae, H., 2009. Modeling the dynamics and control of transmission of *Schistosoma japonicum* and *S. mekongi* in Southeast Asia. Korean J. Parasitol. 47, 1–5.

Jolly, M., Bazillio, R., Audebaud, G., Brumpt, V., Sophinn, B., 1970a. Existence au Cambodge d'un foyer de bilharziose humaine, dans la région de Kratié. II. Enquête épidémiologique. Résultats préliminaires. Med. Trop. (Mars) 30, 462–471.

Jolly, M., Bazillio, R., Audebaud, G., Brumpt, V., Sophinn, B., 1970b. Premières recherches épidémiologiques sur un foyer de bilharziose humaine au Cambodge, dans la région de Kratié. Bull. Soc. Pathol. Exot. Filiales 63, 476–483.

Katz, N., Chaves, A., Pellegrino, J., 1972. A simple device for quantitative stool thick-smear technique in schistosomiasis mansoni. Rev. Inst. Med. Trop. Sao Paulo 14, 397–400.

Keang, H., Odermatt, P., Odermatt-Biays, S., Cheam, S., Degremont, A., Hatz, C., 2007. Liver morbidity due to *Schistosoma mekongi* in Cambodia after seven rounds of mass drug administration. Trans. R. Soc. Trop. Med. Hyg. 101, 759–765.

Keittivuti, B., D'Agnes, T., Keittivuti, A., Viravaidya, M., 1982. Prevalence of schistosomiasis and other parasitic diseases among Cambodian refugees residing in Bang-Kaeng holding center, Prachinburi province, Thailand. Am. J. Trop. Med. Hyg. 31, 988–990.

Kimura, E., 1994. Evaluation of schistosomiasis control in Khong Island, Lao People's Democratic Republic. WP/ICP/PDP/004/RB/94, WHO report, n/d.

Kitikoon, V., 1984. Taxonomy and susceptibilities of molluscan intermediate hosts of human *Schistosoma* in Southeast Asia. Southeast Asian J. Trop. Med. Public Health 15, 462–468.

Kitikoon, V., Schneider, C.R., 1976. Notes on the aquatic ecology of *Lithoglyphopsis aperta*. Southeast Asian J. Trop. Med. Public Health 7, 238–243.

Kitikoon, V., Sornmani, S., Pathammavong, O., 1971. Studies on the size and shape of eggs of *Schistosoma japonicum* at Khong Island, southern Laos. Southeast Asian J. Trop. Med. Public Health 2, 101–102.

Leshem, E., Meltzer, E., Marva, E., Schwartz, E., 2009. Travel-related schistosomiasis acquired in Laos. Emerg. Infect. Dis. 15, 1823–1826.

Li, Y.S., Sleigh, A.C., Ross, A.G., Li, Y., Williams, G.M., Tanner, M., et al., 2000. Two-year impact of praziquantel treatment for *Schistosoma japonicum* infection in China: re-infection, subclinical disease and fibrosis marker measurements. Trans. R. Soc. Trop. Med. Hyg. 94, 191–197.

Li, Y.S., Sleigh, A.C., Li, Y., Tanner, M., Dessein, A., Williams, G.M., et al., 2002. Five-year impact of repeated praziquantel treatment on subclinical morbidity due to *Schistosoma japonicum* in China. Trans. R. Soc. Trop. Med. Hyg. 96, 438–443.

Lin, D.D., Liu, J.X., Liu, Y.M., Hu, F., Zhang, Y.Y., Xu, J.M., et al., 2008. Routine Kato-Katz technique underestimates the prevalence of *Schistosoma japonicum*: a case study in an endemic area of the People's Republic of China. Parasitol. Int. 57, 281–286.

Matsumoto, J., Muth, S., Socheat, D., Matsuda, H., 2002. The first reported cases of canine schistosomiasis mekongi in Cambodia. Southeast Asian J. Trop. Med. Public Health 33, 458–461.

McManus, D.P., Li, Y., Gray, D.J., Ross, A.G., 2009. Conquering 'snail fever': schistosomiasis and its control in China. Expert. Rev. Anti. Infect. Ther. 7, 473–485.

Monchy, D., Dumurgier, C., Heng, T.K., Hong, K., Khun, H., Hou, S.V., et al., 2006. Lésions histologiques hépatiques de la schistosomose due à *Schistosoma mekongi*. À propos de six cas avec hypertension portale sévère opérés au Cambodge. Bull. Soc. Pathol. Exot. 99, 359–364.

Montresor, A., Cong, D.T., Sinuon, M., Tsuyuoka, R., Chanthavisouk, C., Strandgaard, H., et al., 2008. Large-scale preventive chemotherapy for the control of helminth infection in Western Pacific countries: six years later. PLoS Negl. Trop. Dis. 2, e278.

Mott, K.E., 1991. Training course on the diagnosis and control of *S. mekongi* and other helminthic infections. Mission report: 19 to 30 October 1990. LAO/PDP/001, WHO report, n/d.

Mouchet, F., 1995. Malacological data on transmission of *Schistosoma mekongi* in Cambodia. European Conference on Tropical Medicine.

Ohmae, H., Sinuon, M., Kirinoki, M., Matsumoto, J., Chigusa, Y., Socheat, D., et al., 2004. Schistosomiasis mekongi: from discovery to control. Parasitol. Int. 53, 135–142.

Ross, A.G., Vickers, D., Olds, G.R., Shah, S.M., McManus, D.P., 2007. Katayama syndrome. Lancet Infect. Dis. 7, 218–224.

Schneider, C.R., Kitikoon, V., Sornmani, S., Thirachantra, S., 1975. Mekong schistosomiasis. III: a parasitological survey of domestic water buffalo (*Bubalus bubalis*) on Khong Island. Laos. Ann. Trop. Med. Parasitol. 69, 227–232.
Shimada, M., Kato-Hayashi, N., Chigusa, Y., Nakamura, S., Ohmae, H., Sinuon, M., et al., 2007. High susceptibility of *Neotricula aperta* gamma-strain from Krakor and Sdau in Cambodia to *Schistosoma mekongi* from Khong Island in Laos. Parasitol. Int. 56, 157–160.
Sinuon, M., Tsuyuoka, R., Socheat, D., Odermatt, P., Ohmae, H., Matsuda, H., et al., 2007. Control of *Schistosoma mekongi* in Cambodia: results of eight years of control activities in the two endemic provinces. Trans. R. Soc. Trop. Med. Hyg. 101, 34–39.
Sornmani, S., Kitikoon, V., Schneider, C.R., Harinasuta, C., Pathammavong, O., 1973a. Mekong schistosomiasis. 1. Life cycle of *Schistosoma japonicum*, Mekong strain in the laboratory. Southeast Asian J. Trop. Med. Public Health 4, 218–225.
Sornmani, S., Schneider, C.R., Kitikoon, V., 1973b. Life cycle of *Schistosoma japonicum*-like trematode from Khong Island Southern Laos. Southeast Asian J. Trop. Med. Public Health 4, 279.
Sornmani, S., Vivatanasesth, P., Thirachantra, S., 1976. Clinical study of Mekong schistosomiasis at Khong Island Southern Laos. Southeast Asian J. Trop. Med. Public Health 7, 270–281.
Soukhathammavong, P., Sayasone, S., Harimanana, A.N., Akkhavong, A., Thammasack, S., Phoumindr, N., et al., 2008. Three cases of intestinal capillariasis in Lao People's Democratic Republic. Am. J. Trop. Med. Hyg. 79, 735–738.
Steinmann, P., Keiser, J., Bos, R., Tanner, M., Utzinger, J., 2006. Schistosomiasis and water resources development: systematic review, meta-analysis, and estimates of people at risk. Lancet Infect. Dis. 6, 411–425.
Steinmann, P., Utzinger, J., Du, Z.W., Zhou, X.N., 2010. Multiparasitism: a neglected reality on global, regional and local scale. Adv. Parasitol. 73, 21–50.
Stich, A.H., Biays, S., Odermatt, P., Men, C., Saem, C., Sokha, K., et al., 1999. Foci of schistosomiasis mekongi Northern Cambodia: II. Distribution of infection and morbidity. Trop. Med. Int. Health 4, 674–685.
Strandgaard, H., Johansen, M.V., Pholsena, K., Teixayavong, K., Christensen, N.O., 2001. The pig as a host for *Schistosoma mekongi* in Laos. J. Parasitol. 87, 708–709.
Swillen, L., 1990. Report on Field Visit to the Lao People's Democratic Republic. WP/PDV/LAO/PDP/001, WHO report, n/d.
Swillen, L., 1993a. Report on a Field Trip to Khong District: 12 to 29 July 1993. LAO/MAL/002, WHO report, n/d.
Swillen, L., 1993b. Report on a Field Trip to Khong Island: 7 to 11 September 1993. LAO/MAL/002, WHO report, n/d.
Thamkeo, T., Pholsena, K., 2003. Control of schistosomiasis due to *Schistosoma mekongi* in Khong District, 1989–1999. In: Crompton, D.W.T., Montresor, A., Nesheim, M.C., Savioli, L. (Eds.), Control of disease due to helminth infections. World Health Organization, Geneva.
Tournier-Lasserve, C., Audebaud, G., Brumpt, V., Jolly, M., Calvez, F., Mazaud, R., et al., 1970. Existence au Cambodge d'un foyer de bilharziose humaine, dans la rédion de Kratié I. Etude des trois premiers cas cliniques. Med. Trop. (Mars) 30, 451–461.
Urbani, C., Sinoun, M., Socheat, D., Pholsena, K., Strandgaard, H., Odermatt, P., et al., 2002. Epidemiology and control of mekongi schistosomiasis. Acta Trop. 82, 157–168.
Utzinger, J., Booth, M., N'Goran, E.K., Müller, I., Tanner, M., Lengeler, C., 2001. Relative contribution of day-to-day and intra-specimen variation in faecal egg counts of *Schistosoma mansoni* before and after treatment with praziquantel. Parasitology 122, 537–544.
Utzinger, J., Raso, G., Brooker, S., de Savigny, D., Tanner, M., Ornbjerg, N., et al., 2009. Schistosomiasis and neglected tropical diseases: towards integrated and sustainable control and a word of caution. Parasitology 136, 1859–1874.

Vic-Dupont, B.E., Soubrane, J., Halle, B., Richir, C., 1957. Bilharziose à *Schistosoma japonicum* à forme hépato-spléenique révélée par une grande hématemese. Bull. Mem. Soc. Med. Hop. Paris 73, 933–941.
Voge, M., Bruckner, D., Bruce, J.I., 1978. *Schistosoma mekongi* sp. n. from man and animals, compared with four geographic strains of *Schistosoma japonicum*. J. Parasitol. 64, 577–584.
Wang, T.P., Johansen, M.V., Zhang, S.Q., Wang, F.F., Wu, W.D., Zhang, G.H., et al., 2005. Transmission of *Schistosoma japonicum* by humans and domestic animals in the Yangtze River valley, Anhui province, China. Acta Trop. 96, 198–204.
Wang, L., Utzinger, J., Zhou, X.N., 2008. Schistosomiasis control: experiences and lessons from China. Lancet 372, 1793–1795.
Wang, L.D., Chen, H.G., Guo, J.G., Zeng, X.J., Hong, X.L., Xiong, J.J., et al., 2009a. A strategy to control transmission of *Schistosoma japonicum* in China. N. Engl. J. Med. 360, 121–128.
Wang, L.D., Guo, J.G., Wu, X.H., Chen, H.G., Wang, T.P., Zhu, S.P., et al., 2009b. China's new strategy to block *Schistosoma japonicum* transmission: experiences and impact beyond schistosomiasis. Trop. Med. Int. Health 14, 1475–1483.
Wittes, R., MacLean, J.D., Law, C., Lough, J.O., 1984. Three cases of schistosomiasis mekongi from northern Laos. Am. J. Trop. Med. Hyg. 33, 1159–1165.
Yu, J.M., de Vlas, S.J., Jiang, Q.W., Gryseels, B., 2007. Comparison of the Kato-Katz technique, hatching test and indirect hemagglutination assay (IHA) for the diagnosis of *Schistosoma japonicum* infection in China. Parasitol. Int. 56, 45–49.
Zhang, Y.Y., Luo, J.P., Liu, Y.M., Wang, Q.Z., Chen, J.H., Xu, M.X., et al., 2009. Evaluation of Kato-Katz examination method in three areas with low-level endemicity of schistosomiasis japonica in China: a Bayesian modeling approach. Acta Trop. 112, 16–22.
Zhou, X.N., Bergquist, N.R., Leonardo, L., Yang, G.J., Yang, K., Sudomo, M., et al., 2010. Schistosomiasis japonica: research and control. Adv. Parasitol. 72, 145–178.
Zhu, Y.C., Socheat, D., Bounlu, K., Liang, Y.S., Sinuon, M., Insisiengmay, S., et al., 2005. Application of dipstick dye immunoassay (DDIA) kit for the diagnosis of schistosomiasis mekongi. Acta Trop. 96, 137–141.

CHAPTER 8

Elimination of Lymphatic Filariasis in Southeast Asia

Mohammad Sudomo,* **Sombat Chayabejara,**[†] **Socheat Duong,**[‡] **Leda Hernandez,**[§] **Wei-Ping Wu,**[¶] and **Robert Bergquist**[#]

Contents

* Ecology and Health Status Research and Development Centre, National Institute of Health Research and Development, Ministry of Health, Jakarta, Indonesia

† Chairman, Southeast Asian Regional Program Review Group (RPRG), Suanluang, Bangkok, Thailand

‡ National Centre for Parasitology, Entomology, and Malaria Control, Phnom Penh, Cambodia

§ Infectious Disease Office, National Center for Disease Prevention and Control, Department of Health, Manila, Philippines

¶ National Institute of Parasitic Diseases, Chinese Center for Disease Control and Prevention, Shanghai, People's Republic of China

\# Ingerod, Brastad, Sweden

Advances in Parasitology, Volume 72
ISSN 0065-308X, DOI: 10.1016/S0065-308X(10)72008-X

Abstract

Approximately 15 million people with lymphatic filariasis (LF) live in Southeast Asia. *Wuchereria bancrofti* (transmitted by the *Mansonia* and *Anopheles* vectors), *Brugia malayi* and *Brugia timori* (both transmitted by *Culex quinquefasciatus*) are the filarial species in this region. The endemic countries are: Cambodia, Lao People's Democratic Republic, the Philippines, Indonesia, Thailand and Timor-Leste, which have all agreed to eliminate transmission of the disease by 2020. The public health interventions with respect to LF are based on the 1997 World Health Assembly resolution (WHA 50.29) which recommends elimination of the disease through mass drug administration (MDA) using diethylcarbamazine (DEC) and albendazole. The drugs are generally donated and as governments contribute 60–90% of the operational costs, MDA is deemed to be comparatively inexpensive for local administrations in relation to other public health programmes. So far, elimination has been accomplished only in the People's Republic of China (P.R. China) and this achievement is therefore described here in some detail. Resurgences have occurred but they have been successfully dealt with. Historically, the endemic areas in P.R. China covered 16,514 townships (or urban sub-districts), situated in 864 counties (or cities) in 14 provinces (or autonomous regions or municipalities). The total population at risk of infection in all endemic areas of P.R. China was originally 342 million.

8.1. INTRODUCTION

Globally, 110–120 million people suffer from lymphatic filariasis (LF). *Wuchereria bancrofti* affects about 100 million people in Africa, India, Southeast Asia, the Pacific islands, South America and the Caribbean, while *Brugia malayi* and *Brugia timori* affect about 12 million people in Southeast Asia (http://www.dhpe.org/infect/Lymphfil.html). All three species are prevalent in the countries discussed here. The infection can be asymptomatic or it can present with fever and/or local swellings. It is well known because of its chronic complications such as lymphoedema, hydrocele and kidney damage which arise due to obstructions of the lymphatic system.

Bancroftian filariasis, principally transmitted by the vector *Culex quinquefasciatus*, is the most common infection in continental Asia, while *Brugia* infections, transmitted by *Mansonia* and *Anopheles* mosquitoes, dominate in the Indonesian archipelago. LF has been eliminated in the People 's Republic of China (P.R. China) but the vectors remain and they therefore require vigilant surveillance to ensure that the disease does not re-emerge. In P.R. China, the vectors of Bancroftian LF reside in two geographically separate areas around latitude N 32°; *Cx. pipiens pallens* is found north of this divide and *Cx. pipiens fatigans* is found south of it. The Brugian LF vector *Anopheles hircanus sinensis* is distributed all over the formally endemic provinces, and *An. anthropophagus* (which was not distinguished from *An. hircanus sinensis* before 1957) is generally restricted to areas south of latitude N 33° (Sun, 1988).

The endemic areas in Southeast Asia include Cambodia, Indonesia, Lao People's Democratic Republic (Lao PDR), the Philippines, Thailand, Timor-Leste and Vietnam. Control programmes with the goal of achieving elimination by 2020 are in progress in all these countries. Interventions aimed at eliminating LF are based on a World Health Assembly resolution (WHA 50.29), adopted at the 50th WHA in 1997 (http://www.filariasis.org/pdfs/WHA_Resolution_50_29.pdf), which urges member states to interrupt transmission of the parasite through mass drug administration (MDA) using diethylcarbamazine citrate (DEC) and albendazole, or ivermectin and albendazole, once a year for a period of 4–6 years (Ottesen, 2006; WHO, 2002). Although substantial progress has been recorded wherever the strategy has been implemented, elimination has so far only been accomplished in P.R. China where the disease has, however, resurged in some situations (Sunish et al., 2002), thus emphasising the need for long-term commitment and reliable surveillance. Although P.R. China is no longer regarded as endemic, it is included here because the rich experience accumulated over six decades of control activity leading up to elimination can be drawn upon for the remaining work in the region.

An estimated 700 million people live in areas endemic for LF in Asia (including Bangladesh, Cambodia, India, Indonesia, Lao PDR, Maldives, Myanmar, Nepal, Sri Lanka, Thailand, Timor-Leste, Vietnam), approximately 60 million of whom harbour microfilariae or suffer from the chronic manifestations of the infection. This represents 64% of the global burden of LF (http://www.searo.who.int/EN/Section10/Section2096_10588.htm). Based on this information, together with data available from 'The Global Alliance to Eliminate Lymphatic Filariasis' (GAELF; http://www.filariasis.org/pdfs/GAELFnumbers6_13.pdf) and the 'Directors of Health Promotion and Education' (DHPE), Washington, DC, USA (http://www.dhpe.org/infect/Lymphfil.html), it can be estimated that the endemic areas of Southeast Asia account for approximately a quarter of the global burden, that is around 15 million people.

GAELF (http://www.filariasis.org/) is a public–private partnership that was created in 2000 to assist with the advocacy, resource mobilisation, and programme implementation of the elimination of LF. It brings together national Ministries of Health (MoHs), the World Health Organization (WHO), commercial companies, international development agencies, international donor foundations, non-governmental organizations (NGOs), academic institutions, and local communities. GlaxoSmithKline (GSK) and Merck & Co., Inc. have pledged all the drugs necessary to achieve elimination—valued at more than US $ 1 billion, it is the largest drug donation so far for any disease. GAELF co-ordinates, supports, and supervises the local Programmes for the Elimination of Lymphatic Filariasis (PELF) which operates in all endemic countries with the aim of achieving elimination of LF transmission by 2020. There are two approaches to achieve this aim: the distribution of DEC-fortified cooking salt to the entire population of the endemic area for 1 or 2 years, or MDA, the administration of a combination of DEC and albendazole to the entire at-risk population, once a year for 5 or 6 consecutive years. Additional interventions to prevent disability and skin infections, are also part of the elimination programme, which includes education on regular washing, skin care, and timely use of antibiotics (Montresor et al., 2008).

In many areas, the LF elimination efforts are hampered by a dearth of up-to-date information about the situation, in particular regarding the cost of the MDA needed to interrupt transmission. Governments normally contribute most (60–90%) of the operational costs and an economic study, finding that the costs, per person treated, range from US$ 0.06 to US$ 2.23 (Goldman et al., 2007), concluded that MDA is comparatively inexpensive in relation to most other public health programmes. The recognition that areas endemic for LF are also commonly the poorest (Galvez Tan, 2003) opens the way to reduce poverty along with inequalities in health care. The global, multi-stakeholder alliance working towards making all endemic countries free of new LF cases by 2020 is thus not a completely vertical approach but also presents an opportunity to make a contribution to poverty reduction through sustainable development.

8.2. EXPERIENCE GAINED FROM THE LF ELIMINATION PROGRAMME IN P.R. CHINA

In 2007, WHO officially approved the application from the Government of P.R. China MoHs, declaring that LF had been eliminated as a public health problem in P.R. China after having been endemic there for thousands of years (MoH, 2007). The first to report the disease in the form of elephantiasis was Meadows (1871), who documented the diagnosis in a patient in Ningbo prefecture, Zhejiang province. Manson (1872, 1877) wrote several case reports in which he demonstrated *W. bancrofti* microfilariae (MF) in the blood and showed their nocturnal periodicity, as well as proving that the disease was transmitted by a mosquito vector, in this case, *Cx. pipiens fatigans*. Lee (1926), Feng (1933), and Hu (1937) showed that LF was endemic in large areas of the provinces of Jiangsu,

Zhejiang and Fujian and reported the existence of *B. malayi*. Their writings advanced the idea that *An. hircanus sinensis* was the vector of *B. malayi* and that *Cx. pipiens fatigans* and *Cx. pipiens pallens* the vectors of *W. bancrofti*.

8.2.1. The former endemic areas

Blood sampling from large numbers of people carried out from the 1950s up to 1980, together with previous mosquito surveys, sheds light on the former distribution of LF (Shi and Sun, 1999). The endemic areas were found to extend from Sanya city in Guangdong province (now in Hainan province), in the South (latitude 24°10′N) to Leling county, Shandong province, in the North (latitude 37°48′ N), and from the Zhoushan archipelago in the East (longitude 122°30′E) to Yaan city, Sichuan province, in the West (approximately longitude 130°W). The endemic areas covered 16,514 townships (or urban sub-districts), in 864 counties (or cities), in 14 provinces (or autonomous regions or municipalities) with an estimated total population of 342 million (Table 8.1, Fig. 8.1).

Before the control programme was initiated, there were close to 31 million people with LF in the country, 25.6 million of them had microfilaremia (MF), 17.4 million with the Bancroftian type, and 8.2 million

TABLE 8.1 Distribution of human lymphatic filaria species in P.R. China 1959–1980

Name of province/ municipality	Number of endemic counties	Number of counties with filarial species		
		W. bancrofti	*B. malayi*	Both species
Shandong	74	74	0	0
Henan	71	42	1	28
Hubei	69	10	47	12
Anhui	82	28	14	40
Jiangsu	71	64	0	7
Shanghai	10	5	2	3
Zhejiang	67	3	40	24
Jiangxi	75	9	33	33
Fujian	68	16	24	28
Guangdong	62	61	1	0
Hainan	18	18	0	0
Guangxi	68	60	6	2
Hunan	55	39	10	6
Guizhou	47	21	25	1
Sichuan	14	0	14	0
Chongqing	13	13	0	0
Total	864	463	217	184

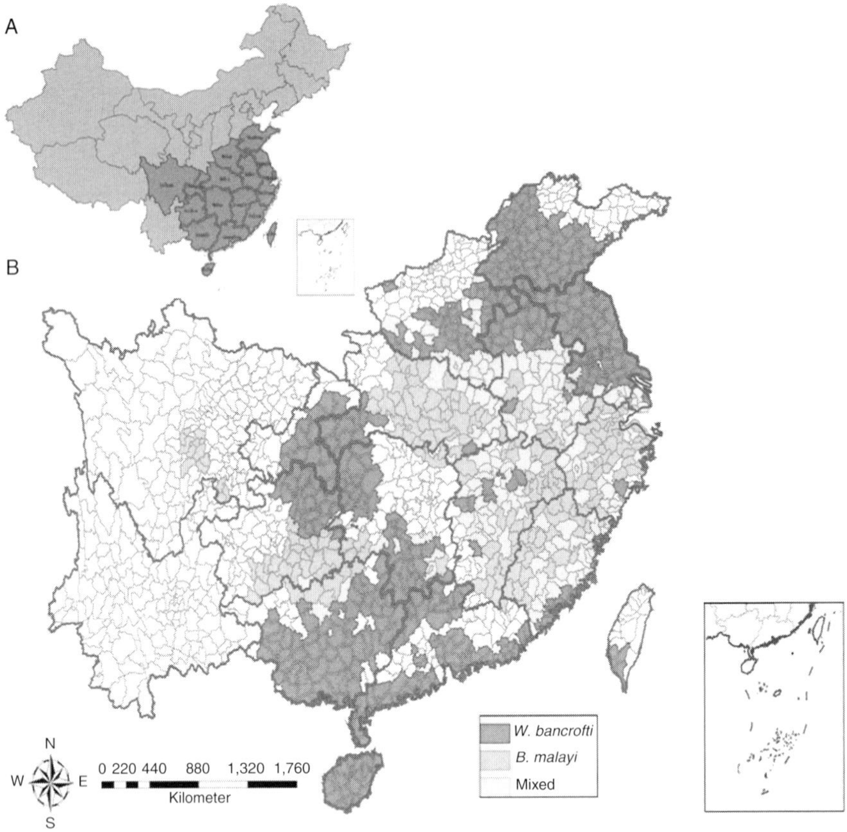

FIGURE 8.1 Distribution map of the original, LF-endemic areas in P.R. China at the provincial level (A) with a blow-up to show the county level (B).

with Brugian infection. About 5.4 million of people suffered from chronic LF (4.6 million due to Bancroftian and 0.8 million due to Brugian infection). In general, the prevalence of microfilariae (MF) was higher among males than females, which may have been due to increased mosquito exposure. In addition, the MF rate and the prevalence of chronic LF tended to increase with age and then decrease after a peak in middle age.

The MF prevalence decreased gradually with distance from highly endemic foci of transmission, and buffer zones were commonly observed between endemic and non-endemic areas (Fig. 8.1B). Surveys, carried out in the 1950s in the provinces of Shaanxi, Shanxi and Hebei, on the northern border of the endemic area, found no LF cases. Also, most of the counties in Henan province, adjacent to the Shanxi, Shaanxi and Hebei provinces, were found to be non-endemic. The same situation was seen in

Yunnan, the mountainous, mainly subtropical province along the southwestern border of the country. Surveys carried out in the central, southern, and western parts of Yunnan from 1960 to 1962 did not find any MF cases, nor could any locally acquired filarial infection be demonstrated, even though the climatic conditions there are suitable for the mosquito vector. The entire province of Yunnan was therefore considered non-endemic, as were the western districts of Guizhou province, bordering Yunnan's north-eastern parts. In Guangxi province, east of Yunnan, only one endemic county (Baise) was found and it had a non-endemic buffer zone towards Funing county in Yunnan. In Sichuan, the province to the north, only one endemic county was found (Junlian). As a result, the western border of LF transmission was considered to pass through the western part of the Sichuan and Guizhou provinces.

In summary, the national survey delineated the area of endemicity and showed that it coincided with the agricultural areas of the central and southeastern part of the country, home to about 80% of the population according to the national population census data (MoH, 1984). Although LF was also found in urban areas, it was mainly limited to the suburbs. For example, in a 1970 survey of Shanghai covering 114,700 persons, only 91 had MF and all of these cases were shown to be imported. In another survey, carried out a year later, 331 of the 1,845,000 urban residents of Guangzhou municipality showed MF. Again, all these cases were found to have been be imported. At the same time, the survey showed that the MF rate was 1.6% in the suburbs of Guangzhou (3034 of 192,732 people surveyed). In the rural areas, the MF rate was the highest among village dwellers, lower among 'market town' residents, and the lowest in residents of the local capital. For example, the positive rates in the villages, market towns, and local capitals in the western part of Hunan province, were 4.3%, 0.47% and 0.03%, respectively. A similar situation was seen in the Shucheng county of Anhui province, where the MF rates were 23.1% and 6.1% in the villages and local capitals, respectively. In the region of Fujian province, where Brugian LF was epidemic, the rate was 7.7% in the villages and 4.5% in the local capitals, while in places endemic for Bancroftian LF, the figures were 6.7% and 2.6%, respectively.

8.2.2. The control strategy

During the long campaign against LF, three important manuals outlining how the work should proceed were issued by the MoH (MoH, 1959, 1984). The control activities benefited from a cohesive network that operated at the national level as well as at the province, county, town, and administrative village levels. The work was carried out over 50 years and based on one professional institution at the national level, 16 institutions at the provincial level, 864 filariasis control units at the county level and more than 16,000 'grass-root' organisations at the local level. Thus, a large number of people were involved and the filariasis control effort helped to cultivate and sharpen the skills of many dedicated public health workers. It was understood early on that reducing the infection source (human MF) would be an important step, given that studies had shown transmission to be relatively low and had demonstrated that there were no non-human reservoirs, neither for *W. bancrofti* nor for *B. malayi* (Feng, 1962). In addition, the effectiveness of DEC against both the MF and the adult worms was documented (Chen, 1955; Li et al., 1990).

Starting in 1956, the National Programme of Agricultural Development was initiated throughout P.R. China with the objective to achieve what was called 'basic elimination' of LF. This meant repeated mass blood surveys and selective treatment of infected persons in areas considered to be endemic (Sun, 1988). To that end, the local governments of the different endemic provinces/autonomous regions/municipalities brought leaders and professionals together for mass campaigns, linked pilot studies with large-scale schemes, integrated LF control with similar campaigns for other major diseases, and carried out epidemiological surveys and treatment campaigns in pilot projects across large areas. At this time, the first pilot survey and treatment sites were established in epidemic areas with particularly high disease burdens. As activities entered a period of rapid, stable development in the late 1980s, the objective to achieve 'basic elimination' of LF in the whole country was proposed (MoH document, 1988). The control strategy was designed with an emphasis on reducing the source of infection, that is, the presence of microfilariae. This strategy proved effective and when the process for independent checks and evaluations to verify progress was standardised, the control work accelerated further. The objective of achieving 'basic elimination' throughout the entire country was eventually realised in 1994.

Health education, including raising awareness of the necessity of control, was a central component of the LF control programme. This approach consisted of messages delivered through newspapers, radio, posters and leaflets, as well as through slide shows and films at community meetings. Patients were also encouraged to discuss their experience with the disease. Vector control was not systematically applied, but pesticide (DDT) spraying, use of insecticide-impregnated bed nets, and environmental modification were adopted in combination with general health campaigns.

P.R. China was the first country to adopt DEC-fortified salt (MoH document, 1981) and Chinese research demonstrated its feasibility, effectiveness and safety, as well as the low frequency of adverse reactions (Shandong Institute of Parasitic Diseases, 1975). The salt, containing a 0.3% concentration of DEC, was used for MDA and continued for

3–6 months. The advantage of this approach was that side effects were kept to a minimum and compliance was therefore never a problem. The main approach, however, was to screen for MF, and to follow this up with 3–7-day courses of DEC tablets at 4.2 g/kg (*sic*) body weight, with at least a 1-month interval between each course. The following scheme to control the source of infection was used at different periods of time as follows:

- Before 1970, repeated mass blood examination and selective treatment of infected persons with DEC tablets as described earlier was implemented in all areas considered to be endemic.
- From the late 1960s up until the year 1990, MDA for the entire at-risk population, began to be implemented first in high-risk endemic villages and in neighbouring areas. People in hypo-epidemic areas of Bancroftian filariasis, as well as meso-epidemic and hypo-epidemic areas of Brugian filariasis, were subjected to large-scale blood surveys and selective treatment.
- Later, DEC-fortified salt was prescribed and gradually spread nationwide, in some areas starting as early as the 1970s. This approach was continued until 1994 and implemented in meso-epidemic, hyper-endemic, and super-epidemic areas of Bancroftian filariasis as well as in hyper-epidemic and super-epidemic areas of Brugian filariasis. The extent of the need for DEC salt treatment was determined according to surveys targeting the populations of the remaining endemic areas as well as people living in the neighbourhood of MF cases. DEC tablets were used to treat MF cases found in the surveys.

In the 1950–1960 period, the MF-positive rate of the population in the endemic areas of the whole country was 5.7% on average, while it had decreased to 0.001% in 2001–2005. The prevalence of chronic LF was 2% before the control programme started but had decreased to 0.04% in the 2001–2005 survey. Studies were also carried out on the relationship between MF density at the population level and the prevalence rate of infected mosquitoes (He et al., 1982). By 1994, control of all endemic counties had been achieved and the criteria for 'basic elimination' had been reached. To verify this, three levels of assessment were adopted:

- self-assessment at the county level;
- assessment of each county by provincial health authorities; and
- assessment of each province by the MoH.

Cluster sampling carried out before 1994 showed that, in the administrative villages control units in 855 of 864 endemic countries/cities in the entire country, positive MF rates were never greater than 1%. The conclusion that 'basic elimination' had been achieved was reached after 8.56 million people had been examined by blood slide in the 855 counties, and 8776 MF-positive cases had been discovered, corresponding to an average rate of 0.1%. In the remaining nine counties and cities, confirmation that the goal of the MF rate $<1\%$ had been reached was based on surveys and recorded data evaluated by the national expert team.

8.2.3. Surveillance in the pre-elimination period

After Shandong had met the criteria for 'basic elimination'—the first province to do so—nationwide surveillance was started in 1983. The main task in this initial period of surveillance was to detect and clear the residual sources of infection (Li and Shi, 1986; Shandong Institute of Parasitic Diseases, 1981). Every county was asked to be vigilant regarding areas that could possibly be harbouring infected people. Follow-up testing, treatment of former MF cases and clearance of residual infectious foci was undertaken to consolidate the achievements of previous control efforts.

When LF had been brought under control in most parts of the country, the national Government issued a document entitled 'Scheme for Evaluation of Basic Elimination of Lymphatic Filariasis' (MoH document, 1988), which outlined the type of surveillance to be followed when most endemic counties had reached the objective of 'basic elimination'. The approach was co-ordinated by the MoH, and implemented by the provincial Health Departments. The MoH's Department of Disease Control formulated surveillance plans and technical schemes, while a 'National LF Guide Team' was formed and charged with managerial tasks such as data collection and analysis, co-ordination of information, communication and discussion. In accordance with MoH requirements, local health sectors and professional institutions prepared detailed local action plans for the implementation and supervision of control activities. This approach was instituted in all filariasis-endemic counties and included cross-sectional surveillance, longitudinal surveillance, and surveillance of the migrant populations based on the following requirements:

- the number of parasitological surveillance townships should exceed 30% of the total endemic townships, and the sampled people in the blood survey should exceed 3% of the total endemic population in the county;
- vector surveillance should be performed in more than three parasitological surveillance townships; the sample size for *Cx. quinquefasciatus* and *Cx. pallens* should be over 3000, while that of *An. sinensis* and *An. anthropophagus* should be over 1000; and
- serological surveillance should be instituted following antifilarial antibody titers using the indirect fluorescent antibody test (IFAT) or the enzyme-linked immunosorbent assay (ELISA).

In order to understand the development of the endemic foci over time, longitudinal surveillance was conducted by observing the situation in one pilot city at the prefecture level in each endemic province. In each pilot prefecture (sample villages with a population of 1000–2000 persons where the MF rate in the previous survey had been >3% and where the intensity of infection had also been high) vector surveillance, combined with parasitological and serological diagnosis, were performed and compared with previous results. People were not treated unless MF was found, but all blood samples were checked every 1 or 2 years until negative. All negative results were verified by follow-up testing at least three times. For all residents in the sample villages aged 1 year or above, blood was examined once every 2 years until the MF had disappeared. The methods for vector surveillance and serological surveillance were same as described for the cross-sectional surveillance.

Surveillance of the migrant populations was carried out by parasitological and serological testing. All MF cases found were treated with DEC tablets and if the MF rate was higher than expected, blood surveys were carried out, both in people's original and current places of residence.

8.2.4. Assessment of LF elimination

After control interventions had been carried out, the average MF rate was ≤1.7% in areas endemic for *W. bancrofti* and ≤1.6% in areas endemic for *B. malayi* (Shi, 1994). The MF rate, as well as the infection rate of filarial larva in the mosquito vector, continued to drop gradually and transmission tended to cease when the average density of MF in the blood fell below 10 MF/60 μl in residual cases. These results demonstrate that the criterion of 'basic elimination', that is an MF rate below 1%, was consistent with transmission interruption. Elimination was declared when it could be demonstrated that there were no human cases with MF and no human filarial larva in the vector. In the end, the term LF elimination was defined as the elimination of all sources of infection and the interruption of transmission in the endemic areas. After the criteria of 'basic elimination' had been met—with the exception of a few remaining endemic foci that required additional treatment—and residual infected persons were gradually becoming free from MF, it was felt that complete elimination of LF would be feasible after another decade of vigilant surveillance and treatment of all cases found. Based on the evidence available in 1994, the MoH issued two draft documents: 'Criteria for verification of LF elimination' and 'Verification of LF elimination' (Shi and Sun, 1999). These documents specified the criteria and procedures for verifying LF elimination and accelerated the progress towards complete elimination. After testing the outlined procedures for a few years, the MoH and the National

Committee of Criteria Standardization formally issued the 'Criteria of LF Elimination' in January, 2006 (Sun et al., 2006).

After assessment by the provincial health administrative sector showing that the county, or district, had achieved and sustained the criteria of 'basic elimination' for at least 10 years, it would be declared free of LF when the following criteria had also been met:

- no signs of MF in any resident person;
- any remaining chronic LF cases identified and treated;
- no human filarial larvae in local mosquitoes; and
- all primary records and statistical data with respect to investigation, surveillance, and assessment kept in good order.

8.2.5. Surveillance in the post-elimination period

During the consolidation stage of the advances made towards the elimination of LF, the MoH issued a document outlining how to avoid any resurgence of the infection (MoH document, 2001) and monitoring and surveillance became more important (Pan et al., 1993). The MoH document called for monitoring of any area with risk factors such as remaining, residual MF cases, imported MF cases, or recent previous MF cases. Since 2004, all LF cases are reported via a network reporting system to ensure that all cases have been investigated and individually verified.

In the period from 1987 to 1988, after the MoH assessment had confirmed that the criteria for 'basic elimination' had been met in each province, only a few villages in four counties/cities in the country were still foci of residual filarial transmission with MF rates above 1%.

From 1980 to 2004, a total of 82 longitudinal surveillance sites were established, 45 of which were subjected to long-term observation. No new, chronic LF cases emerged and residual MF cases turned gradually negative within 10 years. The longest interval recorded for *W. bancrofti* MF to disappear was 9 years, while for *B. malayi* the longest interval was only 5 years. The MF rate decreased year by year in all longitudinal surveillance sites, no new infected cases were found and the filarial mosquito infection rate decreased gradually. After up to 8 years of surveillance in some places, no more infected mosquitoes were found. Assessments were conducted all over P.R. China from 1994 to 2006. By 2006, all 16 endemic provinces had passed the criteria established for elimination starting with the Guangxi and Zhuang autonomous regions in 1995 and ending with Anhui province in February, 2006. Nevertheless, even after the disease had seemingly been eliminated, surveillance continued in areas of possible, suspected disease, and focused particularly on migrant labourers coming back from endemic countries. The web-based 'National Reporting System of Communicable Disease

Surveillance' (http://www.10.254.254.229/) was set up in 2004 and LF is still part of the reporting system.

Between 1984 and 2005, a nationwide survey of migrant populations took place in all provinces, autonomous regions, and municipalities. Out of 363,500 people investigated, 419 people were found to be MF positive. However, all of these infections were detected before 1992. The results showed that MF cases among migrant populations decreased gradually after these areas had met the criteria of basic elimination. No more cases of MF were found from 1993 onwards. In addition, a total of 12,037 previous MF cases from nine provinces were subjected to repeated blood testing between 2001 and 2005 without finding any MF.

From 1996 to 2005, further surveillance of potential risk factors was carried out in 261 counties in several provinces and autonomous regions, testing a total of 835,700 people by blood examination without detecting any microfilaria. Some counties also conducted vector surveillance in which 175,200 mosquitoes were dissected and found negative with respect to human filarial infection.

8.2.6. Risk of re-emergence

As P.R. China has joint borders with several still endemic areas and many Chinese guest workers travel between countries, the emergence of imported cases is a possibility. There is also a risk that cases occasionally remain undetected. For example, on August 14, 2007, through the National Reporting System mentioned above, one filariasis case was reported by the Fuyang town hospital, Fuchuan county, Guangxi Autonomous region. The patient had been a resident worker in Guangdong province since 2005 but after the onset of symptoms (fever and scrotal swelling) in August 2007, he returned home and was admitted at the local hospital in Fuyang town where Bancroftian MF was detected by blood microscopy. Taking into consideration the fact that the symptom of scrotal swelling normally develops very slowly, more than 10 years after the primary infection, the investigation focused on the local village of this pilot case, as well as surrounding villages in Fuchan county and villages in neighbouring counties in Hunan province. A few additional MF cases were found (Duan et al., 2008; Li et al., 2008). In tracing the infection focus, another few cases were found among migrant labourers from the village who had also worked in Guangdong province (Zhang et al., 2008). All in all, 19 MF-positive cases were found and in two natural villages, namely Ganshang and Yinshan in Changtang administrative village, Chaodong township, Fuchuan county, Guangxi Autonomous region, which was therefore regarded as a residual focus of Bancroftian filariasis. All these infected cases were subsequently treated.

8.3. ELIMINATION IN COUNTRIES WITH LIMITED OR LOW-LEVEL PREVALENCE

8.3.1. Thailand

The endemic areas are located along the western border of the country and in the South. Thailand has currently a population of 63 million and is administratively divided into 76 provinces, 926 districts, and 7424 cantons with 76,865 villages. *B. malayi*, transmitted by the *Mansonia* mosquito species, is endemic in the southern part of the country, while *W. bancrofti*, transmitted by mosquitoes of the *Aedes niveus* group, is endemic in the western border provinces. Small-scale filariasis control was initiated in 1961 and then gradually expanded to cover all areas endemic for *B. malayi* in the southern provinces. The control activities were later extended to areas endemic for *W. bancrofti* in the western border provinces. Only a few small endemic foci in 336 sub-villages with altogether 123,000 people at risk have been reported. These foci, which are scattered over 11 provinces, were included in the LF Elimination Programme in 2002 (Fig. 8.2).

By 2007, 10 provinces were deemed free of LF transmission and therefore excluded from MDA. The elimination strategy is, however, maintained in the Narathiwat province where the infection is caused by the nocturnal, sub-periodic *B. malayi*, which is not yet under control. However, night blood surveys carried out in the endemic areas of Narathiwat during 2008 revealed an MF rate of only 0.02%. It is anticipated that elimination of LF in this province should soon be achieved making it possible to interrupt MDA after the 2009 round of chemotherapy (Table 8.2).

With regard to people at an advanced stage of the disease, the disability prevention and control arm of the elimination programme handles 200–300 cases of lymphoedema per year. The number of cases continues to fluctuate around this figure, but is eventually expected to decrease and disappear. The criteria adopted by the Thai LF Elimination Programme are based on the rapid-format, immunochromatographic test (ICT) for circulating filarial antigens (Weil et al., 1997). Survey results covering more than 80% of all children aged 2–6 show an MF rate that varies between 0% and 1% in the *B. malayi* endemic areas (Table 8.3).

8.3.2. Cambodia

LF caused by *W. bancrofti* is a major public health problem in the northern part of Cambodia (Fig. 8.3). The National Centre for Parasitology, Entomology, and Malaria Control (CNM), and the MoH jointly monitor and control the disease. Initial activities aiming at LF elimination began in 1999–2000 and were followed by the establishment of a national task force

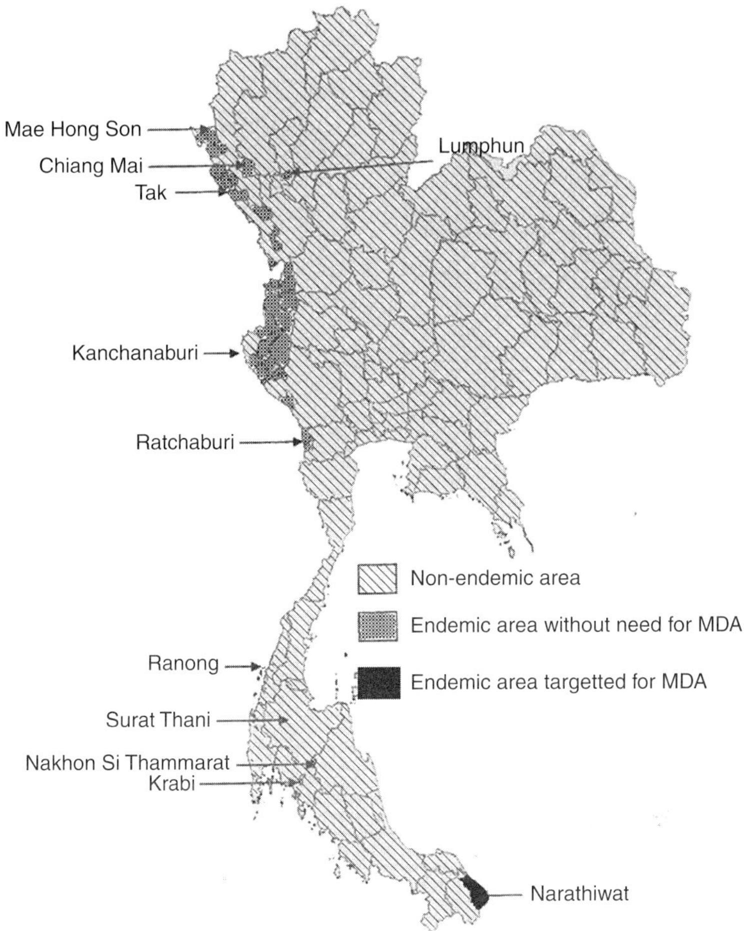

FIGURE 8.2 Thai areas endemic for LF in 2008 by province.

in 2003 (WHO/WPRO, 2007). Mapping of the endemic areas, using the ICT test as well as blood film examinations, was completed in 2004. The great advantage with the ICT approach is that the test, unlike the classic MF blood test, does not have to be performed with blood collected during the night.

The population at risk amounted to just over half a million (502,982) when the programme was initiated. LF was found to be endemic in four of 24 provinces and this area was organised into implementation units (IU) as recommended by the elimination programme. As prevalence was less than 1% in two of these provinces (Siem Reap and Preah Vihear), the IUs were designed to coincide with the districts which resulted in 19 IUs.

TABLE 8.2 Overview of anti-lymphatic filarial drug distribution (MDA) in Thailand

Year	Number of provinces targeted	Population covered	People treated	Reported drug coverage (%)
2002	11	122,811	114,665	93.4
2003	11	139,296	116,911	83.9
2004	11	150,843	125,891	83.5
2005	11	167,194	144,252	86.3
2006	11	166,647	113,380	68.0
2007	1	74,113	61,776	83.4
2008	1	79,267	77,805	95.5

Out of these 19 IUs, four were found to be endemic. All in all, the IUs (that could thus consist of both whole provinces and districts) add up to six endemic IUs out of 41 IUs in the whole country (Table 8.3). Initial case findings by the MoH have so far resulted in the identification of 58 cases of lymphoedema (men and women) and 20 cases of hydrocele scattered throughout the four endemic provinces (Table 8.4). The majority of these patients are taken care of under the disability alleviation component of the elimination programme.

MDA, using DEC and albendazole as recommended by WHO (filariasis fact sheet), was begun in 2005 in the endemic areas. Drug distribution is carried out in schools, pagodas, and villages as well as by door-to-door visits. The drugs are being administered to the entire population of the endemic area for 5–6 consecutive years. The MDA programme for the elimination of LF was begun in 2005 in the two provinces Rattanakiri and Stung Treng, and in six districts in the two provinces Siem Reap and Preah Vihear.

The first round of MDA was conducted in 2005 in all endemic IUs in the four provinces. With the assessment surveys verifying that the coverage figures range between 79% and 90% depending on the IU investigated, it can be concluded that the overall coverage of the population at risk has so far been satisfactory. Furthermore, MF surveys carried out in sentinel sites indicate a 100% reduction of the rates of MF in all IUs after two rounds of MDA.

To reduce cost and to increase efficiency, existing government structures, and personnel are used for drug distribution. For example, with regard to interventions in the four provinces where soil-transmitted helminths (STH) and LF are co-endemic, the timing of albendazole and DEC distribution for LF is organised to fit in with mebendazole (used to treat STH) distribution in such a way that the interval between treatments

TABLE 8.3 Results of night blood/ICT LF surveys between 2002 and 2008 in Thailand

		2002			2003			2004			2005			2006			2007			2008		
Province	Type of survey	No. Exam	No. Pos.	% Pos.	No. Exam	No. Pos.	% Pos.	No. Exam	No. Pos.	% Pos.	No. Exam	No. Pos.	% Pos.	No. Exam	No. Pos.	% Pos.	No. Exam	No. Pos.	% Pos.	No. Exam	No. Pos.	% Pos.
Tak	NBS	4242	3	0.07	3834	9	0.23	5980	15	0.25	5455	0	0	4276	0	0						
	ICT	46	0	0	754	0	0.00				386	0	0	4186	0	0						
	ICT (2–6 years)													4409	0	0	1497	0	0	1181	0	0
Mae Hong Son	NBS	2122	9	0.41	52	1	1.9	591	0	0	290	0	0									
	ICT				1733	5	0.3	947	0	0	368	0	0	359	0	0						
	ICT (2–6 years)													1369	0	0	609	0	0	562	0	0
Kanchanaburi	NBS							4008	0	0	3546	0	0	5699	0	0						
	ICT										547	6	1.09	1821	0	0						
	ICT (2–6 years)																1193	0	0	578	0	0
Chiangmai	NBS							159	0	0	326	0	0	658	0	0						
	ICT (2–6 years)													373	0	0	325	0	0			
Lumphun	NBS				655	0	0	735	0	0	623	0	0									
	ICT													653	0	0						
	ICT (2–6 years)													396	0	0	468	0	0			
Ratburi	ICT							404	0	0	460	0	0	510	0	0						
	ICT (2–6 years)													200	0	0	206	0	0			
Ranong	ICT							282	0	0	431	0	0	414	0	0						
	ICT (2–6 years)																414	0	0			
Suratthani	NBS	478	5	1.04	454	0	0	475	0	0	478	2	0.4	1246	0	0	91	0	0			
	NBS (2–6 years)													277	0	0				125	0	0
Nakhon Sri	NBS	609	0	0	557	0	0	741	2	0.27	672	0	0	412	0	0						
Thammarat	NBS (2–6 years+													45	0	0	71	0	0			
Krabi	NBS	403	0	0	382	0	0	470	0	0	362	0	0	384	0	0						
	NBS (2–6 years)													48	0	0	56	0	0			
Narathiwat	NBS	10,498	51	0.48	10,859	27	0.23	9493	19	0.2	8318	28	0.33	8166	7	0.08	21,287	15	0.07	18,681	5	0.02
	NBS (2–6 years}																					

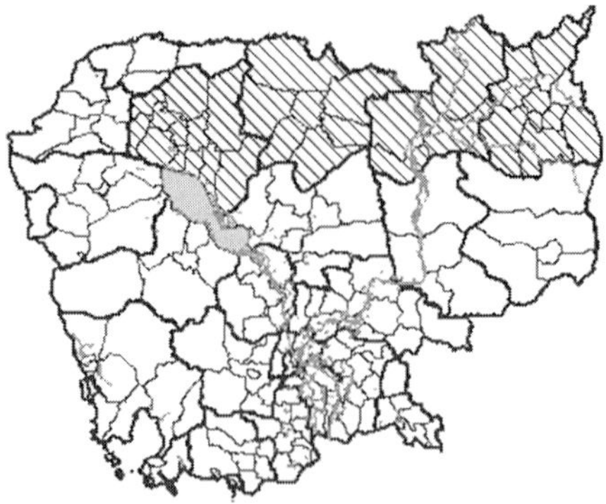

FIGURE 8.3 Map of Cambodia showing the provinces (shaded) where MDA for LF is conducted.

TABLE 8.4 The prevalence of MF according to ICT and/or night blood testing in six provinces in Cambodia

Province	2001	2004	2005	2006
Stung Treng	1053 (0.4%)	Not done	500 (0.8%)	1015 (0%)
Rattanakiri	601 (2.8%)	Not done	500 (1.8%)	985 (0%)
Siem Reap	Not done	2	515 (0%)	978 (0%)
Angkor chum	No done	2	520 (0%)	996 (0%)
Varin	1	?	535 (0%)	987 (0%)
Preah Vihea	917 (0.2%)	?	535 (0%)	1002 (0%)

complies with the WHO's recommendations. In addition, 'Self-Care Patient Guides' and 'Patient Kits' were developed and distributed to all patients and health staff at the community level. Short training courses focusing on the diagnosis and acute treatment of LF are conducted at the health facilities in the communities.

8.3.3. Lao PDR

After the first case of LF was described in Lao PDR in 1925, very few cases were reported before the initiation of the National LF control (NLFC) in 2003. Between 2003 and 2005 two national surveys were carried out in 14 provinces involving 30 districts, without any LF cases being found among the 9,286 people examined (WHO/WPRO, 2007). A third national survey

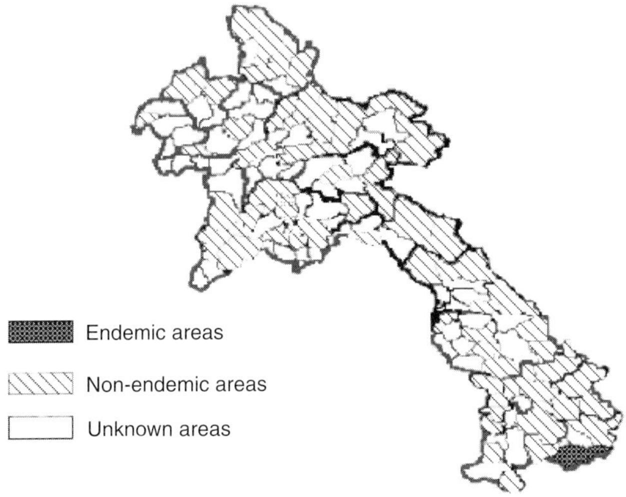

FIGURE 8.4 Map of Lao PDR showing the LF endemic areas of 2007 (based on WHO/WPRO Report, (WP) 2007/ICP/MVP/1.2/001).

took place in 2007. In this survey, which involved six districts in three provinces, four human cases were found by ICT testing in Phouvong district, Attapu province (Fig. 8.4). These cases were treated on an individual base and no MDA campaigns have been instituted in the country (WHO/WPRO, 2007). A special survey covering over 10,000 individuals living in this area was started in 2008 because of these four cases (Montresor et al., 2008), but to this day no further cases have been reported. Full-scale mapping is under way, but of 140 IUs, the results so far categorise only one as endemic and 57 as non-endemic, while 82 are still unknown (WHO/WPRO, 2007).

8.3.4. Vietnam

B. malayi is the predominant cause of LF in Vietnam accounting for 80–95% of all cases in the country. However, the disease in the South is caused by *W. bancrofti* which, in contrast to *B. malayi*, is localised to a few foci. In the period between 1960 and 1975 the infection rate in the north was 6% on average, gradually reducing to 2% during the period 1976–2002, while the rate in the south has varied between 0.4% and 13.3% over the period 1977–2000 (WHO/WPRO, 2007) (Fig. 8.5). At present, the total estimated number of elephantiasis patients in the country is about 5,000.

The elimination programme started in 2003 and has made good progress, especially with regard to the increasing number of courses aiming to

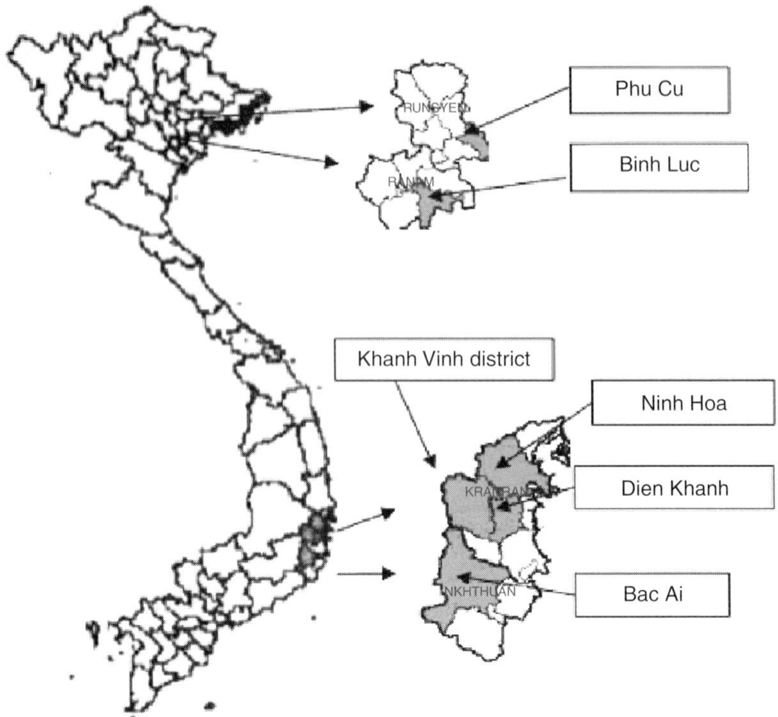

FIGURE 8.5 Map of Vietnam showing the endemic areas (shaded) of LF as of 1977 (based on WHO/WPRO Report, (WP) 2007/ICP/MVP/1.2/001).

teach self-care to patients with elephantiasis (12 courses in 2005 as compared to 27 courses in 2006). The feedback 6 months after course completion showed that patients felt that life had improved for them and they had gained increased levels of self-confidence. In addition, leaflets and posters giving information about LF have been distributed and the media have been relied upon to spread knowledge to as many as possible. Annual knowledge, attitudes and practices (KAP) surveys indicate that the number of people who know about LF, its complications and its treatment is increasing steadily (WHO/WPRO, 2007)

MDA was first initiated in six IUs at the district level and implemented by door to door visits and gatherings in public places. In these six IUs treatment coverage above 90% has been achieved and three rounds of MDA have brought down the MF rates in sentinel sites and spot check sites. 675,000 individuals at risk in six districts in the Red River delta and the Quang Binh province are currently being targeted for drug treatment (Montresor et al., 2008).

8.4. THE ELIMINATION PROGRAMME IN INDONESIA AND TIMOR LESTE

8.4.1. Indonesia

Three nematode species cause LF in Indonesia: *W. bancrofti*, *B. malayi* and *B. timori*. The disease is not only a major cause of disability in the country, but also a question of social stigmatization and of psychological and economic reduction of life opportunities. LF is thus a major part of the public health burden in the country. The disease is distributed throughout the country and exists in all provinces. The overall prevalence appears to be slowly decreasing but endemic foci still exist in urban, rural, and remote areas. LF has disappeared totally in many areas, both with and without intervention, but in others it has increased and new foci have appeared. This is mostly due to environmental changes and population movement. Recent survey results show that suspected chronic cases exist in all provinces. These chronic cases were found in 231 of the 336 districts investigated. An overview of the situation in the endemic districts is shown in Table 8.5 and Fig. 8.6. A total of 316 districts are still endemic, with a total population of approximately 119 million.

The Indonesian MoH recognises LF as a significant health problem as it leads to social and economic deprivation, especially among people who are poor and marginalised. The MoH, in abiding WHA resolution 50.29, is committed to the elimination of LF as a public health problem by the year 2020. The rationale is that reduction or elimination of transmission by MDA, especially in children, will protect future generations from LF. To achieve elimination the following plan was developed:

- *Goal*: To eliminate LF as a public health problem and significantly reduce the number of people living in absolute poverty by the year 2020.
- *Objectives*: To reduce and eliminate LF transmission, reduce and prevent disability in affected individuals, deworm the endemic populations (through MDA using albendazole), and strengthen health services by instituting a successful elimination programme.
- *Approach*: Disability prevention and transmission interruption directed at the population at risk, aiming to reduce the MF load in the community to a level at which LF transmission cannot be sustained. The interruption of transmission will be measured by examining infection in children born after the launch of the elimination programme.

The strategy adopted for the interruption of transmission is MDA, based on the effectiveness of a single dose of 6 mg/kg body weight of

TABLE 8.5 Current distribution of LF in Indonesia

	Number of MDA implementation units (IU)				
Region/province	Number of districts	Endemic districts	Population	Non-endemic districts	Uncertain districts
NAD	23	23	4,377,852	None	None
North Sumatera	28	28	12,236,363	None	None
West Sumatera	19	19	4,549,563	None	None
South Sumatera	15	15	7,234,617	None	None
Riau	11	11	4,608,263	None	None
Jambi	10	10	2,730,655	None	None
Bangka Belitung	7	7	1,047,958	None	None
Riau Kepulauan	6	6	1,198,526	None	None
Bengkulu	9	9	1,602,648	None	None
Lampung	11	11	7,541,977	None	None
West Kalimantan	14	14	4,163,246	None	None
East Kalimantan	14	14	2,978,531	None	None
South Kalimantan	13	13	3,261,727	None	None
Central Kalimantan	14	14	1,941,178	None	None
DKI Jakarta	6	1	1,943,473	None	5
Banten	7	5	10,804,940	None	2
West Jawa	25	14	24,169,785	None	11
Central Jawa	35	6	5,445,590	3	26
East Jawa	38	–	–	None	38
DI Jogjakarta	5	–	–	None	5
Bali	9	–	–	None	9
North Sulawesi	13	–	–	None	13
Central Sulawesi	10	10	2,436,739	None	None
South Sulawesi	23	3	648,062	None	20
Southeast Sulawesi	13	11	2,537,584	None	2
West Sulawesi	5	5	1,144,118	None	None
Gorontalo	6	6	961,390	None	None
East Nusa Tenggara	20	16	4,451,708	None	4
West Nusa Tenggara	9	–	–	None	9
Maluku	10	8	1,202,763	None	2
North Maluku	8	8	782,840	None	None
West Papua	9	9	607,706	None	None
Papua	26	20	2,016,067	None	6
Total	471	316	118,625,869	3	152

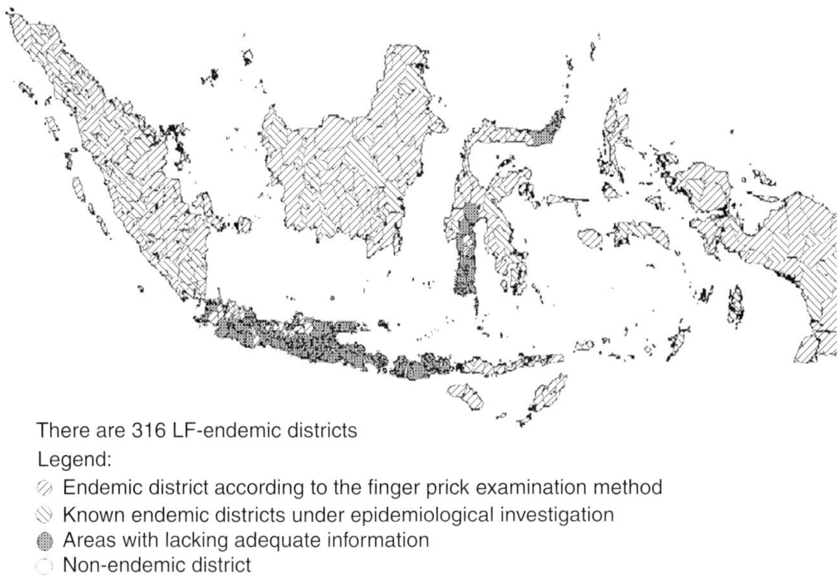

FIGURE 8.6 Distribution of LF in Indonesia in 2008.

DEC in clearing MF and on its sustained effect over a period of at least 1 year (http://www.who.int/mediacentre/factsheets/fs102/en/). The addition of albendazole (400 mg) enhances this effect and the drug also acts on intestinal helminths, which are usually highly endemic in areas of LF endemicity. Specifically, the strategy involves a single dose of DEC and a single dose of albendazole annually for all in the endemic areas, together with the provision of relief to people with chronic LF manifestations. For example, treatment is provided to prevent acute episodes of adenolymphangitis attacks, as well as advice on basic hygiene and the application of topical antifungal and antibiotic creams.

In areas with no previous existing data, staff at health centres receive training on elimination strategies and on the implementation of programme activities started in 2001. Surveys (mapping) are also carried out to assess endemicity or non-endemicity of LF in these areas. MDA has been carried out on an annual basis in endemic populations, beginning in 2002 with the trial use of DEC-fortified salt in communities in certain endemic areas. Health education and advocacy programmes aimed at social mobilisation are ongoing within the programme, while evaluation and surveillance are integral parts of elimination efforts, which will continue until the objectives have been achieved. Important direct benefits of the programme to the national health system include:

- improved reproductive and sexual health;
- improved child and maternal health and development (through the additional effect of albendazole on intestinal parasites);
- improved national capacity of health care delivery;
- increased involvement and opportunities for NGOs in health delivery;
- improved drug distribution; and
- integration with other health sector activities.

8.4.2. Timor Leste

There are 14 regions in Timor Leste with a total population of just above 1 million according to the latest census (2005) (Table 8.6). Public health staff in Timor Leste are struggling to contain many different infectious diseases and to improve the general health situation in the country. A national family planning policy and programme is underway as the 2006 Health Statistics Report indicated that skilled health personnel attend only 27% of all child births.

Historically, *B. timori* is considered to be the most prevalent cause of filarial disease, accounting for about 95% of cases, but LF due to *W. bancrofti* and *B. malayi* also exists. The only known vector of *B. timori* is *An. barbirostris* which breeds in clean water flowing from fresh water springs and which has a particular affinity to irrigated rice-paddy fields.

TABLE 8.6 The MF prevalence rate of lymphatic filariasis in Timor-Leste

No.	Region	Estimated population 2007	MF prevalence (%) 2002	MDA
1	Aileu	46,755	0	–
2	Ainaro	61,609	7.6	–
3	Baucau	116,366	12.5	–
4	Bobonaro	95,013	17.1	–
5	Covalima	61,371	3.4	–
6	Dili	177,127	5.6	2005
7	Emera	119,651	5.6	–
8	Lautem	66,267	5.1	–
9	Liquica	66,381	6.8	2005
10	Manatuto	42,046	15.0	2005
11	Manufahi	53,186	27.0	–
13	Oecusse	66,569	3.3	2005
14	Viqueque	75,291	15.0	–
Total		1,047,632	10.6	–

All 14 regions are endemic for LF and so far only four have been subjected to treatment programmes, that is Dili, Liquica, Oecusse and Manatutu, with a total population of approximately 320,000 people. An integrated LF elimination, STH treatment and yaws eradication programme was successfully launched in February, 2005 in one district and scaled up to cover all four districts later in the same year. The once annual occurrence of MDA using DEC and albendazole is expected to continue for 5–6 years until interruption of LF transmission is achieved. Additionally, children aged 2–16 years receive another dose of albendazole after 6 months, whilst those who are 6 months to 2 years old receive a single dose of pyrantel (11 mg/kg bodyweight), an anti-nematodal tetrahydropyrimidin derivate.

8.5. THE ELIMINATION PROGRAMME IN THE PHILIPPINES

Mapping of the country's disease burden due to *W. bancrofti* and *B. malayi* identified 42 endemic areas and 38 non-endemic areas, with an average MF prevalence of 9.7% in 1998 (WHO/WPRO, 2007). An analysis of cumulative prevalence data available from the Department of Health (DoH) indicated the persistence of LF in each of the three major island groups. LF is thus endemic in most of the southern half of the Philippines with the exception of the islands of Bohol, Cebu, and the northern half of Negros (Fig. 8.7). Luzon is generally free from the disease which is only established in the southernmost part of the island. Kron et al. (2000) summarised the prevalence data before the elimination programme started reviewing host, parasite, and vector (*An. poecilius, An. flavirostris, M. bonnea*, and *M. uniformis*) characteristics relevant to the design and implementation of disease control initiatives.

For practical reasons, the provinces have been designated as IUs, except in the cities, where the IUs cover the same jurisdiction as the districts. MDA, based on combination therapy using DEC and albendazole, was initiated in 2000 in pilot areas, but the programme officially started in 2001. It was scaled up in the succeeding years thanks to increased budget allocations, finally covering almost the entire at-risk population. The DoH has created an LF elimination database which facilitates the generation of reports at all levels of implementation. Through the intervention by the DoH, a master list for MDA and a drug inventory are available. Means have also been made available for surveillance leading to the strengthening of multi-sectoral partnerships with both local and international partners. Also available are the means for the establishment of an action plan, health promotion and social mobilization (DoH).

The MDA campaigns were formally integrated with the deworming campaign in 2006 and there is now a clear association between coverage (low, medium and high) and the degree of MF reduction. Of 36 sites with

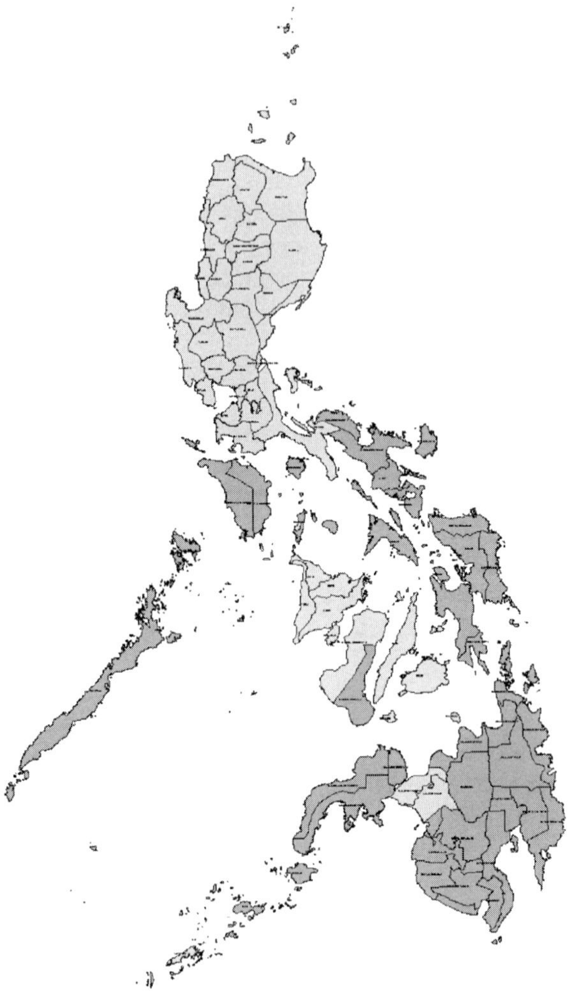

FIGURE 8.7 The darker areas show the distribution of LF in the Philippines in 2008 (based on WHO/WPRO Report, (WP) 2007/ICP/MVP/1.2/001).

known baseline MF rates, 26 (72%) showed decreased MF rates after four rounds of MDA. Ten sites (28%) showed increased MF rates. As for the impact of MDA on the level of circulating antigens, only two of 21 municipalities (9.5%) registered a positive case according to the ICT card test. The results of surveys taken in the areas where MDA had been carried out, showed that only two sites had increased MF rates, while the majority of the sites had lower rates—39 survey sites out of 41 recorded decreased MF rates (WHO/WPRO, 2007). In addition, after conducting lot quality assurance sampling (LQAS) in 2009, testing 3000 school entrants in each IU, two provinces were found to have reached the elimination level defined as MF rates less than 1%, and antigen rates, less than 1% according to the ICT card test. Filter paper tests were also done to validate the results of the LQAS. However, even if two of the 42 endemic provinces were recently able to interrupt MDA distribution, the Philippines still has the largest population at risk from LF in the region (approximately 30 million). Although some disability data are available, actual information on the overall disability situation needs to be attained through further study.

The main problems faced by the LF elimination programme are the lack of ICT cards for surveillance at the sentinel sites, the delays in drug shipment and the travelling expenses of local health workers during MDA implementation and rapid assessment surveys. In addition, there is a direct relationship between LF prevalence and poverty, which is illustrated by the fact that 30 of 39 provinces with a poverty index below the national average are endemic for LF (Galvez Tan, 2003).

The LF elimination programme was integrated with the STH control programme in 2006. However, integration with other programmes has proven difficult in politically unstable areas of Mindanao, especially in the autonomous region in muslim Mindanao, where approximately more than 2 million people are at risk for LF. Still, the United Nations Children's Fund (UNICEF) and the WHO Programme for Expanded Immunization (EPI) have teamed up in some areas and helped integrate MDA with routine immunization programmes wherever feasible. In addition, 'good village health' programmes have been regularly visiting households to monitor the implementation of the LF programme for more than two decades (WHO/WPRO, 2007).

8.6. CONCLUSIONS

The creation of GAELF has shown that it is possible to bring different organisations and donations together under one umbrella to co-ordinate and streamline global activities aiming at eliminating LF transmission by 2020. Although there seems to be no doubt that post-transmission disease (advanced disease with disability) will linger for at least another generation in all countries that have once been endemic, successful interruption of transmission and surveillance will ensure that no new cases will appear. The long-term plans, however, must take this aspect (which is very similar to that with the post-transmission disease of schistosomiasis) into account.

It is noteworthy that filariasis control in P.R. China owes its success to sustained co-operation between all levels involved in the process, over a period exceeding 50 years. This can only be explained by the early recognition of the disease's enormous significance in public health and economic terms, the commitment to a working strategy and the political will to maintain the elimination programme for the long term. However, the success depended also on the availability of an effective drug treatment, intersectoral collaboration, and community participation. The fact that outbreaks have occurred in the 14 years since basic control was achieved also underlines the fact that success depends on a functioning surveillance programme, which continues to operate long after transmission has ceased.

In the still endemic countries, progress has mostly been satisfactory, leading to lower numbers of infected people and to interrupted transmission. In four of the countries covered in this review, Cambodia, Lao PDR, Thailand, Vietnam, and in some IUs in the Philippines, most of the geographical surface and administrative areas are already free from LF and there are strong reasons to believe that the goal of elimination will be reached by 2020 as planned.

REFERENCES

Chen, Z., 1955. Observations on the treatment of 2096 cases of filariasis with diethylcarbamazine. Chin. J. Int. Med. 3, 592–603.

Duan, J., Zhou, S., Jiang, R., Lin, J., He, Z., Tang, G., et al., 2008. An epidemiological investigation of filariasis in the region of Jiangyong county near to residual epidemic focus. J. Pathogen. Biol. 3, 849–851.

Feng, L., 1933. A comparative study of the anatomy of Microfilaria *malayi Brug*, 1927 and Microfilaria *bancrofti Cobbold*, 1877. Chin. Med. J. 47, 1214–1246.

Feng, L., 1962. Filariasis and its control problems. Chin. Med. J. 48, 265–271.

Galvez Tan, J.Z., 2003. The elimination of lymphatic filariasis: a strategy for poverty alleviation and sustainable development—perspectives from the Philippines. Filaria J. 2, 12.

Goldman, A.S., Guisinger, V.H., Aikins, M., Amarillo, M.L., Belizario, V.Y., Garshong, B., et al., 2007. National mass drug administration costs for lymphatic filariasis elimination. PLoS Negl. Trop. Dis. 1, e67.

He, S., Zhang, J.Y., Liu, H.Y., Chang, S.K., Xu, Z.G., Li, F.B., et al., 1982. Relationship between microfilaria rate, microfilaria density in population and infective rate of mosquito vector in bancroftion filariasis. Chin. J. Epidemiol. 3, 297–299.

Hu, S.M.K., 1937. A brief survey of filariasis in Foochow and Futsing regions, southern China. Chin. Med. J. 52, 571–578.

Kron, M., Walker, E., Hernandez, L., Torres, E., Libranda-Ramirez, B., 2000. Lymphatic filariasis in the Philippines. Parasitol. Today 16, 329–333.

Lee, C., 1926. Filariasis investigations in the province of Kiang Su, China. Trans. R. Soc. Trop. Med. Hyg. 20, 279–287.

Li, X., Shi, Z., 1986. Surveillance in areas where filariasis has been basically eliminated. Chin. J. Parasitol. Parasit. Dis. 4, 290–291.

Li, X., Pan, S.X., Gan, Y.C., 1990. Observations on the Effect of Selective Treatment with DEC and Combination with DEC-Medicated Salt for Whole Peoples. Papers of Filariasis Control and Research in China, Fuzhou. Fujian Publishing House of Science and Technology, Fuzhou, pp. 265–268.

Li, X.M., Yang, Y.C., Huang, K.L., Xu, H.B., Xie, Z.Y., Mai, F.Z., et al., 2008. Discovery of a residual focus of Bancroftian filariasis after declaration of its transmission interruption in Guangxi. Chin. J. Parasitol. Parasit. Dis. 26, 404–408.

Manson, P., 1872. Elephantiasis scroti. China Customs Med. Rep. 1, 24.

Manson, P., 1877. Further observations on *Filaria sanguinis hominis*. China Customs Med. Rep. 2, 1.

Meadows, R., 1871. Report on the health of Ningpo. China Customs Med. Rep. 1, 35.

MoH, 1959. Manual of Prevention and Control in Filariasis. The People's Medical Publishing House, Beijing, pp. 42–44.

MoH, 1984. Manual of Filariasis Control. The People's Medical Publishing House, Beijing, pp. 154–161.

MoH, 2007. National Report for Elimination of Lymphatic Filariasis in China. The People's Medical Publishing House, Beijing, pp. 1–15.

MoH document, 1981. Technical Scheme of Filariasis Control. Wei Fang Zi No. 72.

MoH document, 1988. Scheme for Evaluation of Basic Elimination of Lymphatic Filariasis. Wei Fang Zi No. 54.

MoH document, 2001. To Further Enhance the Surveillance and to Reach the Goal of Elimination of Lymphatic Filariasis. Wei Ban Ji Kong Fa No. 12.

Montresor, A., Cong, D.T., Sinuon, M., Tsuyuoka, R., Chanthavisouk, C., Strandgaard, H., et al., 2008. Large-scale preventive chemotherapy for the control of helminth infection in Western Pacific countries: six years later. PLoS Negl. Trop. Dis. 2, e278.

Ottesen, E.A., 2006. Lymphatic filariasis: treatment, control and elimination. Adv. Parasitol. 61, 395–441.

Pan, S., Lv, X.G., Xie, Z.Y., Mai, F.Z., Li, H.Y., Yang, X.C., et al., 1993. Long-term surveillance after basic elimination of bancroftian filariasis. Chin. J. Parasitol. Parasit. Dis. 11, 21–24.

Shandong Institute of Parasitic Diseases, 1975. Experimental observation of DEC-medicated salt on the efficacy of filariasis control. China Prev. Med. J. 55, 316–318.

Shandong Institute of Parasitic Diseases, 1981. Field surveillance in the regions after basic elimination of filariasis. China Prev. Med. J. 15, 236–237.

Shi, Z.J., 1994. Study on the transmission threshold of filariasis. Chin. J. Parasitol. Parasit. Dis. 12, 1–6.

Shi, Z.J., Sun, D.J., 1999. Fifty years' experiences on control of lymphatic filariasis in China. Chin. J. Parasitol. Parasit. Dis. 17, 267–270.

Sun, D.J., 1988. Filariasis: Historical Experience on Preventive Medicine of New China, Vol. 3. The People's Medical Publishing House, Beijing, pp. 332–348.

Sun, D.J., Wu, W.P., Duan, J.H., 2006. Criteria of LF Elimination GB20048-2006). The People's Medical Publishing House, Beijing.

Sunish, I.P., Rajendran, R., Mani, T.R., Munirathinam, A., Tewari, S.C., Hiriyan, J., et al., 2002. Resurgence in filarial transmission after withdrawal of mass drug administration and the relationship between antigenaemia and microfilaraemia—a longitudinal study. Trop. Med. Int. Health 7, 59–69.

Weil, G.J., Lammie, P.J., Weiss, N., 1997. The ICT Filariasis Test: a rapid-format antigen test for diagnosis of bancroftian filariasis. Parasitol. Today 13, 401–404.

WHO, 2002. Lymphatic Filariasis: The Disease and Its Control. Fifth Report of the WHO Expert Committee on Filariasis. WHO, Geneva, Switzerland.

WHO/WPRO, 2007. Sixth Mekong Plus Workshop for Lymphatic Filariasis Programme Managers. Ha Noi, Viet Nam, 24–26 April 2007. (WP)2007/ICP/MVP/1.2/001). Report Series Number: RS/2007/GE/12(VTN).

Zhang, X.C., Huang, S.Y., Deng, Z.H., Ou, Z.Y., Wu, W.P., Luo, X.C., et al., 2008. Follow-up survey on the imported cases of lymphatic filariasis in Guangdong province. Chin. J. Parasitol. Parasit. Dis. 26, 409–411.

CHAPTER 9

Combating *Taenia solium* Cysticercosis in Southeast Asia: An Opportunity for Improving Human Health and Livestock Production

A. Lee Willingham III,[*] **Hai-Wei Wu,**[†,‡] **James Conlan,**[§,¶] and **Fadjar Satrija**[#]

Contents

[*] WHO/FAO Collaborating Center for Research and Training on Neglected and Other Parasitic Zoonoses, Section for Parasitology, Health and Development, Department of Veterinary Disease Biology, Faculty of Life Sciences, University of Copenhagen, Frederiksberg C, Denmark

[†] Department of Pathogen Biology, Nanjing Medical University, Nanjing, Jiangsu Province, People's Republic of China

[‡] Center for International Health Research, Rhode Island Hospital, Providence, Rhode Island, USA

[§] National Animal Health Centre, Department of Livestock and Fisheries, Ministry of Agriculture and Forestry, Luangprabang Road, Vientiane, Lao People's Democratic Republic

[¶] World Health Organization Collaborating Centre for the Molecular Epidemiology of Parasitic Infections, School of Veterinary and Biomedical Sciences, Murdoch University, Murdoch, WA, Australia

[#] Department of Animal Diseases and Veterinary Public Health, Faculty of Veterinary Medicine, Bogor Agricultural University, Jl. Agatis Kampus IPB Darmaga, Bogor, Indonesia

Advances in Parasitology, Volume 72
ISSN 0065-308X, DOI: 10.1016/S0065-308X(10)72009-1

Abstract

Cysticercosis caused by the zoonotic pork tapeworm *Taenia solium* is emerging as a constraint for the nutritional and economic well-being of small-holder farming communities in many underdeveloped areas of Southeast Asia. It occurs mainly in impoverished regions with inadequate sanitation, poor pig management practices and lack of meat inspection and control. Neurocysticercosis, the most serious form of the disease, is considered the most common parasitic infection of the human nervous system and the most frequent preventable cause of epilepsy in the developing world. Although theoretically easy to control and declared eradicable, *T. solium* taeniosis/cysticercosis remains a neglected disease. There is a lack of information and awareness of the burden and transmission of the disease at the regional and global level, partially explained by the unavailability of good quality diagnostic tools in field-applicable formats. These factors are further compounded by a lack of validated simple and sustainable intervention packages as part of integrated helminth control programmes. To date, *T. solium* taeniosis/cysticercosis has not been eliminated from any region by a specific programme in Southeast Asia, and no national control programmes are yet in place except in parts of the People's Republic of China. The presence, distribution, public health importance and economic relevance of cysticercosis need to be better documented in Southeast Asia in order to bring it to the attention of affected communities, decision-makers and funding bodies. A number of proven cost-effective intervention tools for combating cysticercosis appear to be available but need to be field validated. The Regional Network for Asian Schistosomiasis and Other Helminth Zoonoses ($RNAS^+$) serves as an important regional 'driving force' for managing research, capacity building, knowledge and stakeholder engagement essential for controlling cysticercosis in the Southeast Asian region while ensuring that research efforts are integrated with regional needs for surveillance and control.

9.1. INTRODUCTION

Cysticercosis is emerging as a public health and agricultural problem of concern in Southeast Asia, particularly in lesser developed areas where pigs are raised for consumption under traditional husbandry practices.

The infection is caused by the cestode helminth *Taenia solium*, commonly referred to as the "pork tapeworm". It is a zoonotic disease that forms larval cysts in humans and pigs that can lead to epilepsy and death in humans, makes pork unsafe to eat and reduces the market value of pigs. It occurs where sanitation is poor, meat inspection is inadequate and pigs range freely, and is thus strongly associated with poverty and smallholder pig farming. The current state of knowledge concerning *T. solium* infections in Asia has recently been reviewed confirming the emergence of cysticercosis as a threat to economic productivity and human health in many areas of the Southeast Asian region (Ito et al., 2004; Rajshekhar et al., 2003).

T. solium taeniosis/cysticercosis transmission is dependent on a two-host life cycle involving pigs and humans (life cycle presented in Fig. 9.1; distribution map in Fig. 9.2). Humans acquire taeniosis (adult tapeworm infection) when eating raw or undercooked pork contaminated with cysticerci, the larval form of *T. solium*. When ingested, the cysticerci evaginate and attach to the wall of the small intestine and, within approximately two months, develop into adult tapeworms that can grow to more than 3 m long (Flisser, 1994). *T. solium* has a head (scolex) armed with a double row of hooks and four suckers. Its body (strobila) consists of several hundred segments, or proglottids, each containing about 50,000–60,000 eggs (Flisser, 1994; Pawlowski and Murrell, 2000). The most distal proglottids (usually 1–5 daily) detach from the worm (singly or in groups) when their eggs have matured and pass out into the environment with the human host's faeces. These eggs can then in turn infect the same (auto-infection) or other humans through faecal–oral transmission, as well as pigs if they are ingested following direct contact with tapeworm carriers, through ingestion of infected faecal matter or from consuming water or food contaminated with human faeces. In developing countries, pigs are often allowed to roam free and, in the absence of sanitation facilities, being coprophagic they eat human faeces that may contain tapeworm eggs. In some countries, however, human faeces are fed directly to pigs (Flisser, 1988; Pouedet et al., 2002; Shey-Njila et al., 2003). Ingested eggs result in cysticerci that migrate to different parts of the human and pig bodies (e.g. muscles, eyes and brain) via the circulatory system and form cysts resulting in cysticercosis.

A principal site of migration in humans is the central nervous system (CNS), which has been reviewed elsewhere in volume 72 of the *Advances in Parasitology* (Lv et al., 2010). In brief, human neurocysticercosis (NCC) occurs when the cysts develop in the brain. It is considered to be the most common parasitic infection of the human nervous system and the most frequent preventable cause of epilepsy in the developing world (Del Brutto et al., 2001; Román et al., 2000). The clinical manifestations of NCC vary, with seizures being the most common presentation of

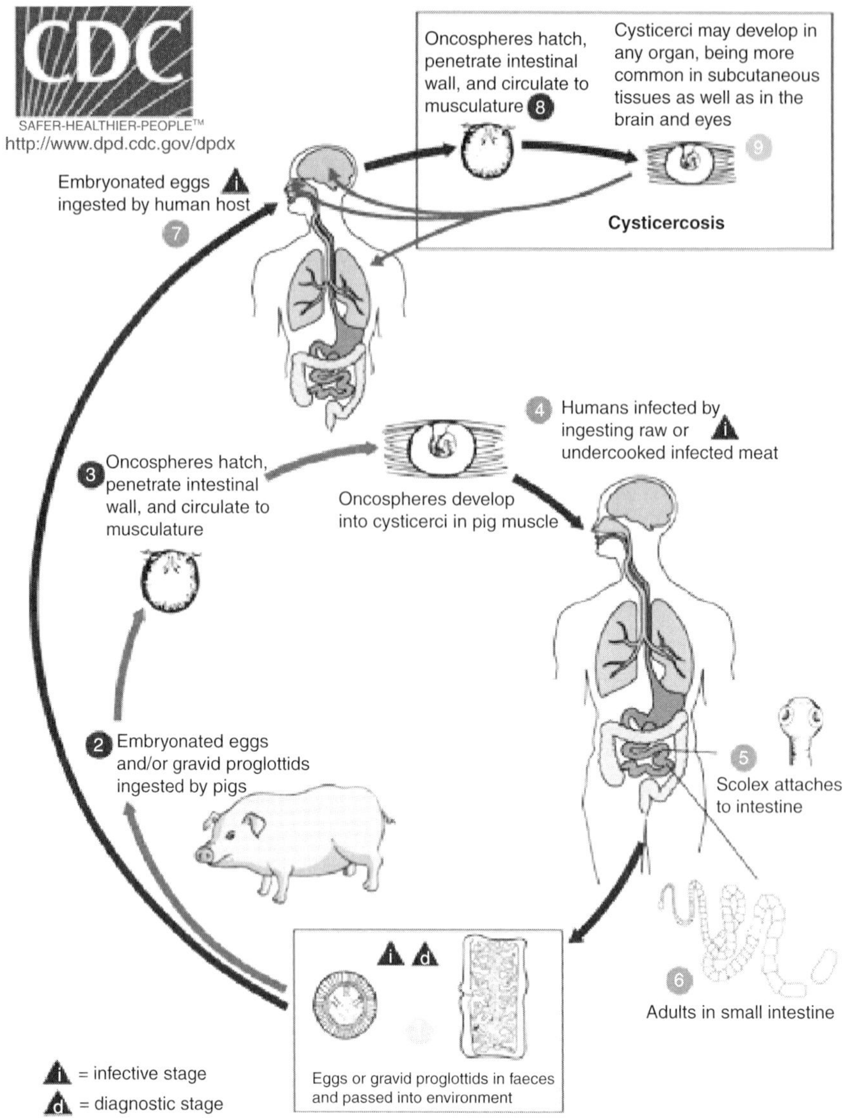

FIGURE 9.1 Cysticercosis is caused by ingestion of eggs shed in the faeces of a human tapeworm carrier ①. Pigs and humans become infected by ingesting eggs or gravid proglottids ②, ⑦. Humans are infected either by ingestion of food contaminated with faeces or by auto-infection. In the latter case, a human infected with adult *T. solium* can ingest eggs produced by that tapeworm, either through faecal contamination or, possibly, from proglottids carried into the stomach by reverse peristalsis. Once eggs are ingested, oncospheres hatch in the intestine ③, ⑧ invade the intestinal wall, and migrate to striated muscles, as well as the brain, liver and other tissues, where they develop into cysticerci ⑨. In humans, cysts can cause serious sequellae if they localise in the brain, resulting in neurocysticercosis. The parasite life cycle is completed, resulting in human tapeworm infection, when humans ingest undercooked pork containing cysticerci ④. Cysts evaginate and attach to the small intestine by their scolex ⑤. Adult tapeworms develop, up to 2–7 m in length and produce less than 1000 proglottids, each with approximately 50,000 eggs) and reside in the small intestine for years ⑥ (adapted from the U.S. Centers for Disease Control and Prevention website, www.cdc.gov).

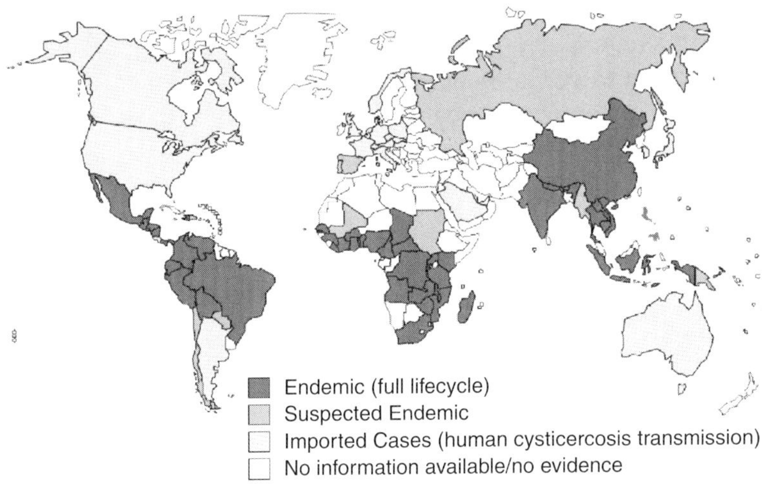

FIGURE 9.2 Global distribution of *T. solium* cysticercosis/taeniosis by country based on Román et al. (2000) and updated by recent published and anecdotal information concerning occurrence of porcine cysticercosis and human taeniosis and cysticercosis cases (provided by WHO/FAO Collaborating Centre for Parasitic Zoonoses, Faculty of Life Sciences, University of Copenhagen, Denmark).

symptomatic NCC, affecting from 69% to 96% of cases (Bern et al., 1999; Carpio and Hauser, 2002). Seizures can be acute symptomatic, occurring singly or in clusters, or they can be recurrent (epilepsy). Neurocysticercosis is reported to cause between 20% and 50% of all late-onset epilepsy cases in endemic countries (Bern et al., 1999; Campbell and Farrell, 1987; Carpio and Hauser, 2002; del Brutto et al., 2005; Preux and Druet-Cabanac, 2005) and is also reported to be a common cause of juvenile epilepsy in certain areas (Gaffo et al., 2004; Grill et al., 1996; Mafojane et al., 2003; Rosenfeld et al., 1996; Shasha and Pammenter, 1991; Thomson, 1993). In addition to seizures and epilepsy, NCC can manifest with severe chronic headaches, blindness, hydrocephalus, meningitis, symptoms due to space-occupying CNS lesions, dementia and even death (Garcia et al., 2003; Richards et al., 1985; Sorvillo et al., 2004, 2007; Townes et al., 2004).

The incubation period of NCC is unknown (due to the lack of cohort studies) and infected people may remain asymptomatic for months to years. The *T. solium* cysts are very effective at evading the hosts' immune system such that viable cysts with little or no inflammatory reaction are usually not associated with symptoms (White et al., 1997). It is when cysts are recognised by the host following spontaneous degeneration or after drug treatment that an inflammatory reaction occurs usually resulting in clinical symptoms. Oedema around calcified cysticercal granulomas has also been found to cause symptoms (Nash and Patronas, 1999;

Nash et al., 2001, 2004). The duration of NCC-associated symptoms and the proportion of these cases that will fully recover from their symptoms with or without treatment remain ill-defined.

People who are not engaged in pig production or those who do not consume pork are also at risk of cysticercosis if they ingest *T. solium* eggs after coming into direct or indirect contact with tapeworm carriers' faeces (e.g. shaking hands, sexual practices, contaminated water/food). For example, there have been reports of orthodox Jews in North America and Muslims in the Middle East, all banned from eating pork for religious reasons, being infected from their domestic helpers who were tapeworm carriers originally from endemic countries (Al Shahrani et al., 2003; Hira et al., 2004; Schantz et al., 1992). Vegetarians in India have been found to be at high risk of infection from tapeworm-infected food preparers (Rajshekhar et al., 2003), while in Vietnam, there have been reports suggesting a link between cysticercosis and the use of human faeces and 'wastewater' for fertilising crops (Willingham et al., 2003). *Taenia* spp. eggs have also been recovered from several varieties of vegetables and fruits available in local markets in endemic areas (Sorvillo et al., 2004). Everyone in endemic areas should thus be concerned about cysticercosis irrespective of cultural, religious and/or consumption practices. Development workers from non-endemic countries sent to work in endemic countries have also become infected (Leutscher and Andriantsimahavandy, 2004).

Although the life cycle of *T. solium* is generally considered to only involve humans and pigs, dogs have also been found to harbour *T. solium* cysts and may possibly play a role in transmission in areas of the world where dog meat consumption is practised such as in parts of Southeast Asia (e.g. People's Republic of China (P.R. China), Indonesia, Thailand, Vietnam) (Buback et al., 1996; Ito et al., 2002a,b, 2004; Jauregui and Marquez-Monter, 1977; Okolo, 1986a,b). Ito et al. (2004) have suggested that canine cysticercosis could be an important, under-recognised factor influencing *T. solium* transmission in Asia and its potential role should be investigated.

There are other *Taenia* tapeworms infecting humans, *T. saginata* and *T. asiatica*. Unlike *T. solium*, however, there have been no reports of metacestodes (cysticerci) of these other species infecting humans. The morbidity associated with adult tapeworm infections of these species is mild (Flisser et al., 2005). Pigs are also the intermediate host for *T. asiatica* and *T. hydatigena*, with the cysticerci developing in the liver and other visceral organs such as the lungs (*T. asiatica*) or on/in the liver, omentum and mesenteries (*T. hydatigena*). Humans are not normally infected with *T. hydatigena*. *T. hydatigena* and *T. asiatica* complicate porcine cysticercosis surveillance efforts as they may be misidentified as *T. solium* cysticerci during meat inspection or may cause cross-reactions in immunodiagnostic tests. Co-infections of *Taenia* species in both humans and pigs have been documented but the frequency of occurrence is unclear and inter-specific competition between these different species in co-endemic areas may play a role in moderating transmission (Anantaphruti et al., 2007; Conlan et al., 2009).

Pig production is central to the livelihoods of many marginalised and resource-poor communities in Southeast Asia, which has one of the highest concentrations of free-ranging pigs in the world. Asia accounts for the largest share (about 43%) of global pig output, with 78% of these pigs produced under mixed crop-livestock small-holder farmers (Groenewold, 2004). Major concentrations of pig production are in southern P.R. China, Vietnam, Thailand and the Philippines (FAO, 2006). Consumption of pork and production of pigs in the region exhibited a significant increase between 1990 and 2002 and are expected to increase further through 2020, with pork being the largest component of meat consumed except in the Islamic countries of Indonesia and Malaysia (Costales, 2006, Delgado, 2003). Increased consumption of pork can improve the incomes of poor farmers in developing countries, as in-depth field studies of rural households in Asia show that the rural poor get a higher share of their income from livestock than do better-off rural people. Thus, a pig can provide a key income supplement for asset-poor farmers if they do not encounter major marketing constraints (Delgado, 2003).

Pigs infected with *T. solium* may harbour thousands of cysts, making the pork from these animals unsafe to eat, often resulting in total condemnation of the pig's carcass, leading to serious economic loss for farmers and traders alike. Pig traders aware of the disease may detect infection during a pre-purchase examination and then refuse to buy a suspect pig. Farms and whole communities may become stigmatised when they are known for selling contaminated meat and/or infected pigs. Usually, a pig carcass infected with cysticercosis is totally condemned or sold at a decreased price. In P.R. China, the amount of pork discarded in the whole country due to cysticercosis annually has been estimated at 200 million kg with a value of more than US$ 120 million (Ito et al., 2003a). There is the additional risk that condemned pig carcasses are sold at reduced prices, putting lower-income consumers at a higher risk of infection. Moderately and lightly infected pigs are, however, the most important animals for continued *Taenia* transmission, as detection of cysts in these animals at inspection is unlikely. The sensitivity of detecting viable cysts by meat inspection or tongue palpation is highly variable and, generally speaking, very low (Dorny et al., 2004).

Cysticercosis has multiple impacts in that infection of humans affects their health, social and family life and productivity, it results in the removal of an important source of protein due to condemnation of pig carcasses, and can reduce the household income of farmers as an obstacle to marketing of pigs and pork (Carabin et al., 2005). The disease can therefore be a constraint to the improvement of the lives and livelihoods of small-holder farming communities. Efforts to comprehensively assess the global burden of cysticercosis are currently ongoing, whereby both the health and agricultural impacts of the disease are given equal consideration (Carabin et al., 2004, 2005, 2006; Praet et al., 2009). Initial results of a global burden assessment indicate a serious impact of cysticercosis on the public health and agricultural systems of endemic countries. However, a full assessment of the burden of disease has been hampered by a lack of quality epidemiological and cost information for many endemic countries including those of Southeast Asia.

9.2. *T. SOLIUM* INFECTIONS IN SOUTHEAST ASIA

T. solium cysticercosis has been reported in Vietnam, Cambodia, Lao People's Democratic Republic (Lao PDR), Thailand, P.R. China, the Philippines and specific regions of Indonesia (Bali and Papua) (Conlan et al., 2008; Dorny et al., 2004; Erhart et al., 2002; Ito et al., 2003a, 2003b; Margono et al., 2001; Rajshekhar et al., 2003; Salim et al., 2009; Singh and Prabhakar, 2002; Somers et al., 2006, 2007; Sovyra, 2005; Subahar et al., 2001; Willingham et al., 2003). In most of these countries, few if any systematic, structured community-based epidemiological surveys have been conducted. Regardless, the evidence gathered thus far (i.e. published and anecdotal reports) indicates that the disease is widespread in the region. In addition to *T. solium*, which causes human cysticercosis, *T. saginata* and *T. asiatica* are also known to be present in the Southeast Asia region and thus must be considered when conducting surveys and surveillance activities (Ito et al., 2003a).

9.2.1. Thailand

Few cases of *T. solium* cysticercosis/taeniosis have been reported in the literature in Thailand. Before the availability of sero-diagnostic tests, less than 500 cases of human cysticercosis were detected mostly by biopsy or imaging during the 40-year period 1965–2005, with cases of NCC reported more than sub-cutaneous cysticercosis (Waikagul et al., 2005). A provincial hospital in northern Thailand has reported finding solitary cysticercosis granulomas in 110 (11%) of 972 patients, with seizure disorder seen in the period 1994–1997 (Yodnopaklow and Mahuntussanapong, 2000). A recent study conducted during 2002–2005 using multiplex polymerase chain reaction (PCR) on human stool samples determined that 11 (45.8%) of 24 *Taenia*-infected patients in western Thailand harboured *T. solium* tapeworms in an area bordering Myanmar where consumption of raw or undercooked pork is common (Anantaphruti et al., 2007).

9.2.2. Lao PDR

There are a few anecdotal and case reports of NCC in Lao PDR, although sero-positivity of the human population has been estimated to be 10%. It should be noted, however that sample size and diagnostic test used to determine this figure are unknown (Singh and Prabhakar, 2002). A recent study on risk factors for epilepsy did not confirm any direct relation between epilepsy and cysticercosis serology as none of the epileptics included in the study were found to be sero-positive, but the sample size ($n = 31$) was considered too small to make any conclusions (Tran et al., 2007). An unpublished pilot survey of porcine cysticercosis conducted in a Louangprabang province slaughterhouse in northern Lao PDR in 2003 estimated the prevalence to be 1.7% based on 25 of 1497 pig carcasses being condemned for cysticercosis, however, speciation of the parasite cysts was not conducted (Conlan et al., 2008).

9.2.3. Cambodia

Like Lao PDR, there are few anecdotal and case reports of human cysticercosis in Cambodia, although sero-positivity of the human population has also been estimated to be 10%. Since sample size and diagnostic test used to determine this figure are unknown, care is indicated in interpreting this figure (Singh and Prabhakar, 2002). A recent survey for porcine cysticercosis based on carcass inspection at four slaughterhouses in Phnom Penh, where pigs were brought from 29 districts in nine provinces, indicated that 47 (10.9%; 95% confidence interval (CI): 8.1–17.2%) of 432 randomly selected pig carcasses harboured *T. solium* cysticerci (Sovyra, 2005). The prevalence ranged from 7.4% to 15.7% for the four slaughterhouses. Nearly half ($n = 212$) of the pigs examined came from intensive farms where the pigs are kept confined indoors. None of the intensively raised pigs was found to be infected, whereas 35 (25.5%; 95% CI: 18.5–33.7%) of 137 outdoor, free-raised pigs and 12 (14.5%; 95% CI: 7.7–23.9%) of 83 mixed indoor/outdoor-raised pigs were found infected. Positive pigs were detected from eight of the nine provinces supplying pigs, with prevalence ranging from 5.3 to 36.4%.

9.2.4. Vietnam

A review of the status of *T. solium* cysticercosis in Vietnam concluded that the disease is a serious health problem in the country, but more studies are needed to estimate the true prevalence and disease burden as most of the information is based on hospital and slaughterhouse data (Willingham et al., 2003). Community-based surveys on cysticercosis in Vietnam have only recently been conducted indicating important foci in rural villages in the northern part of the country. In Bac Ninh province, a serological survey indicated that 12 (5.7%) of 210 persons had circulating *T. solium* antigens, with 9 of these persons confirmed to have cysticercosis by CT scanning (Erhart et al., 2002). In Bac Kan province, 16 (5.3%) of 303 persons tested had circulating *T. solium* antigens (Somers et al., 2006). Recently, 65 *Taenia* tapeworms collected from patients seen at a referral hospital in Hanoi were submitted for morphological examination and molecular testing and 6.2% of these were determined to be *T. solium*, whereas 55.4% were *T. asiatica* and the remaining 38.5% were *T. saginata* (Somers et al., 2007). Interestingly, a 1993 survey at a Hanoi hospital indicated that 30% of cysticercosis patients also had taeniosis, suggesting auto-infection, although the species of tapeworm was unknown (Willingham et al., 2003). The consumption in Vietnam of traditional dishes using raw pork is considered to be a major risk factor for taeniosis (Dorny et al., 2004). A post-mortem survey of pigs slaughtered in southern Vietnam coming from 12 different provinces indicated that 8 (0.9%) of 891 had porcine cysticercosis (Huan, 1998).

9.2.5. Indonesia

Cysticercosis caused by *T. solium* has been found endemic in several areas of Indonesia, including Papua (formerly Irian Jaya) and Bali, and to a lesser extent in Eastern Island province (Timor and Flores Islands), Samosir Island of North Sumatra and Sulawesi. Recent surveys suggest that the incidence of *T. solium* cysticercosis has decreased substantially in Bali, whereas Papua is considered to have one of the highest human cysticercosis prevalences in the world (Simanjuntak et al., 1997; Suroso et al., 2006; Wandra et al., 2006a,b). In particular, Jayawijaya district of Papua has been found to be an important focus of cysticercosis following reports of high prevalence of epileptic seizures and a high number of case reports of burns related to seizuring people falling into open fires (Wandra et al., 2000; Margono et al., 2006). A serological survey in the rural area of Assologaima, Jayawija district indicated that 46 (48%) of 96 people have antibodies to *T. solium* cysts by enzyme-linked immunosorbent assay (ELISA) (Subahar et al., 2001; Wandra et al., 2000, 2003), while a serological survey using Western Blot and ELISA in Kama village of Jayawijaya district indicated that 28 (32%) of 58 persons had antibodies to *T. solium* cysticerci and five (8.6%) of 58 persons were found to have *T. solium* taeniosis by copro-antigen testing and confirmed by purgation and molecular testing (Margono et al., 2003). Also in Kama village, 50 (70.4%) of 71 pigs and seven (10.9%) of 64 dogs were also found to be sero-positive for antibodies against *T. solium* cysticerci (Ito et al., 2002b; Subahar et al., 2001). More recently, a sero-epidemiologic survey based on three-stage stratified cluster sampling was conducted in 2007 in

Jayawijaya and three other districts, that is, Paniai, Pegunungan Bintang and Puncak Jaya, in the central highlands of Papua. Anti-cysticercosis and anti-taeniosis antibodies were measured in 2931 people using recombinant T24 and recombinant ES33 as measures of cysticercosis and *T. solium* taeniosis exposures, respectively. Prevalence of cysticercosis and taeniosis was found to be high in the flat areas of Papua in Jayawijaya and Paniai districts, 20.8% and 29.2% for cysticercosis and 7% and 9.6% for taeniosis, respectively (Salim et al., 2009). Prevalence was relatively low in the hilly areas of Papua in Pegunungan Bintang and Puncak Jaya districts, 2% and 2% for cysticercosis and 1.7% and 10.7% for taeniosis, respectively (Salim et al., 2009). A slaughterhouse survey was conducted in the traditional market of Wamen, Jayawijaya district, whereby 27 (77%) of 35 pigs slaughtered were found to be infected with porcine cysticercosis (Maitindom, 2008).

In Bali, a serological survey indicated that 10 (13.5%) of 74 persons having epileptic seizures were sero-positive for antibodies to *T. solium* cysticerci, while 6 (5.2%) of 115 persons specifically from the village of Pamesan were found to be sero-positive for anti-*T. solium* cysticerci antibodies (Margono et al., 2001; Sutisna et al., 1999). A recent slaughterhouse survey of 108 pigs slaughtered in East Flores district did not find any cysticercosis infections in areas where sporadic human taeniosis cases have been reported (Saleh, 2010).

9.2.6. P.R. China

The emergence of cysticercosis as a public health problem in P.R. China was recognised by the government many years ago such that surveillance and intervention measures for taeniosis/cysticercosis were conducted in several areas of the country as far back as the 1970s. In some endemic areas (e.g. Heilongjiang, Jilin, Henan, and Fujian provinces), mass screening and treatment for taeniosis carriers, treatment of cysticercosis patients and pigs, and enhancement of meat inspection and population education programmes have been conducted (Li et al., 2007). *T. solium* infections were included in the 'National Investigation of Human Parasitic Diseases' conducted in 1990 which indicated that cysticercosis was reported in all provinces, municipalities and autonomous regions of mainland P.R. China (Xu et al., 1999). The national survey was conducted again in 2004, whereby 553 (0.58%) of 96,008 people surveyed had antibodies to *T. solium* cysticerci (Ministry of Health, P.R. China, 2005). The highest sero-positive proportion among occupational groups was among farmers and herdsman (2.51%), while among ethnic groups, the highest prevalence based on anti-cysticerci antibody detection were among the Bai (2.66%) and Miao (1.05%) minorities (Ministry of Health, P.R. China, 2005). In addition, 983 (0.28%) persons of 356,629 tested by coprology were positive for infection with *Taenia* spp., with a very high prevalence detected in Tibet (21.1%), where the number of taeniosis cases accounted for 87% of the national total (Li et al., 2006; Ministry of Health, P.R. China, 2005).

The three species of *Taenia* known to infect humans (i.e. *T. solium*, *T. saginata* and *T. asiatica*) have been found to co-exist in P.R. China and the high prevalence of taeniosis in Tibetans has been determined to be predominantly due to *T. saginata* based on the results of molecular studies (Li et al., 2006; Wang and Bao, 2003). The impact of cysticercosis in P.R. China has been estimated to be at least 3–6 million human cysticercosis cases and US$ 121 million of annual economic loss in national pork production due to porcine cysticercosis (Chen et al., 2004; Xu, 2002). The status of *T. solium* infections in P.R. China was recently reviewed by Li et al. (2007), with special attention to evidence available from the highly endemic areas in the northeast, north, central, northwest and especially southwest regions of the country.

In the northeast, Heilongjiang, Jilin and Liaoning provinces have previously been considered highly endemic for *T. solium* infections, but long-term control measures instituted by the government have succeeded in lowering the prevalence in that region (Li et al., 2007). Hospital records from Jilin province indicate that 4504 cysticercosis cases were identified during the period 1987–1994 (Liu et al., 1997), while serological surveys conducted in Heilongjiang province based on indirect haemagglutination test (IHA) during the period 1993–1994 indicated that 2.29–4.32% of those surveyed had anti-*T. solium* cysticerci antibodies (Ji et al., 1996; Li et al., 1996). Infection of human taeniosis in Dalian district of Liaoning was reported to decrease from 0.72% in 1980 to 0.039% in 1995 (Li et al., 1996), while another study in the province during 1995–1997 indicated that 38 (0.049%) and 27 (0.035%) of 78,274 persons surveyed tested positive for taeniosis and cysticercosis, respectively (Li et al., 1998).

A 1992 survey of 43,220 persons conducted in the northern provinces of Shanxi, Hebei, and Inner Mongolia indicated that 328 (0.76%) were sero-positive for anti-*T. solium* cysticerci antibodies. In addition, 351 (0.81%) of those surveyed were reported to be epileptic and of these 102 (29.1%) were found to be sero-positive for antibodies to *T. solium* cysticerci (Wei et al., 1994). An epidemiological survey conducted at 10 study sites in five cities in Inner Mongolia during 1996–1998 found that 441 (10.8%) of 4092 individuals were sero-positive by IHA for antibodies against *T. solium* cysticerci and 33 (0.81%) of these persons were confirmed to have taeniosis by routine coprology (Zhang et al., 2000).

T. solium infections have also been detected in the northwest region of P.R. China. An epidemiological survey performed during 1997–1998 in Huzhu county of Qinghai province detected 4 (0.39%) of 1024 persons to have taeniosis by Kato-Katz thick smear examination, while 159 (14.7%) of

1081 people were sero-positive by ELISA testing for antibodies against *T. solium* cysticerci (Wu et al., 2001). A more extensive survey was conducted in eastern Qinghai province between 2002 and 2004 which indicated that 5 (0.08%) and 97 (1.64%) of 5943 people were positive for taeniosis and antibodies against *T. solium* cysticerci by routine coprology and ELISA testing, respectively (Wu et al., 2005).

In addition, taeniosis/cysticercosis has been reported to be widely distributed in the central region, including Anhui, Henan, Hunan and Shandong provinces, but control measures instituted by the government have apparently substantially reduced the prevalence of *T. solium* infections (Li et al., 2007). A survey in Shandong province during 1997–2000 indicated prevalence of taeniosis and cysticercosis to be 0.048% and 0.057%, respectively (Liu et al., 2002), in comparison with prevalence of 0.30% and 0.71% for the same infections, respectively, during the early 1990s in the same area (Cao et al., 1995). A 2001 survey of 1480 people conducted in a mining area of southern Anhui province indicated that 14 (0.95%) were sero-positive for anti-*T. solium* cysticercus antibodies, while 12 (0.81%) were confirmed through coprology to be *Taenia* carriers (Wang, 2002).

T. solium infections remain prevalent in the less developed southwest provinces of Sichuan, Yunnan and Guizhou, especially among minority populations such as the Yi, Bai and Miao groups who have a fondness for consuming raw pork, a practice which has now been adopted by the majority Han population in the region as well (Fang et al., 1995). Juvenile neurocysticercosis has also been noted as a problem in the region (Guo et al., 2002; Liu and Mao, 2004). *T. saginata* and *T. asiatica* infections are co-endemic in areas of the region (Li et al., 2006; Wang and Bao, 2003), thus the results of taeniosis surveys must be considered carefully since routine coprology cannot distinguish between eggs of the three species. During the period 1991–1996, 1086 cases of human cysticercosis were recorded in the Affiliated Hospital of the Dali Institute of Schistosomiasis Prevention and Control in Yunnan province, originating from 12 counties of Dali prefecture, with ethnic Bai (59.2%) and Han Chinese populations (34.8%) as the dominant patient groups (Luo and Zhao, 1998). Results from a 1993 community-based survey in an ethnic Yi community of Xide county of Liangshan prefecture of Sichuan province indicated that of 1542 individuals surveyed, 62 (4.0%) reported a history of expulsion of *Taenia* proglottids, eight (0.5%) presented with sub-cutaneous nodules and 112 (7.3%) were sero-positive for anti-*T. solium* cysticercus antibodies (Zhou et al., 1993). A parasitological survey of the Bai population in Dali and Eryuan counties in Dali prefecture in 1992–1993 indicated that 233 (16.6%) of 1406 individuals had taeniosis detected by coprology (Fu et al., 1994; Fang et al., 1995). A more recent community-based survey conducted in 2000 in an ethnic Yi community in Dali prefecture in Yunnan province showed that 42 (34.7%) of 121 human faecal samples were positive for taeniosis by coprology, with frequent consumption of raw pork being strongly related to infection (Fang et al., 2002). While a 2005 survey of 500 human volunteers in Waduo Tibetan Township, Yajiang County, Ganze Tibetan prefecture in mid-west Sichuan province found 20 people (4.0%) to have anti-*T. solium* cysticercus antibodies by ELISA, with a higher prevalence (16.4%) noted in epileptics compared to non-epileptics (2.0%) (Li et al., 2006).

A recent community-based survey among 3220 people living in 35 randomly selected villages in Eryuan county, Yunnan province indicated a sero-prevalence for cysticercosis of 18.5% (95% CI: 17.2–19.9%) based on ELISA for IgG antibodies against *T. solium* cysticerci, while 3.5% (95% CI: 2.9–4.2%) of the same people were positive for taeniosis by Kato-Katz examination of their faeces (Steinmann et al., 2007). Taeniosis infection and sero-positivity for antibodies against cysticerci were particularly prominent in the poor with no or only basic education, living at altitudes ≥2150 m. (Steinmann et al., 2007). In general, 13.5% of the least poor families lacked sanitation facilities, however, among the poorest families, this increased to 86.3%. Raw pork and raw beef were consumed by 90.0% and 25.9% of the participants, respectively, with raw pork consumption being equally common in the Han and Bai populations and across all socio-economic strata. The higher prevalence of taeniosis infection and cysticerci-specific antibodies in the poorer population strata and in mountainous areas could be related to the lack of proper sanitation and a higher prevalence of small-holder pig farming than in more affluent areas (94.9% vs. 62.3%) (Steinmann et al., 2007).

Surveys in all three southwestern provinces indicate porcine cysticercosis to be a widespread problem. A post-mortem long-term survey of pigs conducted during the period 1990–1995 in nine districts of Guizhou province indicated that 328 (7.6%) of 4292 pig carcasses harboured *T. solium* cysts, with the highest prevalence of 12.1% recorded in pigs raised by ethnic Yi, while an ante-mortem serological survey of porcine cysticercosis in the same province indicated that 357 (13.7%) of 2599 pigs were positive for anti-*T. solium* cysticercus antibodies (Qian et al., 1998). In Yunnan province, a post-mortem survey of pig carcasses conducted in 12 counties of Dali prefecture during the period 1990–1995 showed that 11,754 (1.3%) of 871,699 pigs were inspected to be positive for cysticercosis (Wei, 1997). While in Sichuan province, inspection of pig carcasses at Liangshan Prefectural slaughterhouse in 2001 showed that 291 out of 40,791 pigs slaughtered (0.7%) had *T. solium* cysticerci compared to 137 of 29,331 (0.5%) inspected in the year 1990 (Zhou et al., 1993). Dogs raised for consumption in the region have also been detected with *T. solium* cysticerci by post-mortem examination (Zhang and Xu, 1998).

9.2.7. The Philippines

To our knowledge, there are no published reports of systematic, community-based surveys on cysticercosis in the Philippines. However, anecdotal and case reports of both human and porcine cysticercoses suggest that it is endemic. A sero-prevalence survey of human cysticercosis in Macanip, Leyte in the Eastern Visayas conducted on 497 youths and young adults indicated that 24.6% (95% CI: 20.8–28.6%) had antibodies against *T. solium* cysticerci (Xu et al., 2010).

9.2.8. Malaysia

Malaysia has a mostly Muslim population and cysticercosis cases are infrequent, however, a recent sero-prevalence study conducted in a rural population, Ranau village, Sabah, indicated that 3 (2.2%) of 135 people sampled had antibodies to *T. solium*, indicating exposure to the parasite (Noor Azian et al., 2006). Increasing cases of NCC are also being detected in immigrant workers (Arasu et al., 2005).

9.2.9. Myanmar

There are no recently published studies concerning cysticercosis in Myanmar (formerly Burma); however, anecdotal reports and case studies of people originally from Myanmar being infected suggest that the disease is endemic. A serological survey found 6% of the human population of Myanmar having antibodies against *T. solium* cysticerci (Coker-Vann et al., 1981).

9.3. CYSTICERCOSIS—AN ERADICABLE DISEASE

Cysticercosis caused by *T. solium* has been targeted as one of only six potentially eradicable diseases by the International Task Force for Disease Eradication (ITFDE, 1993). The characteristics of *T. solium* that make it vulnerable to eradication are presented in Table 9.1. In 2003, a reconvened International Task Force for Disease Eradication II (ITFDE II) considered the status of *T. solium* cysticercosis and as a result, strengthened its recommendations that cysticercosis is a potentially eradicable disease (ITFDE II, 2003). To date, however, no infection has been eliminated from any region by a specific programme and no national control programmes are yet in place, therefore demonstrating the need for intervention studies to verify outcomes and thus provide the 'proof-of-principle' (ITFDE II, 2003). Recommendations of the ITFDE II include:

TABLE 9.1 The following characteristics of *T. solium* make it vulnerable to eradication (ITFDE, 1993; Schantz et al., 1993)

- The life cycle requires humans as its definitive host
- Tapeworm infection in humans is the only source of infection for pigs, the natural intermediate hosts
- Domestic pigs, the intermediate hosts, can be managed
- No significant wildlife reservoir exists
- Practical intervention is available in the form of chemotherapy for human taeniosis and porcine cysticercosis with safe and effective drugs

- demonstration of effective control or elimination of *T. solium* transmission on a national scale would probably be the greatest single stimulus to further action against cysticercosis/taeniosis;
- a programme strategy that includes multiple interventions in flexible mass or targeted approaches would probably have the greatest chance of success;
- economic factors should be considered in designing any control programme, given the importance of domestic pig husbandry to affected local subsistence economies in endemic areas;
- there is a need to better understand the burden and transmission of the disease at the global level; and
- the impact of parasitic disease control programmes (e.g. schistosomiasis, soil-transmitted helminthiasis) involving the large-scale distribution of praziquantel and albendazole on the cysticercosis/taeniosis situation in areas where the diseases are co-endemic should be evaluated.

The issue of cysticercosis of the CNS has also been discussed at the 56th World Health Assembly (WHA) in May 2003 (WHO, 2003). The WHA secretariat's report strongly encouraged national authorities to set up surveillance and reporting systems and adopt a more active approach towards prevention and control of the diseases through further research and trials of intervention methods (WHO, 2003). An integrated, intersectoral approach to surveillance, prevention and control combining simple tools was promoted by the report for long-term success with regard to substantially reducing the disease burden in endemic areas as well as enhancing food safety and increasing economic benefits for small-holder pig farmers (Engels et al., 2003; WHO, 2003). Since cysticercosis is generally related to poverty and its associated manifestations, all strategies to control the disease must consider costs and locally available resources.

T. solium is potentially eradicable through surveillance and available interventions, but such feasibility needs to be demonstrated in a sizable geographic area (ITFDE, 1993). Chief obstacles to eradication of *T. solium* cysticercosis and taeniosis include the need for simpler and more accurate diagnostic tests for humans and pigs, the unavailability of drugs for treating human taeniosis and porcine cysticercosis (i.e. praziquantel, niclosamide and oxfendazole) in endemic areas, and a general lack of awareness and appreciation of the presence and impact of the disease by the affected communities as well as those in positions who could assist them in combating the problem. Thus far there is no evidence that eradication of *T. solium* is feasible and recommendable within a reasonable time frame (Engels et al., 2003). Alternatively, it is important to define a simple package of interventions that can be routinely conducted utilising existing services and structures in the endemic countries. These interventions must give an optimal, long-term return in terms of reducing the burden of cysticercosis by providing appropriate and sustainable control of the disease and should be validated through intervention research (Table 9.2).

9.4. SURVEILLANCE, PREVENTION AND CONTROL

The ITFDE recommendation on the eradicability of cysticercosis is based in part on the availability of tools to both detect and treat cysticercosis/taeniosis cases (Dorny et al., 2003). Several options are available for detection of human cysticercosis including biopsy of sub-cutaneous cysts, immunodiagnosis (antibody or parasite antigens in serum samples) and imaging techniques (e.g. radiography, CT and MRI scanning). For human taeniosis, the low specificity and sensitivity of routine coprology are complimented by the availability of a copro-antigen test (Allan et al., 1990)

TABLE 9.2 "Best bet" options for prevention and control of taeniosis/cysticercosis

1. Core 'rapid impact' measures
    - Identify areas of *T. solium* transmission
    - Treatment of humans for taeniosis
    - Mass treatment/vaccination of pigs
2. Relatively easy and inexpensive supportive measures
    - Community education
    - Improved sanitation—ending open defecation
3. Measures requiring more fundamental societal changes
    - Improved meat inspection, control and handling
    - Better pig management—no free-roaming

for detecting parasite materials in the faeces which indicates tapeworm infection but not that it is specifically *T. solium* (it also detects *T. saginata* and *T. asiatica* tapeworm infections) as well as a taeniosis immunoblot assay (EITB-T) which indicates that a person has had a *T. solium* tapeworm but not necessarily a current active infection (Wilkins et al., 1999) and PCR multiplex for identifying tapeworms at species level (Li et al., 2006; Yamasaki et al., 2004). Human tapeworm infections can be treated with either praziquantel or nicolosamide, whereas albendazole and praziquantel can be used to treat human cysticercosis cases. Detection of cysticercosis in pigs includes rapid lingual examination for cysts (inexpensive but low sensitivity), immunodiagnostic tests for detecting antibodies (variable specificity and sensitivity) or parasite antigens (very sensitive but low specificity in Asia) in living pigs and post-mortem inspection at slaughter (specific but very low sensitivity) (reviewed in Willingham and Engels, 2006). One dose of the drug oxfendazole has been found to cure porcine cysticercosis though it takes 3 months or more for the cysts to disappear (Gonzalez et al., 1996; Liu et al., 2003; Sikasunge et al., 2008). Guidelines for surveillance, prevention and control of cysticercosis/taeniosis have been published by the WHO, the Food and Agriculture Organization (FAO) and the World Organization for Animal Health (OIE) (Gemmell et al., 1983; Murrell, 2005).

One of the main obstacles to control and eliminate *T. solium* infections is the lack of reliable epidemiological data on cysticercosis and taeniosis which could be overcome through the institution of surveillance systems for the diseases. Taeniosis and cysticercosis do not lead to sudden large-scale international outbreaks of disease and therefore would not constitute an appropriate subject for international notification. Rather, it would be more appropriate for national authorities to establish national surveillance and reporting of cysticercosis and taeniosis as part of a routine system (WHO, 2003). Epidemiological studies have demonstrated clustering of NCC cases around individuals infected with a *T. solium* tapeworm (Garcia et al., 1999), it may be appropriate therefore to have public health follow-up of cysticercosis cases (NCC and/or sub-cutaneous nodules), including screening of household contacts, to identify tapeworm carriers (transmission foci) to be treated and removed as potential sources of further infection. Surveillance of cysticercosis in pigs has been proposed as a practical, inexpensive and sensitive method for indirectly assessing human risk and monitoring and evaluating the effectiveness of community-based control programmes (Gonzalez, 2002). However, pigs may not go through the formal slaughterhouse system, especially if they are suspected by the farmers or pig traders to be infected with cysticercosis and thus community-based surveys should be utilised to provide a more realistic assessment (Cysticercosis Working Group in Peru, 1993; Gonzalez et al., 1990). A proven effective way to assess changes in the intensity of environmental contamination with *T. solium* eggs is to bring in 'sentinel' pigs from non-endemic areas that can be serologically tested periodically which, depending on the cost, may be an effective monitoring tool (Gonzalez, 2002; Sarti et al., 1997). The strength of an epidemiological surveillance system is, however, dependent on the ability of a public health system to detect cases. Developing countries tend to be resource poor and the detection of cysticercosis cases in humans and pigs can be problematic (e.g. lack of neuro-imaging facilities). This fact is compounded by the limited availability of imperfect diagnostic tests.

Only tapeworm carriers and infected pigs are important in terms of transmission of *T. solium* infections and are thus the targets for prevention and control. Individuals with NCC are a health concern but not important for transmission unless they are also infected with a *T. solium* tapeworm. Thus, to be effective and sustainable, a practical, cost-effective combination of simple interventions targeting both the intermediate and definitive hosts should be considered (Garcia, 2002; Lightowlers, 1999). Any selected combination of interventions would need to ensure community co-operation and incorporate economic incentives to ensure sustainability. The appropriateness and justification for undertaking such interventions need to be first verified through 'rapid epidemiological assessment' of the targeted communities to secure the evidence-base on the public health and/or economic relevance of cysticercosis in order to ensure the commitment of local and national decision-makers for implementing the proposed solutions (Engels et al., 2003). Engagement of stakeholders from the various relevant sectors and interested parties, including veterinary and medical workers, should be promoted from the outset to help ensure success.

Sustainable control programmes for *T. solium* infections must aim to both decrease the supply of infected meat to consumers and prevent environmental contamination with parasite eggs. *T. solium* carriers are extremely potent sources of cysticercosis, endangering everyone coming in contact with them, including themselves. Reduction of human taeniosis by detection and treatment of human tapeworm carriers or by mass treatment of the whole population with praziquantel or niclosamide has proven effective for reducing environmental contamination of the parasite in the short term. However, these attempts only had temporary success due to the continued presence of susceptible intermediate hosts and the movement of human tapeworm carriers into the targeted communities. Continuous maintenance and intensive monitoring and surveillance would therefore be required to remain effective (Allan et al., 1997; Cruz et al., 1989; Garcia, 2002). Appropriate surveillance mechanisms should be implemented whereby new cases of NCC or porcine cysticercosis are reported to national authorities in order to facilitate identifying and treating sources of tapeworm eggs, that is, tapeworm carriers and any persons having close contact with them (Román et al., 2000). Since infective eggs of *T. solium* can be expelled following treatment, there is a theoretical risk of a temporary increase in human and porcine cysticercoses during taeniosis treatment campaigns, if disposal of human stools is not carefully controlled. A study in Mexico found that porcine cysticercosis nearly doubled one year after mass human chemotherapy which did not take into consideration the need for safe disposal of faeces post-treatment (Keilbach et al., 1989).

Local populations in endemic areas rarely understand the relationship between cysticercosis in pigs and taeniosis in humans and thus lack knowledge and incentive to change behaviour that facilitates transmission. Efforts to educate villagers at schools, village meetings and on an individual basis have been successful in terms of teaching villagers the life cycle of *T. solium*, the connection between infected pigs and themselves or others getting cysticercosis, and how to improve hygiene, sanitation and pig management practices to reduce the risk of infection (Keilbach et al., 1989; Sarti et al., 1997). However, these initiatives solely based on education have not been shown to dramatically change behaviours affecting transmission and/or risk factors, although in some situations, environmental contamination appears to have decreased following educational campaigns (Sarti et al., 1997). A recent study in northern Tanzania assessing the effectiveness of health and pig management education for combating cysticercosis based on the PRECEDE-PROCEED planning model (Green and Kreuter, 1999) whereby active participation of members of the target community affected by *T. solium* infections systematically analyse factors in the community influencing transmission and then plan, implement and evaluate evidence-based interventions for reducing transmission of the parasite led to a 20% reduction in household consumption of infected pork and a 43% decrease in the incidence of porcine cysticercosis (Ngowi et al., 2007a, 2008, 2009). It is generally accepted that education should be an integral part of any control programme due to the long-term effect of acquired knowledge on the sustainability of intervention efforts as it creates demand for change (Ngowi et al., 2007a, 2009; Sarti et al., 1997). Health and pig managements' education intervention has been shown to have a significant financial benefit to small-holder pig farmers in Tanzania, resulting in their improved economic well-being regardless of plausible changes in costs and benefits in pig production as well as the incidence rate of porcine cysticercosis (Ngowi et al., 2007b).

Interventions focused on the pig population will not only control any further infections of humans in the village, but also by potentially increasing the value of the pigs (i.e. increasing their marketability and value if free from cysticercosis) it will act as an economic incentive and lead to increased compliance with other control activities, such as human treatment and education. Intervention studies in Peru involving concurrent intensive chemotherapy of people and pigs indicate that it is possible to block transmission and eliminate the parasite from communities if the treatment regimen is maintained and a surveillance system is in place to counter the movement of human tapeworm carriers or infected swine into the treated communities (Garcia, 2002). Better market prices for treated pork and access to the formal marketing system will be strong incentives for farmers to treat their pigs, helping to ensure community co-operation. However, in order to improve the commercial value of pork, its appearance should be clean and similar to non-infected meat. Thus, the availability of oxfendazole as a proven effective drug for curing pigs eventually eliminating the cysts with the added benefit of resistance to further infection provides strong incentives for small pork producers to comply with control measures (Gonzalez et al., 1996, 1997, 2001). Such an incentive-based means of having farmers treat their pigs with oxfendazole in Southeast Asia will require traders and a large proportion of consumers having a good understanding of the *T. solium* transmission pathways, so they are able to see the benefit of paying more for pork. This then links directly back to the importance of effective community education programmes. Vaccines against *T. solium* infection may one day make treatment of pigs unnecessary, providing a very useful tool for helping to combat cysticercosis especially if they have both preventive and therapeutic effects (Lightowlers, 2003; Sciutto et al., 2002). An important factor with regard to their potential effectiveness and actual usefulness, the ability of the vaccines to protect young piglets directly or indirectly through sows prior to birth, is currently being assessed through controlled field trials. Much attention is needed with regard to how these tools can actually be utilised by communities in endemic areas to ensure compliance since they may not be affordable for many small-holder pig keepers. There again the economic incentives of prevention may overcome the compliance issue if the farmers are made aware of the benefits compared to the costs.

Transmission of *T. solium* infections can be blocked if the sale and consumption of infected pork are prevented by slaughterhouse meat inspection and confiscation of infected pig carcasses (Joshi et al., 2003). Unfortunately in many endemic countries, national pork inspection guidelines may be inadequate and little attention may be paid to the porcine cysticercosis issue, thus leading to low detection of infected carcasses especially in countries where pig rearing and pork consumption have only recently become popular (Boa et al., 2002; Phiri et al., 2003). Policies concerning confiscation of infected pig carcasses must be strategic since confiscation without payment to the pig's owner may lead to the establishment of clandestine markets and un-official slaughtering establishments for pigs infected with *T. solium*. In Peru where pigs are confiscated without payment to the pig's owner, over 50% of the pigs are slaughtered illegally (Cysticercosis Working Group in Peru, 1993). In addition to enforcing meat inspection, cooking and freezing of pork can also break the parasite's life cycle. Cysticerci are killed best by cooking pork to at least 60 °C or until it loses its pink colour (Pawlowski and Murrell, 2000) or alternatively, pork can be frozen at −5°C for 4 days, −15°C for 3 days or −24°C for 1 day to kill the cysts (Sotelo et al., 1986). Refrigeration of pork at temperatures about 0 °C does not affect the parasite.

Targeting slaughterhouses as the primary intervention fails to influence the husbandry practices which occur before the pigs are brought to market (Lekule and Kyvsgaard, 2003). Pig keeping is popular among small-holder farmers in large part due to minimum inputs required in order to get a good return on their investment. By allowing a pig to roam freely, it is able to supplement its diet with local garbage and human and other faeces, thus helping to keep the community clean and saving the farmer from having to buy expensive feeds. Confining pigs results in major capital inputs from the farmers for proper housing and feeding. Control strategies must consider these potential costs and the economic incentives that will be required for different pig-rearing practices to be adopted (Lekule and Kyvsgaard, 2003). There are instances of new crops being introduced into communities which made it economically advantageous to keep pigs confined or tethered in order to prevent them from consuming the crops, thereby reducing or eliminating pigs having access to human faeces and subsequently reducing the burden of cysticercosis in the pig population (Gonzalez et al., 2003; M.E. Boa, Sokoine University of Agriculture, Tanzania).

9.5. CONCLUSIONS AND RECOMMENDATIONS

Cysticercosis/taeniosis remains a neglected disease in much of Southeast Asia due to lack of information and awareness about the extent and burden of the problem, suitable diagnostic and management capacity and appropriate prevention and control strategies. As with other neglected tropical diseases, ethnic minorities might be at a particularly high risk of cysticercosis/taeniosis (Schratz et al., 2010). Hence, the public health and economic relevance of cysticercosis and its impact on especially marginalised populations and link with poverty need to be better documented in order to convincingly bring it to the attention of affected communities, decision-makers and potential investors. All aspects of cysticercosis in Southeast Asia must be considered in order to make responsible decisions on whether and how to best combat the disease. Such considerations include distribution, prevalence and economic impact, transmission dynamics, the availability of appropriate tools for understanding and combating cysticercosis, the ability to use them in a cost-effective manner and the availability of sustained resources and political will to undertake surveillance and control activities (Colley, 2000). Such an evidence-base is essential for making appropriate and relevant policies as well as setting priorites at the national and regional levels. Political will is a key factor for sustainability and depends on decision-makers understanding the burden of cysticercosis, its impact on health and agricultural systems, its impact overall on development and affected populations demanding action.

It is the responsibility of all stakeholders involved to forge active links between the findings of researchers and those seeking to implement methodologies in disease surveillance and control. Sustainable prevention and control of cysticercosis can be facilitated by bringing together a multidisciplinary coalition of researchers from human medical, social, veterinary, agricultural and environmental sciences as well as national, regional and international institutes to address the major obstacles for combating the disease. These include, among other issues (i) characterising the disease, its risk factors and societal impact; (ii) increasing capacity for identifying and managing cysticercosis and taeniosis cases; (iii) identifying and validating appropriate and sustainable 'best bet' prevention and control strategies; and (iv) promoting collaboration among the various relevant stakeholder groups. Such a coalition of researchers and public health professionals should be linked with appropriate national and regional initiatives on related issues such as parasitic/tropical/zoonotic diseases, epilepsy, sanitation, food safety and livestock development.

The creation of an enabling environment for integration of research activities with control needs should facilitate a thorough understanding and sustainable reduction in the burden of cysticercosis. Formation of a regional working group for combating cysticercosis aimed at promoting communication, collaboration, coordination and sustainability is an effective way to bring together a variety of stakeholders to promote and facilitate advocacy and networking, set regional priorities (i.e. regional action plan), ensure that research efforts are integrated with regional needs for surveillance and control and engage with investors. The Regional Network for Asian Schistosomiasis and Other Helminth Zoonoses (RNAS$^+$) has recently expanded its mandate to include responsibilities for planning, implementing, monitoring and evaluating activities regarding cysticercosis research, training, surveillance, prevention and control based on regional needs and priorities (Conlan et al., 2009; Zhou et al., 2008; see Table 9.3). RNAS$^+$, provided proper technical and financial support, will be an important regional 'driving force' for managing research, capacity building and knowledge management essential for effectively combating cysticercosis in the Southeast Asia region.

TABLE 9.3 Research needs for *Taenia* in Southeast Asia as suggested by Conlan et al. (2009)

Immunological

1. Development of rapid, sensitive and specific point-of-care tests for human taeniosis that is capable of differentiating the three related species *T. solium*, *T. saginata* and *T. asiatica*.
2. Development of sensitive and specific tests for the detection of viable *Taenia* infections of pigs that is able to differentiate and semi-quantify intensity of infection of *T. solium*, *T. hydatigena* and *T. asiatica*.
3. Development of tests capable of identifying pigs with immunity to the pre-encystment phase of infection.

Epidemiological and ecological

1. Development of a comprehensive understanding of the epidemiological and ecological parameters influencing *Taenia* transmission dynamics, including:
   a. Effects of inter-specific crowding in the definitive host on egg production and biotic potential.
   b. Infection pressure of *T. solium* and *T. asiatica* from human tapeworm carriers.
   c. Infection pressure of *T. hydatigena* from dogs.
   d. Age-intensity profiles of the three *Taenia* species infecting pigs and *T. saginata* in cattle and buffalo.
   e. Regional approaches to understanding the socio-ecological risk factors for taeniosis and cysticercosis.
   f. Regional approach to understanding the pig and pork trade networks and associated risks.
2. Characterise passive and acquired immunities of pigs to *T. hydatigena* and *T. asiatica*.
3. Investigate the immunological interactions of the three *Taenia* species infecting pigs.
4. Develop a regionally focused ecological model of *T. solium* cysticercosis and taeniosis.

Prevention and control

1. Regional assessment of the burden of disease resulting from human neurocysticercosis.
2. Regional assessment of the socio-economic impact of *T. solium* cysticercosis in pigs.
3. Develop, implement and assess effectiveness of control programmes that take an ecological perspective.

ACKNOWLEDGEMENTS

The authors wish to thank Dr. Sukwan Handali of the U.S. Centers for Disease Control and Prevention in Atlanta, Georgia, USA; Professor Xiao-Nong Zhou of the National Institute of Parasitic Diseases, China CDC, Shanghai, P.R. China and Ms. Tiao-Ying Li of Sichuan Institute of Parasitic Diseases in Chengdu, Sichuan province, P.R. China for their assistance in preparing this chapter.

REFERENCES

Al Shahrani, D., Frayha, H.H., Dabbagh, O., Al Shail, E., 2003. First case of neurocysticercosis in Saudi Arabia. J. Trop. Pediatr. 49, 58–60.

Allan, J.C., Avila, G., Garcia-Noval, J., Flisser, A., Craig, P.S., 1990. Immunodiagnosis of taeniasis by coproantigen detection. Parasitology 101, 473–477.

Allan, J.C., Velasquez-Tohom, M., Fletes, C., Torres-Alvarez, R., Lopez-Virula, G., Yurrita, P., et al., 1997. Mass chemotherapy for intestinal *Taenia solium* infection: effect on prevalence in humans and pigs. Trans. R. Soc. Trop. Med. Hyg. 91, 595–598.

Anantaphruti, M.T., Yamasaki, H., Nakao, M., Waikagul, J., Watthanakulpanich, D., Nuamtanong, S., et al., 2007. Sympatric occurrence of *Taenia solium, T. saginata*, and *T. asiatica*, Thailand. Emerg. Infect. Dis. 13, 1413–1416.

Arasu, K., Khairul, A., Waran, V., 2005. Neurocysticercosis an uncommon intra-cerebral infection in Malaysia. Med. J. Malaysia 60, 514–516.

Bern, C., Garcia, H.H., Evans, C., Gonzalez, A.E., Verastegui, M., Tsang, V.C.W., et al., 1999. Magnitude of the disease burden from neurocysticercosis in a developing country. Clin. Infect. Dis. 29, 1203–1209.

Boa, M.E., Kassuku, A.A., Willingham, A.L., Keyyu, J.D., Phiri, I.K., Nansen, P., 2002. Intensity, distribution and density of *Cysticercus cellulosae* by muscle groups and organs in naturally infected local slaughter pigs in Mbulu district of Tanzania. Vet. Parasitol. 106, 155–164.

Buback, J.L., Schulz, K.S., Walker, M.A., Snowden, K.F., 1996. Magnetic resonance imaging of the brain for diagnosis of neurocysticercosis in a dog. J. Am. Vet. Med. Assoc. 208, 1846–1848.

Campbell, G.D., Farrell, V.J., 1987. Brain scans, epilepsy and cerebral cysticercosis. S. Afr. Med. J. 72, 885–886.

Cao, W., Xu, J., Gao, C., 1995. Epidemiological survey on *Taenia solium* and *Cysticercus cellulosae* infection in Shandong province, China. Chin. J. Parasit. Dis. Control 8, 168–172.

Carabin, H., Budke, C., Cowan, L.D., Nash, T., Willingham III, A.L., Torgerson, P.R., 2004. Assessing the burden of cysticercosis and echinococcosis. In: Willingham, A.L., Schantz, P. M. (Eds.), Assessing the burden of *Taenia solium* cysticercosis and echinococcosis. Vet. Parasitol. Vol. 125. Elsevier, The Netherlands, pp. 184–186.

Carabin, H., Budke, C.M., Cowan, L.D., Willingham 3rd, A.L., Torgerson, P.R., 2005. Methods for assessing the burden of parasitic zoonoses: echinococcosis and cysticercosis. Trends Parasitol. 21, 327–333.

Carabin, H., Krecek, R.C., Cowan, L.D., Michael, L., Foyaca-Sibat, H., Nash, T., et al., 2006. Estimation of the monetary burden of *Taenia solium* cysticercosis in Eastern Cape Province, South Africa. Trop. Med. Int. Health 2, 906–916.

Carpio, A., Hauser, W.A., 2002. Prognosis for seizure recurrence in patients with newly diagnosed neurocysticercosis. Neurology 59, 1730–1734.

Chen, Y.D., Xu, L.Q., Zhou, X.N., 2004. Distribution and disease burden of cysticercosis in China. Southeast Asian J. Trop. Med. Public Health 35 (Suppl.), 231–239.

Coker-Vann, M.R., Subianto, D.B., Brown, P., Diwan, A.R., Desowitz, R., Garruto, R.M., et al., 1981. ELISA antibodies to cysticerci of *Taenia solium* in human populations in New

Guinea, Oceania, and Southeast Asia. Southeast Asian J. Trop. Med. Public Health 12, 499–505.
Colley, D., 2000. Parasitic diseases: opportunities and challenges in the 21st century. Mem. Inst. Oswaldo Cruz 95 (Suppl. 1), 79–87.
Conlan, J., Khounsy, S., Inthavong, P., Fenwick, S., Blacksell, S., Thompson, R.C., 2008. A review of taeniasis and cysticercosis in the Lao People's Democratic Republic. Parasitol. Int. 57, 252–255.
Conlan, J.V., Vongxay, K., Fenwick, S., Blacksell, S.D., Thompson, R.C., 2009. Does interspecific competition have a moderating effect on *Taenia solium* transmission dynamics in Southeast Asia? Trends Parasitol. 25, 398–403.
Costales, A., 2006. Pig systems, livelihoods and poverty: current status, emerging issues, and ways forward. Food and Agriculture Organization of the United Nations Pro-Poor Livestock Policy Initiative, Research Report 06–10, pp. 1–25..
Cruz, M., Davis, A., Dixon, H., Pawlowski, Z.S., Porano, J., 1989. Operational studies on the control of *Taenia solium* taeniasis/cysticercosis in Ecuador. Bull. World Health Organ. 67, 401–407.
Cysticercosis Working Group in Peru, 1993. The marketing of cysticercotic pigs in the sierra of Peru. Bull. World Health Organ. 71, 223–228.
Del Brutto, O.H., Rajshekar, V., White Jr., A.C., Tsang, V.C., Nash, T.E., Takayanagui, O.M., et al., 2001. Proposed diagnostic criteria for neurocysticercosis. Neurology 57, 177–183.
Del Brutto, O.H., Santibáñez, R., Hidrovo, L., Rodríguez, S., Dìaz-Calderón, E., Navas, C., et al., 2005. Epilepsy and neurocysticercosis in Atahualpa: a door-to-door survey in rural coastal Ecuador. Epilepsia 46, 583–587.
Delgado, C.L., 2003. Rising consumption of meat and milk in developing countries has created a food revolution. J. Nutr. 133 (Suppl. 2), 3907S–3910S.
Dorny, P., Brandt, J., Zoli, A., Geerts, A.T., 2003. Immunodiagnostic tools for human and porcine cysticercosis. Acta Trop. 87, 79–86.
Dorny, P., Phiri, I.K., Vercruysse, J., Gabriel, S., Willingham III, A.L., Brandt, J., Victor, B., Speybroeck, D., Berkvens, D., 2004. A Bayesian approach for estimating values for prevalence and diagnostic test characteristics of porcine cysticercosis. Int. J. Parasitol. 34, 569–576.
Engels, D., Urbani, C., Belotto, A., Meslin, F., Savioli, L., 2003. The control of human (neuro) cysticercosis: which way forward? Acta Trop. 87, 177–182.
Erhart, A., Dorny, P., Van De, N., Vien, H.V., Thach, D.C., Toan, N.D., et al., 2002. *Taenia solium* cysticercosis in a village in northern Viet Nam: seroprevalence study using an ELISA for detecting circulating antigen. Trans. R. Soc. Trop. Med. Hyg. 96, 270–272.
Fang, W., Lian, Z.Q., Fang, C., 1995. Epidemiological survey on taeniasis/cysticercosis in Bai populations from Louyi village of Dali prefecture, Yunnan province. Chin. J. Parasit. Dis. Control 8, 199.
Fang, W., Sheng, X.L., Luo, T.P., Fang, C.H., Xiong, S.L., Yang, G.Y., et al., 2002. Survey on *Taenia solium* in Yi populations from Houshan village of Dali prefecture, Yunnan province, China. Chin. Prev. Med. 3, 7.
FAO, 2006. FAOSTAT Statistical Database. Food and Agriculture Organization. http://faostat.fao.org/default.htm (accessed: 15 January 2010).
Flisser, A., 1988. Neurocysticercosis in Mexico. Parasitol. Today 4, 131–137.
Flisser, A., 1994. Taeniasis and cysticercosis due to *Taenia solium*. In: Sun, T. (Ed.), Progress in Clinical Parasitology. CRC Press, New York, pp. 77–116.
Flisser, A., Vázquez-Mendoza, A., Martiñez-Ocaña, J., Gómez-Colín, E., Sánchez-Leyva, R., Medina-Santillán, R., 2005. Evaluation of a self-detection tool for tapeworm carriers for use in public health. Am. J. Trop. Med. Hyg. 72, 510–512.
Gaffo, A.L., Guillen-Pinto, D., Campos-Olazabal, P., Burneo, J.G., 2004. Cysticercosis as the main cause of partial seizures in children in Peru. Rev. Neurol. 39, 924–926.

Garcia, H.H., Gilman, R.H., Gonzalez, A.E., Pacheco, R., Verastegui, M., Tsang, V.C., 1999. Human and porcine *Taenia solium* infection in a village in the highlands of Cusco, Peru. Acta Trop. 73, 31–36.

Garcia, H.H., 2002. Effectiveness of an interventional control program for human and porcine *Taenia solium* cysticercosis in field conditions. Johns Hopkins University, Baltimore, Maryland (PhD Dissertation, p. 227).

Garcia, H.H., Gonzalez, A.E., Evans, C.A.W., Gilman, R.H., 2003. *Taenia solium* cysticercosis. Lancet 362, 547–556.

Gemmell, M., Matyas, Z., Pawlowski, Z., Soulsby, E.J.L., Larralde, C., Nelson, G.S., et al., 1983. Guidelines for surveillance, prevention and control of taeniasis/cysticercosis, VPH/83.49. World Health Organization, Geneva.

Gonzalez, A.E., 2002. Control of *Taenia solium* with porcine chemotherapy. In: Singh, G., Prabhakar, S. (Eds.), *Taenia solium* Cysticercosis. From Basic to Clinical Science. CABI Publishing, Wallingford, United Kingdom, pp. 431–435.

Gonzalez, A.E., Cama, V., Gilman, R.H., Tsang, V.C., Pilcher, J.B., Chavera, A., et al., 1990. Prevalence and comparison of serologic assays, necropsy, and tongue examination for the diagnosis of porcine cysticercosis in Peru. Am. J. Trop. Med. Hyg. 43, 194–199.

Gonzalez, A.E., Garcia, H.H., Gilman, R.H., Gavidia, C.M., Tsang, V.C., Bernal, T., et al., 1996. Effective, single-dose treatment of porcine cysticercosis with oxfendazole. Am. J. Trop. Med. Hyg. 54, 391–394.

Gonzalez, A.E., Falcon, N., Gavidia, C., Garcia, H.H., Tsang, V.C., Bernal, T., et al., 1997. Treatment of porcine cysticercosis with oxfendazole: a dose-response trial. Vet. Rec. 141, 420–422.

Gonzalez, A.E., Gavidia, C., Falcon, N., Bernal, T., Verastegui, M., Garcia, H.H., et al., 2001. Protection of pigs with cysticercosis from further infections after treatment with oxfendazole. Am. J. Trop. Med. Hyg. 65, 15–18.

Gonzalez, A.E., Garcia, H.H., Gilman, R.H., Tsang, V.C., 2003. Control of *Taenia solium*. Acta Trop. 87, 103–109.

Green, L.W., Kreuter, M.W., 1999. Health Promotion Planning: An Education and Environmental Approach, 3rd edition Mayfield, Mountain View, California.

Grill, J., Rakotomalala, W., Andriantsimahavandy, A., Boisier, P., Guyon, P., Roux, J., et al., 1996. High prevalence of serological markers of cysticercosis among epileptic Malagasy children. Ann. Trop. Paediatr. 16, 185–191.

Groenewold, J.P., 2004. Classification and Characterization of World Livestock Production Systems: Update of the 1994 Livestock Production Systems with Recent Data. FAO AGAL, Rome.

Guo, G., Li, J.H., Wu, J.W., Qiu, X.L., 2002. Report on one human case of cysticercosis. J. Guiyang Med. Coll. 27, 91.

Hira, P.R., Francis, I., Abdella, N.A., Gupta, R., Ai-Ali, F.M., Grover, S., et al., 2004. Cysticercosis: imported and autochthonous infections in Kuwait. Trans. R. Soc. Trop. Med. Hyg. 98, 233–239.

Huan, L.V., 1998. Parasitic helminths in pigs in several southern provinces and preventative measures. Eco. Sci. Technol. Manag. Mag. 1, 5–7.

International Task Force for Disease Eradication (ITFDE), 1993. Recommendations of the International Task Force for Disease Eradication. Morb. Mortal. Weekly Rep 42 (RR-16), 1–46.

International Task Force for Disease Eradication II, 2003. Summary of the Fourth Meeting of the ITFDE II, April 16, 2003. http://www.cartercenter.org/documents/1367.pdf (accessed: 15 January 2010).

Ito, A., Putra, M.I., Subahar, R., Sato, M.O., Okamoto, M., Sako, Y., et al., 2002a. Dogs as alternative intermediate hosts of *Taenia solium* in Papua, Irian Jaya), Indonesia confirmed by highly specific ELISA and immunoblot using native and recombinant antigens and mitochondrial DNA analysis. J. Helminthol. 76, 311–314.

Ito, A., Sako, Y., Nakao, M., Nakaya, K., 2002b. Neurocysticercosis in Asia: serology/in humans and pigs. In: Craig, P., Pawlowski, Z. (Eds.), Cestode Zoonoses: Echinococcosis and Cysticercosis. IOS Press, Amsterdam, pp. 25–31.

Ito, A., Nakao, M., Wandra, T., 2003a. Human taeniasis and cysticercosis in Asia. Lancet 362, 1918–1920.

Ito, A., Urbani, C., Qui, J.M., Vuitton, D.A., Qui, D.C., Heath, D.D., et al., 2003b. Control of echinococcosis and cysticercosis; a public health challenge to international cooperation in China. Acta Trop. 86, 3–17.

Ito, A., Wandra, T., Yamasaki, H., Nakao, M., Sako, Y., Nakaya, K., et al., 2004. Cysticercosis/taeniasis in Asia and the Pacific. Vector-Borne Zoonotic Dis. 4, 95–107.

Jauregui, P.H., Marquez-Monter, H., 1977. Cysticercosis of the brain in dogs in Mexico City. Am. J. Vet. Res. 38, 1641–1642.

Ji, K., Tong, S., Liu, Y., 1996. Serological epidemiological surveys on cysticercosis in humans in Haerbin region of Heilongjiang province, China. Chin. J. Parasit. Dis. Control 9, 313.

Joshi, D.D., Maharjan, M., Johansen, M.V., Willingham 3rd, A.L., Sharma, M., 2003. Improving meat inspection and control in resource-poor communities: the Nepal example. Acta Trop. 87, 119–127.

Keilbach, N.M., de Aluja, A.S., Sarti-Gutierrez, E., 1989. A programme to control taeniasis-cysticercosis *T. solium*: experiences in a Mexican village. Acta Leidensia 57, 181–189.

Lekule, F.P., Kyvsgaard, N.C., 2003. Improving pig husbandry in tropical resource-poor communities and its potential to reduce risk of porcine cysticercosis. Acta Trop. 87, 111–117.

Leutscher, P., Andriantsimahavandy, A., 2004. Cysticercosis in Peace Corps volunteers in Madagascar. N. Engl. J. Med. 350, 311–312.

Li, Y., Wu, F., Zhang, F., 1996. The first survey on cysticercosis in humans in Nangang Region of Heilongjiang province, China. Disease Monitor 11, 25.

Li, F., Xu, J., Sun, T., Chen, X., Lv, Q., Gu, H., 1998. Epidemiological surveys on taeniasis/cysticercosis in humans in Liaoning province. China. Chin. Public Health 14, 227–228.

Li, T.Y., Craig, P.S., Ito, A., Chen, X.W., Qiu, D.C., Qiu, J.M., et al., 2006. Taeniasis/cysticercosis in a Tibetan population in Sichuan province, China. Acta Trop. 100, 223–231.

Li, T.Y., Ito, A., Craig, P.S., Chen, X.W., Qiu, D.C., Zhou, X.N., et al., 2007. Taeniasis/cysticercosis in China. Southeast Asian J. Trop. Med. Public Health 38 (Suppl.), 1–9.

Lightowlers, M.W., 1999. Eradication of *Taenia solium* cysticercosis: a role for vaccination of pigs. Int. J. Parasitol. 29, 811–817.

Lightowlers, M.W., 2003. Vaccines for prevention of cysticercosis. Acta Trop. 87, 129–135.

Liu, J.X., Mao, B.Y., 2004. Analysis of 53 neurocysticercosis children cases. Sichuan Med. J. 25, 886–887.

Liu, X., Zhao, Z., Wan, G., Fu, B., Li, G.P., Chen, X.X., et al., 2002. An epidemiological survey on taeniasis/cysticercosis in Shandong province, China. Chin. J. Parasitol. Parasit. Dis. 20, 25–28.

Liu, Y.J., Li, Q.Z., Hao, Y.H., 2003. Morphological changes to early stage *Taenia solium* cysticerci following oxfendazole treatment. Vet. J. 165, 73–77.

Luo, T.P., Zhao, Y.J., 1998. Analysis of 1086 cysticercosis cases in Dali prefecture, Yunnan province. J. Pract. Parasit. Dis. 6, 87–88.

Lv, S., Zhang, Y., Steinmann, P., Zhou, X.N., Utzinger, J., 2010. Helminth infections of the central nervous system occurring in Southeast Asia and the Far East. Adv. Parasitol. 72, 351–408.

Mafojane, N.A., Appleton, C.C., Krecek, R.C., Michael, L.M., Willingham 3rd, A.L., 2003. The current status of neurocysticercosis in eastern and southern Africa. Acta Trop. 87, 25–33.

Maitindom, F.D., 2008. Study on porcine cysticercosis among pigs sold in the Jibama market, Jayawijaya district, Papua. Graduate School, Bogor Agricultural University, Bogor (Masters' Thesis).

Margono, S.S., Subahar, R., Hamid, A., Wandra, T., Sudewi, S.S., Sutisna, P., et al., 2001. Cysticercosis in Indonesia: epidemiological aspects. Southeast Asian J. Trop. Med. Public Health 32, 79–84.

Margono, S.S., Ito, A., Sato, M.O., Okamoto, M., Subahar, R., Yamasaki, H., et al., 2003. *Taenia solium* taeniasis/cysticercosis in Papua, Indonesia in 2001: detection of human worm carriers. J. Helminthol. 77, 39–42.

Margono, S.S., Wandra, T., Swasono, M.F., Murni, S., Craig, P.S., Ito, A., 2006. Taeniasis/cysticercosis in Papua, Irian Jaya, Indonesia. Parasitol. Int. 55, S143–S148.

Ministry of Health, P.R. China, 2005. Report on the National Survey of Current Situation of Major Human Parasitic Diseases in China. National Institute of Parasitic Diseases, China CDC, Shanghai pp. 1–33.

Murrell, K.D. (Ed.), 2005. WHO/FAO/OIE Guidelines for the Surveillance, Prevention and Control of Taeniosis/Cysticercosis. Office International des Epizooties, Paris.

Nash, T.E., Patronas, N.J., 1999. Edema associated with calcified lesions in neurocysticercosis. Neurology 53, 777–781.

Nash, T.E., Pretell, J., Garcia, H.H., 2001. Calcified cysticerci provoke perilesional edema and seizures. Clin. Infect. Dis. 33, 1649–1653.

Nash, T.E., Del Brutto, O.H., Butman, J.A., Corona, T., Delgado-Escueta, A., Duron, R.M., et al., 2004. Calcific neurocysticercosis and epileptogenesis. Neurology 62, 1934–1938.

Ngowi, N.A., Mlangwa, J.E.D., Carabin, H., Mlozi, M.R.S., Kassuku, A.A., Kimera, S.I., et al., 2007a. Financial efficiency of health and pig management education intervention in controlling porcine cysticercosis in Mbulu District, northern Tanzania. Livestock Research for Rural Development 19, http://www.cipav.org.co/lrrd/lrrd19/5/ngow19062.htm (article #62).

Ngowi, H.A., Tolma, E.L., Kassuku, A.A., Mlozi, M.R.S., Mlangwa, J.E.D., Carabin, H., et al., 2007b. Using the PRECEDE model to plan a health promotion strategy for control of *Taenia solium* infections in northern Tanzania. Int. J. Health Promot. Educ. 45, 41–48.

Ngowi, H.A., Carabin, H., Kassuku, A.A., Mlozi, M.R.S., Mlangwa, J.E.D., Willingham 3rd, A.L., 2008. A health-education intervention trial to reduce porcine cysticercosis in Mbulu District, Tanzania. Prev. Vet. Med. 85, 52–67.

Ngowi, H.A., Mlangwa, J.E.D., Mlozi, M.R.S., Tolma, E.L., Kassuku, A.A., Carabin, H., et al., 2009. Implementation and evaluation of a health-promotion strategy for control of *Taenia solium* infections in northern Tanzania. Int. J. Health Promot. Educ. 47, 24–34.

Noor Azian, M.Y., Hakim, S.L., Sumiati, A., Norhafizah, M., 2006. Seroprevalence of cysticercosis in a rural village of Ranau, Sabah, Malaysia. Southeast Asian J. Trop. Med. Public Health 37, 58–61.

Okolo, M.I., 1986a. Cerebral cysticercosis in rural dogs. Microbios 47, 189–191.

Okolo, M.I., 1986b. Observations on *Cysticercus cellulosae* in the flesh of rural dogs. Int. J. Zoonoses 13, 286–289.

Pawlowski, Z., Murrell, K.D., 2000. Taeniasis and cysticercosis. In: Hui, Y.H., Sattar, S.A., Murrell, K.D., Nip, W.K., Stanfield, P.S. (Eds.), Foodborne Disease Handbook. second ed. Viruses, Parasites, Pathogens and HAACP. Vol. 2. Marcel Dekker, Inc., New York, pp. 217–227.

Phiri, I.K., Ngowi, H., Afonso, S.M.S., Matenga, E., Boa, M., Mukaratirwa, S., et al., 2003. The emergence of *Taenia solium* cysticercosis in Eastern and Southern Africa as a serious agricultural problem and public health risk. Acta Trop. 87, 13–23.

Pouedet, M.S.R., Zoli, A.P., Nguekam, L., Vondou, L., Assana, E., Speybroeck, N., et al., 2002. Epidemiological survey of swine cisticercosis in two rural communities of West-Cameroon. Vet. Parasitol. 106, 45–54.

Praet, N., Speybroeck, N., Manzanedo, R., Berkvens, D., Nsame Nforninwe, D., Zoli, A., et al., 2009. The disease burden of *Taenia solium* cysticercosis in Cameroon. PLoS Negl. Trop. Dis. 3, e406.

Preux, P.M., Druet-Cabanac, M., 2005. Epidemiology and aetiology of epilepsy in sub-Saharan Africa. Lancet Neurol. 4, 21–31.

Qian, D.X., Peng, Y.H., Zeng, H., 1998. Epidemiological study on porcine cysticercosis in Guizhou province. Chin. J. Vet. Parasit. Dis. 6, 29–30.

Rajshekhar, V., Joshi, D.D., Doanh, N.Q., De, N.V., Zhou, X.N., 2003. *Taenia solium* taeniosis/cysticercosis in Asia: epidemiology, impact and issues. Acta Trop. 87, 53–60.

Richards, F.O., Schantz, P.M., Ruiz-Tiben, E., Sorvillo, F.J., 1985. Cysticercosis in Los Angeles County. JAMA 254, 3444–3448.

Román, G., Sotelo, J., Del Brutto, O., Flisser, A., Dumas, M., Wadia, N., et al., 2000. A proposal to declare neurocysticercosis an international reportable disease. Bull. World Health Organ. 78, 399–406.

Rosenfeld, E.A., Byrd, S.E., Shulman, S.T., 1996. Neurocysticercosis among children in Chicago. Clin. Infect. Dis. 23, 262–268.

Saleh, U.S.A., 2010. Study on Cysticercosis in Pig Meat at Traditional Slaughtering Facilities and its Relationship with Public Health in East Flores District—Eastern Islands province. Graduate School, Bogor Agricultural University, Bogor Masters' Thesis.

Salim, L., Ang, A., Handali, S., The Cysticercosis Working Group in Papua, Tsang, V.C.W., 2009. Seroepidemiologic survey of cysticercosis–taeniasis in four central highland districts of Papua, Indonesia. Am. J. Trop. Med. Hyg. 80, 384–388.

Sarti, E., Flisser, A., Schantz, P.M., Gleizer, M., Loya, M., Plancarte, A., et al., 1997. Development and evaluation of a health education intervention against *Taenia solium* in a rural community in Mexico. Am. J. Trop. Med. Hyg. 56, 127–132.

Schantz, P.M., Moore, A.C., Munoz, J.L., Hartman, B.J., Schaefer, J.A., Aron, A.M., et al., 1992. Neurocysticercosis in an orthodox Jewish community in New York City. N. Engl. J. Med. 327, 692–695.

Schantz, P.M., Cruz, M., Sarti, E., Pawlowski, Z., 1993. Potential eradicability of taeniasis and cysticercosis. Bull. Pan Am. Health Organ. 27, 397–403.

Schratz, A., Fernanda Pineda, M., Reforma, L.G., Fox, N.M., Anh, T.L., Cavalli-Sforza, L.T., et al., 2010. Neglected diseases and ethnic minorities in the Western Pacific region: exploring the links. Adv. Parasitol. 72, 79–107.

Sciutto, E., Fragoso, G., Manoutcharian, K., Gevorkian, G., Rosas-Salgado, G., Hernández-Gonzalez, M., et al., 2002. New approaches to improve a peptide vaccine against procine *Taenia solium* cysticercosis. Arch. Med. Res. 33, 371–378.

Shasha, W., Pammenter, M.D., 1991. Sero-epidemiological studies of cysticercosis in school children from two rural areas of Transkei, South Africa. Ann. Trop. Med. Parasitol. 85, 349–355.

Shey-Njila, O., Zoli, P.A., Awah-Ndukum, J., Nguekam, J.P., Assana, E., Byambas, P., et al., 2003. Porcine cysticercosis in village pigs of northwest Cameroon. J. Helminthol. 77, 351–354.

Sikasunge, C.S., Johansen, M.V., Willingham 3rd, A.L., Leifsson, P.S., Phiri, I.K., 2008. *Taenia solium* porcine cysticercosis: viability of cysticerci and persistency of antibodies and cysticercal antigens after treatment with oxfendazole. Vet. Parasitol. 158, 57–66.

Simanjuntak, G.M., Margono, S.S., Okamoto, M., Ito, A., 1997. Taeniasis/cysticercosis in Indonesia as an emerging disease. Parasitol. Today 13, 321–323.

Singh, G., Prabhakar, S., 2002. *Taenia solium* Cysticercosis. From Basic to Clinical Science. CABI Publishing, Wallingford, United Kingdom.

Somers, R., Dorny, P., Nguyen, V.K., Dang, T.C., Goddeeris, B., Craig, P.S., et al., 2006. *Taenia solium* taeniasis and cysticercosis in three communities in north Vietnam. Trop. Med. Int. Health 11, 65–72.

Somers, R., Dorny, P., Geysen, D., Nguyen, L.A., Thach, D.C., Vercruysse, J., et al., 2007. Human tapeworms in north Vietnam. Trans. R. Soc. Trop. Med. Hyg. 101, 275–277.

Sorvillo, F.J., Portigal, L., DeGiorgio, C., Smith, L., Waterman, S.H., Berlin, G.W., et al., 2004. Cysticercosis mortality in California. Emerg. Infect. Dis. 10, 465–469.

Sorvillo, F., DeGiorgio, C., Waterman, S.H., 2007. Deaths from cysticercosis, United States. Emerg. Infect. Dis. 13, 230–235.

Sotelo, J., Rosas, N., Palencia, G., 1986. Freezing of infested pork muscle kills cysticerci. JAMA 256, 893–894.

Sovyra, T., 2005. Prevalence of porcine cysticercosis, trichinellosis in slaughter pigs of Cambodia. Chiang Mai University and Freie Universität, Chiang Mai, Thailand and Berlin, Germany (Masters' Thesis, pp. 125).

Steinmann, P., Zhou, X.N., Li, Y.L., Li, H.J., Chen, S.R., Yang, Z., et al., 2007. Helminth infections and risk factor analysis among residents in Eryuan county, Yunnan province, China. Acta Trop. 104, 38–51.

Subahar, R., Hamid, A., Purba, W., Wandra, T., Karma, C., Sako, Y., et al., 2001. *Taenia solium* infection in Irian Jaya (west Papua), Indonesia: a pilot serological survey of human and porcine cysticercosis in Jayawijaya district. Trans. R. Soc. Trop. Med. Hyg. 95, 388–390.

Suroso, T., Margono, S.S., Wandra, T., Ito, A., 2006. Challenges for control of taeniasis/cysticercosis in Indonesia. Parasitol. Int. 55, S161–165.

Sutisna, I.P., Fraser, A., Kapti, I.N., Rodriguez-Canul, R., Widjana, D.P., Craig, P.S., et al., 1999. Community prevalence study of taeniasis and cysticercosis in Bali, Indonesia. Trop. Med. Int. Health 4, 288–294.

Thomson, A.J.G., 1993. Neurocysticercosis—experience at the teaching hospitals of the University of Cape Town. S. Afr. Med. J. 83, 332–334.

Townes, J.M., Hoffmann, C.J., Kohn, M.A., 2004. Neurocysticercosis in Oregon, 1995–2000. Emerg. Infect. Dis. 10, 508–510.

Tran, D.S., Odermatt, P., Le Oanh, T., Huc, P., Phoumindr, N., Ito, A., et al., 2007. Risk factors for epilepsy in rural Lao PDR: a case-control study. Southeast Asian J. Trop. Med. Public Health 38, 537–542.

Waikagul, J., Dekumyoy, P., Anantaphruti, M.T., 2005. Taeniasis, cysticercosis and echinococcosis in Thailand. Parasitol. Int. 55, S175–S180.

Wandra, T., Subahar, R., Simanjuntak, G.M., Margono, S.S., Suroso, T., Okamoto, M., et al., 2000. Resurgence of cases of epileptic seizures and burns associated with cysticercosis in Assologaima, Jayawijaya, Irian Jaya, Indonesia, 1991–95. Trans. R. Soc. Trop. Med. Hyg. 94, 46–50.

Wandra, T., Ito, A., Yamasaki, H., Suroso, T., Margono, S.S., 2003. *Taenia solium* cysticercosis, Irian Jaya, Indonesia. Emerg. Infect. Dis. 9, 884–885.

Wandra, T., Depary, A.A., Sutisna, P., Margono, S.S., Suroso, T., Okamoto, M., et al., 2006a. Taeniasis and cysticercosis in Bali and North Sumatra, Indonesia. Parasitol. Int. 55, S155–160.

Wandra, T., Sutisna, P., Dharmawan, N.S., Margono, S.S., Sudewi, R., Suroso, T., et al., 2006b. High prevalence of *Taenia saginata* taeniasis and status of *Taenia solium* cysticercosis in Bali, Indonesia, 2002–2004. Trans. R. Soc. Trop. Med. Hyg. 100, 346–353.

Wang, K., 2002. A study on taeniasis/cysticercosis in a mineral area of south Anhui province, China. Anim. Health 18, 597–599.

Wang, Z., Bao, H., 2003. Identification of *Taenia saginata* by mtCOI in four areas of Yunnan and Guizhou provinces. Chin. J. Parasitol. Parasit. Dis. 21, 20–23.

Wei, X.Y., 1997. Analysis of the infectious status of 3 species of zoonotic parasitic diseases in swines via postmortem inspections in Dali prefecture, Yunnan province. Chin. J. Vet. Parasit. Dis. 5, 22–23.

Wei, G.Z., Xie, S.P., Pang, S.Q., Wang, Y.J., Di, Y.H., Gao, W.R., 1994. A seroepidemiological survey on cysticercosis in humans in north China. Chin. J. Neurol. 5, 268–271.
White Jr., A.C., Robinson, P., Kuhn, R., 1997. *Taenia solium* cysticercosis: host–parasite interactions and the immune response. Chem. Immunol. 66, 209–230.
WHO, 2003. Control of Neurocysticercosis. Report of the Secretariat, Fifty-sixth World Health Assembly. Document A56/10. World Health Organization, Geneva.
Wilkins, P.P., Allan, J.C., Verastegui, M., Acosta, M., Eason, A.G., Garcia, H.H., et al., 1999. Development of a serologic assay to detect *Taenia solium* taeniasis. Am. J. Trop. Med. Hyg. 60, 199–204.
Willingham 3rd, A.L., Engels, D., 2006. Control of *Taenia solium* cysticercosis/taeniosis. Adv. Parasitol. 61, 509–566.
Willingham III, A.L., De, N.V., Doanh, N.Q., Cong, L.D., Dung, T.V., Dorny, P., et al., 2003. Current status of cysticercosis in Vietnam. Southeast Asian J. Trop. Med. Public Health 34 (Suppl.), 35–50.
Wu, X.H., Wu, Y.H., Guo, Z.X., Han, X.M., Ning, G., He, D.L., et al., 2001. An epidemiological survey on taeniasis/cysticercosis in Huzhu county of Qinghai province, China. Chin. J. Parasit. Dis. Control 14, 9–10.
Wu, X.H., He, D.L., Lin, B.R., Zhang, J.X., Liu, P.Y., Liu, H.Q., et al., 2005. An epidemiological survey on taeniasis/cysticercosis in eastern Qinghai province, China. Chin. J. Parasit. Dis. Control 18, 384–386.
Xu, L., 2002. Losses from main parasitic diseases in western region, China. Chin. J. Parasit. Dis. Control 15, 1–3.
Xu, L.Q., Jiang, Z.X., Zhou, C.H., Zhang, X.Q., Ren, Z.X., Chang, J., et al., 1999. The investigation of cysticercosis's distribution in China. Chin. J. Prev. Care Parasit. Dis. 12, 30–32.
Xu, J.M., Acosta, L.P., Hou, M., Manalo, D.L., Jiz, M., Jarilla, B., et al., 2010. Sero-prevalence of cysticercosis in children and young adults living in a helminth endemic community in Leyte, the Philippines. J. Trop. Med. (doi: 10.1155/2010/603174; in press).
Yamasaki, H., Allan, J.C., Sato, M.O., Nakao, M., Sako, Y., Nakaya, K., et al., 2004. DNA differential diagnosis of taeniasis/cysticercosis by multiplex PCR. J. Clin. Microbiol. 42, 548–553.
Yodnopaklow, P., Mahuntussanapong, A., 2000. Single small enhancing CT lesion in Thai patients with acute symptomatic seizures: a clinico-radiological study. Trop. Med. Int. Health 5, 250–255.
Zhang, C., Xu, Y.Z., 1998. Infection with cysticercosis in dogs. Sichuan Animal Husbandry Vet. Sci. 2, 31.
Zhang, B., Huo, S.L., Qiqige, S., 2000. Epidemiology investigation of cysticercosis in Nei Monggol Autonomous Region, China. Chin. J. Zoonoses 16, 106–108.
Zhou, G.X., Zhong, G.H., Wang, S.Y., Jiang, M.X., Kang, Y., 1993. Epidemiological survey on *Taenia solium* and cysticercosis in Xide county, Sichuan province. J. Pract. Parasit. Dis. 1, 25–28.
Zhou, X.N., Ohta, N., Utzinger, J., Bergquist, R., Olveda, R.M., 2008. RNAS$^+$: a "win-win" collaboration to combat neglected tropical diseases in Southeast Asia. Parasitol. Int. 57, 243–245.

CHAPTER 10

Echinococcosis with Particular Reference to Southeast Asia

Donald P. McManus

Contents

Abstract

Echinococcosis is a zoonosis caused by adult or larval cestodes belonging to the genus *Echinococcus* (family Taeniidae). The two major species of medical and public health importance are *E. granulosus* and *E. multilocularis*, which, respectively, cause cystic echinococcosis (CE) and alveolar echinococcosis (AE). Both CE and

Molecular Parasitology Laboratory, Queensland Institute of Medical Research, Brisbane, Australia

Advances in Parasitology, Volume 72
ISSN 0065-308X, DOI: 10.1016/S0065-308X(10)72010-8

AE are serious and severe diseases, the latter especially so, with high fatality rates and poor prognosis if managed incorrectly. A number of recent reports indicate that CE and AE are of increasing public health concern and that both can be regarded as emerging or re-emerging diseases. This review discusses aspects of the biology, life-cycle characteristics, aetiology, and the global and Southeast Asian regional distribution and transmission of the *Echinococcus* organisms, and covers the epidemiology, clinical features, treatment and diagnosis of the diseases they cause. The current countermeasures available for the control and prevention of AE and CE, including the development of animal vaccines for the latter, are also reviewed. *E. granulosus* still has a wide geographical distribution although effective control against CE has been achieved in some regions. *E. multilocularis* is more problematic as the primary transmission cycle is almost always sylvatic so that efficient and cost-effective control of AE remains a formidable challenge. Chemotherapy has facilitated less invasive surgical management of CE and AE. Nevertheless, as will be emphasised, there is a clear need for new advances in the prevention and control of both these neglected diseases.

10.1. INTRODUCTION

Echinococcosis is a zoonosis caused by adult or larval tapeworms (cestodes) belonging to the genus *Echinococcus* (family Taeniidae). Larval infection (hydatid disease; hydatidosis) is characterised by long-term growth of metacestode (hydatid) cysts in the intermediate host. Three forms of echinococcosis are recognised clinically: cystic echinococcosis (CE) caused by *E. granulosus*, alveolar echinococcosis (AE) caused by *E. multilocularis* and polycystic echinococcosis caused by *E. vogeli* or *E. oligarthrus*. Until 2005, only these four *Echinococcus* species were recognised, but *E. shiquicus*, present in small mammals from the Tibetan Plateau (Xiao et al., 2005), and *E. felidis* from the African lion (Hüttner et al., 2008, 2009) have now been identified, although their zoonotic transmission potential is unknown. Relatively few human polycystic echinococcosis cases have been reported, all in Central and South America, so as this review focuses on Southeast Asia, only *E. granulosus* and *E. multilocularis* will be considered further.

Human CE is the most common presentation and accounts for the majority of the estimated 2–3 million global cases with human AE causing around 0.3–0.5 million cases (all in the northern hemisphere) (Budke et al., 2006a; Craig et al., 2007). CE and AE are both serious life-threatening diseases, the latter especially so, with a high fatality rate and poor prognosis if careful clinical management is not carried out. The global burden, as assessed by disability-adjusted life years (DALYs), for human CE was recently estimated to be 285,000 and an annual economic loss of US$ 194 million, which is more than that for onchocerciasis and almost the same as that for human African trypanosomiasis (Budke et al., 2006a). In untreated or inadequately treated AE, mortality is >90% within 10–15 years of diagnosis (Torgerson et al., 2008). The mortality rate from CE (about 2–4%) is lower than that from AE, but it may increase considerably if medical treatment and care are inadequate (Brunetti et al., 2010). The socio-economic impact of CE is also considerable (Batelli, 2009).

Comprehensive accounts of the biology, biochemistry, life-cycle characteristics, parasite–host relationships, *in vitro* culture and aetiology of *Echinococcus* are available (Alvite and Esteves, 2009; Craig et al., 2003, 2007; Eckert and Deplazes, 2004; Eckert et al., 2001a,b; McManus, 2009; McManus et al., 2003; Moro and Schantz, 2009; Siracusano et al., 2009; Spiliotis and Brehm, 2009; Thompson, 2008; Thompson and McManus, 2001; Vuitton et al., 2009), so only a brief description is presented here. A recent issue published in *Experimental Parasitology* (August, 2008, vol. 119, issue 4,) entitled 'Experimental Studies in Echinococcosis' should be consulted for further recent progress in experimental aspects of research on echinococcosis and hydatid disease. As well, a major and important review of the diagnosis, treatment and management of CE and AE, written under the aegis of the World Health Organization-Informal Working Group on Echinococcosis (WHO-IWGE), is available (Brunetti et al., 2010).

10.1.1. The parasites

The life cycles of *E. granulosus* and *E. multilocularis* are illustrated in Fig. 10.1.

10.1.1.1. E. granulosus

Following ingestion, *Echinococcus* eggs hatch in the intestine and the released embryos (oncospheres) penetrate through the mucosa and pass in the circulation to various internal organs' sites where development of cysts occurs. Hydatid cysts of *E. granulosus* develop mainly in the liver and lungs of humans and other intermediate hosts as unilocular fluid-filled bladders. The range of intermediate host species involved depends on the infecting strain of *E. granulosus* (see below), regional or local differences in the availability of the various intermediate host species and other factors (Eckert et al., 2001a). Since the life cycle relies on carnivores eating infected herbivores, humans are usually a 'dead-end' for the parasite, although this is not always the case (MacPherson, 1983). An important feature of the biology of *E. granulosus* is the fact that it comprises a number of intra-specific variants or strains that exhibit considerable variation at the genetic level (McManus and Thompson, 2003; Thompson and McManus, 2001, 2002). The term strain is used to describe variants that differ from other

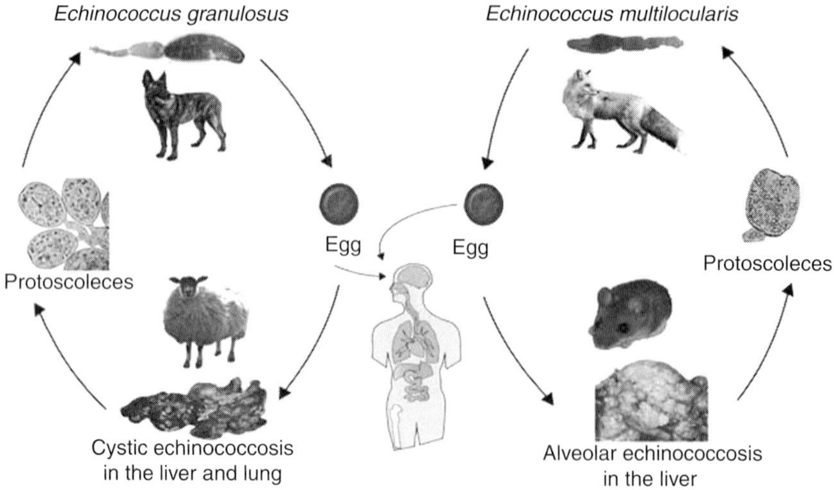

FIGURE 10.1 Life-cycles of *E. granulosus* and *E. multilocularis* (modified from McManus et al., 2003).

groups of the same species in gene frequencies or DNA sequences, and in one or more characters of actual or potential significance to the epidemiology and control of echinococcosis (McManus and Simpson, 1985; McManus and Thompson, 2003; McManus et al., 1985; Rishi and McManus, 1987; Thompson and McManus, 2001, 2002).

To date, analyses of mitochondrial DNA sequences have identified 10 distinct genetic types (genotypes G1–10). This categorisation closely follows the pattern of strain variation emerging based on biological characteristics. As a result of DNA-based phylogenetic studies and other criteria, taxonomic revision of *E. granulosus* has been proposed: the G1 (sheep strain) genotype is the prototypical species of *E. granulosus* and the G4 (horse strain) and G5 (cattle strain) genotypes are distinct species designated *E. equinus* and *E. ortleppi*, respectively (Le et al., 2002; McManus and Thompson, 2003; Nakao et al., 2007; Pednekar et al., 2009; Saarma et al., 2009; Thompson, 2008; Thompson and McManus, 2002). The DNA analysis has provided compelling evidence that *Echinococcus* species began to diverge probably during the Miocene, following the diversification of large mammals (Nakao et al., 2007).

The extensive variation in nominal *E. granulosus* may influence life-cycle patterns, host specificity, development rate, antigenicity, transmission dynamics, sensitivity to chemotherapeutic agents and pathology. It might therefore have implications for the design and development of vaccines, diagnostic assays and drugs affecting control. This issue will be discussed further later when considering the extensive genetic variability in the complete coding DNA sequence of the EG95 vaccine that has shown high levels of protection against *E. granulosus*; this variation may influence host specificity and vaccine efficacy.

10.1.1.2. E. multilocularis

Adult worm infections of *E. multilocularis* are generally perpetuated in a sylvatic cycle (Fig. 10.1) with wild carnivores—mainly red fox (*Vulpes vulpes*) and arctic fox (*Alopex lagopis*)—regarded as the most important definitive hosts. Domestic dogs and, rarely, cats can also harbour the tapeworm and may be involved in a synanthropic cycle. Small mammals (usually microtine and arvicolid rodents or *Ochotona* spp.) act as intermediate hosts. The metacestode of *E. multilocularis* is a tumour-like, infiltrating structure consisting of numerous small vesicles embedded in stroma of connective tissue. The metacestode mass usually contains a semisolid matrix rather than fluid (Pawłowski et al., 2001). The sylvatic cycle probably accounts for most human infections although in some AE-endemic areas, notably in the People's Republic of China (P.R. China), it seems that the domestic dog probably has an important role in zoonotic risk (Craig et al., 2007). It is unclear how much cats, if at all, contribute to human transmission. As with *E. granulosus*, it is thought that humans become exposed to *E. multilocularis* by handling infected definitive hosts, or by ingestion of food contaminated with eggs. Coprophagic flies and other animals may serve as mechanical vectors of the eggs of both species (Eckert et al., 2001a).

In contrast to *E. granulosus*, there is remarkable genetic homogeneity within *E. multilocularis* specimens isolated from different geographical regions based on the analysis of classical coding and non-coding DNA targets (Haag et al., 1997; Nakao et al., 2009, 2010; Rinder et al., 1997). Use of the tandemly repeated multi-locus microsatellite EmsB can provide a more sensitive genetic tool with a high power of discrimination to enable the detection of genetic diversity at regional and local geographical scales in order to provide a better understanding of the epidemiology of *E. multilocularis* (Knapp et al., 2009) and *E. granulosus* (Maillard et al., 2009). For example, application of EmsB profiles as tools for the genetic characterisation of both *E. multilocularis* and *E. granulosus* could allow tracking back the history of a human infection, one of the main challenges in epidemiological studies of AE (Knapp et al., 2009) and CE (Maillard et al., 2009). Whether this microsatellite approach, however, will lead to the design of new strategies for the control of echinococcosis awaits further investigation.

10.2. CLINICAL FEATURES

10.2.1. Cystic echinococcosis

The initial phase of primary infection with *E. granulosus* is always asymptomatic. Small cysts not inducing major pathology may remain asymptomatic for many years, if not permanently. The latent period of CE is unclear but probably lasts for many months to years. The infection may become symptomatic if the cysts either rupture or exert a mass effect. Recurrence (secondary CE) can occur following surgery on primary cysts or if there is spontaneous or trauma-induced cyst rupture and the release of protoscoleces and/or small cysts, which can grow into larger cysts (Eckert and Deplazes, 2004). CE has been reported to present for medical attention in subjects ranging in age from younger than 1 year to older than 75 years. Even though infections may be acquired in childhood, most cases of liver and lung cysts become symptomatic and are diagnosed in adult patients because of the slowly growing nature of echinococcal cysts (Moro and Schantz, 2009). Up to 60% of all CE cases may be asymptomatic—although an unknown proportion may become symptomatic.

Certain occupations such as farm labourers and animal herders are, not surprisingly, associated with an increased risk of CE (Craig, 1997). Over 90% of cysts occur in the liver, lungs or both. Symptomatic cysts have been reported occasionally (2-–3% each) in the kidney, spleen, peritoneal cavity, and the skin and muscles, but rarely in the heart, brain, vertebral column and ovaries (1% or less each) (Craig, 1997; Pawłowski et al., 2001). Presenting symptoms of CE are highly variable (Ammann and Eckert, 1996). Presenting features reflect not only the involved organ, but also the size of the cyst(s) and their position within the organ, the mass effect within the organ and upon surrounding structures, and complications relating to cyst rupture and secondary infection.

Manifestations of systemic immunological responses may be evident in response to cyst leakage or rupture. Common cyst complications include rupture into the biliary tree with secondary cholangitis, biliary obstruction by daughter cysts or extrinsic compression, intra-cystic and/or subphrenic abscess formation, intra-peritoneal rupture (with or without anaphylaxis), rupture into the bronchial tree and development of a bronchobiliary fistula. Anaphylaxis appears to complicate 10% of all intra-peritoneal ruptures, with the remaining patients developing multiple intra-peritoneal cysts (Pawłowski et al., 2001).

10.2.2. Alveolar echinococcosis

AE typically presents later than CE. Cases of AE are characterised by an initial asymptomatic incubation period of 5–15 years duration and a subsequent chronic course (Bresson-Hadni et al., 2008). Untreated or inadequately managed cases have high fatality rates. The peak age group for clinical presentation is from 50 to 70 years in Europe and Japan. The sex distribution is approximately equal. The metacestode develops almost exclusively in the liver in humans (99% of cases) as well as in natural intermediate hosts. The right lobe is involved most frequently, involvement of the porta hepatis or multiple lobes being less frequent. Parasitic lesions in the liver can vary from small vesicles of a few millimetres in size to large (15–20 cm in diameter) areas of infiltration.

Extra-hepatic primary disease is very rare (1% of cases) (Bresson-Hadni et al., 2008; Pawłowski et al., 2001; Sato et al., 1993). Thirteen percent of cases present as multi-organ AE where metacestodes proliferate tumour-like, leading to infiltration of the lungs, spleen or brain in addition to the liver. One-third of cases present with cholestatic jaundice, one-third present with epigastric pain and the remainder present with vague symptoms like weight loss or fatigue, or are noted to have incidental hepatomegaly (McManus et al., 2003; Sato et al., 1993).

10.3. DIAGNOSIS

Early diagnosis of CE and AE can provide significant improvements in the quality of the management and treatment of both diseases. In most cases, the early stages of infection are asymptomatic, so methods that are relatively easy to use and that are cheap are required for large-scale screening of populations at highest risk.

10.3.1. Cystic echinococcosis

The definitive diagnosis for most human cases of CE is by physical imaging methods, such as radiology, utrasonography (US), computed axial tomography (CT scanning) and magnetic resonance imaging (Pawłowski et al., 2001). Abdominal US is the most widely used imaging technique for CE because of its widespread availability and usefulness for defining number, site, dimensions and vitality of cysts (Moro and Schantz, 2009). The WHO expert group on echinococcosis has produced an international classification of ultrasound images of CE which, in principle, should be used whenever US is done (WHO, 2003). Encouraging results have been obtained with portable US in a series of recent field surveys of CE (Moro and Schantz, 2009). There is an urgent need to improve the imaging diagnosis of lung cysts, which could be amenable to screening, and the development of an imaging technique (or any other approach, including serology), to assess parasite viability and/or to assess the progression of CE (and AE).

Immunodiagnosis complements the clinical picture and informative reviews on recent advances in the field for both CE and AE are available (Bart et al., 2007; Carmena et al., 2007; Ito et al., 2007; Li et al., 2004; Reiter-Owona et al., 2009; Tappe et al., 2009; Zhang and McManus, 2006; Zhang et al., 2003). The approach is useful not only in primary diagnosis but also for follow up of patients after surgical or pharmacological treatment (Ben Nouir et al., 2009). Serology can also be applied to aid population studies and epidemiological surveys of CE and AE in endemic regions (Torgerson and Deplazes, 2009).

Available diagnostic methods depend mainly on detection of specific IgG serum antibodies in suspected cases or in individuals enrolled in mass screening programmes. Liver cysts appear to elicit a better immune response than lung cysts. The enzyme-linked immunosorbent assay (ELISA), the indirect haemagglutination antibody assay (IHAT), latex agglutination test (LAT) and immunoblot test (IB) are the most commonly used immunologic methods. The immunofluorescence antibody test (IFAT) and arc-5 immunoelectrophoresis (IEP) are also used. Hydatid cyst fluid (HCF) antigens are the usual source of antigenic material for immunodiagnosis of CE. Along with HCF, the lipoproteins antigen B and antigen 5, the major components of HCF, are widely used in current assays for immunodiagnosis of CE. Some other antigens, such as the 32-kDa calcium-binding *E. granulosus* recombinant antigen EpC1, have shown some promise, although poor sensitivity can limit serological performance in some field settings (Gavidia et al., 2008). Serological techniques are never 100% sensitive and specific, and some CE patients might not produce a measurable antibody response. Cross-reactivity with antigens from other parasites, notably other taeniid cestodes, is a major problem. Overall, CE serology may be improved by combining several defined antigens (including synthetic peptides), and by the design of new *E. granulosus*-specific peptides that react with otherwise false-negative sera (Craig et al., 2007). As the number of available diagnostic molecules grows, it will be important to undertake a multi-centre comparative standardised study of native, recombinant, and peptide antigens for diagnosis of human CE (and AE). It will also be informative in future to undertake longitudinal follow-up studies of human seropositivity in CE-endemic regions using these defined antigens, and to determine the extent, variability and reason for long-term serial antibody responses in ultrasound-negative people (Craig et al., 2007).

Detection of circulating cytokines in serum may be useful in the follow up of patients with CE (Amri et al., 2008). Further, this can be combined with reverse transcriptase-polymerase chain reaction (RT-PCR) to determine mRNA expression of cytokines in peripheral blood mononucleocytes (PBMC) to complement the biological assays in follow up. Detection of circulating *E. granulosus* antigens in sera is less sensitive than antibody detection but may be relevant as a method for post-surgical follow up of patients, and for monitoring the growth dynamics and/or the activity of cysts.

Molecular identification methods for direct detection of *E. granulosus* nucleic acids in clinical samples by the use of the PCR combined with direct sequencing of nuclear or mitochondrial genes provide a highly sensitive and subjective approach that can provide exquisite levels of specificity for unambiguous identification purposes, particularly in areas where AE and CE co-exist (Li et al., 2008; Yang et al., 2006c). The necessity of fairly sophisticated laboratory equipment and the high cost of the molecular reagents required for the analysis preclude routine use these methods in many endemic areas.

Compared with investigations in humans, relatively little research has been directed towards the development of immunodiagnostic techniques for *E. granulosus* infection in domesticated animals such as sheep and cattle (Zhang and McManus, 2006). Currently, diagnosis of CE in intermediate hosts is based mainly on necropsy procedures. Accurate serological diagnosis of CE infection in livestock is difficult due to serological cross-reactions with several other species of taeniid cestodes including *Taenia hydatigena* and *T. ovis*. Furthermore, natural intermediate host animals produce very poor antibody responses to infection compared with the relatively high levels of specific antibody seen in human infection.

In sheep, the principal intermediate host of *E. granulosus* in most endemic regions of the world, antibodies to various antigens including antigen 5 are detectable in the sera of some, but not all infected sheep ('non-responders'). As with human CE, detection of circulating antigen does not appear to be useful for diagnostic purposes. An extensive study by Kittelberger et al. (2002) showed that a crude *E. granulosus* protoscolex preparation (ProtELISA) was the most effective for detection of infection in sheep by ELISA. Though useful for the detection of the presence of infected sheep on a flock basis, its relatively poor sensitivity precluded the identification of individual animals infected with *E. granulosus*. This is an area that requires renewed research efforts, although the sensitivity/'non-responder' issue may be insurmountable.

10.3.2. Alveolar echinococcosis

The diagnosis of AE is based on similar findings and criteria as in CE. These include case history, clinical findings, morphological lesions identified by imaging techniques, PCR or immunofluorescence/immunohistochemistry and immunodiagnosis. A WHO clinical classification for AE staging by imaging (the PNM system; P = parasitic mass in the liver, N = involvement of neighbouring organs, and M = metastasis) is available (Kern et al., 2006). Like CE, serodiagnosis of AE provides a complementary role to other procedures in early detection of the infection. The methods are similar to those used for CE with serological tests for antibody detection being generally more reliable for AE than CE.

AE is a very serious disease with a high fatality rate so that early detection is paramount in order that successful management and treatment can commence. Tests using Em2, a species-specific native antigen isolated from the metacestode of *E. multilocularis* and the Em2^{plus}-ELISA, a combination of Em2 with a recombinant protein designated II/3–10, have proved particularly valuable (Hänle et al., 2009). The Em2^{plus}-ELISA has been commercialised for clinical diagnosis of AE and for population screening (Ito et al., 2007). Other useful diagnostic molecules applicable in immunoblot and/or ELISA include an 18-kDa antigen (Em18) that can differentiate active from inactive AE, recombinant Em13 and Em10 and a purified alkaline phosphatase (pAP) from *E. multilocularis* metacestodes (Ito et al., 2007). Both Em2^{plus}-ELISA and Em18 in an immunoblot format have been used for long-term follow-up monitoring of AE patients after pharmacological treatment. Em18 has been shown to be a fragment of Em10, being the product of its degradation by cysteine protease. Recombinant Em18 (derived from (349)K to (508)K of Em10) shows promise in immunoblotting assays and ELISA for detection of AE, and may prove especially useful for epidemiological surveys. Two recent advances include the development of an immunochromatographic test (ICT) with recombinant Em18 for diagnosis of AE (Sako et al., 2009), and a dot immunogold filtration assay (DIGFA) with multiple native antigens for rapid serodiagnosis of both human AE and CE (Feng et al., 2010). Such simple, rapid tests can be used for clinical diagnosis, as well as in conjunction with US for mass screening in CE- and AE-endemic areas (Feng et al., 2010).

Direct detection or amplification of *E. multilocularis* nucleic acids in clinical samples is useful for the primary diagnostic identification of parasite materials in biopsied specimens from suspected infected patients, and also for the assessment of the viability of parasite samples after chemotherapy or other treatment (Zhang and McManus, 2006). As with CE, the costs of reagents and the requirement for a well-equipped laboratory restrict use of the approach in endemic areas.

Purgation with arecoline compounds and necropsy of the small intestine are two diagnostic methods that have been extensively used in dogs. Necropsy is the method of choice for foxes and other final hosts. Two main immunodiagnostic approaches have been developed for the diagnosis of *E. granulosus* and *E. multilocularis* infection in definitive hosts, namely ELISA-based assays for specific serum antibody and detection of parasite products (coproantigens) in faeces. Coproantigens may be detectable early in the course of both *E. granulosus* and *E. multilocularis* infections (Craig et al., 2007; Hülsmeier et al., 2010; Lahmar et al., 2009; Nonaka et al., 2008b). DNA amplification has also shown potential in diagnosis of echinococcoses by development of stool-based PCR (copro-PCR) tests for both species-specific and strain-specific pre-patent and patent detection of adult worm infections (Boufana et al., 2008; Craig et al., 2007; Lahmar et al., 2009). The coproantigen ELISA has the potential for replacing arecoline purgation or necropsy examinations for field application, and the copro-PCR is a valuable method for confirmation of positive coproantigen results and for diagnosis in individual animals.

10.4. TREATMENT

10.4.1. Cystic echinococcosis

Asymptomatic hepatic CE is common in endemic regions and up to 75% of subjects may remain symptom free for more than 10 years. Cysts may expand, become septate or calcify when subjects are followed by serial ultrasound. Community-based studies using screening ultrasound have identified an increased frequency of asymptomatic hepatic CE compared to similar studies of patients presenting for medical attention. Treatment should be reserved for symptomatic lesions or those affecting vital anatomical structures.

10.4.1.1. Surgery

Surgery has been the mainstay of therapy for large cysts, those that are superficial and likely to rupture, infected cysts and those in vital anatomical locations or exerting significant mass effect. Surgery may be impractical in patients with multiple cysts in several organs or where technical expertise and/or facilities are inadequate. Reported recurrence rates range from 2% to 25%. The advent of effective pre-operative chemotherapy has reduced the requirement for aggressive surgical procedures. There is a need for multi-centre prospective evaluation of surgical procedures and an evaluation of the added modalities of drug treatment given before and after surgery.

10.4.1.2. Puncture, aspiration, injection and reaspiration technique

The puncture, aspiration, injection and reaspiration (PAIR) technique was introduced in the mid-1980s (Pawłowski et al., 2001). The cyst is punctured under ultrasound guidance, as much cyst fluid is aspirated as possible, a protoscolicide (e.g. 95% ethanol) is injected and cyst contents are reaspirated 15–20 min later. PAIR should only be performed on patients with chemotherapeutic cover to minimise the risk of secondary CE. Experience of this technique in children and pregnant women is lacking. PAIR is best performed on liver cysts ≥ 5 cm in diameter that are anechoic, or multiseptate, or multiple and >5 cm each. PAIR has been used in cases that have relapsed after surgery. It is contraindicated for superficial or inaccessible cysts, cysts that are calcified, solid, or have communication with bile ducts. PAIR with albendazole or mebendazole chemotherapy has been shown to be as effective as pericystectomy for hepatic CE with lower post-procedure morbidity and shorter hospital stay (Smego et al., 2003).

10.4.1.3. Chemotherapy

The benzimidazole compounds—albendazole and mebendazole—have been the cornerstone of chemotherapy for CE (Capan et al., 2009; Hemphill and Müller, 2009; McManus et al., 2003; Stamatakos et al., 2009; Vuitton, 2009). The two drugs bind to beta tubulin causing disruption of microtubule-based processes, although other targets including energy metabolism may also be involved (Cumino et al., 2009). Albendazole (10 mg/kg in divided doses, usually 400 mg, twice daily) therapy results in the disappearance of up to 48% of cysts and a significant reduction in size of a further 24%. Mebendazole (40–50 mg/kg per day in three divided doses) is less efficacious than albendazole for CE. Because of limited toxicological data, albendazole was originally administered in three to six 4-week cycles with intervals of 14 days. However, more recent data suggest that continuous treatment achieves equivalent or improved efficacy with no increased adverse effect. Cyst non-viability increases with duration of therapy; from 72% of cysts non-viable after 1 month to 94% of cysts non-viable after 3 months of therapy. Usual adverse events include nausea, hepatotoxicity, neutropenia (which may not be reversible) and occasional allopecia.

Praziquantel has been used (25 mg/kg/day) with albendazole for combined treatment of CE and has shown improved efficacy over albendazole alone. Flubendazole either separately or in combination with ivermectin may be effective in CE therapy (Ceballos et al., 2009; Elissondo et al., 2009). Oxfendazole may also prove to be an adequate treatment for human and animal CE (Gavidia et al., 2009). Chemotherapy should not be used during pregnancy, and in subjects with chronic hepatic diseases or bone marrow depression (Pawłowski et al., 2001).

10.4.1.4. Focused ultrasound as a therapeutic option

High-intensity focused ultrasound (HIFU) is a new technique that can cause cell death and tissue necrosis by focusing high-energy ultrasonic waves on a single location, and it has attracted recent interest as a non-invasive therapy particularly for cancer treatment. Zou et al. (2009) showed that HIFU caused a highly damaging effect on protoscoleces of *E. granulosus*, inhibited their growth both *in vitro* and *in vivo*, and could be a possible therapeutic option for CE. The main advantages of HIFU over conventional therapies is that it is non-invasive, it does not require percutaneous puncture or canulation of the hydatid cysts of *E. granulosus* and the procedure is guided by real-time imaging. This approach could potentially yield a better treatment for CE with a high efficacy and low morbidity, and should be further encouraged.

10.4.2. Alveolar echinococcosis

Radical surgery has been the historical cornerstone of treatment for AE. Early diagnosis of AE can result in a reduced rate of unresectable lesions and reduces the requirement for radical surgery. Perioperative and long-term 'adjuvant' chemotherapy with albendazole (doses up to 20 mg/kg/day) has been associated with increased survival compared with historical controls (McManus et al., 2003). Liver transplantation has been performed on some AE patients with a successful outcome (Mantion et al., 2008; Moray et al., 2009). Albendazole is only parasitostatic against the *E. multilocularis* metacestode and chemotherapy should be continued for at least 2 years after surgery. Indeed, a major issue for patients with AE (and CE) is the longevity of albendazole treatment and the dilemma as to when treatment can be stopped as there is no method currently available to determine when this decision should be made. Combined therapy of albendazole with transfer factor (TF) (Dvoroznáková et al., 2009) or the anti-tumour compound 2-methoxyestradiol (Spicher et al., 2008a) have yielded encouraging results in mice but await clinical testing.

10.4.3. New drugs for CE/AE

Strategies that are currently being employed to identify novel chemotherapeutical treatment options for both CE and AE include *in vitro* and *in vivo* testing of broad-spectrum anti-infective drugs or drugs that interfere with unlimited proliferation of cancer cells (Hemphill and Müller, 2009). Other avenues include the selection of novel drugs that interfere with parasite signalling machinery, and the application of *in silico* approaches by employing available *Echinococcus* genome information to search for suitable targets for compounds of known mode of action (Hemphill and Müller, 2009).

The pyridinyl imidazoles have been identified as a novel class of anti-*Echinococcus* compounds and EmMPK2—a member of the mitogen-activated protein kinase (MAPK) family—as a promising target for the development of drugs against AE (Gelmedin et al., 2008). Other potential drug targets in *Echinococcus* include thioredoxin-glutathione reductase (Bonilla et al., 2008), amino acid transporters (Camicia et al., 2008), and EmABP, from *E. multilocularis*, which is likely involved in cholesterol metabolism and uptake (Bernthaler et al., 2009). The antimalarials dihydroartemisinin and artesunate have also shown some *in vitro* effect on larvae of both *E. multilocularis* and *E. granulosus* (Spicher et al., 2008b), and warrant further investigation.

10.5. GLOBAL DISTRIBUTION OF ECHINOCOCCOSIS

E. granulosus has a worldwide geographic range occurring on all continents including circumpolar, temperate, subtropical and tropical areas, and in at least 100 countries (Eckert and Deplazes, 2004; Eckert et al., 2001b). The highest prevalences are found in parts of Eurasia (e.g. the Mediterranaean region, the Russian Federation and adjacent independent states and P.R. China), Africa (northern and eastern regions) and South America; the actual prevalence can be sporadic to high and only a few countries can be regarded as being free of the parasite (Eckert et al., 2001b).

E. multilocularis has an extensive geographical range in the northern hemisphere, including endemic regions in central Europe, most of northern and central Eurasia (extending eastwards to Japan) and parts of North America (Eckert et al., 2001b). The parasite has been reported in at least 30 countries, including Russia, Kazakhstan, and other parts of Central Asia, P.R. China, parts of Europe and North America (Eckert and Deplazes, 2004).

10.5.1. Distribution in Southeast Asia

10.5.1.1. Overview

As in many other regions of the world, it is very difficult to determine or even estimate the total numbers of human CE and AE cases in Southeast Asia. This is because of the long asymptomatic period (usually >5 years), the difficulty in diagnosis, poor record keeping, failure of patients to seek health care for a chronic condition, and also poor access to medical facilities especially for remote communities. Nevertheless, it is clear that for this region *E. granulosus* and *E. multilocularis* are most highly prevalent in P.R. China (Craig, 2004a,b; Vuitton et al., 2003; Wang et al., 2008). The full extent of echinococcosis as a public health problem in P.R. China is described in detail later.

Cases of CE in humans and animals, apparently acquired locally, have been reported occasionally from Vietnam, the Philippines, Indonesia, Malaysia, Thailand, and Lao People's Democratic Republic (Lao PDR) but nothing is known of the epidemiology of *E. granulosus* in these settings (Craig, 2004a; Eckert et al., 2001b; Schantz et al., 1995). Sporadic cases of *E. granulosus* were reported in humans and animal intermediate hosts in Japan through the 1970s but there is no contemporary information on the details of transmission cycles (Schantz et al., 1995). Human CE is extremely rare in Korea although echinococcal cysts in pigs and cattle are reportedly common in certain areas (Schantz et al., 1995).

E. multilocularis is also endemic to northern Japan (Eckert et al., 2001b). Increasing fox populations, the increasing encroachment of foxes into urban areas and other factors such as spill over of *E. multilocularis* infection from wild carnivores to domestic dogs and cats, point to a new public health hazard associated with AE. *E. multilocularis* is believed to have been introduced into Japan through infected red foxes translocated to Rebun Island, north-west of Hokkaido, from islands in the middle Kuriles from 1924 to 1926, in order to control the vole population (Eckert et al., 2001a). On Rebun Island, 131 human cases of AE were diagnosed between 1937 and 1989. Another outbreak occurred about 1960 in eastern Hokkaido, followed by the spread of *E. multilocularis* to central and western parts of the island. Between 1981 and 1991, the parasite spread from approximately 8% to 90% of the area of Hokkaido. Infected foxes in urban areas represent a new risk factor for humans (Lagapa et al., 2009). Pet dogs and cats may also serve as an infection source to humans in Japan (Nonaka et al., 2008a, 2009).

10.5.1.2. Echinococcosis in P.R. China

Both CE and AE are highly endemic over large areas of the north-western provinces and autonomous regions of P.R. China (Fig. 10.2), where it is estimated that >500,000 cases of human echinococcosis occur, one-third

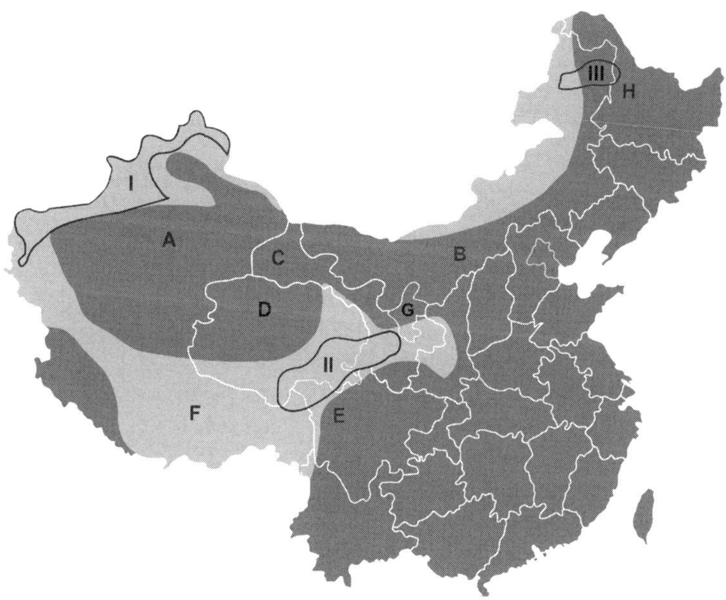

FIGURE 10.2 Areas of highest endemicity for *E. granulosus* and *E. multilocularis* in P.R. China (modified from Craig, 2004b; Wang et al., 2008). Shaded areas indicate *E. granulosus*-endemic regions; circled areas (I, II, and III) indicate foci for *E. multilocularis*. Eight autonomous regions and provinces are shown: Xinjiang Uygur autonomous region (A), Inner Mongolia autonomous region (B), Gansu province (C), Qinghai province (D), Sichuan province (E), Tibet autonomous region (F), Ningxia Hui autonomous region (G), and Heilongjiang province (H).

in children (Craig, 2004a; Craig et al., 2008; Ito et al., 2003). More DALYs are lost due to this disease in P.R. China than any other world region (Budke et al., 2006a). The first human CE case was reported in P.R. China in 1905. At least 35,000 CE cases have been treated surgically in P.R. China since the 1950s, although this figure reflects only symptomatic cases that had access to treatment (availability of health care and/or financial ability to pay) (Craig, 2004a). Human AE was first described in P.R. China in the 1950s (Craig, 2004a).

Of P.R. China's 33 provinces, autonomous regions and municipalities, at least 20 are considered to be endemic for *E. granulosus* and at least five for *E. multilocularis* (Craig, 2004a, 2006; Craig et al., 2008; Eckert et al., 2001b; 2009; Li et al., 2010; Schantz et al., 2003; Vuitton et al., 2003; Wang et al., 2008; Yang et al., 2008a). Those provinces or autonomous regions with the highest risk for *Echinococcus* infection, that is Xinjiang, Qinghai, Sichuan, Gansu and Ningxia, are also co-endemic for both human CE and AE. In addition, significant numbers of CE cases occur in the Tibet autonomous region, Shaanxi province and Inner Mongolia, but AE case reports for these areas are not clear or unknown (Wang et al., 2008). A number of cases of mixed CE and AE infections have also been identified in some patients in co-endemic areas of Xinjiang Uygur autonomous region, Ningxia Hui autonomous region and from Ganze Tibetan autonomous prefecture (Sichuan province) (Craig et al., 2008; Wang et al., 2008; Yang et al., 2008a, 2009a).

The highest prevalence of echinococcosis in the world has been reported to be in the eastern Tibetan Plateau, a newly recognised endemic region in P.R. China for *Echinococcus* spp. (Craig et al., 2008; Tiaoying et al., 2005). The overall prevalence (2.5%) was highest in Tibetan communities in the Tibet autonomous region and in north-western Sichuan and Qinghai provinces (these latter regions form part of the eastern Tibetan Plateau) (Craig et al., 2008; Yu et al., 2008). In Shiqu county of Ganze Tibetan autonomous prefecture, there was 12.9% prevalence for CE or AE in persons surveyed by ultrasound (with serologic confirmation) with a burden of more than 50,000 DALYs lost (Budke et al., 2004).

Echinococcosis is also a serious problem in Ningxia. In order to assess the extent and prevalence of AE and CE there, information was collected by examining hospital surgical and clinical records, and active community case detection of asymptomatic/early stage cases and patient follow up using questionnaire analysis, US examination and serology (Yang et al., 2005b, 2006a,b,c,d,e,f, 2007, 2008a,b). The results of these surveys indicated that CE was present throughout Ningxia, whereas AE cases occurred only in three confluent mountainous counties (Haiyuan, Xiji, and Guyuan) in the south where the average echinococcosis annual incidence was 7 per 100,000 persons compared with 1 per 100,000 persons in the north. The overall echinococcosis prevalence in south Ningxia, as assessed by US and serology, was 3.6% (mean for AE, 2%; mean for CE, 1.6%), with the highest prevalence occurring in Xiji (2% for CE, 2.5% for AE), indicating a variable distribution among the communities. These studies emphasised the severe public health issue that the disease presents in poor rural areas. There are reports of human cases of simultaneous echinococcosis and tuberculosis in Ningxia (Yang et al., 2009b), but the extent of the co-infection in this and other parts of P.R. China remains to be determined.

Extensively developed livestock husbandry maintains stable transmission cycles of *E. granulosus* in P.R. China where nomadic or seminomadic pastoralism is an important risk factor, especially in western and northwestern areas where livestock pastoralism is a major industry (Craig, 2004a,b). These sheep-farming communities harbour the highest prevalence of CE (Craig, 2004a,b), emphasising the public health significance of the sheep–dog cycle and, supported by DNA genotyping, the sheep strain (G1 genotype) of *E. granulosus* in human transmission in P.R. China (Craig et al., 2008; Heath et al., 2005; Li et al., 2005, 2008; Ma et al., 2008; Wang et al., 2008; Yang et al., 2005a, 2006e, 2009a). However, other life-cycle patterns involving domestic dogs and ungulates (camels, goats, cattle, yaks and pigs) (Wang et al., 2008) also occur in P.R. China, and the camel strain (G6 genotype) has been identified in camels from Xinjiang (Zhang et al., 1998). Wild animals can be involved in sylvatic cycles although, generally, their zoonotic importance is minimal compared with the domestic cycles. High rates of infection in dogs, kept in large populations for pastoralism and cultural and religious reasons, have also been reported in west and central P.R. China (Craig, 2004a,b; Yang et al., 2009a). Dogs are often fed by herdsmen with offal from the lungs and livers from sheep and yaks during slaughtering seasons. Because of their close relationship with local people, dogs are without question the most important definitive hosts transmitting *E. granulosus* to humans in P.R. China as in other parts of the world (Eckert et al., 2001a; Han et al., 2009; Yang et al., 2009a; Zhang et al., 2009; Zhao et al., 2009).

CE has been detected in wild species including blue sheep (*Pseudois nayaur*), black-lipped pika (*O. curzoniae*), and Tibetan gazelles (*Procapra picticaudata*) (Craig, 2004a,b; Wang et al., 2008). DNA genotyping and histological examination has shown natural infection of the ground squirrel, *Spermophilus dauricus/alashanicus*, with *E. granulosus* (Yang et al., 2009c). The wolf (*Canis lupus*) is an excellent wild definitive host of *E. granulosus* throughout its northern hemisphere range (Rausch, 2003) and wolf populations are present in sustainable numbers in parts of the Tibetan Plateau, the adjacent mountainous areas, and in Xinjiang (Craig, 2004b). Foxes are also known definitive hosts of *E. granulosus*, but it has not been determined which of the three fox species present in P.R. China, the red fox (*V. vulpes*), the Tibetan fox (*V. ferrilata*) or the Corsac fox (*V. corsac*), acts as the main definitive host (Wang et al., 2008).

The population dynamics of small mammal intermediate hosts appears to be a key factor influencing the transmission of *E. multilocularis* in P.R. China (Danson et al., 2003, 2004; Giraudoux et al., 2006; ; Raoul et al., 2006; Wang et al., 2006b). Overgrazing, deforestation and climate change have dramatically degraded the quality of the grassland in many areas of western P.R. China, resulting in optimal habitats and increased population densities of fauna including pikas (*Ochotona* spp.), voles (*Microtus* spp.), mole rats (*Myospalax baileyi*), gerbils (*Meriones* spp.), ground squirrels (*Spermophilus* spp.) and steppe lemmings (*Eolagurus* and *Lagurus* spp.), all suitable intermediate hosts for *E. mutlilocularis* (Craig, 2006; Wang et al., 2008). High density of intermediate host species has been shown to correlate significantly with heavy infection burden in foxes and dogs, resulting in increased AE prevalence in humans (Craig, 2006; Craig et al., 2000; Viel et al., 1999). In P.R. China, foxes (*V. vulpes*, *V. ferrilata*) are the main definitive hosts of *E. multilocularis* with prevalence as high as 60% in Sichuan province, although the domestic dog (5–15% prevalence) appears also to be a significant host of zoonotic importance (Budke et al., 2006b; Craig, 2006).

10.5.1.3. Risk factors for *Echinococcus* transmission in P.R. China

Human activities affecting the transmission pattern of echinococcosis have been reported worldwide, with *Echinococcus* infection rates generally being significantly different between males and females, and among different age groups. Several studies in P.R. China in the provinces of Sichuan, Qinghai and Ningxia have shown higher infection rates in females than males (Tiaoying et al., 2005; Wang et al., 2006a; Yang et al., 2006d). This is understandable as women are responsible for domestic activities including feeding, herding and milking livestock animals and collecting animal dung for fuel, and hence are more frequently exposed to dogs in these areas. Echinococcosis usually manifests 2–15 years post-infection with non-specific symptoms (Craig, 2004a,b). Consequently, humans may be infected as children, but are diagnosed only when they have become adults. A study in rural communities of southern Ningxia, P.R. China, found no gender-related differences in seroprevalence among children, suggesting an equal chance of exposure to echinococcal egg-contaminated environments (Yang et al., 2008b). The seroprevalence distribution was associated with changes in the ecology of wild hosts for *E. multilocularis* contamination, and with changes in socio-geographic features of the communities for *E. granulosus* contamination (Pleydell et al., 2008).

Human activities affecting the transmission of echinococcosis in P.R. China are usually related to pastoralism and agriculture, which modify the landscape creating better habitats for intermediate host species (e.g. rodents and pikas), thereby increasing the opportunity for spread (Craig et al., 2000; Giraudoux et al., 2006; Pleydell et al., 2008; Wang et al., 2004). A number of studies have shown that pastoralists and agriculturists suffer from the highest CE and AE infection rates due to their close association with foxes/dogs, coupled with a tendency for poor hygiene (Li et al., 2005; Wang et al., 2001, 2004, 2006a). Fencing practices may promote the transmission and maintenance of *E. multilocularis* by changing the small mammal community composition and predator–prey interactions (Wang et al., 2004, 2006a). Increased diversity of suitable intermediate hosts coupled with large populations of dogs in villages appear to be major causes of intensive and stable transmission of *E. multilocularis* around human settlements (Giraudoux et al., 2006). Recently, the Chinese government has initiated a reforestation programme, which may alter the population dynamics of both intermediate and definitive hosts and, consequently, the epidemiology of AE (Wang et al., 2008).

Community surveys and risk factor questionnaire analysis of human AE and CE (Yang *et al.*, 2006d) revealed that key risk factors for infection in Ningxia were age and dog ownership for both CE and AE, and Hui ethnicity and being female for AE; drinking well water decreased the risk for both AE and CE (Table 10.1). Significant risk factors identified for AE cases in other studies include ethnicity (Han, Tibetan, Kazakh, Hui, or Mongol), sex (females are at higher risk), age (>20 years), occupation (agriculture or pastoralism), environment (rural upland grassland/scrubland at an altitude of more than 1500 m above sea level) and dog ownership (Craig et al., 2006). Dogs appear to play a significant role in the transmission of *E. multilocularis* to humans in P.R. China and may be one of the most important risk factors, in combination with landscape/land-use features conducive to maintaining wildlife host populations (Craig et al., 2006). Geographical information system (GIS)-based spatial analysis has revealed a positive correlation between AE prevalence and the proximity of villages to shrub and grassland (Danson et al., 2003, 2006).

The transmission of echinococcosis in P.R. China is clearly complex, involving many animal species, huge remote areas, and various environments which will make effective control programmes difficult to implement.

10.6. EPIDEMIOLOGY AND CONTROL

Exposure to *Echinococcus* eggs may be influenced by occupational and behavioural factors. With *E. granulosus*, acquired immunity in intermediate hosts represents an important density-dependent constraint for transmission but parasite-induced mortality in livestock does not appear to play a role in the regulation of the cycle (Torgerson and Heath, 2003).

TABLE 10.1 Multiple logistic regression analysis of the relationships of dog ownership/livestock ownership and echinococcosis, controlling for potential confounding factors, among participants from three[a] surveyed counties (Guyuan, Longde, Xiji) in Ningxia Hui autonomous region, 2002 and 2003 (after Yang et al., 2006d)

Risk factor	Cystic echinococcosis (CE)		Alveolar echinococcosis (AE)		Combined CE and AE	
	Odds ratio (95% CI[b])	*P*-value[c]	Odds ratio (95% CI)	*P*-value	OR (95% CI)	*P*-value
Exposure variables						
Does not own a dog	0.45 (0.26–0.77)[d]	<0.01	0.54 (0.33–0.89)[d]	<0.05	0.49 (0.34–0.72)[d]	<0.01
Livestock-owner	0.91 (0.42–2.04)	0.81	0.67 (0.28–1.60)	0.36	0.78 (0.43–1.43)	0.41
Other risk factors						
Sex (female)	1.37 (0.83–2.27)	0.22	1.69 (1.06–2.69)[d]	<0.05	1.52 (1.07–2.17)[d]	<0.05
Age <30 years	0.40 (0.19–0.84)[d]	<0.05	0.13 (0.05–0.34)[d]	<0.01	0.24 (0.13–0.43)[d]	<0.01
Ethnicity (Han)	0.72 (0.42–1.24)	0.24	0.53 (0.32–0.88)[d]	<0.05	0.62 (0.42–0.91)[d]	<0.05
Killed animals[e]	1.24 (0.73–2.09)	0.42	1.10 (0.69–1.76)	0.68	1.15 (0.80–1.67)	0.44
Occupation						
Farmer	0.53 (0.18–1.47)	0.09	0.67 (0.20–2.20)	0.51	0.60 (0.27–1.35)	0.22
Student	0.09 (0.009–0.84)[d]	<0.05	0.32 (0.03–3.57)	0.35	0.16 (0.03–0.85)[d]	<0.05

Water supplies						
Others[f]	1.42 (0.39–5.21)	0.59	1.44 (0.49–4.25)	0.50	1.42 (0.59–3.43)	0.44
Tap	1.97 (0.76–5.11)	0.16	0.86 (0.29–2.52)	0.78	1.26 (0.61–2.61)	0.83
Well	0.55 (0.32–0.96)[d]	<0.05	0.37 (0.23–0.59)[d]	<0.01	0.44 (0.30–0.64)[d]	<0.01
Spring	0.69 (0.23–2.04)	0.50	0.70(0.19–2.59)	0.59	0.71 (0.29–1.71)	0.44
Unboiled water	1.11 (0.63–1.96)	0.72	0.78 (0.45–1.35)	0.38	0.94 (0.63–1.42)	0.77
Other risk factors						
Uncooked food	1.10 (0.48–2.54)	0.82	1.90 (0.92–3.92)	0.08	1.48(0.84–2.60)	0.18
No knowledge of *Echinococcus* or echinococcosis	0.16 (0.083–0.32)[d]	<0.01	0.08 (0.04–0.18)[d]	<0.01	0.12 (0.07–0.19)[d]	<0.01
Counties						
Xiji	2.47 (0.30–20.3)	0.40	–	–	3.72 (0.48–28.6)	0.20
Guyan	0.60 (0.06–5.69)	0.65	–	–	1.09 (0.13–8.97)	0.93

[a] The Longde county case numbers were too low to undertake an analysis as a possible risk factor on its own and are therefore not given in the table.
[b] CI = confidence interval.
[c] P-value determined using multiple logistic regression analysis.
[d] Indicates a significant association.
[e] Killed animals included domestic animals and large wild mammals.
[f] Other water supplies that included river water and pool collected water.

In *E. multilocularis*, the natural small mammal intermediate hosts are short-lived, the parasite evades the host immune responses and, generally, but not always, large numbers of protoscoleces are produced in a short period after infection. In contrast, the intermediate hosts of *E. granulosus* are long-lived and early classical studies carried out by David Heath and colleagues (Heath and Lawrence, 1981; Osborn and Heath, 1982) showed that sheep could be immunised against an experimental infection using oncospheres or their secreted products, a characteristic that was utilised subsequently for the development of the promising EG95 vaccine (see below).

The dynamics of *E. multilocularis* transmission are complex, being influenced by many factors that include seasonal fluctuations in the size of fox populations, the dispersal of foxes, involvement of other wild carnivores in the life cycle, the susceptibility and immunity of definitive hosts, worm burdens, pre-patent period and egg production of *E. multilocularis* infections in different definitive hosts, dispersal of eggs and resistance of eggs to environmental factors (Craig et al., 2007). As discussed above, contributions of intermediate hosts and the ecology of small mammalian hosts to the transmission dynamics of *E. multilocularis* are also very important.

Mathematical models of the life cycles of both *E. multilocularis* and *E. granulosus* have been formulated (Heinzmann and Torgerson, 2008; Torgerson, 2006) although these remain to be rigorously tested and verified. The application of satellite remote sensing, GIS and landscape approaches in mammalian ecology to the study of *E. multilocularis* provides a powerful approach to explore spatial relationships between landscape composition and transmission that will allow predictive models of AE risk to be formulated (Pleydell et al., 2008).

Preventative measures that have been used to control *Echinococcus* infections include avoiding contact with dog or fox faeces, hand washing and improved sanitation, reducing dog or fox populations, treating dogs with arecoline hydrobromide, praziquantel, or using praziquantel-impregnated baits, incinerating infected organs and health education. Despite ongoing control efforts, relatively few countries have been able to substantially reduce or eliminate AE or CE. However, there has been notable success in Iceland (elimination in the 1950s), New Zealand (control programme instigated in 1959), Tasmania (1965), the provinces of Neuquen (1970) and Rio Negro (1979) in Argentina, Cyprus (1970) and Chile (1978), where highly effective and sustained CE control programmes have been carried out (Craig et al., 2007). The arecoline-based dog-testing programmes adopted by New Zealand and Tasmania resulted in near elimination of *E. granulosus* within 20–25 years and in both campaigns, transmission to humans almost ceased within about a decade. It has been hypothesised that removal of older animals (sheep, cattle and other husbandry animals) (Torgerson et al., 2009) and stray and unwanted dogs (Zhang et al., 2009) in endemic areas, through culling programmes, could substantially aid in the control of CE.

Control of *E. multilocularis* is especially problematic as the primary cycle is almost always sylvatic and transmission is complicated by a number of epidemiological features discussed earlier. Some progress has been made in recent years and praziquantel baits for control of *E. multilocularis* infections in foxes may prove to be of value (Hegglin et al., 2003). However, the Japanese island of Rebun is the only known instance where *E. multilocularis* has been eliminated from an area where it was previously endemic. This was achieved by eliminating the fox and dog population on the island. Such an approach cannot be carried out in larger areas on ethical and ecological grounds.

10.6.1. Vaccines against *E. granulosus*

The successful CE control programmes show that prevention of transmission to either intermediate or definitive host can reduce or even eliminate the infection in human and livestock populations. So, if either or both hosts could be vaccinated, the effect would be to improve and more rapidly expedite control.

10.6.1.1. Vaccination of intermediate hosts

An *E. granulosus* vaccine would ideally prevent oncosphere development to hydatid cysts in sheep, and thus stop the development of adult gravid tapeworms in dogs. Research on mathematical models of CE control indicate that vaccination of sheep would be an effective control strategy, provided that over 90% vaccine coverage of the sheep population was achieved (Torgerson, 2006). However, the most effective intervention that was revealed by the modelling was a combination of vaccinating sheep and dog anthelminthic treatment. If about 75% vaccine coverage of the sheep population is achieved, anthelminthic treatment of dogs could be reduced to 6-month intervals, while still attaining a high level of control of disease transmission, thereby greatly reducing the cost of a control programme and probably also increasing compliance from dog owners (Torgerson, 2006).

Comprehensive reviews are available of the mechanisms of immunity in echinococcosis, which cover innate and adaptive immunity, immunomodulation and the implications for vaccine development (Amri et al., 2009; Cabezón et al., 2008; Gottstein and Hemphill, 2008; Gottstein et al., 2006; Siles-Lucas et al., 2008; Siracusano et al., 2008a,b; Vuitton et al., 2006; Zhang and McManus, 2006; Zhang et al., 2008). The *Echinococcus* organisms are very complex multi-cellular pathogens. They are highly immunogenic, stimulating pro-inflammatory cellular responses, significant antibody production, and T cell- and other cell-mediated responses in their human and intermediate hosts. An understanding of these immune mechanisms is of fundamental importance for unravelling the underlying host protective responses.

It is clear that host immunity plays a major role in the natural host–parasite relationship in echinococcosis, with this immunity being associated with protective antibodies, a feature that was used to develop the highly immunogenic recombinant vaccine, designated EG95, against *E. granulosus* (Heath and Lawrence, 1996; Lightowlers, 2006). EG95 may be involved in host invasion and is a secreted protein with a GPI anchor and a fibronectin type III (Fn3) domain, upregulated during oncosphere activation, and is probably involved in cell adhesion (Lightowlers, 2006). The vaccine has been shown to confer a high degree of protection against challenge with different geographical isolates of *E. granulosus*, indicating that it could have wide applicability as an effective tool for use in hydatid control campaigns, with the potential to prevent hydatid disease directly through vaccination of humans. However, although some of the immune responses involved in infection have been addressed, including the involvement of Abs, the precise mechanisms underlining protection are largely unknown. Some important unresolved areas of hydatid immunobiology that may inform future vaccine design are presented in Table 10.2. Understanding these mechanisms will benefit researchers working not only on cestode vaccines but also on vaccination against other helminth parasites (Zhang et al., 2008).

It will be important as well to investigate approaches to vaccination against established hydatid cysts both as a treatment option and for use in conjunction with oncosphere vaccines to reduce the time required to break the transmission cycle of the dog–sheep strain (Craig et al., 2007).

Some recent questions have been raised on the potential efficacy of EG95 against variants of *E. granulosus* and discrete *Echinococcus* species. EG95 is encoded by a multi-gene family and amino acid substitutions of the protein have been shown in the G6/G7 genotypes, which may affect the antigenicity/efficacy of the EG95 recombinant antigen against parasites of these genotypes (Chow et al., 2008). Furthermore, extensive sequencing of the complete coding sequence (CDS) of *eg95* genes (CDS) uncovered a large amount of variability (Haag et al., 2009). As the protective EG95 epitopes are conformational (Lightowlers, 2006; Read et al., 2009), a small number of amino acid replacements may affect the efficacy of the vaccine in species other than *E. granulosus* (Haag et al., 2009). However, as the sheep–dog strain of *E. granulosus* (G1 genotype) is responsible for most cases of human CE, the value of the EG95 vaccine should not be unduly compromised.

TABLE 10.2 Unresolved areas of hydatid immunology that may inform improved vaccine design in intermediate hosts (after Zhang et al., 2008)

Required tasks
• Precisely identify the immunoglobulin isotypes involved in protective immunity. • Define the role of T cells as effectors of protective immunity and their regulation. • Unravel the relationship between T cell and B cell responses in protective immunity. • Characterise memory B cell and T cell recognition of protective antigens, including the EG95 vaccine. • Determine the role(s) of antibody (Ab)-dependent cell-mediated immune effector mechanisms such as the involvement of neutrophils and the eosinophil/IgE/mast cell axis and neutrophils with Ab in the killing of the infective larval stage (the oncosphere) contained within the egg. • Evaluate cellular inflammatory responses/cell-mediated immunity, the generation of associated cytokine/chemokines, and the role of regulatory T cells, neutrophils, macrophages, eosinophils, fibrocytes, and NK cells in the early stages of infection. • Determine the involvement of Ab-dependent, complement-mediated lysis (by the classical or alternative pathway) and the role of neutrophils in the immune killing of oncospheres *in vivo*.

A protein containing characteristic fibronectin III domains, related to EM95 (Gauci et al., 2002) (a homologue of EG95), that can induce significant levels of protection against challenge infection with *E. multilocularis* eggs in mice, has been identified in *E. multilocularis* (Merckelbach et al., 2003). Whether this molecule has the potential to form the basis of a practical vaccine for reducing the level of AE in humans in regions of high endemicity remains to be determined, but due to the sylvatic nature of the *E. multilocularis* life cycle, this seems unlikely.

10.6.1.2. Vaccination of definitive hosts

Although the EG95 vaccine against ovine hydatidosis is a reality that now requires innovative delivery strategies (Craig et al., 2007), no similarly effective vaccine exists against canine echinococcosis. This is not because of the lack of potential for application, because such a vaccine for dogs would be of enormous benefit in further reducing the effective period required to stop transmission of *E. granulosus*. Rather, the scarcity of vaccine candidates for immune protection against adult tapeworm infection reflects the lack of research reports on specific immune correlates, the lack of evidence until recently of natural immunity in dogs, and the difficulties and cost in maintaining experimental canids (Craig et al., 2007; Zhang and McManus, 2008). A series of experiments to induce immunity in dogs through vaccination with various components have been carried out (Petavy et al., 2008; Zhang et al., 2006), although there has been stern criticism regarding some of these initial data (Torgerson, 2009). Clearly, these preliminary experiments need to be repeated, confirmed, and extended, but this difficult and dangerous area is important and warrants strong encouragement for the future.

10.7. CONCLUDING REMARKS AND RESEARCH NEEDS

Despite the establishment of extensive and successful control programmes against CE in some countries or regions, *E. granulosus* still has a very wide geographical distribution and the parasite continues to be the cause of substantial morbidity and mortality in many parts of the world. Indeed, recent evidence suggests that CE is a public health problem of increasing concern, persisting or re-emerging in many areas worldwide, causing severe disease and considerable economic loss.

A similar but potentially even more alarming situation prevails with *E. multilocularis* as evidenced by the increasing prevalence of AE, its wider than previously thought distribution and the fact the parasite can readily spread from endemic to non-endemic areas. *E multilocularis* is transmitted mainly within wildlife cycles, with a number of fox species being highly susceptible to infection with the adult tapeworm, and a wide range of rodents (especially microtine voles) and other small mammals can act as intermediate hosts. The greater pathogenicity, treatment difficulty, and higher mortality risk of AE has led to consideration of its control by intervention trials/programmes in a number of endemic areas, including southwest P.R. China (Ito et al., 2003). However, effective methods for control of *E. multilocularis* are not yet available and this adds support to the argument for more efficient prevention measures and early diagnosis of AE.

Chemotherapy has facilitated less invasive surgical management of CE and AE but there is a pressing need for new advances in the prevention of both these neglected diseases to improve prospects for sustainable control programmes (Craig et al., 2007). The research needs and recommendations for effective prevention of echinococcosis transmission are summarised in Table 10.3. As indicated in this review, in P.R. China, both human AE and CE are co-endemic in several western regions, where combined control of both *Echinococcus* species may be warranted (Craig et al., 2007).

TABLE 10.3 Echinococcosis research needs and recommendations (modified from Craig et al., 2007)

Research needs and recommendations
• Measurement of the real burden of cystic echinococcosis disease in South America, Africa, the Mediterranean, and different regions of P.R. China, similar to that recently undertaken for some other areas. Determine mortality and morbidity rates due to echinococcosis generally.
• Sound multi-center prospective evaluation of clinical treatment options for echinococcosis, with a long-term follow up of several years. This is especially needed for surgery, including a comparison of surgical procedures (total cystectomy vs. partial cystectomy), and evaluation of the added values and modalities (drug amount; how long given) of albendazole (with or without praziquantel) given prior to, and following, surgery.
• Large-scale clinical assessment of the drugs flubendazole, either separately or in combination with ivermectin, and oxfendazole in CE therapy. Development of new drugs for cystic and alveolar echinococcosis is a priority.
• Clinical assessment of the use of high-intensity focused ultrasound (HIFU) for treatment of echinococcosis in patients.
• Improve the diagnosis for earlier detection of *Echinococcus* infection. There is a need to improve imaging diagnosis of lung cyst locations, adapted for screening and surveillance.
• Develop a method (e.g. imaging or serology) to assess parasite viability and/or to assess progression potential of both cystic and alveolar echinococcosis.
• Determine the duration required for albendazole treatment of cystic and alveolar echinococcosis. There is a dilemma as to when treatment can be stopped as there is no method currently available to determine when this decision should be made and this is a major issue for patients.
• Undertake a multi-center, comparative, standardised study of native, recombinant, and peptide antigens for diagnosis of human cystic echinococcosis.
• Undertake longitudinal follow-up studies of human seropositivity in CE-endemic regions using defined recombinant antigens. Determine the extent, variability, and reason for long-term serial antibody responses in ultrasound-negative people. As serology on its own is poorly predictive of infection in the field and only of

(continued)

TABLE 10.3 (*continued*)

Research needs and recommendations
limited value to confirm radiological findings, it is necessary to understand, decipher, and dissect the factors affecting serology in human infection.
• Serology in animals is problematical—can this be improved? The sensitivity/'non-responder' issue may be insurmountable as many animals are sero-negative, even with large, viable cysts present.
• Compare the efficacy, sensitivity, and specificity of new copro-DNA tests for CE, and establish strain-specific detection for *E. granulosus* in dogs.
• Research priorities for the EG95 vaccine for ovine echinococcosis include: determining the three-dimensional conformational structure by computer modelling; optimising vaccine delivery with existing established vaccines (e.g. sheep) and carrying out a demonstration programme for hydatid control using EG95 vaccine in sheep, praziquantel dosing of dogs, and health education in different endemic areas. Could the vaccine be developed for human use?
• Investigate approaches for vaccination against established hydatid cysts both as a treatment option and for use in conjunction with oncosphere vaccines to reduce the time required to break the transmission of the dog–sheep cycle.
• Research priorities for dog vaccines against *E. granulosus* include characterising infection dynamics in natural dog populations; expressing adult ES antigens in *Salmonella* and *Vaccinia* vectors; establishing optimum protocols for dog vaccination studies; prototype testing in different settings and endemic areas; developing improved delivery methods using appropriate and acceptable adjuvants; determining the longevity of protection; and determining whether there is an effect against *E. multilocularis* with the caveat that the generally sylvatic nature of the life cycle of this species makes a vaccination approach to control unlikely.
• Guidelines should be developed for consideration of definitions for control of CE, that is what levels of reduction in sheep, dog, and human infections constitute significant effects? Elimination of transmission of *E. granulosus* in a controlled region should be defined. There is a need to standardise robust definitions for many end points such as seropositivity, elimination of disease, and viable/non-viable infection.

ACKNOWLEDGEMENTS

Echinococcosis research in the author's laboratory is supported by the National Health and Medical Research Council of Australia. The author thanks Phil Craig, Hugo Garcia and Dominique Vuitton for valuable suggestions on future areas of echinococcosis research, and Ms Mimi Kersting for kindly providing Fig. 10.2.

REFERENCES

Alvite, G., Esteves, A., 2009. *Echinococcus granulosus* tropomyosin isoforms: from gene structure to expression analysis. Gene 433, 40–49.

Ammann, R., Eckert, J., 1996. Cestodes: *Echinococcus*. Gastroenterol. Clin. N. Am. 25, 655–689.

Amri, M., Mezioug, D., Ait-Aissa, S., Touil-Boukoffa, C., 2008. In vivo IL-12 and IL-8 production in hydatic patients and their possible diffusion in hydatid cysts. Eur. Cytokine Netw. 19, 142–148.

Amri, M., Mezioug, D., Touil-Boukoffa, C., 2009. Involvement of IL-10 and IL-4 in evasion strategies of *Echinococcus granulosus* to host immune response. Eur. Cytokine Netw. 20, 63–68.

Bart, J.M., Piarroux, M., Sako, Y., Grenouillet, F., Bresson-Hadni, S., Piarroux, R., et al., 2007. Comparison of several commercial serologic kits and Em18 serology for detection of human alveolar echinococcosis. Diagn. Microbiol. Infect. Dis. 59, 93–95.

Batelli, G., 2009. Echinococcosis: costs, losses and social consequences of a neglected zoonosis. Vet. Res. Commun. 33 (Suppl. 1), 47–52.

Ben Nouir, N., Gianinazzi, C., Gorcii, M., Müller, N., Nouri, A., Babba, H., et al., 2009. Isolation and molecular characterization of recombinant *Echinococcus granulosus* P29 protein (recP29) and its assessment for the post-surgical serological follow-up of human cystic echinococcosis in young patients. Trans. R. Soc. Trop. Med. Hyg. 103, 355–364.

Bernthaler, P., Epping, K., Schmitz, G., Deplazes, P., Brehm, K., 2009. Molecular characterization of EmABP, an apolipoprotein A-I binding protein secreted by the *Echinococcus multilocularis* metacestode. Infect. Immun. 77, 5564–5571.

Bonilla, M., Denicola, A., Novoselov, S.V., Turanov, A.A., Protasio, A., Izmendi, D., et al., 2008. Platyhelminth mitochondrial and cytosolic redox homeostasis is controlled by a single thioredoxin glutathione reductase and dependent on selenium and glutathione. J. Biol. Chem. 283, 17898–17907.

Boufana, B.S., Campos-Ponce, M., Naidich, A., Buishi, I., Lahmar, S., Zeyhle, E., et al., 2008. Evaluation of three PCR assays for the identification of the sheep strain (genotype 1) of *Echinococcus granulosus* in canid feces and parasite tissues. Am. J. Trop. Med. Hyg. 78, 777–783.

Bresson-Hadni, S., Miguet, J.P., Mantion, G., Giraudoux, P., Vuitton, D.A., 2008. Alveolar echinococcosis: a disease comparable to a slow growing cancer. Bull. Acad. Natl. Med. 192, 1131–1138 (in French).

Brunetti, E., Kern, P., Vuitton, D.A., Writing Panel for the WHO-IWGE, 2010. Expert consensus for the diagnosis and treatment of cystic and alveolar echinococcosis in humans. Acta Trop. 114, 1–16.

Budke, C.M., Jiamin, Q., Zinsstag, J., Qian, W., Torgerson, P.R., 2004. Use of disability adjusted life years in the estimation of the disease burden of echinococcosis for a high endemic region of the Tibetan plateau. Am. J. Trop. Med. Hyg. 71, 56–64.

Budke, C.M., Deplazes, P., Torgerson, P.R., 2006a. Global socioeconomic impact of cystic echinococcosis. Emerg. Infect. Dis. 12, 296–303.

Budke, C.M., Jiamin, Q., Craig, P.S., Torgerson, P.R., 2006b. Modeling the transmission of *Echinococcus granulosus* and *Echinococcus multilocularis* in dogs for a high endemic region of the Tibetan plateau. Int. J. Parasitol. 36, 163–170.

Cabezón, C., Cabrera, G., Paredes, R., Ferreira, A., Galanti, N., 2008. *Echinococcus granulosus* calreticulin: molecular characterization and hydatid cyst localization. Mol. Immunol. 45, 1431–1438.

Camicia, F., Paredes, R., Chalar, C., Galanti, N., Kamenetzky, L., Gutierrez, A., et al., 2008. Sequencing, bioinformatic characterization and expression pattern of a putative amino acid transporter from the parasitic cestode *Echinococcus granulosus*. Gene 411, 1–9.

Capan, M., Keltner, S., Thalhammer, F., Winkler, S., Jäger, W., Zeitlinger, M., et al., 2009. Intra-cystic drug concentration of albendazole sulphoxide in patients with *Echinococcus granulosus* cysts. Am. J. Trop. Med. Hyg. 81, 712–713.

Carmena, D., Benito, A., Eraso, E., 2007. The immunodiagnosis of *Echinococcus multilocularis* infection. Clin. Microbiol. Infect. 13, 460–475.

Ceballos, L., Elissondo, M., Bruni, S.S., Denegri, G., Alvarez, L., Lanusse, C., 2009. Flubendazole in cystic echinococcosis therapy: pharmaco-parasitological evaluation in mice. Parasitol. Int. 58, 354–358.

Chow, C., Gauci, C.G., Vural, G., Jenkins, D.J., Heath, D.D., Rosenzvit, M.C., et al., 2008. *Echinococcus granulosus*: variability of the host-protective EG95 vaccine antigen in G6 and G7 genotypic variants. Exp. Parasitol. 119, 499–505.

Craig, P.S., 1997. Immunodiagnosis of *Echinococcus granulosus* and comparison of techniques for diagnosis of canine echinococcosis. In: Andersen, F., Ouhelli, H., Kachani, M. (Eds.), Compendium on Echinococcosis in Africa and Middle Eastern Countries with Special Reference to Morocco. Brigham Young University Print Services, Provo, Utah, pp. 85–118.

Craig, P.S., 2004a. Epidemiology of echinococcosis in western China. In: Torgerson, P.R., Shaikenov, B. (Eds.), Echinococcosis in Central Asia: Problems and Solutions. Dauir, Zurich, pp. 43–58.

Craig, P.S., 2004b. Epidemiology of echinococcosis in China. Southeast Asian J. Trop. Med. Public Health 35 (Suppl. 1), 1–13.

Craig, P.S., 2006. Echinococcosis Working Group in China. Epidemiology of human alveolar echinococcosis in China. Parasitol. Int. 55 (Suppl.), S221–S225.

Craig, P.S., Giraudoux, P., Shi, D., Bartholomot, B., Barnish, G., Delattre, P., et al., 2000. An epidemiological and ecological study of human alveolar echinococcosis transmission in south Gansu, China. Acta Trop. 77, 167–177.

Craig, P.S., Rogan, M.T., Campos-Ponce, M., 2003. Echinococcosis: disease, detection and transmission. Parasitology 127 (Suppl.), S5–S20.

Craig, P.S., McManus, D.P., Lightowlers, M.W., Chabalgoity, J.A., Garcia, H.H., Gavidia, C. M., et al., 2007. Prevention and control of cystic echinococcosis. Lancet Infect. Dis. 7, 385–394.

Craig, P.S., Li, T., Qiu, J., Zhen, R., Wang, Q., Giraudoux, P., et al., 2008. Echinococcosis and Tibetan communities. Emerg. Infect. Dis. 14, 1674–1675.

Cumino, A.C., Elissondo, M.C., Denegri, G.M., 2009. Flubendazole interferes with a wide spectrum of cell homeostatic mechanisms in *Echinococcus granulosus* protoscoleces. Parasitol. Int. 58, 270–277.

Danson, F.M., Graham, A.J., Pleydell, D., Campos-Ponce, M., Giraudoux, P., Craig, P.S., 2003. Multi-scale spatial analysis of human alveolar echinococcosis risk in China. Parasitology 127, S133–S141.

Danson, F.M., Craig, P.S., Man, W., Shi, D.Z., Giraudoux, P., 2004. Landscape dynamics and risk modelling of human alveolar echinococcosis. Photogramm. Eng. Rem. Sens. 70, 359–366.

Danson, F.M., Giraudoux, P., Craig, P.S., 2006. Spatial modeling and ecology of *Echinococcus multilocularis* transmission in China. Parasitol. Int. 55, S227–S231.

Dvoroznáková, E., Porubcová, J., Sevcíková, Z., 2009. Immune response of mice with alveolar echinococcosis to therapy with transfer factor, alone and in combination with albendazole. Parasitol. Res. 105, 1067–1076.

Eckert, J., Deplazes, P., 2004. Biological, epidemiological, and clinical aspects of echinococcosis, a zoonosis of increasing concern. Clin. Microbiol. Rev. 17, 107–135.

Eckert, J., Deplazes, P., Craig, P., Gemmell, M.A., Gottstein, B., Heath, D., et al., 2001a. Echinococcosis in animals: clinical aspects, diagnosis and treatment. In: Eckert, J., Gemmell, M.A., Meslin, F.-X., Pawlowski, Z.S. (Eds.), WHOI/OIE Manual on Echinococcosis in Humans and Animals: A Public Health Problem of Global Concern. World Organisation for Animal Health, Paris, pp. 72–99.

Eckert, J., Schantz, P.M., Gasser, R.B., Torgerson, P.R., Bessonov, A.S., Movsessian, S.O., et al., 2001b. Geographic distribution and prevalence. In: Eckert, J., Gemmell, M.A., Meslin, F.-X., Pawlowski, Z.S. (Eds.), WHOI/OIE Manual on Echinococcosis in Humans and Animals: A Public Health Problem of Global Concern. World Organisation for Animal Health, Paris, pp. 101–143.

Elissondo, M.C., Ceballos, L., Alvarez, L., Sánchez Bruni, S., Lanusse, C., Denegri, G., 2009. Flubendazole and ivermectin in vitro combination therapy produces a marked effect on *Echinococcus granulosus* protoscoleces and metacestodes. Parasitol. Res. 105, 835–842.

Feng, X., Wen, H., Zhang, Z., Chen, X., Ma, X., Zhang, J., et al., 2010. Dot immunogold filtration assay (DIGFA) with multiple native antigens for rapid serodiagnosis of human cystic and alveolar echinococcosis. Acta Trop. 113, 114–120.

Gauci, C., Merli, M., Muller, V., Chow, C., Yagi, K., Mackenstedt, U., et al., 2002. Molecular cloning of a vaccine antigen against infection with the larval stage of *Echinococcus multilocularis*. Infect. Immun. 70, 3969–3972.

Gavidia, C.M., Gonzalez, A.E., Zhang, W., McManus, D.P., Lopera, L., Ninaquispe, B., et al., 2008. Diagnosis of cystic echinococcosis, central Peruvian Highlands. Emerg. Infect. Dis. 14, 260–266.

Gavidia, C.M., Gonzalez, A.E., Lopera, L., Jayashi, C., Angelats, R., Barron, E.A., et al., 2009. Evaluation of nitazoxanide and oxfendazole efficacy against cystic echinococcosis in naturally infected sheep. Am. J. Trop. Med. Hyg. 80, 367–372.

Gelmedin, V., Caballero-Gamiz, R., Brehm, K., 2008. Characterization and inhibition of a p38-like mitogen-activated protein kinase (MAPK) from *Echinococcus multilocularis*: antiparasitic activities of p38 MAPK inhibitors. Biochem. Pharmacol. 76, 1068–1081.

Giraudoux, P., Pleydell, D., Raoul, F., Que're', J.P., Wang, Q., Yang, Y., et al., 2006. Transmission ecology of *Echinococcus multilocularis*: what are the ranges of parasite stability among various host communities in China? Parasitol. Int. 55, S237–S246.

Gottstein, B., Hemphill, A., 2008. *Echinococcus multilocularis*: the parasite–host interplay. Exp. Parasitol. 119, 447–452.

Gottstein, B., Haag, K., Walker, M., Matsumoto, J., Mejri, N., Hemphill, A., 2006. Molecular survival strategies of *Echinococcus multilocularis* in the murine host. Parasitol. Int. 55 (Suppl.), S45–S49.

Haag, K.L., Zaha, A., Araujo, A.M., Gottstein, B., 1997. Reduced genetic variability within coding and non-coding regions of the *Echinococcus multilocularis* genome. Parasitology 115, 521–529.

Haag, K.L., Gottstein, B., Ayala, F.J., 2009. The EG95 antigen of *Echinococcus* spp. contains positively selected amino acids, which may influence host specificity and vaccine efficacy. PLoS One 4, e5362.

Han, X.M., Wang, H., Cai, H.X., Ma, X., Liu, Y.F., Wei, B.H., et al., 2009. Epidemiological survey on echinococcosis in Darlag County of Qinghai province. Zhongguo Ji Sheng Chong Xue Yu Ji Sheng Chong Bing Za Zhi 27, 22–26 (in Chinese).

Hänle, M.M., Banzhaf, H.M., Forsbach-Birk, V., Kirch, A., Akinli, A.S., Mason, R.A., et al., 2009. Screening methods in alveolar echinococcosis: a follow-up study comparing

Emc- and Emf-ELISA with Em2plus-ELISA and ultrasonography. Epidemiol. Infect. 137, 139–144.

Heath, D.D., Lawrence, S.B., 1981. *Echinococcus granulosus* cysts: early development in vitro in the presence of serum from infected sheep. Int. J. Parasitol. 11, 261–266.

Heath, D.D., Lawrence, S.B., 1996. Antigenic polypeptides of *Echinococcus granulosus* oncospheres and definition of protective molecules. Parasite Immunol. 18, 347–537.

Heath, D.D., Zhang, L.H., McManus, D.P., 2005. Short report: inadequacy of yaks as hosts for the sheep dog strain of *Echinococcus granulosus* or for *E. multilocularis*. Am. J. Trop. Med. Hyg. 72, 289–290.

Hegglin, D., Ward, P.I., Deplazes, P., 2003. Anthelmintic baiting of foxes against urban contamination with *Echinococcus multilocularis*. Emerg. Infect. Dis. 9, 1266–1272.

Heinzmann, D., Torgerson, P.R., 2008. Evaluating parasite densities and estimation of parameters in transmission systems. Parasite 15, 5477–5483.

Hemphill, A., Müller, J., 2009. Alveolar and cystic echinococcosis: towards novel chemotherapeutical treatment options. J. Helminthol. 83, 99–111.

Hülsmeier, A.J., Deplazes, P., Naem, S., Nonaka, N., Hennet, T., Köhler, P., 2010. An *Echinococcus multilocularis* coproantigen is a surface glycoprotein with unique O-gycosylation. Glycobiology 20, 127–135.

Hüttner, M., Nakao, M., Wassermann, T., Siefert, L., Boomker, J.D., Dinkel, A., et al., 2008. Genetic characterization and phylogenetic position of *Echinococcus felidis* (Cestoda: Taeniidae) from the African lion. Int. J. Parasitol. 38, 861–868.

Hüttner, M., Siefert, L., Mackenstedt, U., Romig, T., 2009. A survey of *Echinococcus* species in wild carnivores and livestock in East Africa. Int. J. Parasitol. 39, 1269–1276.

Ito, A., Romig, T., Takahashi, K., 2003. Perspective on control options for *Echinococcus multilocularis* with particular reference to Japan. Parasitology 127 (Suppl.), 159–172.

Ito, A., Nakao, M., Sako, Y., 2007. Echinococcosis: serological detection of patients and molecular identification of parasites. Future Microbiol. 2, 439–449.

Kern, P., Wen, H., Sato, N., Vuitton, D.A., Gruener, B., Shao, Y., et al., 2006. WHO classification of alveolar echinococcosis: principles and application. Parasitol. Int. 55 (Suppl.), S283–S287.

Kittelberger, R., Reichel, M.P., Jenner, J., Heath, D.D., Lightowlers, M.W., Moro, P., et al., 2002. Evaluation of three enzyme-linked immunosorbent assays (ELISAs) for the detection of serum antibodies in sheep infected with *Echinococcus granulosus*. Vet. Parasitol. 110, 57–76.

Knapp, J., Bart, J.M., Giraudoux, P., Glowatzki, M.L., Breyer, I., Raoul, F., et al., 2009. Genetic diversity of the cestode *Echinococcus multilocularis* in red foxes at a continental scale in Europe. PLoS Negl. Trop. Dis. 3, e452.

Lagapa, J.T., Oku, Y., Kaneko, M., Ganzorig, S., Ono, T., Nonaka, N., et al., 2009. Monitoring of environmental contamination by *Echinococcus multilocularis* in an urban fringe forest park in Hokkaido. Jpn. Environ. Health Prev. Med. 14, 299–303.

Lahmar, S., Boufana, B.S., Lahmar, S., Inoubli, S., Guadraoui, M., Dhibi, M., et al., 2009. *Echinococcus* in the wild carnivores and stray dogs of northern Tunisia: the results of a pilot survey. Ann. Trop. Med. Parasitol. 103, 323–331.

Le, T.H., Blair, D., McManus, D.P., 2002. Mitochondrial genomes of parasitic flatworms. Trends Parasitol. 18, 206–213.

Li, J., Zhang, W.B., McManus, D.P., 2004. Recombinant antigens for immunodiagnosis of cystic echinococcosis. Biol. Proced. Online 6, 67–77.

Li, T., Ito, A., Nakaya, K., Qiu, J., Nakao, M., Zhen, R., et al., 2008. Species identification of human echinococcosis using histopathology and genotyping in northwestern China. Trans. R. Soc. Trop. Med. Hyg. 102, 585–590.

Li, T., Chen, X., Zhen, R., Qiu, J., Qiu, D., Xiao, N., et al., 2010. Widespread co-endemicity of human cystic and alveolar echinococcosis on the eastern Tibetan Plateau, northwest Sichuan/southeast Qinghai, China. Acta Trop. 114, 248–256.

Lightowlers, M.W., 2006. Vaccines against cysticercosis and hydatidosis: foundations in taeniid cestode immunology. Parasitol. Int. 55, S39–S43.

Ma, S.M., Maillard, S., Zhao, H.L., Huang, X., Wang, H., Geng, P.L., et al., 2008. Assessment of *Echinococcus granulosus* polymorphism in Qinghai province, People's Republic of China. Parasitol. Res. 102, 1201–1206.

Macpherson, C.N.L., 1983. An active intermediate host role for man in the life cycle of *Echinococcus granulosus* in Turkana. Kenya. Am. J. Trop. Med. Hyg. 32, 397–404.

Maillard, S., Gottstein, B., Haag, K.L., Ma, S., Colovic, I., Benchikh-Elfegoun, M.C., et al., 2009. The EmsB tandemly repeated multilocus microsatellite: a new tool to investigate genetic diversity of *Echinococcus granulosus* sensu lato. J. Clin. Microbiol. 47, 3608–3616.

Mantion, G., Bresson-Hadni, S., Vuitton, D.A., Wen, H., Chapuis, Y., Gillet, M., 2008. Treatment of alveolar echinococcosis: a multidisciplinary task. Bull. Acad. Natl. Med. 192, 1151–1157 (in French).

McManus, D.P., 2009. Reflections on the biochemistry of *Echinococcus*: past, present and future. Parasitology 136, 1643–1652.

McManus, D.P., Simpson, A.J., 1985. Identification of the *Echinococcus* spp. (hydatid disease) organisms using cloned DNA markers. Mol. Biochem. Parasitol. 17, 171–178.

McManus, D.P., Knight, M., Simpson, A.J., 1985. Isolation and characterisation of nucleic acids from the hydatid organisms, *Echinococcus* spp. (Cestoda). Mol. Biochem. Parasitol. 16, 251–266.

McManus, D.P., Thompson, R.C., 2003. Molecular epidemiology of cystic echinococcosis. Parasitology 127, S37–S51.

McManus, D.P., Zhang, W., Li, J., Bartley, P.B., 2003. Echinococcosis. Lancet 362, 1295–1304.

Merckelbach, A., Wager, M., Lucius, R., 2003. Analysis of cDNAs coding for immunologically dominant antigens from an oncosphere-specific cDNA library of *Echinococcus multilocularis*. Parasitol. Res. 90, 493–501.

Moray, G., Shahbazov, R., Sevmis, S., Karakayali, H., Torgay, A., Arslan, G., et al., 2009. Liver transplantation in management of alveolar echinococcosis: two case reports. Transplant. Proc. 41, 2936–2938.

Moro, P., Schantz, P.M., 2009. Echinococcosis: a review. Int. J. Infect. Dis. 13, 125–133.

Nakao, M., McManus, D.P., Schantz, P.M., Craig, P.S., Ito, A., 2007. A molecular phylogeny of the genus *Echinococcus* inferred from complete mitochondrial genomes. Parasitology 134, 713–722.

Nakao, M., Li, T., Han, X., Ma, X., Xiao, N., Qiu, J., et al., 2009. Genetic polymorphisms of *Echinococcus* tapeworms in China as determined by mitochondrial and nuclear DNA sequences. Int. J. Parasitol. 40, 379–385.

Nakao, M., Xiao, N., Okamoto, M., Yanagida, T., Sako, Y., Ito, A., 2010. Geographic pattern of genetic variation in the fox tapeworm *Echinococcus multilocularis*. Parasitol. Int. 58, 384–389.

Nonaka, N., Hirokawa, H., Inoue, T., Nakao, R., Ganzorig, S., Kobayashi, F., et al., 2008a. The first instance of a cat excreting *Echinococcus multilocularis* eggs in Japan. Parasitol. Int. 57, 519–520.

Nonaka, N., Oka, M., Kamiya, M., Oku, Y., 2008b. A latex agglutination test for the detection of *Echinococcus multilocularis* coproantigen in the definitive hosts. Vet. Parasitol. 152, 278–283.

Nonaka, N., Kamiya, M., Kobayashi, F., Ganzorig, S., Ando, S., Yagi, K., et al., 2009. *Echinococcus multilocularis* infection in pet dogs in Japan. Vector Borne Zoonotic Dis. 9, 201–206.

Osborn, P.J., Heath, D.D., 1982. Immunisation of lambs against *Echinococcus granulosus* using antigens obtained by incubation of oncospheres in vitro. Res. Vet. Sci. 33, 132–133.

Pawłowski, Z.S., Eckert, J., Vuitton, D.A., Ammann, R.W., Kern, P., Craig, P.S., et al., 2001. Echinococcosis in humans: clinical aspects, diagnosis and treatment. In: Eckert, J., Gemmell, M.A., Meslin, F.-X., Pawlowski, Z.S. (Eds.), WHOI/OIE Manual on Echinococcosis in Humans and Animals: A Public Health Problem of Global Concern. World Organisation for Animal Health, Paris, pp. 20–71.

Pednekar, R.P., Gatne, M.L., Thompson, R.C., Traub, R.J., 2009. Molecular and morphological characterisation of *Echinococcus* from food producing animals in India. Vet. Parasitol. 165, 58–65.

Petavy, A.F., Hormaeche, C., Lahmar, S., Ouhelli, H., Chabalgoity, A., Marchal, T., et al., 2008. An oral recombinant vaccine in dogs against *Echinococcus granulosus*, the causative agent of human hydatid disease: a pilot study. PLoS Negl. Trop. Dis. 2, e125.

Pleydell, D.R., Yang, Y.R., Danson, F.M., Raoul, F., Craig, P.S., McManus, D.P., et al., 2008. Landscape composition and spatial prediction of alveolar echinococcosis in southern ningxia. China. PLoS Negl. Trop. Dis. 2, e287.

Raoul, F., Que're', J.P., Rieffel, D., Bernard, N., Takahashi, K., 2006. Distribution of small mammals in a pastoral landscape of the Tibetan plateaus (western Sichuan, China) and relationship with grazing practices. Mammalia 70, 214–225.

Rausch, R.L., 2003. Cystic echinococcosis in the Arctic and the Subarctic. Parasitology 127 (Suppl.), S73–S85.

Read, A.J., Casey, J.L., Coley, A.M., Foley, M., Gauci, C.G., Jackson, D.C., et al., 2009. Isolation of antibodies specific to a single conformation-dependant antigenic determinant on the EG95 hydatid vaccine. Vaccine 27, 1024–1031.

Reiter-Owona, I., Grüner, B., Frosch, M., Hoerauf, A., Kern, P., Tappe, D., 2009. Serological confirmatory testing of alveolar and cystic echinococcosis in clinical practice: results of a comparative study with commercialized and in-house assays. Clin. Lab. 55, 41–48.

Rinder, H., Rausch, R.L., Takahashi, K., Kopp, H., Thomschke, A., Löscher, T., 1997. Limited range of genetic variation in *Echinococcus multilocularis*. J. Parasitol. 83, 1045–1050.

Rishi, A.K., McManus, D.P., 1987. Genomic cloning of human *Echinococcus granulosus* DNA: isolation of recombinant plasmids and their use as genetic markers in strain characterization. Parasitology 94, 369–383.

Saarma, U., Jõgisalu, I., Moks, E., Varcasia, A., Lavikainen, A., Oksanen, A., et al., 2009. A novel phylogeny for the genus *Echinococcus*, based on nuclear data, challenges relationships based on mitochondrial evidence. Parasitology 136, 317–328.

Sako, Y., Fukuda, K., Kobayashi, Y., Ito, A., 2009. Development of an immunochromatographic test to detect antibodies against recombinant Em18 for diagnosis of alveolar echinococcosis. J. Clin. Microbiol. 47, 252–254.

Sato, N., Akoi, S., Matsushita, M., Uchino, J., 1993. Clinical features. In: Uchino, Y., Sato, H. (Eds.), Alveolar Echinococcosis of the Liver. Hokkaido University School of Medicine, Sapporo, pp. 63–68.

Schantz, P.M., Chai, J., Craig, P.S., Eckert, J., Jenkins, D., Macpherson, C.N.L., et al., 1995. Epidemiology and control. In: Thompson, R.C.A., Lymbery, A.J. (Eds.), Echinococcosis and Hydatid Disease. CAB, London, pp. 233–331.

Schantz, P.M., Wang, H., Qiu, J., Liu, F.J., Saito, E., Emshoff, A., et al., 2003. Echinococcosis on the Tibetan Plateau: prevalence and risk factors for cystic and alveolar echinococcosis in Tibetan populations in Qinghai province, China. Parasitology 127 (Suppl.), S109–S120.

Siles-Lucas, M., Merli, M., Gottstein, B., 2008. 14-3-3 proteins in *Echinococcus*: their role and potential as protective antigens. Exp. Parasitol. 119, 516–523.

Siracusano, A., Margutti, P., Delunardo, F., Profumo, E., Riganò, R., Buttari, B., et al., 2008a. Molecular cross-talk in host–parasite relationships: the intriguing immunomodulatory role of *Echinococcus* antigen B in cystic echinococcosis. Int. J. Parasitol. 38, 1371–1376.

Siracusano, A., Riganò, R., Ortona, E., Profumo, E., Margutti, P., Buttari, B., et al., 2008b. Immunomodulatory mechanisms during *Echinococcus granulosus* infection. Exp. Parasitol. 119, 483–489.

Siracusano, A., Teggi, A., Ortona, E., 2009. Human cystic echinococcosis: old problems and new perspectives. Interdiscip. Perspect. Infect. Dis. 2009, 474368.

Smego Jr., R.A., Bhatti, S., Khaliq, A.A., Beg, M.A., 2003. Percutaneous aspiration–injection–reaspiration drainage plus albendazole or mebendazole for hepatic cystic echinococcosis: a meta-analysis. Clin. Infect. Dis. 38, 1073–1083.

Spicher, M., Naguleswaran, A., Ortega-Mora, L.M., Müller, J., Gottstein, B., Hemphill, A., 2008a. In vitro and in vivo effects of 2-methoxyestradiol, either alone or combined with albendazole, against *Echinococcus* metacestodes. Exp. Parasitol. 119, 475–482.

Spicher, M., Roethlisberger, C., Lany, C., Stadelmann, B., Keiser, J., Ortega-Mora, L.M., et al., 2008b. In vitro and in vivo treatments of *Echinococcus* protoscoleces and metacestodes with artemisinin and artemisinin derivatives. Antimicrob. Agents Chemother. 52, 3447–3450.

Spiliotis, M., Brehm, K., 2009. Axenic in vitro cultivation of *Echinococcus multilocularis* metacestode vesicles and the generation of primary cell cultures. Methods Mol. Biol. 470, 245–262.

Stamatakos, M., Sargedi, C., Stefanaki, C.H., Safioleas, C., Matthaiopoulou, I., Safioleas, M., 2009. Anthelminthic treatment: an adjuvant therapeutic strategy against *Echinococcus granulosus*. Parasitol. Int. 58, 115–120.

Tappe, D., Frosch, M., Sako, Y., Itoh, S., Grüner, B., Reuter, S., et al., 2009. Close relationship between clinical regression and specific serology in the follow-up of patients with alveolar echinococcosis in different clinical stages. Am. J. Trop. Med. Hyg. 80, 792–797.

Thompson, R.C.A., 2008. The taxonomy, phylogeny and transmission of *Echinococcus*. Exp. Parasitol. 119, 439–446.

Thompson, R.C.A., McManus, D.P., 2001. Aetiology: parasites and life cycles. In: Eckert, J., Gemmell, M.A., Meslin, F.-X., Pawlowski, Z.S. (Eds.), WHO/OIE Manual on Echinococcosis in Humans and Animals: A Public Health Problem of Global Concern. World Organisation for Animal Health, Paris, pp. 1–19.

Thompson, R.C., McManus, D.P., 2002. Towards a taxonomic revision of the genus *Echinococcus*. Trends Parasitol. 18, 452–457.

Tiaoying, L., Jiamin, Q., Wen, Y., Craig, P.S., Xingwang, C., Ning, X., et al., 2005. Echinococcosis in Tibetan populations, western Sichuan Province. China. Emerg. Infect. Dis. 11, 1866–1873.

Torgerson, P.R., 2006. Mathematical models for the control of cystic echinococcosis. Parasitol. Int. 55, S253–S258.

Torgerson, P.R., 2009. Dogs, vaccines and *Echinococcus*. Trends Parasitol. 25, 57–58.

Torgerson, P.R., Deplazes, P., 2009. Echinococcosis: diagnosis and diagnostic interpretation in population studies. Trends Parasitol. 25, 164–170.

Torgerson, P.R., Heath, D.D., 2003. Transmission dynamics and control options for *Echinococcus granulosus*. Parasitology 127, S143–S158.

Torgerson, P.R., Schweiger, A., Deplazes, P., Pohar, M., Reichen, J., Ammann, R.W., et al., 2008. Alveolar echinococcosis: from a deadly disease to a well-controlled infection. Relative survival and economic analysis in Switzerland over the last 35 years. J. Hepatol. 49, 72–77.

Torgerson, P.R., Ziadinov, I., Aknazarov, D., Nurgaziev, R., Deplazes, P., 2009. Modelling the age variation of larval protoscoleces of *Echinococcus granulosus* in sheep. Int. J. Parasitol. 39, 1031–1035.

Viel, J.F., Giraudoux, P., Arbial, V., Bresson-Hadni, S., 1999. Water vole (*Arvicola terrestris*) density as risk factor for human alveolar echinococcosis. Am. J. Trop. Med. Hyg. 61, 559–565.

Vuitton, D.A., 2009. Benzimidazoles for the treatment of cystic and alveolar echinococcosis: what is the consensus? Expert Rev. Anti. Infect. Ther. 7, 145–149.

Vuitton, D.A., Zhou, H., Bresson-Hadni, S., Wang, Q., Piarroux, M., Raoul, F., et al., 2003. Epidemiology of alveolar echinococcosis with particular reference to China and Europe. Parasitology 127 (Suppl.), S87–S107.

Vuitton, D.A., Zhang, S.L., Yang, Y., Godot, V., Beurton, I., Mantion, G., et al., 2006. Survival strategy of *Echinococcus multilocularis* in the human host. Parasitol. Int. 55 (Suppl.), S51–S55.

Vuitton, D.A., Bresson-Hadni, S., Giraudoux, P., Bartholomot, B., Laplante, J.J., Delabrousse, E., et al., 2009. Alveolar echinococcosis: from an incurable rural disease to a controlled urban infection? Presse Med. 39, 216–230 (in French).

Wang, Q., Qiu, J.M., Schantz, P., He, J.G., Ito, A., Liu, F.J., 2001. Investigation of risk factors for development of human hydatidosis among households raising livestock in Tibetan areas of western Sichuan province. Zhongguo Ji Sheng Chong Xue Yu Ji Sheng Chong Bing Za Zhi 19, 93–96.

Wang, Q., Vuitton, D.A., Qiu, J., Giraudoux, P., Xiao, Y., Schantz, P.M., et al., 2004. Fenced pasture: a possible risk factor for human alveolar echinococcosis in Tibetan pastoralist communities of Sichuan, China. Acta Trop. 90, 285–293.

Wang, Q., Qiu, J., Yang, W., Schantz, P.M., Raoul, F., Craig, P.S., et al., 2006a. Socioeconomic and behavior risk factors of human alveolar echinococcosis in Tibetan communities in Sichuan, People's Republic of China. Am. J. Trop. Med. Hyg. 74, 856–862.

Wang, Q., Vuitton, D.A., Xiao, Y., Budke, C.M., Campos-Ponce, M., Schantz, P.M., et al., 2006b. Pasture types and *Echinococcus multilocularis*, Tibetan communities. Emerg. Infect. Dis. 12, 1008–1010.

Wang, Z., Wang, X., Liu, X., 2008. Echinococcosis in China, a review of the epidemiology of *Echinococcus* spp. EcoHealth 5, 115–126.

WHO, 2003. International classification of ultrasound images in cystic echinococcosis for application in clinical and field epidemiological settings. Acta Trop. 85, 253–261.

Xiao, N., Qiu, J., Nakao, M., Yang, W., Chen, X., Schantz, P.M., et al., 2005. *Echinococcus shiquicus* n. sp., a taeniid cestode from Tibetan fox and plateau pika in China. Int. J. Parasitol. 35, 693–701.

Yang, Y.R., Rosenzvit, M.C., Zhang, L.H., Zhang, J.Z., McManus, D.P., 2005a. Molecular study of *Echinococcus* in west-central China. Parasitology 131, 547–555.

Yang, Y.R., Sun, T., Li, Z., Li, X., Zhao, R., Cheng, L., et al., 2005b. Echinococcosis, Ningxia, China. Emerg. Infect. Dis. 11, 1314–1316.

Yang, Y.R., Cheng, L., Yang, S.K., Pan, X., Sun, T., Li, X., et al., 2006a. A hospital-based retrospective survey of human cystic and alveolar echinococcosis in Ningxia Hui Autonomous Region. P.R. China. Acta Trop. 97, 284–291.

Yang, Y.R., Ellis, M., Sun, T., Li, Z., Liu, X., Vuitton, D.A., et al., 2006b. Unique family clustering of human echinococcosis cases in a Chinese community. Am. J. Trop. Med. Hyg. 74, 487–494.

Yang, Y.R., Liu, X.Z., Vuitton, D.A., Bartholomot, B., Wang, Y.H., Ito, A., et al., 2006c. Simultaneous alveolar and cystic echinococcosis of the liver. Trans. R. Soc. Trop. Med. Hyg. 100, 597–600.

Yang, Y.R., Sun, T., Li, Z., Zhang, J., Teng, J., Liu, X., et al., 2006d. Community surveys and risk factor analysis of human alveolar and cystic echinococcosis in Ningxia Hui autonomous region. China. Bull. World Health Organ. 84, 714–721.

Yang, Y.R., Sun, T., Zhang, J.Z., McManus, D.P., 2006e. Molecular confirmation of a case of multiorgan cystic echinococcosis. J. Parasitol. 92, 206–208.

Yang, Y.R., Williams, G.M., Craig, P.S., Sun, T., Yang, S.K., Cheng, L., et al., 2006f. Hospital and community surveys reveal the severe public health problem and socio-economic impact of human echinococcosis in Ningxia Hui autonomous region. China. Trop. Med. Int. Health 11, 880–888.

Yang, Y.R., Craig, P.S., Ito, A., Vuitton, D.A., Giraudoux, P., Sun, T., et al., 2007. A correlative study of ultrasound with serology in an area in China co-endemic for human alveolar and cystic echinococcosis. Trop. Med. Int. Health 12, 637–646.

Yang, Y.R., Craig, P.S., Sun, T., Vuitton, D.A., Giraudoux, P., Jones, M.K., et al., 2008a. Echinococcosis in Ningxia Hui autonomous region, northwest China. Trans. R. Soc. Trop. Med. Hyg. 102, 319–328.

Yang, Y.R., Craig, P.S., Vuitton, D.A., Williams, G.M., Sun, T., Liu, T.X., et al., 2008b. Serological prevalence of echinococcosis and risk factors for infection among children in rural communities of southern Ningxia. China. Trop. Med. Int. Health 13, 1086–1094.

Yang, Y.R., Gray, D.J., Ellis, M.K., Yang, S.K., Craig, P.S., McManus, D.P., 2009a. Human cases of simultaneous echinococcosis and tuberculosis—significance and extent in China. Parasit. Vectors 4, 53.

Yang, Y.R., Liu, T., Bai, X., Boufana, B., Craig, P.S., Nakao, M., et al., 2009b. Natural infection of the ground squirrel (*Spermophilus* spp.) with *Echinococcus granulosus* in China. PLoS Negl. Trop. Dis. 3, e518.

Yang, Y.R., McManus, D.P., Huang, Y., Heath, D.D., 2009c. *Echinococcus granulosus* infection and options for control of cystic echinococcosis in Tibetan communities of western Sichuan Province. China. PLoS Negl. Trop. Dis. 3, e426.

Yu, S.H., Wang, H., Wu, X.H., Ma, X., Liu, P.Y., Liu, Y.F., et al., 2008. Cystic and alveolar echinococcosis: an epidemiological survey in a Tibetan population in southeast Qinghai. China. Jpn. J. Infect. Dis. 61, 242–246.

Zhang, W., McManus, D.P., 2006. Recent advances in the immunology and diagnosis of echinococcosis. FEMS Immunol. Med. Microbiol. 47, 24–41.

Zhang, W., McManus, D.P., 2008. Vaccination of dogs against *Echinococcosus granulosus*: a means to control hydatid disease? Trends Parasitol. 24, 419–424.

Zhang, L.H., Chai, J.J., Jiao, W., Osman, Y., McManus, D.P., 1998. Mitochondrial genomic markers confirm the presence of the camel strain (G6 genotype) of *Echinococcus granulosus* in north-western China. Parasitology 116, 29–33.

Zhang, W., Li, J., McManus, D.P., 2003. Concepts in immunology and diagnosis of hydatid disease. Clin. Microbiol. Rev. 16, 18–36.

Zhang, W., Zhang, Z., Shi, B., Li, J., You, H., Tulson, G., 2006. Vaccination of dogs against *Echinococcus granulosus*, the cause of cystic hydatid disease in humans. J. Infect. Dis. 194, 966–974.

Zhang, W., Ross, A.G., McManus, D.P., 2008. Mechanisms of immunity in hydatid disease: implications for vaccine development. J. Immunol. 181, 6679–6685.

Zhang, W., Zhang, Z., Yimit, T., Shi, B., Aili, H., Tulson, G., 2009. A pilot study for control of hyper-endemic cystic hydatid disease in China. PLoS Negl. Trop. Dis. 3, e534.

Zhao, Y.M., Tong, S.X., Jing, T., Chong, S.G., Cai, X.P., Jing, Z.Z., et al., 2009. Investigation on echinococcosis in animals in Gannan Tibetan autonomous prefecture. Zhongguo Ji Sheng Chong Xue Yu Ji Sheng Chong Bing Za Zhi 27, 27–30 (in Chinese).

Zou, X., Wang, J., Zhao, H., Zhang, J., Wu, W., Ye, B., 2009. *Echinococcus granulosus*: protoscolicidal effect of high intensity focused ultrasound. Exp. Parasitol. 121, 312–316.

CHAPTER 11

Food-Borne Trematodiases in Southeast Asia: Epidemiology, Pathology, Clinical Manifestation and Control

Banchob Sripa,* **Sasithorn Kaewkes,**† **Pewpan M. Intapan,**† **Wanchai Maleewong,**† and **Paul J. Brindley**‡

Contents

* Tropical Disease Research Laboratory (TDR), Department of Pathology, Faculty of Medicine, Khon Kaen University, Thailand
† Department of Parasitology, Faculty of Medicine, Khon Kaen University, Thailand
‡ Department of Microbiology, Immunology and Tropical Medicine, The George Washington University Medical Center, Washington, District of Columbia, USA

Advances in Parasitology, Volume 72
ISSN 0065-308X, DOI: 10.1016/S0065-308X(10)72011-X

Abstract

The food-borne trematodiases are an important group of neglected tropical diseases (NTDs). Over 40 million people are infected with food-borne trematodes and 750 million (>10% of the world's population) are at risk of these NTDs. Here, we review the life cycles, epidemiology, clinical manifestations, pathology and pathogenesis, diagnosis, treatment, and prevention and control of the major food-borne trematodiases in Southeast Asia. We focus particularly on opisthorchiasis caused by *Opisthorchis viverrini* and clonorchiasis caused by *Clonorchis sinensis*, which people contract by ingestion of metacercariae in flesh of raw or undercooked freshwater fishes, on fascioliasis caused by *Fasciola* species, where infection arises from ingestion of metacercariae on water plants such as watercress, and on *Paragonimus* species, the lung flukes, which use freshwater crabs and other crustaceans as intermediate hosts. We also include information on the intestinal flukes *Fasciolopsis buski*, the echinostomes and the so-called 'minute intestinal flukes' of the family Heterophyidae. Ecological information, placing emphasis on reservoir hosts, intermediate snail hosts and secondary hosts where applicable, is also reviewed and research needs are highlighted.

11.1. INTRODUCTION

Food-borne trematodiases are one major group of the so-called neglected tropical diseases (NTDs) worldwide with more than 40 million people infected and 750 million (>10% of the world's population) at risk (Hotez et al., 2008; Keiser and Utzinger, 2005). Over 100 species of food-borne trematodes are known to infect humans. These infections usually occur focally, are still endemic in many parts of the world, particularly Southeast Asia (Graczyk and Fried, 2007). Common clinical important trematodes in this region include *Opisthorchis viverrini*, *Clonorchis sinensis*, *Fasciola* spp., *Paragonimus* spp. and intestinal flukes (Table 11.1) (WHO, 2002). Most trematodiases affect the poor and poorest people in rural areas. Many factors contribute to the high prevalence of these infections, including lack of education, poor recognition of the trematode infections because of their asymptomatic clinical presentation, poverty, malnutrition, a lack of food inspection and poor sanitation (Graczyk and Fried, 2007).

This review highlights on the life cycles, epidemiology, clinical manifestations, pathology and pathogenesis, diagnosis, and prevention and control of the most important trematodiases in Southeast Asia, particularly opisthorchiasis and clonorchiasis. Fascioliasis, one of the clinically important trematodiasis in the region, has been extensively updated in this journal recently (Mas-Coma et al., 2009a). For detailed biology of other trematodes, several recent in-depth reviews are recommended, that is Dorny et al. (2009) and Keiser and Utzinger (2009).

11.2. OPISTHORCHIASIS AND CLONORCHIASIS

The human liver flukes, *O. viverrini*, *O. felineus* and *C. sinensis* remain important public health problems in many parts of the world (Fig. 11.1). *C. sinensis* is widespread in the People's Republic of China (P.R. China), Korea and north Vietnam, while *O. viverrini* is endemic in Southeast Asia, including Thailand, Lao People's Democratic Republic (Lao PDR), Cambodia and central Vietnam. Human infection follows the consumption of raw or undercooked cyprinoid (freshwater) fish habouring infective metacercariae. Recent reports suggested that about 35 million people are infected with *C. sinensis* globally (Keiser and Utzinger, 2005); with up to 15 million human infections in P.R. China alone and another 8–10 million individuals infected with *O. viverrini* in Thailand and Lao PDR (Andrews et al., 2008; Jongsuksuntigul and Imsomboon, 2003; WHO, 1995). More than 600 million people, mainly in Asia, are at risk of infection with these two liver flukes (Keiser and Utzinger, 2005). The infections are associated with hepatobiliary diseases including hepatomegaly, cholangitis, fibrosis of the periportal system, cholecystitis, gallstones and are major aetiological agents of bile duct cancer, cholangiocarcinoma (CCA). *O. viverrini* and *C. sinensis* are classified as Group 1 carcinogens—metazoan parasites that are carcinogenic to humans—by the International Agency for Research on Cancer, World Health Organization (WHO) (Bouvard et al., 2009; IARC, 1994). Therefore, not only do these liver flukes cause pathogenic helminth infections, but they are also carcinogenic in humans in a fashion similar to several other more well-known biological carcinogens, in particular hepatitis viruses, human papilloma virus and *Helicobacter pylori*. The liver fluke endemic area of Khon Kaen,

TABLE 11.1 Food-borne trematodes of medical importance and public health significance in Asia (WHO, 2002)

Family	Genus	Species	Source of human infection	Location in human body
Opisthorchidae	*Clonorchis*	*C. sinensis*	Fish	Liver and biliary system
	Opisthorchis	*O. viverrini*	Fish	Liver and biliary system
Fasciolidae	*Fasciola*	*F. hepatica*	Plants	Liver and biliary system
		F. gigantica	Plants	Liver and biliary system
	Fasciolopsis	*Fas. buski*	Plants	Small intestine
Troglotrematidae	*Paragonimus*	Species complex	Crabs and crayfish	Pleural cavity and lung; occasional brain invasion
Heterophyidae	*Haplorchis*	*H. taichui*	Fish	Mucosa of small intestine
	Metagonimus	*M. yokogawai*	Fish	Mucosa of small intestine

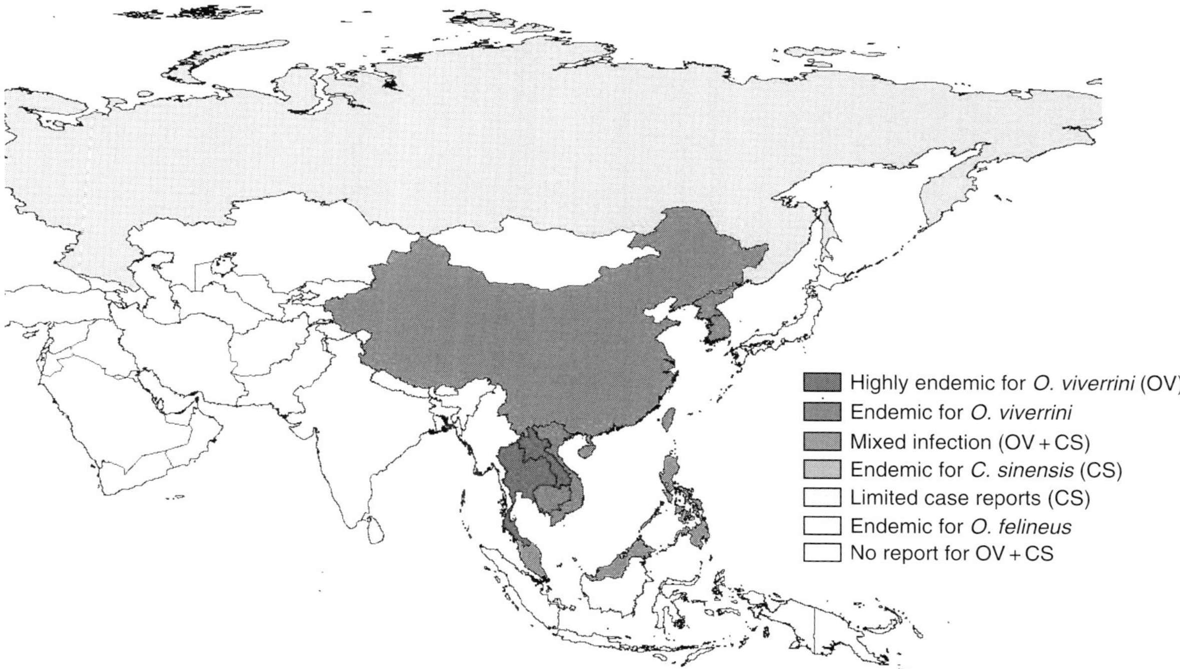

FIGURE 11.1 Geographical distribution of human liver flukes, namely *O. viverrini*, *O. felineus* and *C. sinensis*. The map emphasises the regions where opisthorchiasis and clonorchiasis are endemic in Asia.

Northeast Thailand have reported the highest incidence of the liver cancer in the world (Vatanasapt et al., 1990). In regard to socioeconomic impact, it was estimated 20 years ago that the total direct cost of *O. viverrini* infection to work force (between the age of 15 and 60 years) in Northeast Thailand was US$ 80 million per annum (Loaharanu and Sornmani, 1991). More recently, it has been reported that liver and bile duct cancer, the end-stage consequence of liver fluke disease, ranks number five in Thai males among all diseases with highest number of disability-adjusted life years (DALYs) (Table 11.2) (Sripa and Pairojkul, 2008).

11.2.1. Life cycles

The adult worms of *O. viverrini* and *C. sinensis* inhabit the intra- and extrahepatic biliary system. The life cycle of the two liver flukes is shown in Fig. 11.2. Embryonated eggs containing the miracidium release from gravid worms are passed into the bile and eventually the faecal

TABLE 11.2 Top 10 diseases with high burden (expressed in disability-adjusted life years (DALYs) lost) in Thai population stratified by sex for the year 2004 (Sripa and Pairojkul, 2008)

	Male			Female		
Rank	Disease	DALY ('000)	%	%	DALY ('000)	Disease
1	HIV/AIDS	645	11.3	7.4	313	Stroke
2	Traffic accidents	584	10.2	6.9	291	HIV/AIDS
3	Stroke	332	5.8	6.4	271	Diabetes
4	Alcohol dependence/ harmful use	332	5.8	4.5	191	Depression
5	**Liver and bile duct cancer**	**280**	**4.9**	3.4	142	Ischemic heart disease
6	COPD	187	3.3	3.0	125	Traffic accidents
7	Ischemic heart disease	184	3.2	**3.0**	**124**	**Liver and bile duct cancer**
8	Diabetes	175	3.1	2.8	118	Osteoarthritis
9	Cirrhosis	144	2.5	2.7	115	COPD
10	Depression	137	2.4	2.6	111	Cataracts

Liver and bile duct cancer, highlighted in bold, is mainly resulted from chronic *Opisthorchis* infection.

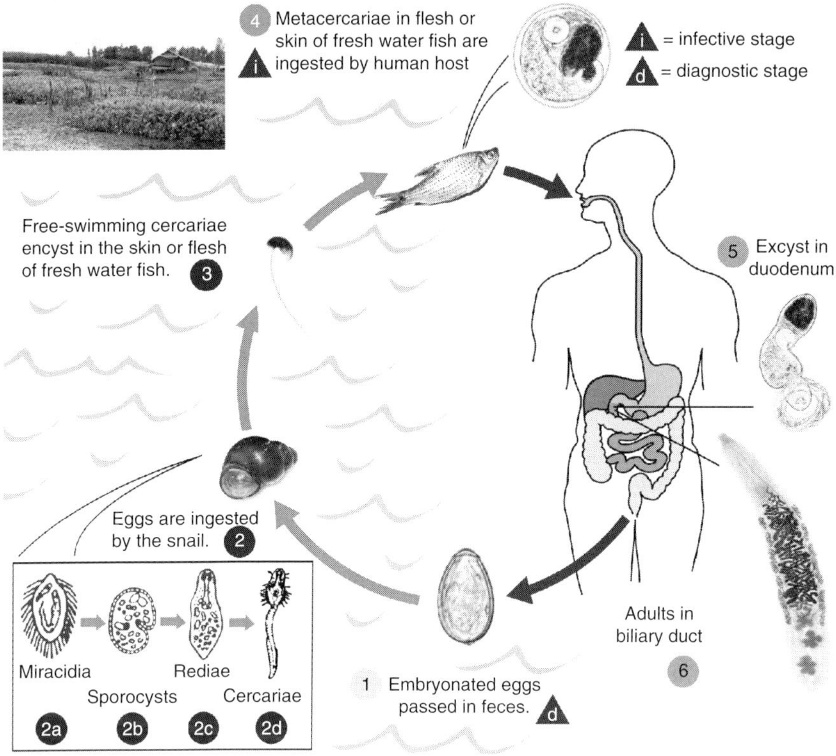

FIGURE 11.2 Life cycle of *O. viverrini* (modified from http://www.dpd.cdc.gov/dpdx/hTML/Frames/M-R/Opisthorchiasis/body_Opisthorchiasis_page1.htm).

stream. After reaching freshwater, these eggs are ingested by *Bithynia* snails and hatch. The miracidia then transform to sporocysts and asexual reproduction occurs giving rise to rediae and, in turn, to cercariae. After escape from the snail, the free-living cercaria attaches to and penetrates the skin of ~18 susceptible species of fish in the family Cyprinidae. Once on and within the skin, the cercariae encysts as metacercariae. Metacercariae are infective to final definitive hosts including humans, dogs and cats when they ingest raw or inadequately cooked fish. After ingestion, the metacercaria is digested by gastric and intestinal juices, respectively. Excysted juvenile flukes at the duodenum then migrate through the ampulla of Vater into the common bile duct and into the intrahepatic bile ducts, where they mature and reproduce. Some flukes can be found in the common bile duct, cystic duct and even in the gallbladder. The adult liver fluke is an hermaphrodite, and can live for several years or even decades.

11.2.2. Epidemiology

11.2.2.1. *Opisthorchis viverrini*

In Southeast Asia, opisthorchiasis has been reported from Thailand, Lao PDR, Cambodia and Vietnam. We are unaware of reports of opisthorchiasis from Myanmar. The first human cases of *O. viverrini* infection were reported in Thailand, nearly a century ago (Leiper, 1915), and the prevalence of *O. viverrini* infection remains high in Thailand nearly a century later. The first systematic investigation on opisthorchiasis in Thailand was reported by Sadun (1955) who described a high prevalence of the infection and its associated morbidities in Northeast Thailand. The prevalence in certain villages reached 100%. The first nationwide survey in 1980–1981 revealed a prevalence of *O. viverrini* infection as follows, Northeast (34.6%), Central (6.3%), the North (5.6%) and the South (0.01%) of Thailand, with an overall prevalence of 14%. Due to the intensive and continuous control activities, the prevalence of infection in Northeast Thailand declined to 15.7% in 2001, and the rate of other areas was as follows: the North (19.3%), Central (3.8%) and the South (0%), with an average prevalence of 9.4% (Jongsuksuntigul and Imsomboon, 2003). However, these nationwide survey data may not reflect the actual situation in local endemic areas in Northeast Thailand where the prevalence can approach 70% (Sripa, 2008). Continuing or re-emerging *O. viverrini* infections in these regions warrants more investigation and control-related resources in these regions.

It is estimated that over 2 million people are infected with *O. viverrini* in Lao PDR (WHO, 1995), mainly in the south of the country. Based on a nationwide survey of primary schoolchildren from 17 provinces and the Vientiane municipality, a national prevalence rate for *O. viverrini* was estimated as 10.9%, from 29,846 participants. Regions along the Mekong River including Khammuane, Saravane or Savannakhet showed higher prevalence of *O. viverrini* (32.2%, 21.5% and 25.9%, respectively) (Rim et al., 2003). More recently, a survey in Saravane district revealed a 58.5% prevalence of *O. viverrini* infection among 814 persons from 13 villages (Sayasone et al., 2007). There are few official reports or published data on *O. viverrini* infection in Cambodia. A small survey in primary schoolchildren from Kampongcham province showed the prevalence of *O. viverrini* of 4.0% from 251 faecal specimens in 2002 (Lee et al., 2002). Recent reports from this province revealed a high prevalence of *O. viverrini* metacercariae in 10 species of freshwater cyprinoids with the infection rate ranging from 2.1% to 66.7% and mean intensities of infection of 1.0–15.0 metacercariae per fish depending on fish species (range: 1–65) (Touch et al., 2009). Vietnam has been reported to be endemic for both *C. sinensis* in the northern part and *O. viverrini* in the central and southern regions. *O. viverrini* infection rates in three endemic southern provinces range from 15.2% to 36.9% (De et al., 2003). Six endemic districts, namely Nui Thanh, Mo Duc, Mhu My, Song Cau, Tuy An and Buon Don are known in central Vietnam (WHO, 2008).

11.2.2.2. *Clonorchis sinensis*

C. sinensis was first reported in 1874 from the bile duct contents of a Chinese carpenter who died in Calcutta, India. However, human clonorchiasis has been documented in P.R. China for more than 2000 years since *C. sinensis* eggs were detected in faecal remains from an ancient corpse buried at the middle stage of the Warring States Period (475–221 BC) in Hubei, P.R. China (Wu et al., 1996). Following the discovery of the causative agent and the disease, *C. sinensis* infections have been reported from many parts of Eastern Asia, Eastern Siberia, Japan, the Republic of Korea, P.R. China, Taiwan and Vietnam. Sporadic cases have been reported in Malaysia, Singapore and the Philippines (IARC, 1994). In P.R. China, *C. sinensis* is endemic in southern (Gaungxi and Guangdong) and northeastern provinces (Heilongjiang) (Lun et al., 2005). A recent national sampling survey in endemic areas of 217,829 individuals, revealed *C. sinensis* infections among 5230 participants (2.4%), and the number of infected persons was estimated to be 12.49 million (Fang et al., 2008). In Southeast Asia, clonorchiasis has been reported in northern Vietnam close to southern P.R. China. An epidemiological survey carried out in 12 out of 61 provinces of Vietnam, showed that *C. sinensis* was prevalent in nine northern provinces with prevalences ranging from 0.2% to 26.0%, mainly in the Red River delta region (De et al., 2003; WHO, 2008). A recent study of 1155 villagers in two communes in northern Vietnam showed a prevalence of *C. sinensis* infection of 26% (Dang et al., 2008). Countries in Southeast Asia other than Vietnam have yet to publish data on the endemicity of clonorchiasis, with the exception of a report of clonorchiasis cases detected by genetic diagnosis (polymerase chain reaction, PCR) in a recent survey in a community in central Thailand (Traub et al., 2009). The infected population may be Vietnamese who migrated to this area in recent times. In any event, this finding can be expected to lead to further investigation on potential molluscan and freshwater fish intermediate hosts and on the extent of the human infections in neighbouring districts.

11.2.3. Clinical manifestations

Most chronic human opisthorchiasis and clonorchiasis cases show few specific signs or symptoms, except an increased frequency of palpable liver, as shown in community-based studies (Rim, 2005; Upatham et al., 1982, 1984). Haematological and biochemical features are generally unremarkable, even in heavy infections (Pungpak et al., 1994). By contrast, ultrasonography, however, reveals a high frequency of gallbladder enlargement, sludge, gallstones and poor function in asymptomatic individuals (Choi et al., 2005; Mairiang et al., 1992, 1993). These gallbladder abnormalities usually resolve to a large extent after treatment with praziquantel, usually within a year or two after treatment (Mairiang et al., 1993). Periductal fibrosis seen as periportal echoes along the intrahepatic biliary trees is a predominant ultrasonographic feature in chronic liver fluke infections (Fig. 11.3) (Choi et al., 2004, 2005; Mairiang et al., 1992). Upon ultrasonographic grading, positive advanced periductal fibrosis (APF) has been observed in chronic opisthorchiasis in >30% of cases (Pungpak et al., 1997). In a recent case–control study, involving 328 men and women with asymptomatic *O. viverrini* infection, we observed that individuals with positive APF significantly showed poor contraction of the gallbladder as measured by difference of the gallbladder length before and after a fatty meal (Sripa et al., 2009). A similar association was also observed between the positive APF and the presence of sludge in the gallbladder. Sludge and stones in the gallbladder from opisthorchiasis or clonorchiasis patients usually contain liver fluke eggs (Rim, 2005; Sripa et al., 2004).

Symptomatic cases of opisthorchiasis and clonorchiasis generally experience pain in the right upper quadrant, diarrhoea, loss of appetite, indigestion and fullness. For opisthorchiasis, Upatham et al. (1982, 1984) found that 5–10% of infected individuals had weakness or malaise, flatulence or dyspepsia and abdominal pain, and 5% had hepatomegaly. Clinical symptoms were related to intensity of the infection. Severe cases may present with weakness, lassitude, weight loss, ascites and oedema. Complications may include cholangitis, obstructive jaundice, intra-abdominal mass, cholecystitis and gallbladder or intrahepatic stones. Such stones are particularly frequent in clonorchiasis (Choi et al., 2008; Rim, 2005).

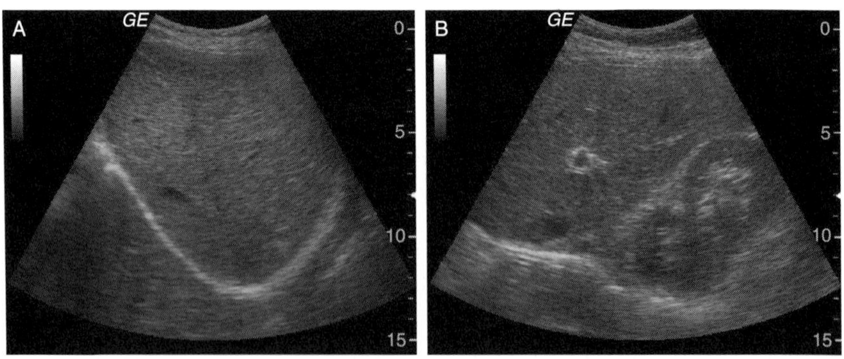

FIGURE 11.3 Ultrasonography of the liver of a patient with chronic opisthorchiasis showing severe periportal echoes along the intrahepatic biliary trees (B) compare to the normal liver (A). (Courtesy of Dr. E. Mairiang).

The most important clinical manifestation of liver fluke infection is an enhanced susceptibility to CCA. Several cross-sectional and case–control studies carried out in Northeast Thailand demonstrated increased risk of CCA in *O. viverrini*-infected individuals. For example, a population-based survey of *O. viverrini* infection in 12,311 adults over age 24 years from 85 villages in northeast Thailand (including patients with varying faecal egg count categories) were selected for ultrasound examination to identify hepatobiliary disease. Fifteen preclinical cases of CCA were diagnosed from a total of 1807 infected people. A five-fold increased risk was calculated for all patients, while heavily infected people may approach a 15-fold risk compared with the uninfected group (Haswell-Elkins et al., 1994). Moreover, an up to 27-fold increased risk has been reported using antibody to the liver fluke in a case–control study in this region (Honjo et al., 2005). For clonorchiasis, similarly, one case–control study in Busan Korea including 41 patients with CCA and 203 cases of hepatocellular carcinoma (HCC) revealed that CCA was significantly correlated with *C. sinensis* eggs in stool, past history of liver flukes, hepatitis history, and a history of heavy consumption of alcoholic beverages (Shin et al., 1996). Similar findings were seen for 185 cases with CCA and matched controls in Korea. Radiologic evidence of *C. sinensis*, history of eating raw freshwater fish, and positive serologic result for *C. sinensis* were found to be related to an increased risk of CCA in this study, with an odds ratio (OR) of up to 8.62 (Choi et al., 2006).

Patients with liver fluke-associated CCA present variable clinical manifestations. Jaundice is the main clinical manifestation that accounts for 60% of a hospital series of opisthorchiasis-related CCA in Northeast Thailand (Mairiang and Mairiang, 2003). The patients may present with (i) obstructive jaundice alone, (ii) obstructive jaundice with fever, or (iii) obstructive jaundice with acute abdominal complications, such as cholangitis, acalculous cholecystitis and generalised bile peritonitis. Non-jaundiced patients may present with dyspeptic pain, anorexia, weight loss, right upper abdominal mass and distant metastasis (Mairiang and Mairiang, 2003; Rim, 2005). Most patients with peripheral CCA or intrahepatic CCA present with palpable liver mass. The mass may be single or multiple and may involve one or both lobes of the liver. The majority of the tumor mass is located in the posterior segment of the right lobe adjacent to the diaphragm (Uttaravichien et al., 1999).

11.2.4. Pathology and pathogenesis

In both infections with *O. viverrini* and *C. sinensis*, pathological consequences of the infection occur mainly in the liver, extrahepatic bile ducts and gallbladder, and have been described in both humans, experimentally infected hamsters and other animal models (for recent reviews, see Rim, 2005; Sripa, 2003; Sripa et al., 2007). The severity of disease is associated with both intensity and duration of infection. Grossly, infected animals or humans show hepatomegaly, dilatation of subcapsular bile ducts and thickend gallbladder. Histopathologic features of opisthorchiasis or clonorchiasis include inflammation, epithelial desquamation, epithelial and adenomatous hyperplasia, goblet cell metaplasia, periductal fibrosis and granuloma formation (Fig. 11.4). In chronic inflammation, infiltration of lymphocytes, monocytes, eosinophils and plasma cells are common. Granulomatous inflammation around the parasite eggs is occasionally observed along the bile ducts of the infected human but is more commonly seen in animal models (Sripa, 2003). Epithelial hyperplasia occurs at early stage through late stage of infection. Adenomatous hyperplasia, and goblet cell metaplasia can be seen in chronic human opisthorchiasis or clonorchiasis but uncommonly in hamsters (Harinasuta et al., 1984; Rim, 2005; Sripa, 2003). Periductal fibrosis is the most prominent histological feature of chronic liver fluke infection.

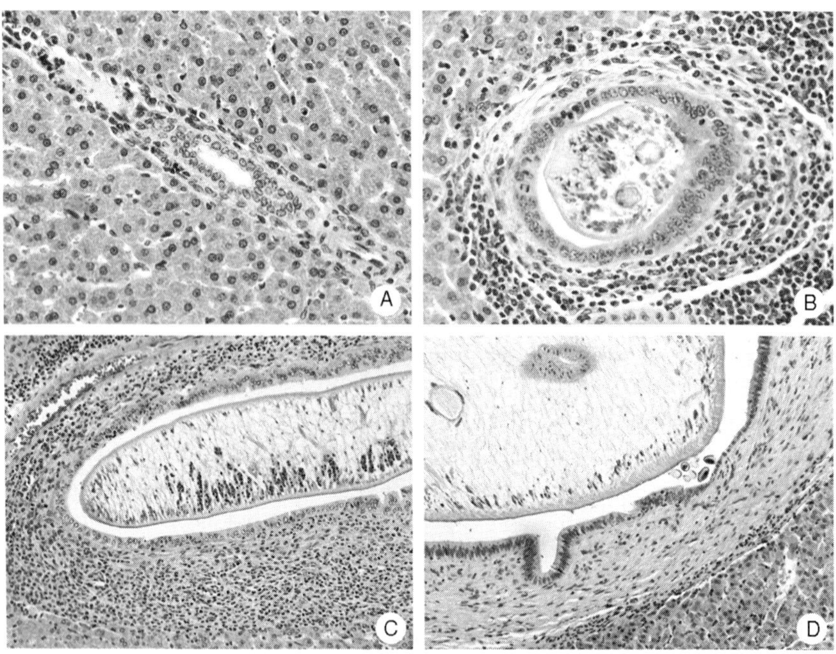

FIGURE 11.4 Histopathology of a normal hamster liver (A), a liver from a hamster 2 weeks after an infection with *O. viverrini* (B), 4 weeks post-infection (C) and 24 weeks post-infection (D). Severe inflammation around the bile ducts and biliary hyperplasia are gradually observed at week 2 to week 4 post-infection (B and C). Periductal fibrosis is a prominent feature of chronic opisthorchasis at week 24 post-infection (D). Haematoxylin-eosin staining (original magnification, 100×).

This corresponds to periportal echoes detected by ultrasonography as mentioned earlier. The pathology of fluke-associated cholecystitis consists of fibrosis, infiltration of mast cells and eosinophils and mucosal hyperplasia of the gallbladder wall (Rim, 2005; Sripa, 2003; Sripa et al., 2003). Gallstone is a rather common complication of liver fluke infection, present in up to 5% of people in *Opisthorchis*-endemic sites (Mairiang et al., 2006). Parasites eggs have been observed in the nidus of stones in the gallbladder and intrahepatic ducts (Fig. 11.5). It has been proposed that poor function of the gallbladder causes calcium/bilirubin precipitation on fluke eggshell, admixed with mucin and other bile constituents and leads to stone formation (Sripa et al., 2004). Perforation of the gallbladder wall is uncommon in liver fluke infection.

Pathogenesis of liver fluke-mediated tissue damage may be directly via mechanical or chemical irritation and/or is immune-mediated (Rim, 2005; Sripa, 2003). Mechanical injury caused by parasite's suckers during feeding activities and migration contributes to biliary ulceration. For the biliary hyperplasia, several *in vitro* experiments provided strong evidence that both liver flukes possess mitogenic factors in their excretory–secretory (ES) products. The metabolic products themselves,

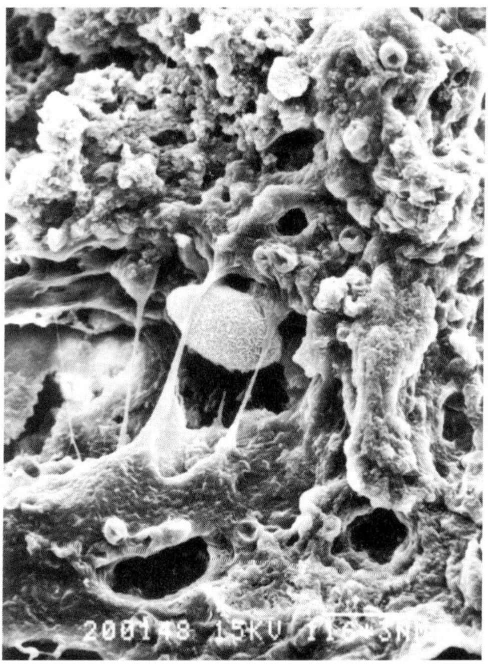

FIGURE 11.5 Scanning electron micrograph (SEM) of a gall stone showing an *Opisthorchis* egg with prominent mush melon eggshell surface at the center of the stone.

apart from inducing host immune responses, may be toxic or interact with the biliary epithelium (Sripa, 2003). Indeed, mouse fibroblasts (NIH-3T3) co-cultured with *O. viverrini* adult worms underwent more than four-fold greater proliferation than control (Thuwajit et al., 2004). Moreover, ES product(s) increased cell proliferation by stimulating the expression of phosphorylated retinoblastoma (pRB) and cyclin D1, the key proteins in driving cells through the G1/S transition point of the cell cycle. Similar experiment undertaken with *C. sinensis* ES products co-cultured with human embryonic kidney epithelial cell line HEK293 revealed that ES products alter the proportion of cells in each stage of the cell cycle and induce HEK293 cell proliferation (Kim et al., 2008). The results showed that ES products alter the proportion of cells in each stage of the cell cycle and induce HEK293 cell proliferation. Human biliary cell lines underwent excessive proliferation upon stimulation with *O. viverrini* soluble ES products from live worms (Sripa, 2003). These studies clearly indicate that metabolic products of *Opisthorchis/Clonorchis* contain mitogen-like activity that can induce cell proliferation. This is in agreement with earlier findings of hyperplasia of biliary epithelial cells in opisthorchiasis or clonorchiasis (Bhamarapravati et al., 1978; Rim, 2005; Sripa and Kaewkes, 2000).

Recently, using a proteomics approach, we identified in ES of *O. viverrini* a homologue of human granulin, a potent growth factor involved in cell proliferation and wound healing. *O. viverrini* granulin, termed *Ov*-GRN-1, was expressed in most parasite tissues, particularly the gut and tegument, and was present in biliary epithelial cells of experimentally infected hamsters. Recombinant *Ov*-GRN-1 stimulated proliferation of murine fibroblasts and induced morphological changes in affected cells. Anti-*Ov*-GRN-1 antibody inhibited *O. viverrini* ES induced proliferation of human CCA cell lines, indicating that *Ov*-GRN-1 is an important growth factor. These findings indicated that liver fluke granulin is involved with the establishment of a tumorigenic environment in the infected liver that may ultimately manifest as CCA (Smout et al., 2009).

For immune-mediated mechanisms, inflammation around the infected bile ducts and periportal areas are mainly in response to liver fluke antigens. Sripa and Kaewkes (2000) demonstrated that *O. viverrini* antigens can be detected in both the parasite and biliary epithelium. The presence of antigens in the biliary epithelium corresponds with severe inflammation even in the small bile ducts, which the fluke cannot inhabit. Severe inflammation can lead to more oxidative DNA damage and genetic alteration. Diffuse nitrative and oxidative DNA damage (8-nitroguanine and 8-oxodG) was reported in biliary epithelium of hamsters infected with *O. viverrini* (Pinlaor et al., 2003), and these DNA lesions still remained in the epithelium at least 180 days post-infection. Moreover, repeated infections with liver fluke result in enhanced biliary DNA damage (Pinlaor et al., 2004). This may be explained by the fact that repeated infection increased inducible nitric oxide synthase (iNOS) expression in the bile duct epithelium. The DNA damage in infected biliary cells is a result of the inflammatory response caused by *O. viverrini* because 8-nitroguanine and 8-oxodG disappeared after praziquantel treatment (Pinlaor et al., 2006). Studies with humans also showed oxidative DNA damage in *O. viverrini*-infected individuals (Thanan et al., 2008). Urinary 8-oxodG levels were significantly higher in *O. viverrini*-infected patients than in healthy subjects. Moreover, urinary 8-oxod G levels in *O. viverrini*-infected patients significantly decreased 2 months after praziquantel treatment. However, anthelminthic treatment with praziquantel may cause deleterious effects on biliary epithelium (Pinlaor et al., 2008). Praziquantel-induced dispersion of parasite antigens produced a marked recruitment of inflammatory cells in infected livers. NF-kappaB and iNOS mRNA expression is significantly elevated in the bile duct epithelium and inflammatory cells. This can cause more oxidative DNA damage of the biliary cells and therefore repeated infections and treatments may enhance cholangiocarcinogenesis (Pinlaor et al., 2008). Increased endogenous production of *N*-nitroso compounds and enhanced hepatic activation of carcinogens have been described (Satarug et al., 1996, 1998) and may establish highly mutagenic conditions for the chronically inflamed and proliferating bile duct epithelium. Together, these pathological conditions form an ideal environment for cancer development in the infected bile ducts (Sripa et al., 2007).

11.2.5. Diagnosis

Diagnosis of opisthorchiasis and clonorchiasis can be accomplished by several approaches. Demonstrations of eggs in faeces, bile or duodenal fluids are the gold standard diagnosis for *O. viverrini* or *C. sinensis* infection. Parasitological examination of faecal samples provides routine diagnosis and is widely used. However, sensitivity and accuracy depend on methods of faecal examination and the expertise of the microscopist. The most frequently used methods to detect eggs in the faeces are the Kato-Katz thick smear, Stoll's dilution and the quantitative formalin ethyl acetate concentration technique (Bergquist et al., 2009; Elkins et al., 1990; Hong et al., 2003; Viyanant et al., 1983). Due to similar morphology of trematode eggs, particulary of the families Opisthorchiidae, Heterohyidae and Lecithodendriidae, microscopy has limitations for diagnosis of opisthorchiasis and clonorchiasis in areas where these trematodes and minute intestinal flukes are co-endemic, including Lao PDR and northern Thailand (Chai et al., 2005; Kaewkes et al., 1991; Radomyos et al., 1994). Immunodiagnostic tests have been developed for *Opisthorchis* and *Clonorchis* infections. Whereas most antigens of these flukes are non-specific and antibodies persist long after treatment, good results have been gained from new serological tests using individual antigens and those detecting isotype-specific antibodies (Wongratanacheewin et al., 2003). Faecal antigen detection by enzyme-linked immunosorbent assays (ELISAs) using monoclonal antibodies against secretory antigens and DNA probes also show promise (Chaicumpa et al., 1991; Sirisinha et al., 1995). However, recent attention has been focused on the detection of egg DNA in faecal specimens by PCR-based approaches, which is effective in the diagnosis of liver fluke infection in experimental animals as well as in humans (Duenngai et al., 2008; Le et al., 2006b; Lovis et al., 2009; Traub et al., 2009; Wongratanacheewin et al., 2001). Further details of trematode diagnosis can be found in other articles in this thematic volume of the *Advances in Parasitology* (Johansen et al., 2010; Lv et al., 2010).

11.2.6. Treatment

Treatment with praziquantel at a single 40 mg/kg oral dose is effective against opisthorchiasis and clonorchiasis. This regimen has been widely used in large-scale control programmes (Jongsuksuntigul and Imsomboon, 2003). Rim (2005) recommended that the most effective regimen, particularly for clonorchiasis, is 25 mg/kg three times over a day (total dose: 75 mg/kg). Adverse events, such as dizziness, vomiting and abdominal pain, occur frequently but are transient and rarely severe. Details of treatment regimens and pharmacodynamics are described elsewhere in volume 73 of the *Advancces in Parasitology* (Keiser and Utzinger, 2010).

11.2.7. Prevention and control

Prevention and control of human liver fluke infection can be facilitated by treatment of human and animal reservoirs (to reduce the excretion of eggs), improved sanitation (to prevent eggs from reaching water sources) and health promotion including information, education and communication (IEC) (to discourage consumption of raw fish and to improve sanitary practices) (Jongsuksuntigul and Imsomboon, 2003; Rim, 2005). Control of snail intermediate hosts by molluscicides is not considered feasible because of widespread distribution of snails, low prevalence of fluke infection of snails even in endemic communities and economic considerations. To be most effective, IEC strategies should be designed and delivered in a culturally sensitive manner with the aim of stimulating behavioural change as well as simply providing information and therefore raising awareness. Targeting young people, for example, school-aged children, may be attractive for long-term control. Large-scale efforts in endemic areas by public health agencies have probably had a major impact on reducing the intensity of infections, although the efficacy and cost-effectiveness remains to be determined. Multisectoral participation among local government, private organizations including non-governmental organizations (NGOs) and the residents of the endemic areas can facilitate sustainable parasite disease control.

11.3. FASCIOLIASIS

There are an estimated 2.4–17 million people worldwide, including Asia, infected with one or both species of the liver fluke *Fasciola*, namely *F. hepatica* and *F. gigantica*, often causing serious acute and chronic morbidity (Mas-Coma et al., 2005, 2009a). The estimated at-risk population is 80 million (Keiser and Utzinger, 2005). In the past, *Fasciola* infections were limited to specific and typical geographical areas, but more recently, this liver fluke has spread throughout the world, especially where sheep and cattle are farmed intensively. Human cases are increasingly reported from Europe, the Americas and Oceania (where only *F. hepatica* is transmitted), and from Africa and Asia (where the two species overlap) (Mas-Coma et al., 2009a). These parasites commonly infect domestic ruminants, particularly sheep, goats and cattle. Humans usually become infected by eating aquatic plants grown in water that is contaminated with faeces from animals harbouring *Fasciola*. With regard to Southeast Asia, particularly in Vietnam, *Fasciola* infections are on the rise (Mas-Coma et al., 2009a; Tran et al., 2001).

11.3.1. Life cycle and transmission

Fascioliasis is a zoonosis, a disease transmissable from animals to humans. Susceptible animal reservoir hosts for *Fasciola* include sheep, pigs, buffaloes, donkeys, horses, goats, dromedaries, camels, rabbits and rodents. Parasite eggs (immature) are passed in the faeces of infected animals or humans and contaminate water. The eggs become embryonated in water, the miracidia release from the eggs and invade a suitable snail intermediate host, including the genera *Galba*, *Fossaria* and *Pseudosuccinea*. In the snail the parasites undergo several developmental stages (sporocysts, rediae and cercariae). The cercariae are released from the snail and encyst as metacercariae on aquatic vegetation or other surfaces. Mammals acquire the infection by eating vegetation containing metacercariae. Humans can become infected by ingesting metacercariae-containing freshwater plants. Evidence also indicates that infection may occur by drinking water contaminated with floating metacercariae and by ingesting metacercariae attached to the surface of food or kitchen utensils washed with water contaminated with floated metacercariae (Mas-Coma et al., 2009a). After ingestion, the metacercariae excyst in the duodenum and migrate through the intestinal wall, the peritoneal cavity, and the liver parenchyma into the biliary ducts, where they develop into adults. In humans, maturation from metacercariae into adult flukes takes approximately 3–4 months. The adult flukes (*F. hepatica*: up to 30 mm by 13 mm; *F. gigantica*: up to 75 mm) reside in the large biliary ducts of the mammalian host.

11.3.2. Epidemiology

Human fascioliasis is at present emerging or re-emerging in many countries, including increases of prevalence and intensity and geographical expansion (Mas-Coma et al., 2009a). Levels of infection depend on the frequency of humans eating plants (mainly watercress in Europe, morning glory in Asia) from water bodies contaminated with animal faeces. Outbreaks of *Fasciola* occur in households and communities, and are often traced to consumption of wild, rather than cultivated, water plants. Infection might also occur from contaminated drinking water or cooking utensils. In most endemic areas, human infection is infrequent, even where prevalence among domestic animals is high. For example, in Southeast Asia, high prevalence of *F. gigantica* has been reported in cattle and buffaloes in areas with large water reservoirs in Thailand (Srihakim and Pholpark, 1991) and Cambodia (Suon et al., 2006). However, whereas sporadic human fascioliasis is documented in the countries (Kachintorn et al., 1988), Mas-Coma and coworkers consider that fascioliasis is an emerging problem in many regions including in higher elevations in Bolivia and other countries in South and Central America (Mas-Coma et al., 2009a).

There is no definite report on the burden of disease of human fascioliasis in Southeast Asia or indeed Asia at large. However, the strikingly increased number of human fascioliasis in Vietnam during the past decade (500 cases from 1998 to 2000) calls for enhanced surveillance (Tran et al., 2001). Fascioliasis occured throughout Vietnam, in both rural and peri-urban areas, particularly in central Vietnam. It has been estimated in 2008 that in previous years, 5000 cases had to be treated annually in 172 districts of 36 endemic provinces (WHO, 2008). The re-emergence of human fascioliasis in Vietnam may be due to climate changes (Mas-Coma et al., 2009b) and/or the genetic changes of *Fasciola* itself. Hybrid and/or introgressed populations of liver flukes bearing genetic material from both *F. hepatica* and *F. gigantica* have been reported in Vietnam from infected cattle and human patients (Le et al., 2008).

11.3.3. Pathology and pathogenesis

The parasites cause considerable mortality in sheep and cattle, and human morbidity, which is dependent on the number of worms and stage of infection. The acute phase occurs during migration of the immature flukes through the liver. Severe pathology results from ingestion of liver tissues by the flukes and destruction of parenchymal tissue, haemorrhage, parasite death and inflammatory responses largely mediated by eosinophils. Repair mechanisms can lead to extensive periportal fibrosis. Radiologic imaging in the acute phase may present with multiple, small, clustered, necrotic cavities or abscesses in the peripheral parts of the liver, showing 'tunnels and caves' sign, reflecting parasite migration in the liver parenchyma (Lim et al., 2008).

The chronic phase, during which parasites are present in the bile ducts, tends to be less severe. Tissue change, including bile duct proliferation, dilatation and fibrosis, is largely caused by mechanical obstruction of the ducts, inflammatory responses and the activity of proline, which the fluke excretes in large quantities. In this phase, the flukes are demonstrated in the intra- and extrahepatic bile ducts and the gallbladder as small intraluminal flat objects, sometimes moving spontaneously. Bile ducts are dilated (Lim et al., 2008; Yesildag et al., 2009). Anaemia may result from blood loss through bile duct lesions. Death can result, especially in sheep and young cattle, as the consequence of haemorrhage into the bile duct (Chen and Mott, 1990).

11.3.4. Clinical features

Fascioliasis can be symptomatic or asymptomatic (Mas-Coma et al., 2005). Symptomatic cases begin approximately 2 months following ingestion of metacercariae. During the acute phase (caused by the migration of the immature fluke through the hepatic parenchyma), manifestations include abdominal pain, hepatomegaly, fever, vomiting, diarrhoea, urticaria and eosinophilia and can last for months. In the chronic phase (caused by the adult fluke within the bile ducts), the symptoms are more discrete and reflect intermittent biliary obstruction and inflammation. Occasionally, flukes have been seen in ectopic locations of infection, including the intestinal wall, lungs, subcutaneous tissue and pharyngeal mucosa (Sithithaworn et al., 2009). Aberrant migration by immature *Fasciola* through the skin in human fascioliasis has been reported in Vietnam (Le et al., 2007; Xuan le et al., 2005).

11.3.5. Diagnosis

Diagnosis of fascioliasis during the adult (chronic) phase can be made by observation of eggs during faecal examination. Eggs can be recovered in the stools or in material obtained by duodenal or biliary drainage. They are morphologically indistinguishable from those of *Fasciolopsis buski*. Differentiation between eggs from *F. hepatica* and *F. gigantica* is also difficult (Valero et al., 2009). False fascioliasis (pseudofascioliasis) refers to the presence of eggs in the stool resulting not from an actual infection but from recent ingestion of infected livers containing eggs. This situation (with its potential for misdiagnosis) can be avoided by having the patient follow a liver-free diet several days before a repeat stool examination (Beaver et al., 1984). Dietary history is helpful for differential diagnosis (Sithithaworn et al., 2009).

Antibody detection tests are useful especially in the early invasive stages, when the eggs are not yet apparent in the stools, or in ectopic fascioliasis as well as for confirmation of chronic fascioliasis when egg production is low or sporadic and for ruling out 'pseudofascioliasis'. Specific antibodies to *Fasciola* may be detectable within 2–4 weeks after infection, which is 5–7 weeks before eggs appear in stool. Current tests for immunodiagnosis of human *Fasciola* infection include ELISAs with ES antigens or purified/recombinant proteins in serum (Dixit et al., 2008; Espinoza et al., 2005; O'Neill et al., 1999). Detection of *Fasciola* antigens in *F. gigantica*-infected mouse serum (Anuracpreeda et al., 2009), and coproantigens in faeces from infected cattle (Estuningsih et al., 2009) and humans (Ubeira et al., 2009) has been reported. The latter using MM3-COPRO method with a new preservative/diluent, CoproGuard, for preservation of *Fasciola* coproantigens is promising with 100% sensitivity and 100% specificity. The use of CoproGuard enhanced coproantigen extraction without affecting the detection limit of the assay even in faecal samples stored at 37 °C up to 120 days (Ubeira et al., 2009).

Diagnosis of fascioliasis can also be done clinically including radiological methods and laparotomy.

11.3.6. Treatment

Unlike infections with other flukes, *F. hepatica* infections do not respond to praziquantel. The drug of choice is triclabendazole with bithionol as an alternative. Triclabendazole at a dose of 10 or 20 mg/kg has been shown to be effective against *Fasciola* infection and without serious adverse events (Keiser et al., 2005). Further details of treatment against fascioliasis are provided elsewhere (Keiser and Utzinger, 2010).

11.3.7. Prevention and control

Ultimate control of *Fasciola* must focus on strategic treatment or immunization of livestock and other herbivorous animals that maintain the life cycle (Dorny et al., 2009; Mas-Coma et al., 2005). Advances in the development of veterinary vaccines are very encouraging; however, it will be several years until a vaccine will be commercially available. Control of the snail intermediate hosts (pulmonate gastropods of the family Lymnaeidae, e.g. species of *Galba*, *Lymnaea* and *Pseudosuccinea*) using molluscicides is not considered practical in most situations. Health education to discourage human consumption of raw wild watercress and other edible water plants may be effective in areas where the disease is prevalent. Increased awareness by clinicians of the problem and its diagnostic difficulties, along with community-based studies assessing seroprevalence, will help quantify the extent to which fascioliasis affects human health (Mas-Coma et al., 2009a).

11.4. PARAGONIMIASIS

Paragonimus spp., the lung flukes, represent one of the most injurious of the food-borne helminths. These flukes cause paragonimiasis in people and other crab-eating mammals in Asia, parts of West Africa, and South and Central America. About 20 million people are infected with lung flukes (WHO, 1995) and an estimated 293 million people are at-risk (Keiser and Utzinger, 2005). There are about 15 species of *Paragonimus* known to infect humans. *P. westermani* infection is the most common elsewhere, while *P. heterotremus* is the aetiologic agent of human paragonimiasis in P.R. China, Lao PDR, Vietnam and Thailand (Blair et al., 1999; Le et al., 2006a; Liu et al., 2008; Maleewong, 2003; Yahiro et al., 2008). Species of *Paragonimus* are reported to infect humans in other places, including *P. africanus* (e.g. Nkouawa et al., 2009) and *P. kellicotti* in North America (Procop, 2009), and their distributions are listed in Table 11.3. *P. miyazakii* may be synonymous with *P. skrjabini* (Chen et al., 2004).

11.4.1. Life cycle and transmission

The life cycle of the lung fluke and its mode of transmission are partially shown in Fig. 11.6 and a photomicrograph of *P. heterotremus* adult worm is depicted in Fig. 11.7. Adult worms, which like all species that cause food-borne trematodiases are hermaphrodites, are about 1 cm in diameter, are fleshy flatworms and have an appearance that is similar to a coffee bean in shape and indeed colour. Pairs of adult worms are not uncommon in the same lesion with the human lung.

11.4.2. Epidemiology

Human paragonimiasis occurs in three endemic focal areas: Asia (P.R. China, Japan, Korea, Lao PDR, Philippines, Vietnam, Taiwan and Thailand), South and Central America (Ecuador, Peru, Costa Rica and Columbia) and Africa (Cameroon, Gambia and Nigeria) (Maleewong,

TABLE 11.3 Species of *Paragonimus* reported in infected human in Asia

	Paragonimus species	Geographical distribution
1.	*P. westermani* Kerbert, 1878	India, Ceylon, Thailand, P.R. China, Taiwan, Japan, etc.
2.	*P. ringeri* Cobbold, 1880[a]	Taiwan
3.	*P. pulmonis* Nakahama, 1883[a]	Japan
4.	*P. pulmonalis* Baelz, 1880[a]	Japan, Korea, Taiwan
5.	*P. skrjabini* Chen, 1959	P.R. China
6.	*P. miyazakii* Kamo, Nishida, Hatsushika, and Tomimura, 1961	Japan
7.	*P. heterotremus* Chen and Hsia, 1964	P.R. China, Thailand, Lao PDR, Vietnam
8.	*P. tuanshanensis* Chung, Ho, Cheng, Tsao, 1964[b]	P.R. China
9.	*P. philippinensis* Ito, Yokogawa, Araki and Kobayashi, 1978[a]	The Philippines
10.	*P. heitungensis* Chung, Hsu, Ho, Kao, Lan and Chiu, 1977	P.R. China

[a] Appears to be identical with *P. westermani*.
[b] Appears to be identical with *P. heterotremus*.

2003). Endemic areas can be identified as the people eat raw, pickled and/ or semi-cooked fresh-water species of crabs, crayfishes and shrimps.

Kung Plah, Kung Ten (raw crayfish salad) and *Nam Prik Poo* (crab sauce) are popular and widely consumed dishes in Thailand. Human paragonimiasis has been reported in at least 10 provinces, and there is evidence that *P. heterotremus* is the major aetiologic agent of human paragonimiasis (Anantaphruti, 2001; Vajarasthira, 1985). The prevalence and intensity among infected inhabitants are slightly lower among males than females (Upatham et al., 1995). The prevalence for both sexes is highest in the 25–29 year-old-age group.

Kinagang, which is semi-cooked freshwater mountainous crabs, are eaten as an appreciated dish in the Philippines. Human diseases are caused by two species, *P. westermani* and *P. philippinensis* (Belizario et al., 1997).

In Vietnam, where people have the habit of eating undercooked crabs, the infection rate of human *Paragonimus* ranged from 6.4% to 7.4% (De et al., 2000). Recently, epidemiological examinations reported that the disease is endemic in northwestern areas, Laichau and neighbouring provinces (Doanh et al., 2007). *P. heterotremus* is the (usual) known aetiological agent of human paragonimiasis in Vietnam (Le et al., 2006a).

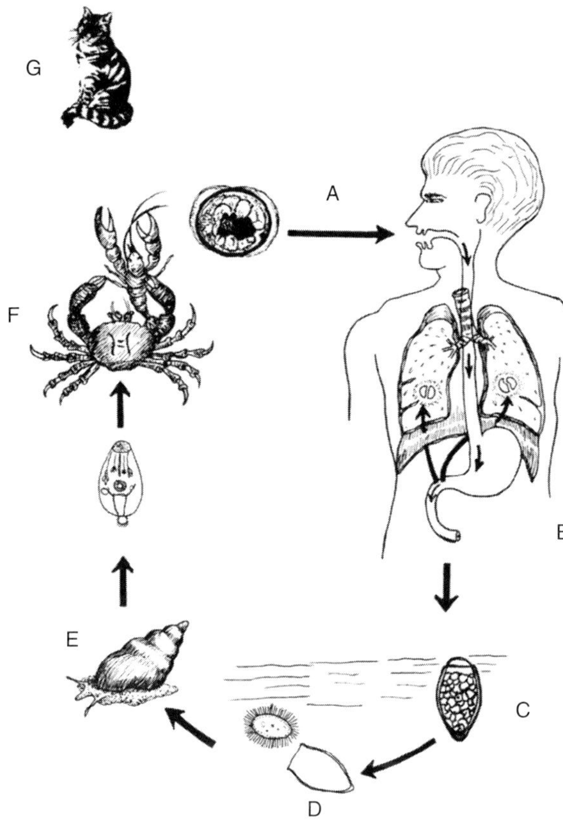

FIGURE 11.6 Life cycle of *Paragonimus* spp. When the metacecariae in infected crustacean hosts are eaten raw or undercooked by the final host, man and mammals especially Felidae and Canidae, (A) the metacercariae excyst in the small intestine and penetrate through the intestinal wall into the abdominal cavity, prior to migration through the sub-peritoneal tissues, the muscle, the liver, the diaphragm, and finally enters the lung where maturation occurs (B). Adult flukes lay eggs, which are coughed up and ejected by spitting with the sputum or swallowed and passed in the faeces (C). In the water, the immature eggs develop into miracidia (D), freely swim and then invade the fresh water snails (E). In the crustacea, such as fresh water crabs (F), crayfish, and shrimp probably acquire the infection by consuming free-living cercariae or eating infected snails containing the fully developed microcercus cercariae. The cercariae then develop into metacercariae, the infective stage. Reservoir hosts including cat, tiger, dog and rodents (G) can be infected by eating the metacercariae.

In Lao PDR, human paragonimiasis was reported from Namback district of Luangprabang province by means of skin tests, sputum studies and identification of *Paragonimus* metacercariae (Song et al., 2008). The people have numerous experiences of eating roast crabs from the field

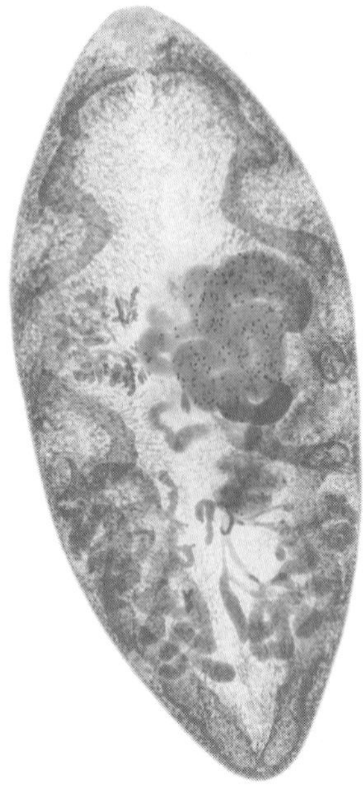

FIGURE 11.7 Morphology of *P. heterotremus* adult worm.

and seasonal crabs (*Tan Cheoy Kouang*) as well as papaya salad (*Tammack Koung*) with crushed raw crabs. Drinking of fresh crab juice as the traditional cure for measles is a known route of infection (Song et al., 2008). This disease is a common cause of persistent pleural effusion in Lao PDR (Vidamaly et al., 2009).

From Myanmar, there was a recent case report of a worker with history of haemoptysis and presence of *P. westermani* eggs in bronchial washings. The patient was born in Myanmar and lived in Malaysia for 2 years before migrating to Australia. The haemoptysis began before the person emigrated from Myanmar (Ibrahim et al., 2008).

11.4.3. Pathology, pathogenesis and clinical manifestations

Pathogenesis ensues because of the migration of the lung form from the gut to the lungs and indeed through not infrequent ectopic migrations to aberrant sites including the brain and subcutaneous sites at the extremities, and toxin and other mediators released by the migratory parasites (Lv et al., 2010). The presence of the flukes in the lung causes haemorrhage, inflammatory reaction with leukocytic infiltration and necrosis of lung parenchyma that gradually proceeds to the development of fibrotic encapsulation except for an opening from the evolving lesion to the respiratory tract to allow the fluke eggs to exit to the outside environment.

There are signs and symptoms that allow characterization of acute and chronic stages of paragonimiasis. In pulmonary paragonimiasis, for example, the most noticeable clinical symptom of an infected individual is a chronic cough with gelatinous, rusty brown, pneumonia-like, blood-streaked sputum. Hemoptysis is commonly induced by heavy work. Pneumothorax, empyema from secondary bacterial infection and pleural effusion might also be presented. When symptoms include only a chronic cough, the disease may be misinterpreted as chronic bronchitis and bronchiectasis or bronchial asthma. Pulmonary paragonimiasis is frequently confused with pulmonary tuberculosis (Liu et al., 2008).

In extrapulmonary paragonimiasis, the symptoms of extrapulmonary lesions vary depending on the location of the fluke, including cerebral paragonimiasis (Lv et al., 2010) and abdominal paragonimiasis.

11.4.4. Diagnosis and treatment

Diagnosis of human paragonimiasis is based on clinical features, as well as on laboratory tests. Definitive diagnosis is established by presentation of *Paragonimus* eggs in the sputa and/or faeces by microscopic examination. Supporting methods include chest X-ray (Fig. 11.8) and immunological tests. Reliable serological tests have been applied for

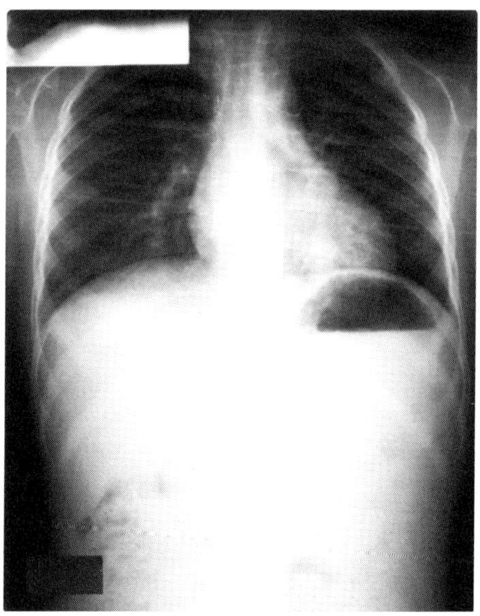

FIGURE 11.8 Chest X-ray, postero-anterior view, of a paragonimiasis patient showing abnormal multiple conglomerated thin wall cystic lesions at left lower lung, retrocardiac region. (Courtesy of Dr. Jaturat Kanpittaya, M.D.).

immunodiagnosis of human paragonimiasis; these include ELISA and immunoblotting-based methods (Maleewong, 2003). Immunoblotting for the detection of IgG4 antibody to ES products of adult *P. heterotremus* provides a sensitive and specific test (Wongkham et al., 2005). Recently, a recombinant protein of a *P. westermani* egg antigen was tested as an ELISA antigen (Lee et al., 2007). This assay offered a highly sensitive and specific assay for serodiagnosis. A PCR for detection of DNA from *Paragonimus* eggs in faeces or sputa has potential in clinical epidemiological studies (Intapan et al., 2005).

The anthelminthic drugs praziquantel and triclabendazole are both recommended by WHO for the treatment of *Paragonimus* infection (Keiser et al., 2005; Liu et al., 2008). Praziquantel given in doses of 25 mg/kg of body weight for 1–3 days produces a cure rate of 70–100% (Maleewong, 2003; Vajarasthira, 1985). Triclabendazole at a dose of 10 mg/kg daily for 3 days results in cure rates of up to 98.5% (Calvopiña et al., 1998; Keiser and Utzinger, 2010).

11.4.5. Prevention and control

The most effective strategy for the control and eventual elimination of paragonimiasis requires the interruption of the parasite-life cycle. Elimination of an intermediate host, such as snails, is difficult to achieve, since they are widespread and a part of the environment. Molluscicides probably also kill fish, a dietary protein source. Environmental sanitation can be carried out successfully by providing latrines and health education in the endemic areas. Changing the habits of no longer consuming raw or semicooked crabs and crayfishes can prevent infections with metacercariae. Cobalt-60 irradiation of crustaceans at a dose of 2.5 kGray can remedy the infectivity of *Paragonimus* metacercariae (Song et al., 1992). Effective treatment is one of the important measures of control. Finally, intersectoral collaboration between the ministries of public health, agriculture, aquaculture, education, and finances could play an effective role in any exertion to control infections (WHO, 1995).

11.5. INTESTINAL FLUKES

The intestinal fluke category comprises a large assemblage of trematode species that induce food-borne parasitic zoonoses. Collectively, these parasites have a major impact on the health and economy in developing countries of the tropics and sub-tropics in Asia, Africa, Europe and the Americas.

11.5.1. Fasciolopsiasis

Fasciolopsiasis is caused by the infection of a giant intestinal fluke, *Fasciolopsis buski* (Beaver et al., 1984). It is classified in the same family (Fasciolidae) as the liver fluke genus *Fasciola* and shares a similar developmental cycle and morphology (Fig. 11.9). However, *Fasciolopsis buski* infection is largely confined to Asian countries, namely southern P.R. China, India, Bangladesh, Thailand, Malaysia, Borneo, Sumatra and Myanmar, and may reach high prevalences within endemic areas. The parasite attaches to the intestinal wall of man and pig. Light infections are asymptomatic or less pathogenic than those of *Fasciola* and more easily diagnosed and treated. Heavy infections can cause severe disease.

11.5.1.1. Life cycle and transmission

The life cycle was first described in pigs by Nakagawa in 1921 and in humans by Barlow in 1925 (Beaver et al., 1984). In contrast to *Echinostoma* spp., the final host range of *Fasciolopsis buski* is limited and many mammals are refractory (Beaver et al., 1984; Rim, 1982b). Humans and pigs

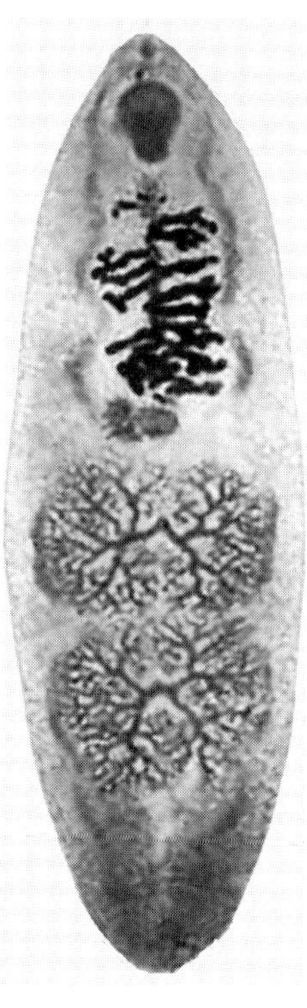

FIGURE 11.9 Morphology of *Fasciolopsis buski* adult worm.

become infected through the consumption of viable metacercariae attached on the seed pods, bulbs, stems or roots of water plants. These include the water caltrops, water hyacinth, water chestnut, water bamboo, lotus, etc. Although metacercariae are not present on the edible seed of these plants, ingestion frequently occurs during removal of pods with the teeth and lips.

Fasciolopsis buski metacercariae excyst in the duodenum and the juvenile worms attach to the duodenal and jejunal wall. The larvae develop to mature adults within 3 months and produce large numbers of eggs (an estimated 10,000–25,000 eggs per worm/day). Eggs are large, yellowish in colour and operculate. If the eggs reach freshwater sources, further development and embryonation occur over 3–7 weeks, then miracidia hatch and penetrate snail intermediate hosts in the family Planorbidae, especially in the genus *Segmentina*, *Hippeutis* and *Gyraulus*. After transformation and asexual multiplication as sporocysts, rediae and cercariae, free-swimming cercariae released from the snails attach and encyst on seed pods or any freshwater plant surface.

11.5.1.2. Epidemiology

Infections in definitive hosts are associated with the consumption of freshwater vegetables. Vegetables cultivated in endemic foci are usually confined to low-lying land where susceptible species of snail hosts abound. In Thailand, infections are endemic in the central region(s), characterised by heavy rainfall and extensive flooding, which leads to faecal contamination of the water (Jaroonvesama et al., 1986; Rim, 1982b; Sadun and Maiphoom, 1953). Using of pig or human faeces for fertilization is associated with endemicity (Weng et al., 1989). The highest prevalence occurs in areas with cultivation or year-round availability of water caltrops and other aquatic vegetation and where people enjoy eating the water chestnuts. Community-based prevalences generally reach 20%, with a typical peak in children aged 10–15 years and little difference between sexes (Graczyk et al., 2001; Handoyo et al., 1987; Manning et al., 1969; Sadun and Maiphoom, 1953). Children are often more frequently and heavily infected than adults since they enjoy gathering and eating water plants during play (Bunnag et al., 1983; Handoyo et al., 1986, 1987; Keiser and Utzinger, 2009).

11.5.1.3. Pathology and pathogenesis

The attachment of parasites on the duodenal or jejunal wall can cause low grading eosinophilia (<35%), where mechanical injury and inflammation lead to ulcer formation (Beaver et al., 1984; Gutierrez, 2000; Rim, 1982b). These ulcers sometimes bleed due to capillary damage and then may lead to petechial bleeding and the formation of intestinal abscesses. In mild infection, it may be associated with lower haematocrit and serum levels of vitamin B_{12}, but no apparent change in other nutrients (Jaroonvesama et al., 1986). This may result from the competitive utilisation of vitamin B_{12} or its impaired absorption from the damaged intestinal mucosa.

Although a low burden of parasites causes little damage, the presence of many (hundreds) flukes is associated with severe pathology and sometimes acute intestinal obstruction in children. Extensive intestinal ulceration may interfere with digestion, and cause malabsorption, leading to severe malnutrition and wasting. Oedema also occurs in long-standing severe cases; it may result from toxic parasite metabolites, allergic reactions or from hypoalbuminaemia secondary to protein and electrolyte imbalance from chronic malabsorption.

11.5.1.4. Clinical manifestations

In general, symptoms are absent or mild, but may include chronic diarrhoea, mild abdominal colic, hunger pains, flatulence, poor appetite, vomiting, eosinophilia and fever (Beaver et al., 1984; Gutierrez, 2000; Rim, 1982b). The abdominal pain may be due to duodenal ulcer caused by mechanical damage. Long-standing severe cases present with ascites or oedema of the eyelid, face, abdomen and legs, anasarca, anaemia, anorexia, weakness and vomiting. Patients may pass stools containing large amounts of undigested material. Deaths have been reported in long-standing heavy infection with intestinal obstruction, as with a Thai girl found at autopsy to harbour 466 worms (Sadun and Maiphoom, 1953).

11.5.1.5. Diagnosis and treatment

Faecal examination is commonly used for laboratory diagnosis. Direct smears, Stoll's dilution, formalin ethyl acetate centrifugation, and Kato-Katz techniques have been used successfully. Differentiation of *Fasciolopsis*, *Fasciola* and echinostome eggs is difficult due to the similarity in both shape and size of the ova (Fig. 11.10), so that a dietary, clinical history and living history in endemic areas should also be considered. Praziquantel is now the drug of choice, with a high efficacy following an oral dose of 25 mg/kg (WHO, 2009). In heavily infected cases, there may be some danger of intestinal obstruction or acute toxicemia with treatment, such that conservative or supportive treatment is advised.

11.5.1.6. Prevention and control

Community-based praziquantel treatment has been used to control infections in Indonesia (Handoyo et al., 1986, 1987). However, migration and rapid reinfection after treatment (prevalence reached pre-treatment levels within 1 year) confounded efforts to control infection by chemotherapy alone.

The use of fermented or boiled, instead of fresh vegetables, for feeding pigs in endemic areas may reduce the chance of transmission since

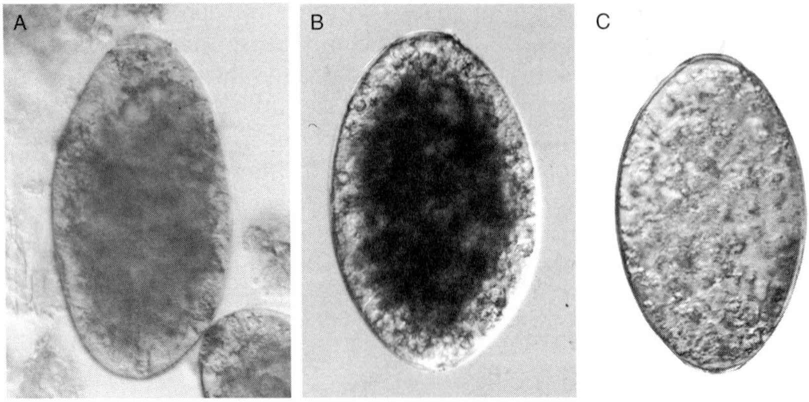

FIGURE 11.10 Egg morphology of *Fasciolopsis buski* (A), *Fasciola* spp. (B) and echinostome (C).

metacercariae are sensitive to both heat and salt. Drying the plants may also be effective. Sterilizing or prohibiting the use of human and pig faeces for fertilizer and improved sanitation would help interrupt the life cycle. Changing the habit of using the teeth to peel vegetables, then boiling for a few seconds, or careful washing after peeling them with hands or knife would reduce human infection. Filtering drinking water may prevent some infections by metacercariae that might be detached from water plants into water in the endemic areas. Health education should help people recognize the problem as well as indicate practical ways to avoid infection, since most infections are mild. Successful control efforts in one Chinese county reduced the prevalence from 76% in 1951 to 24% in 1976 (Weng et al., 1989).

11.5.2. Echinostomiasis

At least 17 species of echinostomes have been recorded in man, and the most common appear to be *E. ilocanum*, *E. revolutum*, *E. malayanum*, *E. echinatum* and *E. hortense* (Beaver et al., 1984; Carney, 1991; Chai and Lee, 2002; Huffman and Fried, 1990; Waikagul, 1991). Although they are considered of minor medical importance, infections with these parasites reach high prevalences in endemic areas. The literature on human infections is limited and has been reviewed (Graczyk and Fried, 1998; Huffman and Fried, 1990; Keiser and Utzinger, 2009; Rim, 1982a).

11.5.2.1. Life cycle and transmission

Echinostomes have a low host specificity with highly variable and wide host range. Humans are infected with echinostomes by the consumption of raw or incompletely cooked freshwater snails, clams, tadpoles and fish harbouring metacercariae. The parasites live in the intestine of the definitive or reservoir hosts, and eggs are excreted in faeces. Small freshwater snails are the first intermediate host. Free-swimming stage cercariae encyst within a second intermediate host, which may be another or the same species of mollusc that act as the first intermediate host, amphibian or fish larva. Aquatic birds, dogs and rats are the most important reservoir hosts of echinostomes.

11.5.2.2. Epidemiology

Most human infections occur in Asia in areas where raw or incompletely cooked molluscs and fish are eaten. Infection is common in Korea, Indonesia, the Philippines, Malaysia, Taiwan and Thailand (Beaver et al., 1984; Carney, 1991; Chai and Lee, 2002; Huffman and Fried, 1990; Keiser and Utzinger, 2009; Radomyos et al., 1982; Rim, 1982a; Tangtrongchitr and Monzon, 1991; Waikagul, 1991). Reported prevalences in endemic communities range from 1% to 50% (Graczyk and Fried, 1998; Phathihutthagon et al., 1984). Infections are most prevalent in poor rural areas and may be clustered in families who prefer raw foods (Bunnag et al., 1983; Graczyk and Fried, 1998; Keiser and Utzinger, 2009).

11.5.2.3. Diagnosis

The large, unembryonated, operculated eggs of echinostomes can be observed in faeces but are difficult to differentiate from those of *Fasciola* and *Fasciolopsis* (Fig. 11.10). Adult worms can be recovered from faeces following expulsion chemotherapy (Radomyos et al., 1982; Waikagul, 1991). This allows for possible differentiation based on morphology, of which the predominant morphology is the circumoral disc and collar spines around the oral sucker. It should be noted that the morphology may be altered by the drug and the durations of purged stool collection (Beaver et al., 1984; Rim, 1982a; Tangtrongchitr and Monzon, 1991; Waikagul, 1991).

11.5.2.4. Pathology, pathogenesis and clinical manifestations

The major pathological lesions of echinostomes are associated with parasite attachment deep between the villi of the jejunal wall. There may be inflammation and ulceration of the mucosa where the parasites locate. However, echinostomes are not highly pathogenic to humans and there are only a few reports of clinical aspects of this infection. While light-infection intensities are asymptomatic, heavy infections may cause diarrhoea, eosinophilia, abdominal discomfort and anorexia. These symptoms apparently do not develop into the life-threatening presentations that are described in some cases of *Fasciolopsis* infection (Gutierrez, 2000; Huffman and Fried, 1990; Rim, 1982a; Toledo et al., 2006).

11.5.2.5. Treatment

Treatment with praziquantel at 25 mg/kg is recommended, due to its broad efficacy, safety and ease of use (Huffman and Fried, 1990; Radomyos et al., 1982; Rim, 1982a).

11.5.2.6. Prevention and control

Prevention can be implemented by health education to discourage the consumption of raw or incompletely cooked molluscs and fish, as for other food-borne trematode infections. However, programmes to control echinostomiasis have had limited success compared to other helminthiases owing to several factors. Among these are the broad specificity for the second intermediate host and the existence of reservoir hosts (Gutierrez, 2000). Moreover, the first intermediate hosts are able to serve as the second intermediate hosts. The presence of low host specificity causes the difficulties to the successful control of the medically important echinostome parasites. This should be kept in mind when designing health promotion strategies.

11.5.3. Heterophyiasis

There are a large number of small or minute intestinal flukes, measuring less than 2.5 mm in length and just visible to the eye, which parasitise man, fish-eating birds and other mammals (Beaver et al., 1984; Waikagul, 1991). These include members of the families Heterophyidae, Lecithodendriidae, Plagiorchiidae, Diplostomidae, Gymnophallidae and Microphallidae. The examination of adults in purged stools after treatment with praziquantel or bithionol has shown that these parasites, previously considered 'rare', may be common and very numerous in people who live in areas where raw fish, aquatic vegetables and/or insect larvae are eaten (Chai et al., 1997, 2000, 2009; Chi et al., 2008; Radomyos et al., 1984, 1998; Sukontason et al., 2005; Velasquez, 1982). Species of *Heterophyes*, *Haplorchis*, *Metagonimus* and *Carneophallus* may cause disease in man (Beaver et al., 1984; Gutierrez, 2000; Velasquez, 1982). Because of the worldwide geographic distribution found only in flukes in the family Heterophyidae, these parasites are covered here under the term 'heterophyids'.

11.5.3.1. Life cycle and transmission

Heterophyes heterophyes, *Metagonimus yokogawai*, *Haplorchis taichui*, *Haplorchis pumilio* and *Stellantchasmus falcatus* are a few of the many heterophyids known to parasitise man (Beaver et al., 1984; Velasquez, 1982; Waikagul, 1991). The first two species are considered to be of most importance from the standpoint of human disease.

Adult heterophyids attach and live deeply embedded in the intestinal mucosa of mammals and birds where they produce embryonated eggs which are excreted in faeces. Due to the lack or non-use of sanitary latrines, eggs in faeces on the ground are washed into water reservoirs. Upon ingestion by a freshwater snail (species of *Melanoides, Semisulcospira* and others), the miracidia hatch out in the digestive tract, penetrate the wall and develop to sporocysts and undergo asexual reproduction to rediae and cercariae which escape back into the water. The free-swimming cercariae penetrate and encyst mainly in muscles of many species of fresh and brackish water fish or shrimps (Waikagul, 1991). Humans become infected while eating fish or shrimps harbouring viable metacercariae, which mature into adults within 5–10 days. An average of 10,000 metacercariae of *M. yokogawai* are found in the sweetfish (*Plecoglossus altivelis*) during the 'eating season' in Korea (Cho et al., 1984).

11.5.3.2. Epidemiology

Heterophyids are mainly found in Asian countries (Japan, Korea, Lao PDR, Vietnam, Thailand, Taiwan, Philippines and P.R. China), Hawaii, Siberia, Turkey and the Balkans (Beaver et al., 1984; Chai et al., 1997, 2000; Chi et al., 2008; Kaewkes, 1995; Radomyos et al., 1994; Sukontason et al., 2005). The use of expulsion chemotherapy to recover adult worms has revealed the large number and remarkable variety of flukes that can be harboured by a person. Food habits and access to rich aquatic fauna are the important factors influencing the rate of human infections.

M. yokogawai infects 1.2% of the Korean population, and is common (5–20% prevalence) in riverside communities where raw sweetfish is commonly eaten (Cho et al., 1984). One study found infection rates to be as high as 29.7%, with a striking difference between males (46.6%) and females (16.3%) (Chai et al., 2000). Over 100,000 adults were found in a person. Large numbers of another species, *Heterophyes nocens*, which utilises brackish water intermediate hosts, was found in 42% of residents from a Korean island and in 75% in some coastal areas (Chai et al., 1997). The prevalent rates may have increased due to the emerging nature of food-borne parasites (Dorny et al., 2009).

11.5.3.3. Pathology, pathogenesis and clinical manifestations

Most infections of heterophyids are asymptomatic or accompanied by mild intestinal discomfort, which may include mucous diarrhoea, colicky pains, intermittent neurasthenia (Beaver et al., 1984; Gutierrez, 2000; Toledo et al., 2006; Velasquez, 1982) induced by the attachment of the flukes and lethargy. These symptoms probably result from mild inflammation with mainly eosinophils, superficial necrosis, hypermucin secretion and bleeding at the site of attachment. Microscopic examination of *H. taichui* infection reveals mucosal ulceration, mucosal and submucosal haemorrhages, fusion and shortening villi, chronic inflammation, and fibrosis of the submucosa (Sukontason et al., 2005).

Symptoms are most frequent in heavy infections, but they subside spontaneously after approximately 1 month, although the flukes remain (Cho et al., 1984). Upon further infection, symptoms may recur, giving rise to occasional episodes of diarrhoea in endemic areas.

An infection with heterophyids may lead to death. Ante-mortem and the post-mortem diagnosis has demonstrated cardiac beriberi and cardiac dilatation. The eggs of heterophyid flukes were found in cardiac muscles of four autopsy cases and an adult in one case. Worms embed deeply in the intestinal wall, activating eosinophil and neutrophil infiltration. The eggs (and sometimes adult worms) may then enter nearby lymphatics or blood vessels and may be transported to other organs, such as the heart, spinal cord or brain, lungs, liver and spleen (Africa et al., 1935; Gutierrez, 2000; Toledo et al., 2006; Velasquez, 1982). Eggs become trapped and elicit granulomatous lesions and fibrosis. Signs of heterophyid myocarditis may include subepicardial oedema, epicardium haemorrhage, fragmentation of muscle fibres, cardiac enlargement, embolism of the capillaries, cough, dyspnea, cyanosis, fatigue, oedema and ascites, palpitation, loss of reflexes and abnormal heart sounds. Eggs or worms in the spinal cord or brain may cause neurological disease, transverse myelitis and loss of sensory and motor function.

11.5.3.4. Diagnosis

Diagnosis is usually based on the recovery of eggs in faeces, but there are many problems due to the similarity of shape and size (Kaewkes et al., 1991). The daily egg output is low (35–45) and light infections (<100 worms) are easily missed. Distinction between species of heterophyids and *Clonorchis* and *Opisthorchis* by egg morphology is difficult. However, several publications have helped establish criteria for differential diagnosis (Ditrich et al., 1992; Kaewkes, 2003; Kaewkes et al., 1991; Lee et al., 1984). Extraintestinal cases of heterophyiasis may be discovered at surgery or autopsy, and then only after careful searching. The recovery of adult worms from post-treatment stools allows a definitive diagnosis, but this procedure is tedious due to their minute size (Kaewkes, 1995; Kaewkes et al., 1991; Radomyos et al., 1984).

11.5.3.5. Treatment

A single dose of 25 mg/kg praziquantel is recommended, as it is highly efficacious (Chai et al., 2000; Velasquez, 1982; Waikagul et al., 2005).

11.5.3.6. Prevention and control

Treatment with praziquantel, combined with health education to encourage thorough cooking of fish and other aquatic animals in order to kill the metacercariae, is important. Further studies are required on the frequency and spectrum of clinical consequences in order to assess the amount of resources that should be provided for control. Although the ability of the parasites to cause fatal disease has been reported, the actual frequency of this has recently received very little attention.

11.6. CONCLUSIONS AND RESEARCH IMPLICATIONS

The food-borne trematodiases not only remain major NTDs in South East Asia and sub-Saharan Africa, throughout much of the developing world, they are emerging and re-emerging, including developed regions, such as *O. felineus* in Western Europe (Armignacco et al., 2008), *P. westermani* in Miyazaki prefecture, Japan (Nakano et al., 2009) and fascioliasis in the Bolivian Altiplano (Parkinson et al., 2007).

There is a need to undertake risk mapping using geographical information systems (GIS) and remote sensing for *O. viverrini*, *C. sinensis*, *F. hepatica*, *F. gigantica* and other important food-borne trematodes in East Asia, particularly in Thailand, Lao PDR, Cambodia and Vietnam to enable effective control measure to be established (Zhou et al., 2009). It is also apparent that more detailed research needs to be undertaken in Vietnam, in particular, on the immediate hosts, climatic factors, and the possibility of hybrid species for *O. viverrini* and *C. sinensis* (Traub et al., 2009).

Indeed, we certainly do not yet have a complete understanding on their pathogenesis, epidemiology including importance of reservoir hosts, molecular biology and immunology. Among obvious examples, how and why *O. viverrini* and *C. sinensis* cause CCA deserves much more attention and resources (Bouvard et al., 2009). Diagnosis often remains problematic, with the example of the difficulty in distinguishing *Opisthorchis*, *Clonorchis* and heterophyiid (minute intestinal fluke) eggs by morphology during stool examination. The development of other, probably molecular techniques to resolve these problems would be welcome and useful. Advances have been made, however, including field-based immunological tested based on recombinant antigens for diagnosis of *F. hepatica* infection (Kasný et al., 2009). It is hoped that advances in transcriptomics and proteomics will aid in development of more specific and sensitive diagnostics for these diseases (Laha et al., 2007; Morphew et al., 2007).

Research into basic biochemical and physiological processes in these flukes can also be expected to enhance our understanding of the host–parasite relationship and the evolution of the food-borne trematodes. Draft genome sequences have recently been reported for two of the major human schistosome species (reviewed in Han et al., 2009). Though less well studied, there is an increasing catalogue of molecular information for *F. hepatica*. Increased information for the other food-borne trematodes including *Opisthorchis* and *Paragonimus* species will deepen our understanding of the evolution and pathogenesis of these infections. Schistosomes employ serine proteases to accomplish infection of human skin. By contrast, *F. hepatica* utilises cysteine proteases (cathepsin L, cathepsin B) to cross the gut and to burrow through the exterior of the liver capsule (McGonigle et al., 2008). As more molecular information become available, it should become feasible to interpret the evolution of protease networks and pathways employed by the different food-borne trematodes during infection and migration, and indeed the role of these enzymes in definitive host species range (Robinson et al., 2008; Stack et al., 2008).

Not only will expanded knowledge on the genomes and proteomes of food-borne trematodes increase our understanding of their fundamental nature and evolution (Brindley et al., 2009), characterisation of the nature and action of secreted proteins of these parasites will provide insights into pathogenesis and disease process. For example, enhanced understanding of the proteins and antigens secreted by *O. viverrini* can be expected to provide insights into liver fluke-induced CCA, and indeed fundamental insights into carcinogenesis at large. In addition, a number of *O. viverrini* such as thioredoxin peroxidase (Suttiprapa et al., 2008), cathepsin F (Pinlaor et al., 2009) and aspartic protease (Suttiprapa et al., 2009) may have potential as intervention target including as vaccine candidates, given recent successes with chemotherapy targeting related enzymes in schistosomes (Abdulla et al., 2007) and with vaccines targeting cathepsin L of *Fasciola* (Kasný et al., 2009; McManus and Dalton, 2006). Indeed, in view of the recent implementation of an acclaimed vaccination of adolescents against papilloma-virus infection to provide protection from cervical cancer (Schiller et al., 2008), there is the tantalizing prospect that vaccination to prevent *O. viverrini* infection could provide protection against another infection-related cancer, liver fluke-induced CCA.

Finally, given that these infections are all food-borne—one has to put the uncooked fish, crab, watercress, etc. in the mouth—we need to enhance our communication to educate the at-risk populations about the dangers in their behaviours. Hence, new techniques need to be developed, including IEC media for populations at risk. Unfortunately, age-old culinary preferences for uncooked dishes such as *koi-pla*, a source of *O. viverrini* infection in Thailand and Lao PDR do not readily allow for this possibility. Moreover, fish farming of grass carp and other susceptible species in ponds that are routinely contaminated by untreated sewage has resulted in the establishment of infection in fish populations at large, which, along with the involvement of animal reservoir hosts, makes control of liver fluke infection even more challenging (Lun et al., 2005; Sripa et al., 2007).

ACKNOWLEDGEMENTS

We gratefully acknowledge support from award number UO1AI065871 from the National Institute of Allergy and Infectious Diseases (NIAID), the Thailand Research Fund (grant no. BRG4580016) and the Thailand-Tropical Diseases Research Programme (T-2, grant number ID 02-2-HEL-05-054). The content of this article is solely the responsibility of the authors and does not necessarily represent the official views of the NIAID or the National Institutes of Health (NIH).

REFERENCES

Abdulla, M.H., Lim, K.C., Sajid, M., McKerrow, J.H., Caffrey, C.R., 2007. Schistosomiasis mansoni: novel chemotherapy using a cysteine protease inhibitor. PLoS Med. 4, e14.

Africa, C., Leon, W.D.E., Garcia, E.Y., 1935. Intestinal heterophyidiasis with cardiac involvement: a contribution to etiology of heart failure. J. Philipp. Islands Med. Assoc. 15, 358–361.

Anantaphruti, M.T., 2001. Parasitic contaminants in food. Southeast Asian J. Trop. Med. Public Health 32, 218–228.

Andrews, R.H., Sithithaworn, P., Petney, T.N., 2008. *Opisthorchis viverrini*: an underestimated parasite in world health. Trends Parasitol. 24, 497–501.

Anuracpreeda, P., Wanichanon, C., Chawengkirtikul, R., Chaithirayanon, K., Sobhon, P., 2009. *Fasciola gigantica*: immunodiagnosis of fasciolosis by detection of circulating 28.5 kDa tegumental antigen. Exp. Parasitol. 123, 334–340.

Armignacco, O., Caterini, L., Marucci, G., Ferri, F., Bernardini, G., Natalini, R.G., et al., 2008. Human illnesses caused by *Opisthorchis felineus* flukes, Italy. Emerg. Infect. Dis. 14, 1902–1905.

Beaver, P.C., Jung, R.C., Cupp, E.W., 1984. Clinical Parasitology, 9th ed. Lea & Febiger, Philadelphia.

Belizario, V., Guan, M., Borja, L., Ortega, A., Leonardia, W., 1997. Pulmonary paragonimiasis and tuberculosis Sorsogon, Philippines. Southeast Asian J. Trop. Med. Public Health 28, 37–45.

Bergquist, R., Johansen, M.V., Utzinger, J., 2009. Diagnostic dilemmas in helminthology: what tools to use and when? Trends Parasitol. 25, 151–156.

Bhamarapravati, N., Thammavit, W., Vajrasthira, S., 1978. Liver changes in hamsters infected with a liver fluke of man, *Opisthorchis viverrini*. Am. J. Trop. Med. Hyg. 27, 787–794.

Blair, D., Xu, Z.B., Agatsuma, T., 1999. Paragonimiasis and the genus *Paragonimus*. Adv. Parasitol. 42, 113–222.

Bouvard, V., Baan, R., Straif, K., Grosse, Y., Secretan, B., Ghissassi, F., et al., 2009. WHO International Agency for Research on Cancer Monograph Working Group. A review of human carcinogens–part B: biological agents. Lancet Oncol. 10, 321–322.

Brindley, P.J., Mitreva, M., Ghedin, E., Lustigman, S., 2009. Helminth genomics: implications for human health. PLoS Negl. Trop. Dis. 3, e538.

Bunnag, D., Radomyos, P., Harinasuta, T., 1983. Field trial on the treatment of fasciolopsiasis with praziquantel. Southeast Asian J. Trop. Med. Public Health 14, 216–219.

Calvopiña, M., Guderian, R.H., Paredes, W., Chico, M., Cooper, P.J., 1998. Treatment of human pulmonary paragonimiasis with triclabendazole: clinical tolerance and drug efficacy. Trans. R. Soc. Trop. Med. Hyg. 92, 566–569.

Carney, W.P., 1991. Echinostomiasis: a snail-borne intestinal trematode zoonosis. Southeast Asian J. Trop. Med. Public Health 22, 206–211.

Chai, J.Y., Lee, S.H., 2002. Food-borne intestinal trematode infections in the Republic of Korea. Parasitol. Int. 51, 129–154.

Chai, J.Y., Kim, I.M., Seo, M., Guk, S.M., Kim, J.L., Sohn, W.M., et al., 1997. A new endemic focus of *Heterophyes nocens*, *Pygidiopsis summa*, and other intestinal flukes in a coastal area of Muan-gun, Chollanam-do. Korean J. Parasitol. 35, 233–238.

Chai, J.Y., Han, E.T., Park, Y.K., Guk, S.M., Kim, J.L., Lee, S.H., 2000. High endemicity of *Metagonimus yokogawai* infection among residents of Samchok-shi, Kangwon-do. Korean J. Parasitol. 38, 33–36.

Chai, J.Y., Darwin, M.K., Lymbery, A.J., 2005. Fish-borne parasitic zoonoses: status and issues. Int. J. Parasitol. 35, 1233–1254.

Chai, J.Y., Han, E.T., Shin, E.H., Sohn, W.M., Yong, T.S., Eom, K.S., et al., 2009. High prevalence of *Haplorchis taichui*, *Phaneropsolus molenkampi*, and other helminth infections among people in Khammouane province, Lao PDR. Korean J. Parasitol. 47, 243–247.

Chaicumpa, W., Ruangkunaporn, Y., Kalambaheti, T., Limavongpranee, S., Kitikoon, V., Khusmith, S., et al., 1991. Specific monoclonal antibodies to *Opisthorchis viverrini*. Int. J. Parasitol. 21, 969–974.

Chen, M.G., Mott, K.E., 1990. Progress in assessment of morbidity due to *Fasciola hepatica* infection: a review of recent literature. Trop. Dis. Bull. 87, R1–R38.

Chen, M.G., Chang, Z.S., Cui, A.L., Blair, D., Zhang, Y.N., Chen, S.H., et al., 2004. DNA sequences of *Paragonimus skrjabini* populations from five provinces in China. Chin. Med. J. 117, 219–224.

Chi, T.T., Dalsgaard, A., Turnbull, J.F., Tuan, P.A., Murrell, K.D., 2008. Prevalence of zoonotic trematodes in fish from a Vietnamese fish-farming community. J. Parasitol. 94, 423–428.

Cho, S.Y., Kang, S.Y., Lee, J.B., 1984. Metagonimiasis in Korea. Arzneimittelforschung 34, 1211–1213.

Choi, D., Hong, S.T., Lim, H., Cho, S.Y., Rim, H.J., Ji, Z., et al., 2004. Sonographic findings of active *Clonorchis sinensis* infection. J. Clin. Ultrasound 32, 17–23.

Choi, M.S., Choi, D., Choi, M.H., Ji, Z., Li, Z., Cho, S.Y., et al., 2005. Correlation between sonographic findings and infection intensity in clonorchiasis. Am. J. Trop. Med. Hyg. 73, 1139–1144.

Choi, D., Lim, J.H., Lee, K.T., Lee, J.K., Choi, S.H., Heo, J.S., et al., 2006. Cholangiocarcinoma and *Clonorchis sinensis* infection: a case-control study in Korea. J. Hepatol. 44, 1066–1073.

Choi, D., Lim, J.H., Lee, K.T., Lee, J.K., Choi, S.H., Heo, J.S., et al., 2008. Gallstones and *Clonorchis sinensis* infection: a hospital-based case-control study in Korea. J. Gastroenterol. Hepatol. 23, 399–404.

Dang, T.C., Yajima, A., Nguyen, V.K., Montresor, A., 2008. Prevalence, intensity and risk factors for clonorchiasis and possible use of questionnaires to detect individuals at risk in northern Vietnam. Trans. R. Soc. Trop. Med. Hyg. 102, 1263–1268.

De, N.V., Cong, L.D., Kino, H., Son, D.T., Vien, H.V., 2000. Epidemiology, symptoms and treatment of paragonimiasis in Sin Ho district, Lai Chau province, Vietnam. Southeast Asian J. Trop. Med. Public Health 31, 26–30.

De, N.V., Murrell, K.D., Cong le, D., Chau le, V., Cam, P.D., Chau, V., et al., 2003. The food-borne trematode zoonoses of Vietnam. Southeast Asian J. Trop. Med. Public Health 34, 12–34.

Ditrich, O., Giboda, M., Scholz, T., Beer, S.A., 1992. Comparative morphology of eggs of the Haplorchiinae (Trematoda: Heterophyidae) and some other medically important heterophyid and opisthorchid flukes. Folia Parasitol. 39, 123–132.

Dixit, A.K., Dixit, P., Sharma, R.L., 2008. Immunodiagnostic/protective role of cathepsin L cysteine proteinases secreted by *Fasciola* species. Vet. Parasitol. 154, 177–184.

Doanh, P.N., Shinohara, A., Horii, Y., Habe, S., Nawa, Y., The, D.T., et al., 2007. Morphological and molecular identification of two *Paragonimus* spp., of which metacercariae concurrently found in a land crab, *Potamiscus tannanti*, collected in Yenbai province, Vietnam. Parasitol. Res. 100, 1075–1082.

Dorny, P., Praet, N., Deckers, N., Gabriel, S., 2009. Emerging food-borne parasites. Vet. Parasitol. 163, 196–206.

Duenngai, K., Sithithaworn, P., Rudrappa, U.K., Iddya, K., Laha, T., Stensvold, C.R., et al., 2008. Improvement of PCR for detection of *Opisthorchis viverrini* DNA in human stool samples. J. Clin. Microbiol. 46, 366–368.

Elkins, D.B., Haswell-Elkins, M.R., Mairiang, E., Mairiang, P., Sithithaworn, P., Kaewkes, S., et al., 1990. A high frequency of hepatobiliary disease and suspected cholangiocarcinoma associated with heavy *Opisthorchis viverrini* infection in a small community in north-east Thailand. Trans. R. Soc. Trop. Med. Hyg. 84, 715–719.

Espinoza, J.R., Timoteo, O., Herrera-Velit, P., 2005. Fas2-ELISA in the detection of human infection by *Fasciola hepatica*. J. Helminthol. 79, 235–240.

Estuningsih, E., Spithill, T., Raadsma, H., Law, R., Adiwinata, G., Meeusen, E., et al., 2009. Development and application of a fecal antigen diagnostic sandwich ELISA for estimating prevalence of *Fasciola gigantica* in cattle in central Java, Indonesia. J. Parasitol. 95, 450–455.

Fang, Y.Y., Cheng, Y.D., Li, X.M., 2008. Current prevalence of *Clonorchis sinensis* infection in endemic areas of China. Chin. J. Parasitol. Parasit. Dis. 26, 81–86 (in Chinese).

Graczyk, T.K., Fried, B., 1998. Echinostomiasis: a common but forgotten food-borne disease. Am. J. Trop. Med. Hyg. 58, 501–504.

Graczyk, T.K., Fried, B., 2007. Human waterborne trematode and protozoan infections. Adv. Parasitol. 64, 111–160.

Graczyk, T.K., Gilman, R.H., Fried, B., 2001. Fasciolopsiasis: is it a controllable food-borne disease? Parasitol. Res. 87, 80–83.

Gutierrez, Y., 2000. Diagnostic Pathology of Parasitic Infections with Clinical Correlations, 2nd ed. Oxford University Press, New York.

Han, Z.G., Brindley, P.J., Wang, S., Chen, Z., 2009. Schistosome genomics: new perspectives on schistosome biology and host parasite interaction. Annu. Rev. Genomics Hum. Genet. 10, 211–240.

Handoyo, I., Ismuljowono, B., Darwis, F., Rudiansyah, 1986. Further survey of fasciolopsiasis in Babirik subdistrict, Hulu Sungei Utara Recency, South Kalimantan province. Trop. Biomed. 3, 119–123.

Handoyo, I., Ismuljowono, B., Darwis, F., Rudiansyah, X., 1987. Evaluation of post-treatment control of fasciolopsiasis in Sei Papuyu village of Babirik subdistrict, Hulu Sungai Utara Regency, South Kalimantan province, Indonesia. Trop. Biomed. 4, 125–127.

Harinasuta, T., Riganti, M., Bunnag, D., 1984. *Opisthorchis viverrini* infection: pathogenesis and clinical features. Arzneimittelforschung 34, 1167–1169.

Haswell-Elkins, M.R., Mairiang, E., Mairiang, P., Chaiyakum, J., Chamadol, N., Loapaiboon, V., et al., 1994. Cross-sectional study of *Opisthorchis viverrini* infection and cholangiocarcinoma in communities within a high-risk area in northeast Thailand. Int. J. Cancer 59, 505–509.

Hong, S.T., Choi, M.H., Kim, C.H., Chung, B.S., Ji, Z., 2003. The Kato-Katz method is reliable for diagnosis of *Clonorchis sinensis* infection. Diagn. Microbiol. Infect. Dis. 47, 345–347.

Honjo, S., Srivatanakul, P., Sriplung, H., Kikukawa, H., Hanai, S., Uchida, K., et al., 2005. Genetic and environmental determinants of risk for cholangiocarcinoma via *Opisthorchis viverrini* in a densely infested area in Nakhon Phanom, northeast Thailand. Int. J. Cancer 117, 854–860.

Hotez, P.J., Brindley, P.J., Bethony, J.M., Pearce, E.J., King, C.H., Jacobson, J., 2008. Helminth infections: the great neglected tropical diseases. J. Clin. Invest. 118, 1311–1321.

Huffman, J.E., Fried, B., 1990. *Echinostoma* and echinostomiasis. Adv. Parasitol. 29, 215–269.

IARC, 1994. Schistosomes, liver flukes and *Helicobacter pylori*. IARC Working Group on the Evaluation of Carcinogenic Risks to Humans. Lyon, 7–14 June 1994. IARC Monogr. Eval. Carcinog. Risks Hum. 61, 1–241.

Ibrahim, M.G., Bunter, R., Rajasooriar, S., Thien, F., 2008. Paragonimiasis: an unusual case of haemoptysis. Med. J. Aust. 188, 734–735.

Intapan, P.M., Wongkham, C., Imtawil, K.J., Pumidonming, W., Prasongdee, T.K., Miwa, M., et al., 2005. Detection of *Paragonimus heterotremus* eggs in experimentally infected cats by a polymerase chain reaction-based method. J. Parasitol. 91, 195–198.

Jaroonvesama, N., Charoenlarp, K., Areekul, S., 1986. Intestinal absorption studies in *Fasciolopsis buski* infection. Southeast Asian J. Trop. Med. Public Health 17, 582–586.

Johansen, M.V., Sithithaworn, P., Bergquist, R., Utzinger, J., 2010. Towards improved diagnosis of zoonotic trematode infections in Southeast Asia. Adv. Parasitol. 73, 171–195.

Jongsuksuntigul, P., Imsomboon, T., 2003. Opisthorchiasis control in Thailand. Acta Trop. 88, 229–232.

Kachintorn, U., Atisook, K., Tesjaroen, S., Lertakyamanee, N., Plengvanit, U., 1988. *Fasciola gigantica*: the second case of human infection in Thailand. J. Med. Assoc. Thai. 71, 451–455.

Kaewkes, S., 1995. The Epidemiology and Taxonomy of Minute Intestinal Flukes in Northeast Thailand. PhD thesis, University of Queensland.

Kaewkes, S., 2003. Taxonomy and biology of liver flukes. Acta Trop. 88, 177–186.

Kaewkes, S., Elkins, D.B., Sithithaworn, P., Haswell-Elkins, M.R., 1991. Comparative studies on the morphology of the eggs of *Opisthorchis viverrini* and lecithodendriid trematodes. Southeast Asian J. Trop. Med. Public Health 22, 623–630.

Kasný, M., Mikes, L., Hampl, V., Dvorák, J., Caffrey, C.R., Dalton, J.P., et al., 2009. Peptidases of trematodes. Adv. Parasitol. 69, 205–297.

Keiser, J., Utzinger, J., 2005. Emerging foodborne trematodiasis. Emerg. Infect. Dis. 11, 1507–1514.

Keiser, J., Utzinger, J., 2009. Food-borne trematodiases. Clin. Microbiol. Rev. 22, 466–483.

Keiser, J., Utzinger, J., 2010. The drugs we have and the drugs we need against major helminth infections. Adv. Parasitol. 73, 197–230.

Keiser, J., Engels, D., Büscher, G., Utzinger, J., 2005. Triclabendazole for the treatment of fascioliasis and paragonimiasis. Exp. Opin. Investig. Drugs 14, 1513–1526.

Kim, Y.J., Choi, M.H., Hong, S.T., Bae, Y.M., 2008. Proliferative effects of excretory/secretory products from *Clonorchis sinensis* on the human epithelial cell line HEK293 via regulation of the transcription factor E2F1. Parasitol. Res. 102, 411–417.

Laha, T., Pinlaor, P., Mulvenna, J., Sripa, B., Sripa, M., Smout, M.J., et al., 2007. Gene discovery for the carcinogenic human liver fluke, *Opisthorchis viverrini*. BMC Genomics 8, 189.

Le, T.H., De, N.V., Blair, D., McManus, D.P., Kino, H., Agatsuma, T., 2006a. *Paragonimus heterotremus* Chen and Hsia (1964), in Vietnam: a molecular identification and relationships of isolates from different hosts and geographical origins. Acta Trop. 98, 25–33.

Le, T.H., De, N.V., Blair, D., Sithithaworn, P., McManus, D.P., 2006b. *Clonorchis sinensis* and *Opisthorchis viverrini*: development of a mitochondrial-based multiplex PCR for their identification and discrimination. Exp. Parasitol. 112, 109–114.

Le, T.H., De, N.V., Agatsuma, T., Blair, D., Vercruysse, J., Dorny, P., et al., 2007. Molecular confirmation that *Fasciola gigantica* can undertake aberrant migrations in human hosts. J. Clin. Microbiol. 45, 648–650.

Le, T.H., De, N.V., Agatsuma, T., Thi Nguyen, T.G., Nguyen, Q.D., McManus, D.P., et al., 2008. Human fascioliasis and the presence of hybrid/introgressed forms of *Fasciola hepatica* and *Fasciola gigantica* in Vietnam. Int. J. Parasitol. 38, 725–730.

Lee, S.H., Hwang, S.W., Chai, J.Y., Seo, B.S., 1984. Comparative morphology of eggs of Heterophyids and *Clonorchis sinensis* causing human infections in Korea. Kisaengchunghak Chapchi 22, 171–180.

Lee, K.J., Bae, Y.T., Kim, D.H., Deung, Y.K., Ryang, Y.S., Kim, H.J., et al., 2002. Status of intestinal parasites infection among primary school children in Kampongcham, Cambodia. Korean J. Parasitol. 40, 153–155.

Lee, J.S., Lee, J., Kim, S.H., Yong, T.S., 2007. Molecular cloning and characterization of a major egg antigen in *Paragonimus westermani* and its use in ELISA for the immunodiagnosis of paragonimiasis. Parasitol. Res. 100, 677–681.

Leiper, R.T., 1915. Notes of the occurrence of parasites presumably rare in man. J. R. Army Med. Corps 24, 569–575.

Lim, J.H., Mairiang, E., Ahn, G.H., 2008. Biliary parasitic diseases including clonorchiasis, opisthorchiasis and fascioliasis. Abdom. Imaging 33, 157–165.

Liu, Q., Wei, F., Liu, W., Yang, S., Zhang, X., 2008. Paragonimiasis: an important food-borne zoonosis in China. Trends Parasitol. 24, 318–323.

Loaharanu, P., Sornmani, S., 1991. Preliminary estimates of economic impact of liver fluke infection in Thailand and the feasibility of irradiation as a control measure. Southeast Asian J. Trop. Med. Public Health 22, 384–390.

Lovis, L., Mak, T.K., Phongluxa, K., Soukhathammavong, P., Sayasone, S., Akkhavong, K., et al., 2009. PCR diagnosis of *Opisthorchis viverrini* and *Haplorchis taichui* infections in a Lao community in an area of endemicity and comparison of diagnostic methods for parasitological field surveys. J. Clin. Microbiol. 47, 1517–1523.

Lun, Z.R., Gasser, R.B., Lai, D.H., Li, A.X., Zhu, X.Q., Yu, X.B., et al., 2005. Clonorchiasis: a key foodborne zoonosis in China. Lancet Infect. Dis. 5, 31–41.

Lv, S., Zhang, Y., Steinmann, P., Zhou, X.N., Utzinger, J., 2010. Helminth infections of the central nervous system occurring in Southeast Asia and the Far East. Adv. Parasitol. 72, 351–408.

Mairiang, E., Mairiang, P., 2003. Clinical manifestation of opisthorchiasis and treatment. Acta Trop. 88, 221–227.

Mairiang, E., Elkins, D.B., Mairiang, P., Chaiyakum, J., Chamadol, N., Loapaiboon, V., et al., 1992. Relationship between intensity of *Opisthorchis viverrini* infection and hepatobiliary disease detected by ultrasonography. J. Gastroenterol. Hepatol. 7, 17–21.

Mairiang, E., Haswell-Elkins, M.R., Mairiang, P., Sithithaworn, P., Elkins, D.B., 1993. Reversal of biliary tract abnormalities associated with *Opisthorchis viverrini* infection following praziquantel treatment. Trans. R. Soc. Trop. Med. Hyg. 87, 194–197.

Mairiang, E., Chaiyakum, J., Chamadol, N., Laopaiboon, V., Srinakarin, J., Kunpitaya, J., et al., 2006. Ultrasound screening for *Opisthorchis viverrini*-associated cholangiocarcinomas: experience in an endemic area. Asian Pac. J. Cancer Prev. 7, 431–433.

Maleewong, W., 2003. *Paragonimus* spp. In: Miliotis, M.D., Bier, J.W. (Eds.), International Handbook of Food-borne Pathogens. Marcel Dekker, Inc., New York, pp. 601–613.

Manning, G., Sukhawat, K., Viyanant, V., Subhakul, M., Lertprasert, P., 1969. *Fasciolopsis buski* in Thailand, with comments on other intestinal parasites. J. Med. Assoc. Thai. 52, 905–913.

Mas-Coma, S., Bargues, M.D., Valero, M.A., 2005. Fascioliasis and other plant-borne trematode zoonoses. Int. J. Parasitol. 35, 1255–1278.

Mas-Coma, S., Valero, M.A., Bargues, M.D., 2009a. *Fasciola*, lymnaeids and human fascioliasis, with a global overview on disease transmission, epidemiology, evolutionary genetics, molecular epidemiology and control. Adv. Parasitol. 69, 41–146.

Mas-Coma, S., Valero, M.A., Bargues, M.D., 2009b. Climate change effects on trematodiases, with emphasis on zoonotic fascioliasis and schistosomiasis. Vet. Parasitol. 163, 264–280.

McGonigle, L., Mousley, A., Marks, N.J., Brennan, G.P., Dalton, J.P., Spithill, T.W., et al., 2008. The silencing of cysteine proteases in *Fasciola hepatica* newly excysted juveniles using RNA interference reduces gut penetration. Int. J. Parasitol. 38, 149–155.

McManus, D.P., Dalton, J.P., 2006. Vaccines against the zoonotic trematodes *Schistosoma japonicum*, *Fasciola hepatica* and *Fasciola gigantica*. Parasitology 133, 43–61.

Morphew, R.M., Wright, H.A., LaCourse, E.J., Woods, D.J., Brophy, P.M., 2007. Comparative proteomics of excretory-secretory proteins released by the liver fluke *Fasciola hepatica* in sheep host bile and during in vitro culture ex host. Mol. Cell. Proteomics 6, 963–972.

Nakano, N., Kirino, Y., Uchida, K., Nakamura-Uchiyama, F., Nawa, Y., Horii, Y., 2009. Large-group infection of boar-hunting dogs with *Paragonimus westermani* in Miyazaki prefecture, Japan, with special reference to a case of sudden death due to bilateral pneumothorax. J. Vet. Med. Sci. 71, 657–660.

Nkouawa, A., Okamoto, M., Mabou, A.K., Edinga, E., Yamasaki, H., Sako, Y., et al., 2009. Paragonimiasis in Cameroon: molecular identification, serodiagnosis and clinical manifestations. Trans. R. Soc. Trop. Med. Hyg. 103, 255–261.

O'Neill, S.M., Parkinson, M., Dowd, A.J., Strauss, W., Angles, R., Dalton, J.P., 1999. Immunodiagnosis of human fascioliasis using recombinant *Fasciola hepatica* cathepsin L1 cysteine proteinase. Am. J. Trop. Med. Hyg. 60, 749–751.

Parkinson, M., O'Neill, S.M., Dalton, J.P., 2007. Endemic human fasciolosis in the Bolivian Altiplano. Epidemiol. Infect. 135, 669–674.

Phathihutthagon, W., Sornmani, S., Imphan, P., Srithabut, P., 1984. Studies on the prevalence and reinfection rate of *Echinostoma* spp. in an irrigated area. J. Parasitol. Trop. Med. Assoc. Thai. 7, 12–16.

Pinlaor, S., Yongvanit, P., Hiraku, Y., Ma, N., Semba, R., Oikawa, S., et al., 2003. 8-nitroguanine formation in the liver of hamsters infected with *Opisthorchis viverrini*. Biochem. Biophys. Res. Commun. 309, 567–571.

Pinlaor, S., Ma, N., Hiraku, Y., Yongvanit, P., Semba, R., Oikawa, S., et al., 2004. Repeated infection with *Opisthorchis viverrini* induces accumulation of 8-nitroguanine and 8-oxo-7, 8-dihydro-2′-deoxyguanine in the bile duct of hamsters via inducible nitric oxide synthase. Carcinogenesis 25, 1535–1542.

Pinlaor, S., Hiraku, Y., Yongvanit, P., Tada-Oikawa, S., Ma, N., Pinlaor, P., et al., 2006. iNOS-dependent DNA damage via NF-kappaB expression in hamsters infected with *Opisthorchis viverrini* and its suppression by the antihelminthic drug praziquantel. Int. J. Cancer 119, 1067–1072.

Pinlaor, S., Prakobwong, S., Hiraku, Y., Kaewsamut, B., Dechakhamphu, S., Boonmars, T., et al., 2008. Oxidative and nitrative stress in *Opisthorchis viverrini*-infected hamsters: an indirect effect after praziquantel treatment. Am. J. Trop. Med. Hyg. 78, 564–573.

Pinlaor, P., Kaepitoon, N., Laha, T., Sripa, B., Kaewkes, S., Morales, M.E., et al., 2009. Cathepsin F cysteine protease of *Opisthorchis viverrini*. PLoS Negl. Trop. Dis. 3, e398.

Procop, G.W., 2009. North American paragonimiasis (caused by *Paragonimus kellicotti*) in the context of global paragonimiasis. Clin. Microbiol. Rev. 22, 415–446.

Pungpak, S., Chalermrut, K., Harinasuta, T., Viravan, C., Schelp, P.F., Hempfling, A., et al., 1994. *Opisthorchis viverrini* infection in Thailand: symptoms and signs of infection—a population-based study. Trans. R. Soc. Trop. Med. Hyg. 88, 561–564.

Pungpak, S., Viravan, C., Radomyos, B., Chalermrut, K., Yemput, C., Plooksawasdi, W., et al., 1997. *Opisthorchis viverrini* infection in Thailand: studies on the morbidity of the infection and resolution following praziquantel treatment. Am. J. Trop. Med. Hyg. 56, 311–314.

Radomyos, P., Bunnag, D., Harinasuta, T., 1982. *Echinostoma ilocanum* (Garrison, 1908) Odhner, 1911, infection in man in Thailand. Southeast Asian J. Trop. Med. Public Health 13, 265–269.

Radomyos, P., Bunnag, D., Harinasuta, T., 1984. Worms recovered in stools following praziquantel treatment. Drug Res. 34, 1215–1217.

Radomyos, P., Radomyos, B., Tungtrongchitr, A., 1994. Multi-infection with helminths in adults from northeast Thailand as determined by post-treatment fecal examination of adult worms. Trop. Med. Parasitol. 45, 133–135.

Radomyos, B., Wongsaroj, T., Wilairatana, P., Radomyos, P., Praevanich, R., Meesomboon, V., et al., 1998. Opisthorchiasis and intestinal fluke infections in northern Thailand. Southeast Asian J. Trop. Med. Public Health 29, 123–127.

Rim, H.J., 1982a. Echinostomiasis. In: Hillyer, G.V., Hopla, C.E. (Eds.), Section C: Parasitic Zoonoses Boca Raton. CRC Press, Florida, pp. 53–69.

Rim, H.J., 1982b. Fasciolopsiasis. In: Hillyer, G.V., Hopla, C.E. (Eds.), Section C: Parasite Zoonoses Boca Raton. CRC Press, Florida, pp. 89–97.

Rim, H.J., 2005. Clonorchiasis: an update. J. Helminthol. 79, 269–281.

Rim, H.J., Chai, J.Y., Min, D.Y., Cho, S.Y., Eom, K.S., Hong, S.J., et al., 2003. Prevalence of intestinal parasite infections on a national scale among primary schoolchildren in Laos. Parasitol. Res. 91, 267–272.

Robinson, M.W., Dalton, J.P., Donnelly, S., 2008. Helminth pathogen cathepsin proteases: it's a family affair. Trends Biochem. Sci. 33, 601–608.

Sadun, E.H., 1955. Studies on *Opisthorchis viverrini* in Thailand. Am. J. Hyg. 62, 81–115.

Sadun, E.H., Maiphoom, C., 1953. Studies on the epidemiology of the human intestinal fluke, *Fasciolopsis buski* (Lankester) in Central Thailand. Am. J. Trop. Med. Hyg. 2, 1070–1084.

Satarug, S., Lang, M.A., Yongvanit, P., Sithithaworn, P., Mairiang, E., Mairiang, P., et al., 1996. Induction of cytochrome P450 2A6 expression in humans by the carcinogenic parasite infection, opisthorchiasis viverrini. Cancer Epidemiol. Biomarkers Prev. 5, 795–800.

Satarug, S., Haswell-Elkins, M.R., Sithithaworn, P., Bartsch, H., Ohshima, H., Tsuda, M., et al., 1998. Relationships between the synthesis of N-nitrosodimethylamine and immune responses to chronic infection with the carcinogenic parasite, *Opisthorchis viverrini*, in men. Carcinogenesis 19, 485–491.

Sayasone, S., Odermatt, P., Phoumindr, N., Vongsaravane, X., Sensombath, V., Phetsouvanh, R., et al., 2007. Epidemiology of *Opisthorchis viverrini* in a rural district of southern Lao PDR. Trans. R. Soc. Trop. Med. Hyg. 101, 40–47.

Schiller, J.T., Castellsague, X., Villa, L.L., Hildesheim, A., 2008. An update of prophylactic human papillomavirus L1 virus-like particle vaccine clinical trial results. Vaccine 26, 53–61.

Shin, H.R., Lee, C.U., Park, H.J., Seol, S.Y., Chung, J.M., Choi, H.C., et al., 1996. Hepatitis B and C virus, *Clonorchis sinensis* for the risk of liver cancer: a case-control study in Pusan, Korea. Int. J. Epidemiol. 25, 933–940.

Sirisinha, S., Chawengkirttikul, R., Haswell-Elkins, M.R., Elkins, D.B., Kaewkes, S., Sithithaworn, P., 1995. Evaluation of a monoclonal antibody-based enzyme linked immunosorbent assay for the diagnosis of *Opisthorchis viverrini* infection in an endemic area. Am. J. Trop. Med. Hyg. 52, 521–524.

Sithithaworn, P., Sripa, B., Kaewkes, S., Haswell, M.R., 2009. Food-borne trematodes. In: Cook, G.C., Zumla, A.I. (Eds.), Manson's Tropical Diseases. 22nd ed. Saunders Elsevier, London, pp. 1461–1476.

Smout, M.J., Laha, T., Mulvenna, J., Sripa, B., Suttiprapa, S., Jones, A., et al., 2009. A granulin-like growth factor secreted by the carcinogenic liver fluke, *Opisthorchis viverrini*, promotes proliferation of host cells. PLoS Pathog. 5, e1000611.

Song, C.C., Duan, Y.F., Shou, G.C., Zhu, H., 1992. Effect of cobalt-60 irradiation on the infectivity of *Paragonimus westermani* metacercariae. J. Parasitol. 78, 869–871.

Song, H.O., Min, D.Y., Rim, H.J., Youthanavanh, V., Daluny, B., Sengdara, V., et al., 2008. Skin test for paragonimiasis among schoolchildren and villagers in Namback district, Luangprabang province, Lao PDR. Korean J. Parasitol. 46, 179–182.

Srihakim, S., Pholpark, M., 1991. Problem of fascioliasis in animal husbandry in Thailand. Southeast Asian J. Trop. Med. Public Health 22, 352–355.

Sripa, B., 2003. Pathobiology of opisthorchiasis: an update. Acta Trop. 88, 209–220.

Sripa, B., 2008. Concerted action is needed to tackle liver fluke infections in Asia. PLoS Negl. Trop. Dis. 2, e232.

Sripa, B., Kaewkes, S., 2000. Localisation of parasite antigens and inflammatory responses in experimental opisthorchiasis. Int. J. Parasitol. 30, 735–740.

Sripa, B., Pairojkul, C., 2008. Cholangiocarcinoma: lessons from Thailand. Curr. Opin. Gastroenterol. 24, 349–356.

Sripa, B., Haswell-Elkins, M.R., Sinawat, P., 2003. Histological analysis of gallbladder diseases in relation to opisthorchiasis in endemic areas of Thailand. Acta Trop. 88, 239–246.

Sripa, B., Kanla, P., Sinawat, P., Haswell-Elkins, M.R., 2004. Opisthorchiasis-associated biliary stones: light and scanning electron microscopic study. World J. Gastroenterol. 22, 3318–3321.

Sripa, B., Kaewkes, S., Sithithaworn, P., Mairiang, E., Laha, T., Smout, M., et al., 2007. Liver fluke induces cholangiocarcinoma. PLoS Med. 4, e201.

Sripa, B., Mairiang, E., Thinkhamrop, B., Laha, T., Kaewkes, S., Sithithaworn, P., et al., 2009. Advanced periductal fibrosis from infection with the carcinogenic human liver fluke *Opisthorchis viverrini* correlates with elevated levels of interleukin-6. Hepatology 50, 1273–1281.

Stack, C.M., Caffrey, C.R., Donnelly, S.M., Seshaadri, A., Lowther, J., Tort, J.F., et al., 2008. Structural and functional relationships in the virulence-associated cathepsin L proteases of the parasitic liver fluke, *Fasciola hepatica*. J. Biol. Chem. 283, 9896–9908.

Sukontason, K., Unpunyo, P., Sukontason, K.L., Piangjai, S., 2005. Evidence of *Haplorchis taichui* infection as pathogenic parasite: three case reports. Scand. J. Infect. Dis. 37, 388–390.

Suon, S., Hol, D., Siek, S., McLean, M., Copeman, B., 2006. Seasonal differences in the incidence of infection with *Fasciola gigantica* in Cambodian cattle. Trop. Anim. Health Prod. 38, 23–28.

Suttiprapa, S., Loukas, A., Laha, T., Wongkham, S., Kaewkes, S., Gaze, S., et al., 2008. Characterization of the antioxidant enzyme, thioredoxin peroxidase, from the carcinogenic human liver fluke, *Opisthorchis viverrini*. Mol. Biochem. Parasitol. 160, 116–122.

Suttiprapa, S., Mulvenna, J., Huong, N.T., Pearson, M.S., Brindley, P.J., Laha, T., et al., 2009. Ov-APR-1, an aspartic protease from the carcinogenic liver fluke, *Opisthorchis viverrini*: functional expression, immunolocalization and subsite specificity. Int. J. Biochem. Cell Biol. 41, 1148–1156.

Tangtrongchitr, A., Monzon, R.B., 1991. Eating habits associated with *Echinostoma malayanum* infections in the Philippines. Southeast Asian J. Trop. Med. Public Health 22, 212–216.

Thanan, R., Murata, M., Pinlaor, S., Sithithaworn, P., Khuntikeo, N., Tangkanakul, W., et al., 2008. Urinary 8-oxo-7, 8-dihydro-2′-deoxyguanosine in patients with parasite infection and effect of antiparasitic drug in relation to cholangiocarcinogenesis. Cancer Epidemiol. Biomarkers Prev. 17, 518–524.

Thuwajit, C., Thuwajit, P., Kaewkes, S., Sripa, B., Uchida, K., Miwa, M., et al., 2004. Increased cell proliferation of mouse fibroblast NIH-3 T3 in vitro induced by excretory/secretory product(s) from *Opisthorchis viverrini*. Parasitology 129, 455–464.

Toledo, R., Esteban, J.G., Fried, B., 2006. Immunology and pathology of intestinal trematodes in their definitive hosts. Adv. Parasitol. 63, 285–365.

Touch, S., Komalamisra, C., Radomyos, P., Waikagul, J., 2009. Discovery of *Opisthorchis viverrini* metacercariae in freshwater fish in southern Cambodia. Acta Trop. 111, 108–113.

Tran, V.H., Tran, T.K., Nguye, H.C., Pham, H.D., Pham, T.H., 2001. Fascioliasis in Vietnam. Southeast Asian J. Trop. Med. Public Health 32, 48–50.

Traub, R.J., Macaranas, J., Mungthin, M., Leelayoova, S., Cribb, T., Murrell, K.D., et al., 2009. A new PCR-based approach indicates the range of *Clonorchis sinensis* now extends to central Thailand. PLoS Negl. Trop. Dis. 3, e367.

Ubeira, F.M., Muino, L., Valero, M.A., Periago, M.V., Perez-Crespo, I., Mezo, M., et al., 2009. MM3-ELISA detection of *Fasciola hepatica* coproantigens in preserved human stool samples. Am. J. Trop. Med. Hyg. 81, 156–162.

Upatham, E.S., Viyanant, V., Kurathong, S., Brockelman, W.Y., Menaruchi, A., Saowakontha, S., et al., 1982. Morbidity in relation to intensity of infection in

Opisthorchiasis viverrini: study of a community in Khon Kaen, Thailand. Am. J. Trop. Med. Hyg. 31, 1156–1163.

Upatham, E.S., Viyanant, V., Kurathong, S., Rojborwonwitaya, J., Brockelman, W.Y., Ardsungnoen, S., et al., 1984. Relationship between prevalence and intensity of *Opisthorchis viverrini* infection, and clinical symptoms and signs in a rural community in north-east Thailand. Bull. World Health Organ. 62, 451–461.

Upatham, E.S., Viyanant, V., Kurathong, S., Vichasri, S., Brockelman, W.Y., Ardsuengnoen, P., 1995. *Paragonimus heterotremus* infection in a community in Saraburi province, central Thailand. J. Sci. Soc. Thailand 21, 1–9.

Uttaravichien, T., Bhudhisawasdi, V., Pairojkul, C., Pugkhem, A., 1999. Intrahepatic cholangiocarcinoma in Thailand. J. Hepatobiliary Pancreat. Surg. 6, 128–135.

Vajarasthira, S., 1985. Paragonimiasis. Proceeding of the 25th Anniversary of the Faculty of Tropical Medicine, Bangkok. pp. 98–104.

Valero, M.A., Perez-Crespo, I., Periago, M.V., Khoubbane, M., Mas-Coma, S., 2009. Fluke egg characteristics for the diagnosis of human and animal fascioliasis by *Fasciola hepatica* and *F. gigantica*. Acta Trop. 111, 150–159.

Vatanasapt, V., Uttaravichien, T., Mairiang, E.O., Pairojkul, C., Chartbanchachai, W., Haswell-Elkins, M., 1990. Cholangiocarcinoma in north-east Thailand. Lancet 335, 116–117.

Velasquez, C.C., 1982. Heterophyidiasis. In: Hillyer, G.V., Hopla, C.E. (Eds.), Section C: Parasitic Zoonoses. CRC Press, Florida, pp. 99–107.

Vidamaly, S., Choumlivong, K., Keolouangkhot, V., Vannavong, N., Kanpittaya, J., Strobel, M., 2009. Paragonimiasis: a common cause of persistent pleural effusion in Lao PDR. Trans. R. Soc. Trop. Med. Hyg. 103, 1019–1023.

Viyanant, V., Brockelman, W.Y., Lee, P., Ardsungnoen, S., Upatham, E.S., 1983. A comparison of a modified quick-Kato technique and the Stoll dilution method for field examination for *Opisthorchis viverrini* eggs. J. Helminthol. 57, 191–195.

Waikagul, J., 1991. Intestinal fluke infections in Southeast Asia. Southeast Asian J. Trop. Med. Public Health 22, 158–162.

Waikagul, J., Watthanakulpanich, D., Muennoo, C., Maipanich, W., Sa-nguankiat, S., Phubampen, S., 2005. Efficacy of benzimidazole carbamate on an intestinal fluke co-infected with nematodes. J. Med. Assoc. Thai. 88, 233–237.

Weng, Y.L., Zhuang, Z.L., Jiang, H.P., Lin, G.R., Lin, J.J., 1989. Studies on ecology of *Fasciolopsis buski* and control strategy of fasciolopsiasis. Chin. J. Parasitol. Parasit. Dis. 7, 108–111.

WHO, 1995. Control of foodborne trematode infections. Report of a WHO Study Group. WHO Tech. Rep. Ser. 849, 1–157.

WHO, 2002. Report of the Joint WHO/FAO Workshop on Food-borne Tramatode Infections in Asia. Ha Noi, Vietnam, 26–28 November 2002.

WHO, 2008. Review on the epidemiological profile of helminthiases and their control in the Western Pacific Region, 1997–2008. World Health Organization, MVP/WPRO, The Western Pacific Region.

WHO, 2009. WHO Model Formulary. In: World Health Organization. WHO Press, Geneva, p. 644.

Wongkham, C., Intapan, P.M., Maleewong, W., Miwa, M., 2005. Evaluation of human IgG subclass antibodies in the serodiagnosis of *Paragonimiasis heterotremus*. Asian Pac. J. Allergy Immunol. 23, 205–211.

Wongratanacheewin, S., Pumidonming, W., Sermswan, R.W., Maleewong, W., 2001. Development of a PCR-based method for the detection of *Opisthorchis viverrini* in experimentally infected hamsters. Parasitology 122, 175–180.

Wongratanacheewin, S., Sermswan, R.W., Sirisinha, S., 2003. Immunology and molecular biology of *Opisthorchis viverrini* infection. Acta Trop. 88, 195–207.

Wu, Z., Guan, Y., Zhou, Z., 1996. Study of an ancient corpse of the Warring States period unearthed from Tomb No. 1 at Guo-Jia Gang in Jingmen City (A comprehensive study). J. Tongji Med. Univ. 16 (1–5), 10.
Xuan le, T., Hung, N.T., Waikagul, J., 2005. Cutaneous fascioliasis: a case report in Vietnam. Am. J. Trop. Med. Hyg. 72, 508–509.
Yahiro, S., Habe, S., Duong, V., Odermatt, P., Barennes, H., Strobel, M., et al., 2008. Identification of the human paragonimiasis causative agent in Lao People's Democratic Republic. J. Parasitol. 94, 1176–1177.
Yesildag, A., Yildiz, H., Demirci, M., Goren, I., Isler, M., 2009. Biliary fascioliasis: sonographic appearance patterns. J. Clin. Ultrasound 37, 26–30.
Zhou, X.N., Lv, S., Yang, G.J., Kristensen, T.K., Bergquist, N.R., Utzinger, J., et al., 2009. Spatial epidemiology in zoonotic parasitic diseases: insights gained at the 1st International Symposium on Geospatial Health in Lijiang, China, 2007. Parasit. Vectors 2, 10.

CHAPTER 12

Helminth Infections of the Central Nervous System Occurring in Southeast Asia and the Far East

Shan Lv,[*,†,‡] **Yi Zhang,**[*] **Peter Steinmann,**[*,†,‡] **Xiao-Nong Zhou,**[*] and **Jürg Utzinger**[†,‡]

Contents

* National Institute of Parasitic Diseases, Chinese Center for Disease Control and Prevention, Shanghai, People's Republic of China
† Department of Epidemiology and Public Health, Swiss Tropical and Public Health Institute, Basel, Switzerland
‡ University of Basel, Basel, Switzerland

Advances in Parasitology, Volume 72
ISSN 0065-308X, DOI: 10.1016/S0065-308X(10)72012-1

Abstract

Although helminth infections of the central nervous system (CNS) are rare, their public health implications must not be neglected. Indeed, several helminth species can cause cerebrospinal infections, especially if humans serve as intermediate or non-permissive host. The diagnosis of cerebrospinal helminthiases is difficult, and the detection of parasites in cerebrospinal fluid is rarely successful. Cerebrospinal helminth infections therefore often remain undetected, and hence prognosis is poor. Increases in tourism and population movements are risk factors for cerebrospinal helminthiases and infections pose particular challenges to clinicians in non-endemic areas. In this review, we focus primarily on food-borne helminthiases that are endemic and often emerging in Southeast Asia and the Far East, namely angiostrongyliasis, gnathostomiasis, sparganosis, paragonimiasis and cysticercosis. Additionally, we discuss neuroschistosomiasis, a disease that is transmitted through human–water contact. For each disease, we describe the pathogen, its transmission route and possible mechanisms for entering the CNS. We also summarise common signs and symptoms, challenges and opportunities for diagnosis, treatment, clinical management, geographical distribution and epidemiology. The adoption of a comprehensive set of diagnostic criteria for different cerebrospinal helminthiases is proposed, including epidemiological history, typical signs and symptoms, neuroimaging and laboratory findings. Finally, risk factors, and research needs for enhanced patient management and population-based control measures are discussed.

12.1. INTRODUCTION

The majority of parasitic worms (helminths) fall into two groups: Nematoda, comprising the nematodes (roundworms), and Platyhelminthes, comprising the trematodes (flukes) and the cestodes (tapeworms) (Muller, 2002). To date, more than 340 helminth species have been identified in parasitic associations with humans, with a fair number of them probably representing cases of pseudoparasitism or accidental infection (Cox, 2002; Crompton, 1999). A few dozen species exert a considerable impact on human health and well-being.

Nematodes are transmitted via soil where their eggs and larvae reside (e.g. *Ascaris lumbricoides*, *Trichuris trichiura* and the hookworms), or by biological vectors such as mosquitoes (e.g. lymphatic filariasis), and intermediate host snails (e.g. angiostrongyliasis), freshwater fish (e.g. gnathostomiasis) and mammals (e.g. trichinellosis). Soil-transmitted helminth infections are the most common nematodes in the world, with particularly high prevalences reported from the tropics and subtropics (Bethony et al., 2006; de Silva et al., 2003; Hotez et al., 2007). Food-borne nematode infections are comparatively rare, but outbreaks are common for some species, such as *Trichinella spiralis* (Liu and Boireau, 2002) and *Angiostrongylus cantonensis* (Lv et al., 2008), and cause considerable morbidity. Many nematode species can invade the central nervous system (CNS) via the bloodstream. Angiostrongyliasis, gnathostomiasis, strongyloidiasis, toxocariasis and baylisascariasis are some of the most common infections of the CNS and the former three are prevalent in Southeast Asia.

With a few exceptions, trematodes rely on aquatic snails as their first intermediate hosts (Gryseels et al., 2006; Keiser and Utzinger, 2009). In the case of food-borne trematodiases, cercariae either encyst on aquatic vegetation, or penetrate the skin of a second intermediate host (e.g. fish and frogs) where they encyst (Keiser and Utzinger, 2009). Humans acquire an infection through the consumption of contaminated raw water plants (*Fasciola* spp.) or insufficiently cooked freshwater fish and other aquatic products. In view of the exponential growth of aquaculture, food-related trematode infections have gained in importance in many parts of the world (Keiser and Utzinger, 2005). With the exception of the lung fluke *Paragonimus*, with one report from the People's Republic of China (P.R. China) indicating that 9.8–19.7% of hospitalised patients had developed cerebrospinal paragonimiasis (Zhao, 1994), other trematodes seldom enter the CNS. Regarding schistosomiasis, it has been reported that the eggs of *Schistosoma japonicum* can lead to CNS involvement (Liu, 1993).

Adult cestodes exclusively parasitise the intestines of their definitive host, while the larvae reside in different locations in the intermediate host. Humans acquire an infection through the consumption of larvae-infested intermediate or paratenic hosts, or become intermediate hosts when accidentally ingesting worm eggs. Some species also rely on direct transmission or vectors. Negative health effects due to adult cestodes are minimal and mainly due to the competition for nutrients. However, larvae often induce severe disease if they end up in an accidental host. Cysticercosis caused by the cysticercus of *Taenia solium* and echinococcosis caused by the metacestodes of *Echinococcus* spp. are the most important human larval cestodiases. Neurocysticercosis (NC), as the most severe form of cysticercosis, is the leading cause of acquired epilepsy (García and Del Brutto, 2005; Roman et al., 2000). Cerebral sparganosis caused by the migration of sparganum of *Spirometra* is relatively rare, but can be of local importance in Southeast Asia and the Far East, and is linked to specific cultural and dietary habits.

The human CNS does not constitute a definitive location for any helminth species but is occasionally and mostly accidentally reached during the migration of helminth larvae and eggs in the human body, especially if humans serve as intermediate or non-permissive hosts. However, some species show neurotropism if they accidentally end up in humans, such as the larvae of *A. cantonensis* and *T. solium*. With a few exceptions of ocular and nasal involvement, almost all angiostrongyliasis cases due to *A. cantonensis* infection involve the CNS (Wang et al., 2008). As many as 91.0% (7889/8674) of all cysticercosis inpatients in the mainland of P.R. China show cerebrospinal involvement (Wang, 2008). Usually, helminths invade the CNS via two routes: either the bloodstream or migration through soft tissue. For the larvae of most nematodes (e.g. *A. cantonensis* and *Toxocara* spp.) and some tapeworms (e.g. *T. solium* and *Echinococcus* spp.) the bloodstream is the main avenue to the CNS. Infrequently, the eggs of *Schistosoma* spp. can also be carried to the CNS via the blood (Gryseels et al., 2006). Larvae of other species may migrate to the CNS along nerves, vessels and muscles (e.g. *Gnathostoma* spp., *Spirometra mansoni* and *Paragonimus westermani*) (Oh, 1968a; Punyagupta et al., 1990).

An infection of the CNS with helminths can be disabling and fatal if left untreated. The diagnosis of cerebrospinal helminthiases is difficult since larvae or worms can seldom be recovered and symptoms are unspecific. Eosinophil cells in the cerebrospinal fluid (CSF) can serve as an indicator for helminth infection of the CNS but they are not necessarily always present over the course of an infection. Neuroimaging techniques can reveal lesions in the CNS, but the manifestations are often non-specific and typical imaging features are lacking in most patients. Therefore, misdiagnosis due to signs and symptoms common for other diseases (e.g. tuberculosis and intracranial cancers) is widespread, particularly outside known endemic areas.

Cerebrospinal helminthiases are often neglected in disease control programmes because they are not a primary clinical form for most helminth infections. However, some emerging risk factors call for more attention to cerebrospinal helminth infections. Large population movements and expanding international tourism place people from non-endemic areas at risk of acquiring a disease and thus pose challenges to clinicians in non-endemic areas (Gushulak and MacPherson, 2004). Immunocompromised individuals (due to AIDS, chronic diseases or use of immunosuppressants) are at a higher risk of cerebral involvement, for example in the case of a *Strongyloides stercoralis* infection (Walker and Zunt, 2005).

In this review, we focus on cerebrospinal helminthiases with particular consideration of those commonly occurring in Southeast Asia and the Far East. Food-borne trematode infections are an emerging public health issue in Southeast Asia and the Far East, partially explained by rapidly expanding aquaculture, and diversification and long-distance distribution of food resources. Angiostrongyliasis, gnathostomiasis, sparganosis and paragonimiasis are typically associated with aquatic products such as freshwater fish, snails, frogs, snakes, crabs and crayfish. Rapidly increasing consumption of pork imposes new risks for cysticercosis, especially in rural areas. Considerable progress has been made in the control of Asian schistosomiasis, but in view of its public health importance and the risk of re-emergence due to climate change, it is also discussed. Key features of the main cerebrospinal helminthiases, including causative agents, risk factors, common signs and symptoms and differential diagnosis are summarised in Table 12.1.

12.2. ANGIOSTRONGYLIASIS

12.2.1. Pathogen

Human angiostrongyliasis is primarily caused by *A. cantonensis* and *A. costaricensis*. The former is also known as rat lungworm and is the most important aetiological agent of eosinophilic meningitis (Graeff-Teixeira et al., 2009). *A. cantonensis* was first discovered in 1933 during the examination of *Rattus norvegicus* (brown rats) and *R. rattus* (black rats) in Guangzhou, P.R. China (Chen, 1935). The first human infection was reported from Taiwan in 1945, but the public health significance was not recognised until the 1960s (Cross, 1987), when the parasite was recovered from a Filipino patient in Hawaii (Rosen et al., 1962) and an epidemic was identified on some Pacific islands (Rosen et al., 1967). *A. costaricensis* mainly causes eosinophilic infiltrations in the intestinal wall, especially the ileocecal region (Loria-Cortes and Lobo-Sanahuja, 1980). Two other species, namely *A. malayiensis* in Southeast Asia and *A. mackerras* in Australia, have been suspected as the causes of neurological lesions in

TABLE 12.1 Summary of main cerebrospinal helminth infections in Southeast Asia and the Far East

Disease	Causative agent(s)	Main occurrence in Eastern Asia	Risk factors	Signs and symptoms	Laboratory findings	Neuroimaging	Main differential diagnosis	Treatment
Angiostrongyliasis	*Angiostrongylus cantonensis* (larva)	P.R. China, Japan, Thailand, Vietnam, etc.	Eating raw or undercooked snails, slugs, frogs, crustaceans and lizards. In Western hemisphere, consumption of raw vegetables contaminated by snail or slug secretions or egg masses	Meningitis (severe headache, nausea, vomiting, neck stiffness, paraesthesia, fever, etc.); meningoencephalitis (headache, pain in trunk); radiculomyelitis (pain in trunk and extremities)	Eosinophilia and larvae in CSF; eosinophilia in peripheral blood	Compatible with meningitis	Gnathostomiasis, cysticercosis, paragonimiasis, schistosomiasis, meningitis caused by tuberculosis, viral meningitis	Chemotherapy (albendazole and mebendazole); anti-inflammatory treatment (corticosteroids)
Neurognathostomiasis	*Gnathostomus spinigerum, G. hispidum, G. nipponicum, G. doloresi* (larva)	Thailand	Eating raw or undercooked fish (swamp eel), frogs, snakes, birds; drinking untreated water	Radiculomyelitis (a sudden radicular pain and/or headache, followed by paralysis of the extremities and/or cranial nerve palsies); encephalitis (headache, disturbance of consciousness and cranial nerve palsies); radiculomyeloencephalitis Manifestation outside CNS: subcutaneous migratory swellings with haemorrhage	Xanthochromia and eosinophilia in CSF, larvae during biopsy; eosinophilia in peripheral blood	Cord enlargement and diffuse high-signal intensity; haemorrhagic tract and scattered deep intracerebral haemorrhage with diffuse, fuzzy white matter lesions in brain	Angiostrongyliasis, sparganosis, schistosomiasis, intraspinal tumor	Surgery; chemotherapy (albendazole and ivermectin); anti-inflammatory treatment (corticosteroids)

Neurocysticercosis	*Taenia solium* (cysticercus)	P.R. China, Indonesia, Malaysia, Thailand, Vietnam, Lao PDR	Eating raw or undercooked vegetables and plant food; contact with tapeworm carriers	Mass effect (seizure); meningoencephalitis (headache, vomiting, diplopia, papilloedema, etc.) Manifestation outside CNS: subcutaneous swellings		A viable cyst presents a ''hole-with-dot''; a degenerating cyst appear as contrast-enhancing rings or nodules surrounded by oedema; a calcified cyst appear as hyperdense dots or areas of subtracted signal	Intracranial tumours, sparganosis, paragonimiasis	Chemotherapy (praziquantel and albendazole); anti-inflammatory treatment (corticosteroids); antiepileptic drugs and surgery
Neruosparganosis	*Spirometra mansoni* (sparganum)	P.R. China, Thailand, Korea, Japan	Eating raw or undercooked frog/tadpole, snake; drinking raw snake blood or bile, or untreated water; using poultice of frog flesh	Seizures, hemiparesis, headache Manifestation outside CNS: subcutaneous migratory swellings	Sparganum during biopsy, eosinophilia in peripheral blood	Tunnel sign and multiple conglomerated ring or bead-shaped enhancements	Metastatic brain tumours	Surgery
Neuroparagonimiasis	*Paragonimus westermani*, *P. skrjabini*, *P. heterotremus*, *P. miyazakii*, *P. ohirai* (worm or egg)	P.R. China, Vietnam	Eating raw or undercooked crab or crayfish	Eosinophilic meningitis (headache, fever, vomiting); seizure, arachnoiditis, mass effects (paralysis) Manifestation outside CNS: subcutaneous migratory swellings, coughing and rusty sputum for a long time	Xanthochromia in CSF; eggs in sputum; eggs or worms during biopsy	Clustered ring-enhancing lesions	Sparganosis, tuberculosis	Chemotherapy (triclabendazole and praziquantel); anti-inflammatory treatment (corticosteroids); surgery

(*continued*)

TABLE 12.1 *(continued)*

Disease	Causative agent(s)	Main occurrence in Eastern Asia	Risk factors	Signs and symptoms	Laboratory findings	Neuroimaging	Main differential diagnosis	Treatment
Neuroschistosomiasis	*Schistosoma japonicum*, *S. mekongi* (egg)	P.R. China, Philippines, Indonesia, Lao PDR, Cambodia	Contact with freshwater in endemic area	Encephalitis and/or meningitis (headache, vomiting, speech disturbances, disorientation, visual abnormality, urinary incontinence, etc.); tumoral form (seizures accompanied by the loss of consciousness; headache, visual abnormality, sensory disturbance, hemiparesis, etc.) Manifestation outside CNS; Katayama syndrome	Eggs in faeces; eggs during biopsy	Multiple clustered, enhanced nodules	Intracranial tumours (brain glioma), epilepsy due to other causes	Chemotherapy (praziquantel); anti-inflammatory treatment (corticosteroids); surgery

humans (Cross, 1987; Prociv et al., 2000). However, thus far, the worms have not been isolated from patients.

Adult *A. cantonensis* worms parasitise the pulmonary arteries and cardiac cavities of rats and release their eggs into the bloodstream. After hatching, the larvae penetrate the capillary walls in the lung tissue and enter the airways. The first-stage larvae (L_1) in the rat sputum are then swallowed and pass the intestine to be released with the faeces. The free larvae enter their mollusk intermediate hosts (i.e. snails or slugs) upon which they develop into third-stage infective larvae (L_3). Various animals (e.g. frogs, shrimps, crabs, fish and lizard) can serve as paratenic hosts in which the infective larvae can live several weeks without further development (Wallace and Rosen, 1966, 1967). When rats ingest intermediate or paratenic hosts harbouring infective larvae, the larvae penetrate the stomach or intestinal walls and migrate through the host body.

A. cantonensis is neurotropic; that means the larvae stay in the CNS where they further grow and develop. Within approximately 4 weeks and after two molts, worms penetrate the cerebral vein and migrate to the heart and pulmonary arteries. Adult worms mate and deposit the first eggs approximately 5 weeks post-infection.

Humans are non-permissive hosts for this nematode. The larvae can invade the human CNS via the bloodstream, but usually fail to pass through the cerebral vessels and enter the pulmonary arteries. In children, the larvae may enter the pulmonary vessels and induce potentially fatal inflammation in the lung, but sexually mature adult worms are seldom found. Infections occur when raw or undercooked freshwater or terrestrial snails and slugs, paratenic hosts or contaminated vegetables are consumed.

12.2.2. Clinical manifestations

A. cantonensis induces inflammation in neural tissues and usually increases eosinophil cell counts, a syndrome known as eosinophilic meningitis. The incubation period of eosinophilic meningitis is variable, ranging from 1 day to several months. In an angiostrongyliasis outbreak that could be linked to the consumption of the terrestrial snail *Achatina fulica*, typical clinical symptoms appeared within 1–6 days (Kliks et al., 1982). However, in a large outbreak which occurred in Beijing in 2006, involving 160 patients, the incubation period in 128 patients (80%) was 7–36 days with a median of 14 days (He et al., 2007). This outbreak was linked to the consumption of *Pomacea canaliculata* snails, a freshwater species. The estimated mean incubation period among 33 patients in a recent outbreak in Dali, P.R. China, which was due to the consumption of raw *P. canaliculata* snails, was 16 days with a range of 3–50 days (Lv et al., 2009a). The latent period was as long as 54 days (standard deviation: 30 days) in an outbreak due to drinking raw vegetable juice (Tsai et al., 2004). These outbreaks indicate that the incubation period might be associated with the number of ingested larvae.

Different clinical manifestations of angiostrongyliasis have been described. Eosinophilic meningitis is the main clinical entity associated with the disease (Sawanyawisuth and Sawanyawisuth, 2008). Other clinical manifestations include eosinophilic meningoencephalitis (Furugen et al., 2006), eosinophilic radiculomyelitis (Schmutzhard et al., 1988), ocular angiostrongyliasis (Sinawat et al., 2008) and, more rarely, nasal (Liu and An, 2000) or pulmonary infections (Li et al., 2001; Lindo et al., 2004). Most infections are self-limiting and recovery is without sequelae (Punyagupta et al., 1975; Yii, 1976). However, illness developing into encephalitis may be fatal (Sawanyawisuth and Sawanyawisuth, 2008). Less than 10% of all patients infected with *A. cantonensis* develop encephalitis, but among them a lack of effective treatment results in high mortality (Sawanyawisuth and Sawanyawisuth, 2008).

Cerebrospinal inflammation and resulting increased intracranial pressure is the primary pathology of angiostrongyliasis. The most common complaint of patients is acute and deteriorating headache as a result of increased intracranial pressure (Graeff-Teixeira et al., 2009). Headache may be accompanied by nausea and vomiting. Approximately 40% of all patients experience neck stiffness and paraesthesia (Wang et al., 2008), which usually lasts for less than 2 weeks and affects different locations (usually the extremities). It has been described as hyperaesthesia, itching or a sensation of worms crawling under the skin (Wang et al., 2008). Less common symptoms include pain in the trunk or extremities, facial paralysis, blurred vision or diplopia. Fever is mostly absent in adults while paediatric patients are often highly febrile (Hwang and Chen, 1991). Children suffer more often from neck stiffness, nausea, vomiting, somnolence and abdominal pain (Hwang and Chen, 1991).

12.2.3. Diagnosis

The recovery of larvae from CSF or the ocular chamber is the definitive proof for human angiostrongyliasis. However, in a recent review of case reports and outbreaks occurring in the mainland of P.R. China between 1979 and 2006, only 16 patients (4.8%) out of a total of 334 cases were parasitologically diagnosed (Lv et al., 2008). In Thailand, none of the 484 cases reported there revealed parasites in the CSF (Punyagupta et al., 1975). The chance of diagnosing a child parasitologically is higher than for adults; the larval recovery rate from CSF by lumbar puncture was as high as 41.5% among paediatric cases in Taiwan (Hwang and Chen, 1991). In another survey involving 125 individuals, 8 out of 9 parasitologically confirmed cases were younger than 8 years (Yii, 1976). A clinical angiostrongyliasis diagnosis is often made based on eating history, clinical symptoms and diagnostic work-up. Specifically, a history of eating freshwater or terrestrial mollusks, paratenic hosts or potentially contaminated vegetables is crucial for clinical diagnosis.

Eosinophilia is an important indicator for helminth infections. An elevated eosinophil cell count (>10% of total white blood cells or >500 cells/μl) in CSF is of specific relevance for angiostrongyliasis due to the frequent involvement of the brain (Lv et al., 2009a; Punyagupta et al., 1970; Slom et al., 2002). However, not each examination of an angiostrongyliasis case shows eosinophilia in the CSF, since the counts may vary over the course of infection (Lv et al., 2009a; Punyagupta et al., 1975). Another diagnostic approach is immunological testing for antibodies or specific antigens from *A. cantonensis* in peripheral blood and CSF (Dorta-Contreras et al., 2005; Slom et al., 2002; Tsai et al., 2001b). Several tests including enzyme-linked immunosorbent assay (ELISA) and immuno-polymerase chain reaction (PCR) have been developed but reported sensitivities and specificities are questionable due to small sample sizes. At present, no commercially available kit for diagnosing angio-strongyliasis is on the market (Wang et al., 2008).

Categorised diagnosis based on the strength of clinical and epidemiological evidence was recently proposed (Lv et al., 2009a). Although *A. cantonensis* is generally regarded as the leading agent for eosinophilic meningitis, other causes must be considered to strengthen differential diagnosis. Hence, thorough diagnostic work-up and differential diagnosis are important in areas such as Southeast Asia and the Far East where special food items (e.g. snails, frogs, snakes and raw fish) are popular and other parasites causing eosinophilic meningitis co-exist. For example, both *A. cantonensis* and *Gnathostoma spinigerum* contributed to an epidemic of eosinophilic meningitis in Thailand (Punyagupta et al., 1975, 1990).

12.2.4. Treatment and clinical management

The severity of human angiostrongyliasis varies from mild and self-limiting to fatal, depending on the parts of the brain involved and the worm burden. The clinical management of angiostrongyliasis includes administration of anthelminthic drugs, supportive measures and sometimes even surgery. Repeated lumbar puncture or mannitol transfusion is employed to relieve symptoms such as severe headache and vomiting by decreasing intracranial pressure (Chotmongkol et al., 2000; Lv et al., 2009a). Surgical removal of worms is the preferred method for the management of ocular angiostrongyliasis (Kumar et al., 2005; Malhotra et al., 2006; Sinawat et al., 2008; Toma et al., 2002).

The suitability of anthelminthics is controversial due to their potential to exacerbate inflammation (Bowden, 1981; Hidelaratchi et al., 2005). Still, albendazole and mebendazole are widely used against *A. cantonensis* in clinical practice (Sawanyawisuth and Sawanyawisuth, 2008). A trend to lower frequency of headache and a shorter mean duration of headache in the treatment group were reported from a randomised placebo-controlled trial assessing the efficacy of albendazole, but the statistical evidence was weak (Jitpimolmard et al., 2007). Two observational studies showed a satisfactory effect of albendazole in the treatment of children (Hwang and Chen, 1991; Lin et al., 2003b). Levamisole is another anthelminthic drug which has been used to treat children with reportedly good efficacy (Hwang, 1997). Thiabendazole showed no appreciable effect when the drug was administered at a dosage of 50 mg/kg/day for 3 days (Kliks et al., 1982). No clinical trial has assessed the efficacy of mebendazole alone. Corticosteroids have been confirmed to be useful, probably by decreasing inflammation (Chotmongkol et al., 2000; Sawanyawisuth and Sawanyawisuth, 2008; Tsai et al., 2004), but many relapses were reported (Sawanyawisuth et al., 2004a; Tsai et al., 2004). Currently, a combination of anthelminthic drugs and corticosteroids is recommended for the treatment of angiostrongyliasis patients (Chotmongkol et al., 2004, 2006).

12.2.5. Geographical distribution and epidemiology

Since 1945 when the first human angiostrongyliasis case was described, over 2800 cases have been documented in the literature; 77% of them in Southeast Asia, P.R. China and Japan (Wang et al., 2008). More than 30 countries or territories, mainly located in tropical and subtropical regions, have been identified as endemic (Kliks and Palumbo, 1992). All countries in Southeast Asia except Myanmar, Brunei and Timor Leste are considered endemic for *A. cantonensis*. Thailand is the most heavily endemic area; more than 1300 cases have been reported since the 1950s (Wang et al., 2008). Today, hundreds of suspected cases are reported every year, especially from northeastern Thailand (Eamsobhana and Tungtrongchitr, 2005). It is estimated that the annual incidence rate is approximately 2 per 100,000 in Thailand (Suankratay et al., 2001). Other countries including Vietnam, Cambodia, Indonesia and Malaysia reported sporadic cases. A total of 382 cases from nine provinces had been identified in the mainland of P.R. China by the end of 2008 (Deng et al., 2007; Lv et al., 2008, 2009a). Fifty-four cases were described in Japan before 2003 and 61.1% of all cases were found on Okinawa (Nawa, 2005). Many of the remaining infections probably originated from Okinawa or outside Japan (Nawa, 2005).

Considerable geographical heterogeneity with regard to prevalence among animal hosts has been found. For instance, two high-prevalence clusters located in Fujian province and Guangxi Zhuang autonomous region in P.R. China were identified when infection rates in *P. canaliculata* were surveyed (Lv et al., 2009b). At a smaller spatial scale, prevalence can decrease with the distance from the centre of the village (Li et al., 2006b). The host specificity of *A. cantonensis* is low. For example, natural infections have been found in 22 mollusk species and 11 different rodents (Lv et al., 2008). The first national survey in P.R. China revealed that *P. canaliculata* and *A. fulica* were the predominant intermediate hosts (Lv et al., 2009b), while *Pila* spp. was identified as the key intermediate host in Thailand (Tesana et al., 2008).

The prevalence of angiostrongyliasis in Southeast Asia and the Far East is strongly associated with eating habits deeply rooted in local culture. Freshwater and terrestrial snails, mainly *Pomacea* spp., *Pila* spp. and *A. fulica*, are the most common source of infection in this region (Lv et al., 2008; Punyagupta et al., 1970; Yii, 1976). Since the terrestrial snail *A. fulica* usually has a higher infection rate and worm burden than freshwater snails, the consumption of *A. fulica* often results in more severe manifestations and higher case numbers (Yii, 1976). Isolated cases are often attributed to freshwater snails (Lv et al., 2008; Tsai et al., 2001a) or terrestrial slugs, frogs and monitor lizards (Li et al., 2006a; Liu et al., 2006; Parameswaran, 2006). Living slugs are sometimes swallowed as part of traditional medicine treatments and might result in severe meningitis (Li et al., 2006a; Liu et al., 2006).

The epidemiological patterns of eosinophilic meningitis due to *A. cantonensis* in Southeast Asia and the south of P.R. China and Japan are changing. For example, the use of snails for rearing domestic animals was widely practiced in Taiwan in the 1970s (Yii et al., 1975) but is declining, and the importance of slugs in traditional medicine is diminishing. However, the spread of invasive snail species, tourism and the consumption of exotic foods have become driving factors in the epidemiology of angiostrongyliasis. The invasion of *P. canaliculata* in P.R. China may serve as an illustration. This freshwater snail was introduced around 1980, and is now well established in southern P.R. China (Lv et al., 2009b). Three quarters of the 382 cases and eight of nine outbreaks (each comprising at least six cases) of cerebral angiostrongyliasis have been attributed to this species (Deng et al., 2007; Lv et al., 2008, 2009a).

Travel is the common route of exposure to *A. cantonensis* for individuals from non-endemic countries (Deng et al., 2007; Malvy et al., 2008; Maretic et al., 2009; Slom et al., 2002; Tsai et al., 2001a). Long-distance food transportation is another important risk factor. The large outbreak in Beijing (non-endemic) in 2006 was attributed to snails imported from an endemic area.

12.3. GNATHOSTOMIASIS

12.3.1. Pathogen

Human gnathostomiasis is caused by the larval migration of at least four *Gnathostoma* species, namely *G. spinigerum*, *G. hispidum*, *G. doloresi* and *G. nipponicum* (Herman and Chiodini, 2009). The most common species parasitising humans is *G. spinigerum* (Rusnak and Lucey, 1993). First discovered in the stomach wall of a tiger that died in a zoological garden in London in 1836 (Graeff-Teixeira et al., 2009), *G. spinigerum* is now recognised as a common stomach parasite of cats and dogs, especially in Southeast Asia (Anderson, 2000). Although the first human case of gnathostomiasis (cutaneous migration) was reported from Thailand as early as 1889 (Herman and Chiodini, 2009), the first case with CNS involvement was only recognised in 1967 (Chitanondh and Rosen, 1967). Today, *G. spinigerum* and *A. cantonensis* are considered the two main agents for eosinophilic meningoencephalitis (Ramirez-Avila et al., 2009), with the mortality caused by the former far exceeding that due to the latter (Boongird et al., 1977; Punyagupta et al., 1990; Schmutzhard et al., 1988).

Adult *G. spinigerum* typically parasitise the stomach wall of carnivorous mammals. Eggs are passed to the environment via faeces and, upon reaching freshwater, hatch within 8–10 days to release L_1 (Rojekittikhun, 2002b). The free larvae are ingested by the first intermediate host, namely water fleas (copepods). They develop into second-stage larvae (L_2) and when infected copepods are ingested by a second intermediate host (e.g. fish, eels, frogs and reptiles), the larvae are released in the intestine and develop into L_3 which then migrate through the tissue and encyst in muscles of their hosts. Infective L_3 can also be passed from one host to another (paratenic host) via predation and scavenging. When ingested by a definitive host, L_3 are released in the gastrointestinal tract from where they migrate to the liver and abdominal cavity. Within approximately 4 weeks they return to the stomach and invade the gastric wall, resembling a tumour with an aperture in the gastric lumen through which eggs are released starting about 100 days post-infection (Miyazaki, 1960).

Humans are non-permissive definitive hosts of *G. spinigerum* and subcutaneous or visceral migrating larvae are more frequently found than adult worms in the stomach wall. The mechanism of migration to the CNS is unclear, but based on the typical clinical picture, migration is likely to occur from nerve roots to the CNS (Boongird et al., 1977). The consumption of insufficiently cooked second intermediate hosts or paratenic hosts probably is the primary source of infection. Thus far, 48 vertebrate species have been found to be naturally infected with *G. spinigerum* in Thailand (Rojekittikhun, 2002b), suggesting a complex transmission route to humans. Drinking freshwater contaminated with infected copepods has also been suggested as a route of infection (Punyagupta et al., 1990; Samarasinghe et al., 2002), in this case rendering humans to become second intermediate hosts rather than definitive hosts. However, it is unclear whether this route is associated with a higher risk of neurognathostomiasis (NG). Direct skin penetration of infective larvae and prenatal transmission have also been suggested (Rusnak and Lucey, 1993).

12.3.2. Clinical manifestations

The incubation period of NG is not known. Unlike the neurotropic *A. cantonensis*, *G. spinigerum* accidentally invades the CNS while the larvae migrate through the human body (Punyagupta et al., 1990). An outbreak of gnathostomiasis revealed that the most common clinical feature (i.e. migratory swellings and creeping eruptions) occurs within 20 days after consumption of raw fish and can repeatedly appear within 10 weeks (Chai et al., 2003). This probably indicates that migration lasts for several weeks and that the CNS can be involved at any time.

The main findings in CNS involvement are radiculomyelitis, radiculomyeloencephalitis and subarachnoid haemorrhage (Boongird et al., 1977; Punyagupta et al., 1990). Typical symptoms are a sudden onset of severe radicular pain and/or headache, followed by paralysis of the extremities and/or cranial nerve palsies (Boongird et al., 1977; Punyagupta et al., 1990). This clinical picture probably reflects the migratory pathway of the parasite, that is entering the spinal cord along nerve roots (Boongird et al., 1977). Radicular pain is extremely sharp, non-shooting or shooting along the nerve root, sometimes accompanied by a burning component. Severe pain can last from half an hour to a few hours and occurs several times each day (Punyagupta et al., 1990). Though not as frequent as in eosinophilic meningitis due to *A. cantonensis*, headache can appear when the cervical and cranial nerve roots are involved, or due to larval migration in cerebral tissue. The degree of paralysis varies from minimal weakness of the extremities to complete paralysis, depending on the migration pathway and the areas involved. Monoplegia, triplegia and quadriplegia have been observed, with paraplegia of lower limbs the most common. Cranial nerve palsies usually occur after paralysis of the extremities, which implies that the parasite tends to migrate from the lower spinal cord towards the brain. Multiple cranial nerve palsies usually indicate a poor prognosis. Urinary retention usually follows radiculomyelitis and radiculomyeloencephalitis.

In addition to pain and paralysis, other symptoms include neck stiffness, paraesthesia, fever, blurred vision and migrating swelling. Cutaneous gnathostomiasis accounts for the majority of patients infected with *Gnathostoma* but is rarely found in NG patients (Boongird et al., 1977;

Punyagupta et al., 1990). Hence, cutaneous migratory swelling is not considered important evidence for diagnosis. However, xanthochromic or bloody spinal fluid is characteristic of NG; more than 60% of all patients experience xanthochromic CSF (Boongird et al., 1977; Punyagupta et al., 1990). Over 12% of all patients with NG die due to extensive damage of vital centres in the brain stem or other complications (Boongird et al., 1977). The hallmark signs of gnathostomiasis are haemorrhagic tracts throughout the spinal cord and cerebral tissue post-mortem (Boongird et al., 1977; Bunnag et al., 1970; Punyagupta et al., 1990).

12.3.3. Diagnosis

Recorded outbreaks of gnathostomiasis following the consumption of raw fish suggest that only few patients present with symptoms associated with cerebrospinal involvement (Chai et al., 2003; Díaz Camacho et al., 2003). NG is diagnosed based on a combination of recent exposure history, symptoms and laboratory findings. A history of eating undercooked freshwater fish (e.g. swamp eels and loaches), frogs, snakes and chicken in endemic areas and drinking untreated water are risk factors for a *Gnathostoma* infection (Punyagupta et al., 1990; Samarasinghe et al., 2002). The typical clinical symptoms of NG mentioned above are essential for diagnosis, but other findings can be equally important. Although migratory swellings in subcutaneous tissue and eyelids only appear in about 4% and 7% of all NG cases respectively (Punyagupta et al., 1990), subcutaneous haemorrhage due to larval migration is characteristic of gnathostomiasis and thus important for differential diagnosis (Herman and Chiodini, 2009). The appearance of red blood cells is the hallmark sign of gnathostomiasis and crucial for diagnosis. Sometimes the larvae can be isolated from creeping eruptions (Chai et al., 2003).

Immunological tests for the diagnosis of NG have been developed (Anantaphruti, 2002), but tests with good sensitivity and specificity are still lacking and cross-reactivity with other parasitic infections remains a problem (Herman and Chiodini, 2009). Serological tests currently available for the diagnosis of gnathostomiasis include an assay based on crude somatic extracts of adult *G. doloresi* worms (Chai et al., 2003; Díaz Camacho et al., 2003), and an immunoblot technique to detect the specific 24-kDa band, which is widely used in Europe (Tapchaisri et al., 1991). However, no commercial reagents are currently available (Herman and Chiodini, 2009). Magnetic resonance imaging (MRI) and computed tomography (CT) are also used for diagnosis. Cord enlargement with diffuse high-signal intensity can indicate spinal gnathostomiasis (Sawanyawisuth et al., 2004b). Haemorrhagic tracts and scattered deep haemorrhage with fuzzy white matter lesions are found in cerebral gnathostomiasis (Sawanyawisuth et al., 2004b, 2009).

The main parasite to consider in differential diagnosis of NG is *A. cantonensis*. Angiostrongyliasis produces similar neurological manifestations, but acute severe radicular pain, signs of spinal cord compression and xanthochromic spinal fluid are uncommon (Ramirez-Avila et al., 2009; Schmutzhard et al., 1988). Freshwater fish may be paratenic hosts of *A. cantonensis* (Wallace and Rosen, 1967), but terrestrial or freshwater snails and slugs are more important sources of infection, especially in Southeast Asia and the Far East (Lv et al., 2008; Punyagupta et al., 1970). Thus, differential diagnosis should always consider the eating history. Another parasitic infection which must be ruled out in differential diagnosis is cerebral sparganosis caused by the sparganum of *Spirometra mansoni*.

12.3.4. Treatment and clinical management

To our knowledge, no effective treatment is available for *Gnathostoma* infections. Surgical removal of the larvae is effective in the management of subcutaneous infections and occasionally NG (Bunyaratavej et al., 2008). Various anthelminthic drugs (e.g. thiabendazole, praziquantel, metronidazole and diethylcarbamazine) and the antimalarial drug quinine have been assessed for their efficacy against gnathostomiasis both in animal studies and in humans, but failed to exhibit appreciable efficacy.

Currently, researchers focus on two widely used anthelminthics, albendazole and ivermectin. Poor absorption generally limits the deployment of albendazole for the treatment of tissue nematodes, but one clinical trial with this drug reported high cure rates in subcutaneous gnathostomiasis. The regimen of 400 mg once or twice daily for 3 weeks effectively reduced the frequency of symptoms and lowered eosinophil counts (Kraivichian et al., 1992). At present, there are insufficient data regarding its use in NG, although complete recovery was reported for some individuals treated with albendazole (Bunyaratavej et al., 2008; Germann et al., 2003). Ivermectin has been reported to be similarly effective as albendazole for the treatment of gnathostomiasis (Kraivichian et al., 2004; Nontasut et al., 2000, 2005). However, the sample sizes of previous studies involving ivermectin were small (17–21 subjects). Larger clinical trials assessing both efficacy and safety are needed. No obvious adverse events were reported but a potential issue is exacerbation of cutaneous symptoms. In a clinical trial, more patients treated with ivermectin than patients receiving albendazole experienced local skin reactions during the first week after drug administration (Kraivichian et al., 2004), raising concerns that ivermectin treatment of patients with ocular and CNS involvement might be unsafe (Herman and Chiodini, 2009).

Corticosteroids have been successfully used to prevent inflammation in cerebrospinal tissue due to angiostrongyliasis and neurocystercercosis

(Chotmongkol et al., 2000; García et al., 2002). One observational study involving gnathostomiasis patients failed to show conclusive results. The symptoms did not significantly improve in 118 out of 162 patients with NG after the administration of oral prednisolone at 40–60 mg daily or intravenous dexamethasone at 5 mg every 4–6 h (Punyagupta et al., 1990). This failure could be partially explained by the fact that irreversible mechanical injury such as tearing and destruction of the nerve tissue and its vascular structures is the major CNS damage caused by *Gnathostoma* spp. (Boongird et al., 1977).

12.3.5. Geographical distribution and epidemiology

Human gnathostomiasis mainly occurs in Southeast Asia, P.R. China, Japan, India, Mexico and Ecuador (Herman and Chiodini, 2009). The highest number of human cases are found in Japan, Thailand, Vietnam and Mexico, from where hundreds of infections are reported every year (Ogata et al., 1998; PAHO, 2003; Rojekittikhun, 2002a). In Japan, a total of 3225 cases were documented between 1911 and 2001, with a peak in the period 1941–1965 (Ando, 2005). No specific figures on human gnathostomiasis in Thailand are available, but the number of cases documented in some hospital-based surveys indicates the relatively common character of this parasite. Overall 528 patients were clinically diagnosed with gnathostomiasis in Siriraj Medical School Hospital during the period 1940–1945 (Rojekittikhun, 2005). Approximately 900 cases were diagnosed in Thailand in 1961, 1962 and 1963 (Rojekittikhun, 2002a). Annually, 300–600 gnathostomiasis patients were admitted to the Hospital for Tropical Diseases affiliated to Mahidol University during 1985–1988, and 100–400 new suspected cases were admitted to the same hospital yearly, starting in 1989 (Rojekittikhun, 2002a). Approximately 60 cases have been reported from the mainland of P.R. China. Since the parasite is highly prevalent among animals, it is conceivable that gnathostomiasis is underestimated in P.R. China, which can be attributed to the unavailability of immunological tests, as well as lack of awareness among clinicians.

The cutaneous form is predominant in human gnathostomiasis and CNS involvement is a rare entity. However, considerable numbers of NG have been found in Thailand. During a 3-year clinical observation in the mid-1960s, 162 patients were presumptively diagnosed with NG (Punyagupta et al., 1990). Similarly, a 5-year study in the early 1970s identified 24 patients with eosinophilic meningitis or radiculomyelitis probably caused by *G. spinigerum* (Boongird et al., 1977). Another 39 cases were reported from the same hospital during 1980–1985 (Schmutzhard et al., 1988). Interestingly, few cases of NG were reported outside Thailand. The following points are offered for consideration. First, thousands of gnathostomiasis cases have been identified in Thailand and thus the number of NG cases should far exceed those in other countries, despite the low frequency of CNS involvement. Second, *G. spinigerum* is the most common species responsible for human cases in Thailand. Compared to other species, *G. spinigerum* tends to migrate deeper into the skin and thus arguably has a higher chance of entering the spinal cord and brain (Ando, 2005; Rojekittikhun, 2005).

Gnathostoma is widely distributed throughout Southeast Asia and the Far East, but the locally predominant species differ between areas. Clearly, *G. spinigerum* is the most common species: about 51.7% of 120 parasitologically diagnosed patients were attributed to *G. spinigerum* in Japan, and all 20 patients from whom adult worms were recovered were parasitised by this species (Ando, 2005). In P.R. China, *G. spinigerum* accounts for approximately 95% of all reported cases. In Thailand, *G. spinigerum* is considered the only cause of human gnathostomiasis although five species have been documented in the country (Rojekittikhun, 2002a). *G. hispidum* and *G. doloresi* are mainly found in Japan and P.R. China. *G. nipponicum* is endemic in Japan. Another species, *G. malaysiae* is the suspected cause of human gnathostomiasis in Malaysia.

The life cycle of *Gnathostoma* spp. can involve numerous animals as intermediate and paratenic hosts, which complicates the route of human infection. In Thailand, for example, 48 vertebrate species were found naturally infected with L_3 of *G. spinigerum* (Rojekittikhun, 2005). Investigations of freshwater fish sold on markets in Thailand, Vietnam and Myanmar showed high *G. spinigerum* infection rates and intensities (Chai et al., 2003; Le and Rojekittikhun, 2000; Rojekittikhun et al., 2002, 2004; Saksirisampant et al., 2002; Sieu et al., 2009; Sugaroon and Wiwanitkit, 2003). Swamp eels (*Monopterus albus*) were identified as the most important host. Studies showed that the infection rate of swamp eels from Thai markets ranged from 10.7% to 44.1% (Rojekittikhun et al., 2002, 2004; Saksirisampant et al., 2002). The highest worm burden observed in one fish was 2583. In southern provinces of Vietnam, the monthly prevalence in swamp eels varied between 0.8% and 19.6% (Sieu et al., 2009). The highest incidence in Southeast Asian countries is associated with the rainy season (Le and Rojekittikhun, 2000; Maleewong et al., 1992; Sieu et al., 2009; Wiwanitkit, 2004). Snakehead fish is the leading source of infection in Japan where 603 cases were attributed to the consumption of this fish (Ando, 2005).

The exponential growth of aquaculture (Keiser and Utzinger, 2005) and the increasing share of freshwater fish produced in local aquaculture ponds across Eastern Asia places many people at risk of gnathostomiasis. The low host specificity means that humans can acquire the infection through a variety of food items, and increasing travelling puts individuals from non-endemic areas at risk of infection (Moore et al., 2003). The percentage of travellers infected with *Gnathostoma* spp. from non-endemic areas is growing (Gorgolas et al., 2003). Embracing local cultural habits, which includes consumption of local delicacies, has become an important trait for many travellers (Herman and Chiodini, 2009). It is therefore not surprising that outbreaks have occurred among non-native populations. Indeed, cases of human gnathostomiasis have been observed among Koreans living in Myanmar (Chai et al., 2003), although few local cases had been reported previously.

It should also be noted that the prevalence of *G. spinigerum* has declined in some regions. In Japan, for example, the prevalence dramatically decreased in the 1970s, and neither larvae nor adult worms from animals have been reported since 1980 (Ando, 2005). On the other hand, more and more gnathostomiasis cases involving other species were reported. Since 1979, a total of 119 human cases caused by *G. hispidum* have been found in Japan, with 75.6% being attributed to loaches imported from P.R. China (Ando, 2005). *G. nipponicum* is only endemic in Japan and, by 2005, a total of 26 human cases had been reported (Ando, 2005). *G. doloresi* has been found in humans only in southern Japan from where 45 cases have been reported (Ando, 2005). Additionally, *G. malaysiae* was found in a Japanese man who consumed raw freshwater shrimps in Myanmar (Nomura et al., 2000).

12.4. CYSTICERCOSIS

A detailed account of the epidemiology and control of *T. solium* cysticercosis/taeniasis is provided elsewhere in volume 72 of the *Advances in Parasitology* (Willingham et al., 2010). Hence, an attempt has been made here to shorten this contribution to a minimum to avoid excessive overlap.

12.4.1. Pathogen

Cysticercosis is caused by cysticerci (larvae) of the swine tapeworm *T. solium*. Cattle and swine tapeworms are among the few helminths already described in ancient times (Del Brutto et al., 1998). Symptoms due to the presence of adult worms in the human small intestine are usually mild, but cysticercosis is a serious disease, recognised in the report of a human case more than 400 years ago (Del Brutto et al., 1998). Differentiation of *T. solium* and *T. saginata* was accomplished in the middle of the nineteenth century (Grove, 1990). The public health importance of NC was emphasised by British scientists in the 1930s, who recognised the disease among soldiers returning from India (Wadia and Singh, 2002).

The life cycle of *T. solium* includes two hosts: humans are the only natural definitive host and pigs act as intermediate host. The adult worms parasitised the upper small intestine of humans and the gravid segments with the eggs are excreted in faeces. When ingested by pigs, the eggs hatch and oncospheres are liberated in their intestine. Oncospheres enter the bloodstream through the intestinal wall, settle in different organs and tissues and develop into cystic larvae (cysticercus). Cysts containing viable larvae are found mainly in skeletal muscles, subcutaneous tissue, eyes and the CNS (Graeff-Teixeira et al., 2009). The cysts reach their maximum size ($\sim$1 cm) within 2–3 months and seldom trigger obvious perilesional inflammation (García and Del Brutto, 2005). Upon ingestion by humans, live cysticerci develop into adult worms within 5–12 weeks (Muller, 2002).

Humans can also serve as accidental intermediate hosts for the parasite if *T. solium* eggs are ingested. The oncospheres penetrate the intestinal walls and are dispersed via the bloodstream throughout the human body. They develop into cysticerci but then usually die, followed by calcification. In immunologically privileged sites such as the CNS and the eyes (García and Del Brutto, 2005), cysticerci remain viable for several years and induce few inflammatory reactions in the surrounding tissues (Carpio, 2002). A lack of adequate sanitation and hygiene behaviour are considered key risk factors for environmental contamination with *T. solium* eggs, and hence drivers for human cysticercosis (García and Del Brutto, 2005). Recent epidemiological studies demonstrate clustering of NC patients around tapeworm carriers (Lescano et al., 2009; Sarti et al., 1994), suggesting direct human-to-human transmission. External and internal autoinfection has also been suggested; 5–50% of all *T. solium* carriers develop cysticercosis (Carpio, 2002) and a high taeniasis prevalence is found among patients with NC (Gilman et al., 2000).

12.4.2. Clinical manifestations

The typical neurological symptoms of NC result from cystic degeneration after a variable but often long incubation period (Carpio, 2002). Although the latent period of NC is difficult to determine, a study among British soldiers returning from India provided an estimate of several years (Mac Arthur, 1934). Symptomatic NC results from a combination of factors, including the amount, stage and location of cysticerci in the nervous system and the host's immune response (García and Del Brutto, 2005). NC can induce virtually any neurological symptoms but seizures (epilepsy) and symptoms related to intracranial hypertension are most commonly found (Del Brutto et al., 1992; Scharf, 1988; Sotelo et al., 1985). Seizures occur in 52–75% of all NC patients admitted to hospital (Guo et al., 2001; Sotelo et al., 1985; Wei et al., 1988; Zhang and Li, 1999), with higher rates among children (Sáenz et al., 2006; Singhi et al., 2000). NC has been recognised as a leading cause of acquired epilepsy (Senanayake and Roman, 1993). Generalised seizures or partial seizures with secondary generalisation are common in adults (Carpio, 2002; Del Brutto et al., 1992; Sotelo et al., 1985), while paediatric cases tend to present with partial seizures (Gogia et al., 2003; Murthy and Yangala, 2000; Ruiz-García et al., 1997; Singhi and Singhi, 2009; Singhi et al., 2000). Seizures generally occur in the degenerative phase of cysticerci due to an inflammatory reaction or in the calcification phase due to perilesional oedema, and can be accompanied by other neurologic symptoms. Most symptoms apart from seizures are transient or mild. For example, in a clinical observation of 1400 cases, 46.1% reported seizures as the initial symptom and 40.1% had seizures with no other symptoms observed (Wei et al., 1988).

Headache is commonly reported, probably as a result of increased intracranial pressure and meningitis. Intracranial hypertension usually causes more severe headache, whereas meningitis often results in moderate headache (Guo et al., 2001). Hydrocephalus secondary to chronic meningitis or ventricular cysticercosis is the main cause of intracranial hypertension (Sotelo et al., 1985; Wei et al., 1988), triggering headache, vomiting, diplopia, papilloedema and even intracranial herniation resulting in death. Compared to adult patients, a lower incidence of headache and intracranial hypertension is seen in children but seizures are more common (Sáenz et al., 2006); 18–32% of all paediatric cases reported headache and 15–32% mentioned vomiting/nausea (Gogia et al., 2003; Rosenfeld et al., 1996; Ruiz-García et al., 1997; Singhi et al., 2000). Less common symptoms in children include cranial nerve palsy, motor neurodeficit, papilloedema, altered mental status, learning disability and behavioural disturbance.

Epidemiological surveys suggest that only a small fraction of the infected population shows symptoms (Diaz et al., 1992; Fleury et al., 2003, 2006; Sanchez et al., 1999). The introduction of neuroimaging techniques such as CT and MRI has revealed a wide spectrum from mild infections in asymptomatic individuals and patients with sporadic seizures to heavy infection and high morbidity, thus changing the perception of NC from a fatal or severe disease to a more variable one (García and Del Brutto, 2005). Recently, several population-based surveys in hyperendemic areas showed that 7–9% of all asymptomatic residents presented one or several calcified intraparenchymal brain lesions in CT scanning (Fleury et al., 2003, 2006). Most asymptomatic cases identified by CT scan had single calcified lesions compatible with NC, probably due to low infection intensity and rapid death of the cysticercus caused by the host's immune system (García and Del Brutto, 2005).

12.4.3. Diagnosis

In the absence of highly sensitive and specific diagnostic assays, a set of diagnostic criteria for NC has been proposed, including epidemiological risk factors, typical symptoms, neuroimaging results and serological tests, as well as the results of trial therapy (Del Brutto et al., 2001). Living in, or frequent travel to endemic areas, is an important risk factor. Consumption of certain dishes, such as chicharrones in Latin America and pork lawar in Southeast Asia are risk factors for the disease (Fang, 2002; García et al., 1998; Ito et al., 2005). Although up to 50% of all seizures in developing countries may be linked to NC, many other causes must be considered in differential diagnosis (Senanayake and Roman, 1993). Non-invasive diagnostic techniques such as neuroimaging and immunoserological assays have greatly improved diagnosis (White, 2000). The images of lesions vary depending on the larval stages and examination techniques. MRI is more accurate than CT, but the latter is more widely available in low-income countries. The typical image of a viable cyst presents as a ''hole-with-dot'', with the scolex as a bright nodule within the cyst (Del Brutto et al., 2001). Degenerating cysts appear as contrast-enhancing rings or nodules surrounded by areas of brain oedema (García and Del Brutto, 2005). At this stage, the scolex is not usually seen but improved imaging techniques such as diffusion-weighted MRI may still visualise the scolex in degenerating cysts (García and Del Brutto, 2005). Calcified cysts appear as punctate hyperintense dots in CT scans, or as areas of subtracted signal in MRI visualizations.

A host of serological assays to detect specific antibodies have been developed. Recently, an enzyme-linked immunoelectrotransfer blot (EITB) with purified glycoprotein antigens has been confirmed to be sensitive if used on serum samples or CSF (Tsang et al., 1989; Wilson et al., 1991). An advantage of EITB is that its sensitivity in serum samples is equal to or higher than that in CSF samples (García et al., 1991). Although the reported specificity and sensitivity of EITB are 100% and 98%, a shortcoming is that ~30% of the patients with a single brain cysticercus may test negative (Prabhakaran et al., 2004). Serological assays may also fail to detect calcified cysts (Fleury et al., 2003; Schantz et al., 1994).

12.4.4. Treatment and clinical management

The treatment of NC is complicated by the evolving stage and location of the parasite. Interventions include anthelminthic drugs, anti-inflammatory drugs, antiepileptic drugs (AEDs) and surgery (Nash et al., 2006). Praziquantel and albendazole are most commonly used in the treatment of NC (Nash et al., 2006). Praziquantel shows satisfactory efficacy and is well tolerated at a dose of 50 mg/kg/day for 15 days (García et al., 2002). Regimens with variable doses and duration have also proven efficacious (Bittencourt et al., 1990). Albendazole was initially recommended at a dose of 15 mg/kg/day for 1 month (Sotelo et al., 1990). Subsequent studies showed that at the same doses, the treatment duration could be shortened to 1 week or even 3 days without compromising on efficacy (Del Brutto et al., 1992; Sotelo et al., 1988). A comparison between praziquantel and albendazole produced conflicting results, but albendazole appeared to be generally more efficacious than praziquantel (Sotelo et al., 1990). Current evidence favours anthelminthic therapy in patients with viable or degenerating cysts in the brain parenchyma or in the subarachnoidal space at the convexity of the cerebral hemispheres (Del Brutto et al., 2006). Thus far, the role of anthelminthic drugs in the management of ventricular cysts has not been adequately studied.

Corticosteroids as an anti-inflammatory agent are recommended in the treatment of active NC manifesting as encephalitis, angiitis or chronic meningitis, and if subarachnoidal cysts are present. Antiseizure treatment including AEDs is important for all epileptic patients (Nash et al., 2006), in addition to antiparasitic therapy which apparently also plays a role in reducing the frequency of seizures (Del Brutto et al., 1992; García et al., 2004). Many patients remain seizure-free while under AED treatment, but suffer relapses after drug discontinuation, indicating that the intracranial cysticerci are permanent substrates for seizures and may be re-activated when the inhibitory influence of AEDs is withdrawn (Nash et al., 2004). Prognostic factors associated with seizure recurrence include the development of parenchymal brain calcifications, and the presence of recurrent seizures and multiple brain cysts before the onset of therapy (Del Brutto, 1994).

Surgical treatment of NC has lost prominence, especially since the advent of efficacious, safe and inexpensive anthelminthic drugs. However, it still plays an important role in relieving acute intracranial hypertension secondary to ventricular cysticerci or single huge cysts (Colli et al., 1986). Shunt dysfunction is the main problem in these cases and thus shunt placement and cyst removal are the main interventions. However, shunt failure rates are high and secondary meningitis may occur (Colli et al., 1986, 2002). It was suggested that the failure rate might be lowered through concurrent administration of antiparasitic drugs or steroids (Del Brutto and Sotelo, 1990; Martinez et al., 1995; Suastegui Roman et al., 1996). Recently, less invasive procedures such as endoscopic resection have been used to remove ventricular cysts (Bergsneider, 1999; Cudlip et al., 1998; Neal, 1995), resulting in less sequelae than open surgery (Bergsneider et al., 2000).

12.4.5. Geographical distribution and epidemiology

T. solium infections including taeniasis and cysticercosis are a global public health problem. Highly endemic areas are located in Latin America, Asia (mainly P.R. China and India) and sub-Saharan Africa (Carpio, 2002). Cysticercosis is a common zoonotic infection in P.R. China where

T. solium infections have been reported from 29 provinces (Xu et al., 1999b). Most cases are clustered in the northeast (Heilongjiang, Jilin and Liaoning provinces), centre (Henan, Hebei and Shandong provinces) and southwest (Yunnan province and Guangxi Zhuang autonomous region) of the country. A systematic review suggests that the average prevalence of *T. solium* infection was 0.11% (range: 0.05–15%) in endemic areas, with an estimated total number of *T. solium* carriers of 1.26 million (Chen et al., 2004). The prevalence of cysticercosis ranged from 0.14% to 3.2% and the estimated number of cysticercosis cases was 3–6 millions (Chen et al., 2004). The second national survey on important human parasitic diseases carried out in P.R. China, between 2001 and 2004 indicated that the seroprevalence was 0.55% across all tested populations (Wang, 2008). Seropositives were found in 25 out of 31 provinces covered in this survey. A retrospective survey in the hospitals of 23 endemic provinces identified 11,196 cysticercosis inpatients during the period 1991–2001 (Wang, 2008). Yunnan, Hebei and Heilongjiang provinces accounted for 77.9% of all hospital cases, and NC was predominant with a prevalence of 91.0%.

Taeniasis and cysticercosis are moderately endemic in Southeast Asia (Carpio, 2002). In Indonesia, *T. solium* infections are limited to the non-Muslim population in north Sumatra, Bali and Irian Jaya (Simanjuntak et al., 1997). Up to 51% of all Christians and animists in some localities of Irian Jaya harboured *T. solium* (Margono et al., 2003). A recent community-based study on cysticercosis showed that 2.2% of the study participants had been exposed to *T. solium* in Malaysia (Noor Azian et al., 2006). Human cysticercosis is also endemic in northern Vietnam where 100–150 patients are admitted to specialised hospitals every year (Dorny et al., 2004). The seroprevalence of cysticercosis is less than 6% (Dorny et al., 2004; Erhart et al., 2002; Somers et al., 2006). About 0.2–7.2% of the residents harboured tapeworms (Willingham et al., 2003). In Thailand, the prevalence of taeniasis is lower than 1%, but in the north of the country, the prevalence can be as high as 5.9%. Since the mid-1960s, less than 500 cases were diagnosed in Thailand. Immunoserological assays revealed a higher prevalence of cysticercosis, but *T. saginata* was the dominant *Taenia* species in the country (Waikagul et al., 2006). In Lao People's Democratic Republic (Lao PDR), several surveys conducted over the past 20 years found a prevalence of human taeniasis ranging from 0% to 14.0% (Conlan et al., 2008). Few data regarding *T. solium* infection in human populations are available from Cambodia and Myanmar.

Human cysticercosis has been identified as an eradicable parasitic disease, but current global efforts are unsatisfactory, and hence control, let alone local elimination and eradication, will be difficult to achieve in the near future (Pawlowski et al., 2005). In P.R. China, *T. solium* infection was listed as a national priority for control as early as 1956 (Xu et al., 1999a). Nationwide control programmes, including stricter meat inspection and improving sanitary conditions, were implemented in the following decades. Today, 200,000 tons of pork meat are rejected each year due to cysticerci, an annual loss of 1 billion Chinese Yuan (about US$ 121 million) (Ito et al., 2003). However, the situation in many rural areas has not markedly changed with pigs raised and slaughtered under traditional husbandry practices. This is especially true in remote areas with little transportation infrastructure (Steinmann et al., 2007). Consumption of raw pork is closely associated with the endemicity of *T. solium*. For example, up to 80% of all raw pork bought on local markets was used to prepare the local favourite dish "shengpi" of thin-sliced raw pork in some villages of Dali prefecture in P.R. China (Fang et al., 1995). In some rural areas of southwest P.R. China, latrines are uncommon and pigs roam freely (Steinmann et al., 2008), conditions facilitating the transmission of *T. solium* between humans and pigs. In other areas, latrines are available but fresh human faeces are used to fertilize crops ("night soil") (Willingham et al., 2003). Indeed, *Taenia* eggs have been recovered from a variety of vegetables and fruits available in local markets in endemic areas (Kozan et al., 2005). Thus, improving sanitary conditions, pig husbandry practices, meat inspection and health education is considered decisive for breaking the transmission cycle and to render cysticercosis control sustainable.

12.5. SPARGANOSIS

12.5.1. Pathogen

Human sparganosis is caused by the sparganum of *Spirometra* spp. Human ocular sparganosis was described in the book "Compendium of Medical Herbs" as early as 1596. The first case of *Spirometra mansoni* was isolated as a sparganum from a man in P.R. China in 1882. The adult *Spirometra mansoni* was first described in 1929, when adult worms were successfully isolated from the intestines of experimentally infected animals (Faust et al., 1929). Six years later, Mueller discovered a similar species in Syracuse cats in the United States and temporarily named it *Diphyllobothrium mansonoides* (Mueller, 1935). Subsequent studies showed that this species was morphologically different from *Spirometra mansoni* and variations in its life history were noted, leading to the establishment of a new species, *Spirometra mansonoides* (Mueller, 1935, 1974). Their pathogenicities are similar and, today, they are considered to be responsible for most human sparganosis cases in Asia and the Americas, respectively (Holodniy et al., 1991). In 1918, Takeuchi reported the first case of neurosparganosis (NSP) (Takeuchi, 1918). It is estimated that 3.2% of all patients develop NSP (Wu, 2005).

The life cycle of *Spirometra* is complex and involves three hosts. Adult worms dwell in the intestine of carnivores such as cats and dogs. Their eggs are passed in the faeces and hatch in freshwater, releasing L_1, the coracidia. These larvae are consumed by *Cyclops* spp. (the first intermediate host), in which they develop into L_2, the procercoids. When infected *Cyclops* spp. are consumed by a second intermediate host such as frogs, the larvae penetrate the bowel wall of the new host and migrate to various organs and tissues where procercoids develop into spargana. A variety of paratenic hosts are known; many amphibians, reptiles and even mammals were found to be naturally infected with spargana. It proved difficult to identify their route of infection and both ingestion of *Cyclops* and preying on frogs have been proposed. Once the second intermediate host or paratenic host is consumed by a cat or dog, the spargana develop into adult tapeworms in their intestine within approximately 3 weeks. Adult worms then live for up to 3–4 years.

Humans can become accidental definitive hosts, second intermediate hosts or paratenic hosts. Adult worms parasitising the intestine of humans are rare and result in few health problems. However, spargana can invade any organs or tissues and thus are medically more significant. The migration route of spargana to the CNS is not known but a sparganum may accidentally migrate through the foramina of the skull base and vertebral column along the loose connective tissue surrounding vessels and nerves. Humans are infected in three main ways; firstly, by drinking water containing infected *Cyclops* spp.; secondly, by ingesting the flesh of second intermediate or paratenic hosts harbouring spargana, usually in the form of raw or undercooked meat; and thirdly, by applying the flesh or skin of infected intermediate hosts as a poultice to an open wound, whereby the sparganum can directly invade human tissues. Other transmission routes are rare. Ocular sparganosis may be attributable to direct contact with contaminated water (Leon et al., 1972) and trans-placental infection has also been hypothesised (Chen, 1983).

12.5.2. Clinical manifestations

The incubation period of NSP is variable but generally long. Two studies on NSP indicate an incubation period between 1 and 30 years (Kim et al., 1996; Song et al., 2007). However, estimating the incubation period is difficult since the exposure to the parasite can often not be identified. The incubation period of subcutaneous sparganosis is easier to determine because of the obvious migrating swellings. It is estimated to range between 1 day and several months (Chen et al., 2002; Huang, 2003; Lin et al., 2002).

Clinical manifestations of NSP depend on the regions involved. Seizures, hemiparesis and headache are the most common symptoms.

Approximately 84% of all patients with NSP experience a long history of seizures (Chang et al., 1992). The duration of symptoms is variable, ranging from 2 weeks to 24 years (median: 36 months) (Kim et al., 1996). Most patients present with generalised tonic convulsion, followed by motor weakness of the extremities. Long-term clinical manifestations often tend to be associated with generalised cognitive dysfunction and generalised degenerative changes in white matter, suggesting a chronic progressive inflammatory disease (Kim et al., 1996). Interestingly, NSP and subcutaneous swelling seldom occur simultaneously, which is probably linked with the observation that humans are usually infected by only one or a few spargana. Death is a rare outcome of NSP but can occur in the absence of appropriate treatment.

Involvement of the spinal cord is less frequent than cerebral manifestations. Symptoms depend on the location of the lesions; a typical clinical picture is back pain followed by progressive weakness of lower limbs (Fung et al., 1989; Kudesia et al., 1998; Liu, 2006; Wu et al., 1990). At an early stage, patients may experience repeated light fever for several months (Fung et al., 1989; Kudesia et al., 1998). Incontinence is not unusual in spinal sparganosis (Fung et al., 1989; Liu, 2006; Wu et al., 1990). At a later stage, patients may suffer from degeneration or loss of sensation such as pain and temperature in affected regions (Fung et al., 1989; Zhao et al., 1998).

12.5.3. Diagnosis

The definitive diagnosis of NSP is based on the discovery of a sparganum in the brain or spinal cord. In most cases, parasites are found during surgery or upon autopsy. Preoperative diagnosis of NSP can be made based on a combination of factors such as exposure history, clinical manifestations and findings from physical examination and laboratory tests. Although the exposure is complex, some specific behavioural traits are indicative (e.g. eating raw frogs, tadpoles and snakes or drinking snake bile and blood). These risk factors are present in some populations in the Far East and Southeast Asia, as is the practice of applying poultices made of frog flesh to open wounds.

There are no specific neurological symptoms indicative of NSP. Headaches, seizures, paraesthesia, hemiparesis and homonymous hemianopsia have been reported and depend upon the location of the worms as well as the amount of granulation tissue. Cytological examinations are usually normal. Eosinophilia is not always present in NSP, probably because most patients experience a long illness course and degenerated worms are enclosed by inflammatory granuloma. The neuroimaging findings are not specific but still provide important information. CT characteristics of NSP include (i) unilateral involvement; (ii) extensive or multifocal areas of low density along white matter fascicles, with ipsilateral ventricular dilatation and localised cortical atrophy; (iii) nodular or irregular enhancement with spotty calcification; and (iv) change in the location of enhancing nodules on sequential scans (Chang et al., 1992). Recent studies showed that MRI (particularly contrast enhancement MRI) was superior to CT. The most important findings were the tunnel sign and multiple conglomerated ring or bead-shaped enhancements on MRI (Song et al., 2007).

Immunological assays for NSP have been developed and ELISA detecting sparganum-specific IgG antibodies have been widely used. Kim et al. (1984) reported the performance of serum ELISA for diagnosing individual patients. The study showed high sensitivity and specificity (100% and 95.7%, respectively), but there was cross-reactivity between *Spirometra* spp. and *Taenia* spp. Recent studies confirmed the value of immunological assays for diagnosis and showed that there was an agreement between serum- and CSF-derived antibodies (Chang et al., 1987; Kim et al., 1996; Song et al., 2007).

NSP is difficult to distinguish from brain tumours based on symptoms and neuroradiological findings. The majority of all patients are misdiagnosed as having a metastatic brain tumour (Fung et al., 1989). NSP should be considered whenever a patient has an unusual history incompatible with brain tumour, especially in sparganosis-endemic areas. Metastatic brain tumours often have a mass effect and compress the ventricle, while sparganosis seldom has a mass effect but is associated with adjacent ventricular dilation. Additionally, sparganosis shows the unique image of tunnel sign on post-contrast MRI (Song et al., 2007). Diagnosis can be complicated by larval migration (Eom and Kim, 2009; Kim et al., 2007) and the proliferative form (Lo et al., 1987).

12.5.4. Treatment and clinical management

To our knowledge, there is no treatment available against sparganosis and, thus far, no systematic evaluation of anthelminthic drugs has been performed. Anecdotal clinical data indicate that praziquantel was unable to kill live larvae or otherwise benefit patients who had not undergone surgery (Kim et al., 1996). Hence, surgery is the only option to improve the condition of patients with NSP. A prospective study showed that fair to excellent outcomes could be expected for patients from whom live worms or granuloma with degenerative worms had been completely removed. Improvement was only poor in patients who did not receive surgical removal and those in whom a granuloma with a degenerating worm had been incompletely removed (Kim et al., 1996).

12.5.5. Geographical distribution and epidemiology

Over 1400 human sparganosis cases have been reported from at least 39 countries (Qiu and Qiu, 2009), including imported cases related to international travel and migration. On a global scale, most cases are reported from the Far East, including P.R. China, Japan and the Republic of Korea (Korea) where *Spirometra mansoni* is endemic. Before 1998, 632 cases had been documented in P.R. China (Xu et al., 1999b), and over 100 cases were reported in the following years (Wu et al., 2007). Some 470 cases have been described in Japan (Kimura et al., 2003). A literature review documented 63 cases in Korea during the period 1917–1971 (Cho et al., 1975), and many sporadic cases have been reported thereafter. Southeast Asia is moderately endemic. Thirty-four cases have been described in Thailand (Wiwanitkit, 2005), and several cases have been reported from Indonesia, where the causative agent might be a species other than *Spirometra mansoni* (Margono et al., 2007). Only a few cases of sparganosis were reported from Vietnam, but case reports among Vietnamese emigrants and a deeply rooted tradition of eating frogs suggest the disease is endemic (Vortel et al., 1995).

NSP is uncommon; only five cases were identified among 34 sparganosis patients in Thailand (Wiwanitkit, 2005). Two out of 63 cases presented with spinal lesions in Korea (Cho et al., 1975). Less than 5% (18/542) of all cases in the mainland of P.R. China showed CNS involvement (Xu et al., 1999b). Recently, the number of reported CNS sparganosis increased in P.R. China (Wu et al., 2007), perhaps explained by advanced diagnostic tools that are more likely to reveal helminths in the CNS. Indeed, along with the wider application of non-invasive neuroimaging techniques such as CT and MRI, more accurate diagnosis of intracranial helminth infections has become possible (Song et al., 2007; White, 2000). However, a real increase in the number of NSP cannot be ruled out and might be associated with shifts in dietary habits and the involvement of new host species.

Consumption of frogs and snakes are recognised risk factors, but infections due to other animals may be under-diagnosed. *Spirometra mansoni* in pigs is not uncommon in P.R. China, with infections reported from at least 12 provinces (Wu, 2005). *Spirometra mansoni* is found in frogs from both tropical and temperate regions in P.R. China. The natural infection rate is variable, ranging from 3.2% to 100% (Qiu and Qiu, 2009), with an average sparganum burden of 2–7 per frog. Several frog species are important intermediate hosts, but the predominant species differs between locations. For example, *Rana nigromaculata* is the main host in western Guangdong province (Li et al., 2009), whereas *R. limnecha* is the predominant intermediate host in Fujian province (Wu and Lin, 2001). Frogs sold on local markets were also found to be infected. Recent investigations showed infection rates of 58.4–66.5% among frogs in markets in Guangzhou (Qi et al., 2008; Wu et al., 1997), 18.7% in Guiyang and 17.5%

in Ningbo (Wu et al., 2007; Ye et al., 2005). Snakes are an other important sources of infection. Since snakes prey on frogs, the infection rate among snakes is high. For instance, individuals of all seven snake species examined in a survey were infected by this parasite and the overall prevalence was 47.6% (Huang et al., 1990).

Social and economic development is impacting on risk factors, and hence the distribution of sparganosis. Enhanced access to clean water lowers the risk of infection, and consumption of raw tadpoles and frogs for medical purposes or applying frog flesh poultice to open wounds has lost in popularity with the availability of western medicine. However, in some rural and mountainous areas, beliefs prevail that frogs and tadpoles can treat some illnesses such as skin or oral ulcer, fever and open wounds (Qiu and Qiu, 2009). A recent clinical observation showed that all 13 sparganosis patients from Henan province in central P.R. China had acquired their infection by eating live tadpoles; the average number of tadpoles eaten by individual patients was 96 (range: 6–300) (Lin et al., 2008). Among them were 10 cases aged less than 12 years. A subsequent survey revealed that 36.6% (145/396) of the habitants of a single village had eaten live tadpoles as a local remedy to cure illnesses (Lin et al., 2008). A review of 378 human sparganosis cases in 1994 showed that 54.0% of the patients had applied frog flesh poultice (Zhao, 1994). The percentage dropped to 19.2% in 2007 (Wu et al., 2007). Contrasting with the use of frogs in traditional medicine, the consumption of frogs and snakes appears to be increasingly popular, although they are usually adequately cooked. A recent review showed that 34.6% of 104 sparganosis patients from P.R. China had a history of eating frogs or snakes (Wu et al., 2007). New risk factors have been described; consumption of raw snake blood and snake bile is increasingly popular in some areas and several cases of sparganosis were attributed to this behaviour (Lin et al., 2003a).

12.6. PARAGONIMIASIS

Comprehensive reviews pertaining to the epidemiology, clinical manifestations and control of food-borne trematodiases, including paragonimiasis, are available (Keiser and Utzinger, 2009; Sripa et al., 2010). Hence, the current section is kept as short as possible.

12.6.1. Pathogen

Pulmonary paragonimiasis is caused by adult *Paragonimus* worms, whereas cerebrospinal involvement can occur during worm migration. More than 50 species and subspecies of *Paragonimus* have been described (Blair et al., 1999), eight of which are major causes of human paragonimiasis (Murrell and Fried, 2007). Five species, namely *P. westermani*, *P. heterotremus*, *P. miyazakii*, *P. ohirai* and *P. skrjabini*, are endemic in Southeast Asia and the Far East. The most important species is *P. westermani*. The first case of neuroparagonimiasis (NP) was described in 1887 after two adult worms were recovered from the brain of a patient (Oh, 1968a). The percentage of NP relative to the total number of paragonimiasis cases varies between different areas. In P.R. China, the percentage among hospitalised patients ranged from 9.8% to 19.7% (Zhao, 1994).

Details of the life cycle of *Paragonimus* spp. have been described elsewhere (Keiser and Utzinger, 2009; Sripa et al., 2010). In brief, adult worms live encapsulated in the lungs of mammals (e.g. humans, cats and dogs). The eggs are deposited into bronchial secretions and eliminated via sputum or swallowed and excreted in faeces. Miracidia are released after 2 weeks of embryonation once eggs have reached freshwater bodies. Larvae penetrate the first intermediate host snail (*Melania* spp.), and ultimately develop into cercariae. Crustaceans (e.g. crabs and crayfish) serve as second intermediate hosts, which become infected via direct penetration of cercariae or ingestion of infected mollusks. Cercariae then encyst and develop into metacercariae. Mammals acquire an infection through consumption of infected crustaceans that are not or insufficiently cooked. Metacercariae excyst in the small intestine and migrate through the intestinal wall to reach the abdominal cavity, enter the abdominal wall, and migrate to the pleural cavity. Typically, two maturing worms pair in the pleural cavity and move into the parenchyma of the lungs where a fibrous cyst develops and then mate and produce eggs.

Unlike in the case of angiostrongyliasis, gnathostomiasis, cysticercosis and sparganosis, humans are permissive definitive hosts for *Paragonimus* and worms migrate along a mostly defined route to their final destination, the lung. NP develops if worms accidentally migrate through the soft tissues along the vessels of the neck and via the jugular foramen into the CNS (Oh, 1968a).

12.6.2. Clinical manifestations

Pulmonary symptoms usually appear after an incubation period of at least 11 days and up to 6 weeks (Cui et al., 1998; Owatari et al., 1994). Cerebral involvement is not common in paragonimiasis and determining the incubation period of NP proved difficult, not least due to frequent exposure in endemic areas. A series of studies on paediatric patients indicates that the incubation period ranges from 1 month to 3 years (Cheng, 2004; Dai, 1997; Yin, 1997).

NP may present with a number of different symptoms, including eosinophilic meningitis, arachnoiditis, mass lesions, visual disturbances and seizures. Most patients experience an insidious onset of symptoms, but a few suffer from acute meningitis (Li et al., 1996; Yin, 1997). About one-third of the NP patients report a history of meningitis, usually mild, transient and self-limiting (Oh, 1968a). The predominant manifestations are fever, headache and vomiting, as well as neck stiffness and Kernig's sign. The duration of meningitis is variable from 3 days to 15 weeks. Interestingly, 45% of patients with recurrent meningitis recovered spontaneously. Some patients may only present discrete headache (Li et al., 1996). Seizures are common and found in 16–87.8% of patients with NP (Cheng, 2004; Dai, 1997; Huang, 2000; Li et al., 1996). Other symptoms include visual disturbances, motor weakness and sensory disturbance. Ophthalmologic involvement was reported in three-quarters of these patients and hemiparesis, hemihypaesthesia and menigeal signs were also found. Another frequent finding is a worsened mental status. Specific disturbances include personality changes, a decline in intellectual function, disorientation and depressed consciousness. A declining mental status was seen in approximately 70% of all patients (Kusner and King, 1993).

The average incidence of spinal paragonimiasis in CNS infections ranges from 2.9% to 13.3% (Moon et al., 1964; Oh, 1968b, 1969). The typical clinical picture of spinal paragonimiasis is a long history of coughing and rusty sputum, followed by radicular pain. Subsequently, patients experience progressive motor weakness and sensory loss in the lower extremities and often urinary and faecal incontinence.

12.6.3. Diagnosis

NP patients show both neurological and pulmonary symptoms, with the former preceding the latter in one-third of the patients (Oh, 1968a). Thus, a history of pulmonary paragonimiasis (i.e. coughing and rusty sputum) is indicative for NP. Common symptoms such as seizures and progressive weakness in the extremities are additional useful indicators. While consumption of freshwater or land crabs and crayfish is common worldwide, specific risk factors such as eating "drunk" crabs and using crab juice are important for differential diagnosis at a local scale. The definitive diagnosis of paragonimiasis relies on the discovery of the worm during biopsy or its eggs in sputum or faeces. However, the diagnosis of NP is difficult since many patients do not present active pulmonary manifestations at the time of hospital admission (Higashi et al., 1971; Oh, 1968a). Eosinophilia in peripheral blood has limited value in the diagnosis of NP because only 43.8–62.5% of the patients present eosinophilia, mainly at the acute stage involving meningitis and in pulmonary paragonimiasis (Moon et al., 1964; Oh, 1968a). The eosinophil cell count in the CSF can be elevated when acute meningitis occurs, but it is usually unchanged in the case of chronic meningitis or single spinal involvement (Higashi et al., 1971; Moon et al., 1964; Oh, 1968a,b).

Several immunologic assays and gene probes have been developed and are considered equivalent or even better than microscopic detection of parasite eggs (Maleewong, 1997). Today, imaging techniques play an important role for diagnosis. X-ray and more recently CT and MRI have been used, and findings of clustered ring-enhancing lesions, seen in approximately half of all early cerebral paragonimiasis cases, are suggestive of NP (Cha et al., 1994).

The diagnosis of NP is complicated by the presence of pulmonary changes due to tuberculosis (de Leon and Piad, 2005; Doanh et al., 2005) and NP can be confused with tuberculosis meningitis (Sharma, 2005). Distinguishing features are the acute onset and relatively mild nature of *Paragonimus* meningitis, compared to the gradual onset and more severe neurologic deficits seen in tuberculosis meningitis. Analysis of CSF shows an elevated cell count, increased pressure and elevated protein in 75% of the cases, and a depressed glucose level in 55%. Of note, in 80% of all NP patients, eosinophils constituted between 5% and 90% of the total CSF leukocytes.

12.6.4. Treatment and clinical management

Cerebrospinal involvement is rare and usually accompanied by pulmonary paragonimiasis. Although the mechanism of cerebrospinal involvement is unknown, treatment of pulmonary paragonimiasis should be an integral part of treating NP. Chemotherapy using praziquantel and triclabendazole has been recommended by WHO and is reviewed elsewhere in this thematic volume of the *Advances in Parasitology* (Keiser and Utzinger, 2010). In brief, recommended treatment regimens of praziquantel are either 25 mg/kg/day for 2 consecutive days or a single 40 mg/kg oral dose. Triclabendazole is recommended at a dose of 20 mg/kg/day in two divided doses given on 1 day. At present, triclabendazole is only registered in few countries, but efforts are underway by WHO to make the drug more widely available (Keiser and Utzinger, 2009). Bithionol had been widely used before praziquantel became available but cure rates are low-to-moderate (50–60%) and adverse events are common (Chen et al., 2001).

Surgical removal of the cysts or granulomas is the treatment of choice for NP, resulting in moderate to marked improvement (Moon et al., 1964). Treatment failure may occur if cysts and affected tissues are incompletely removed or diffuse atrophy of the cord is present (Higashi et al., 1971; Moon et al., 1964). Recurrence due to persisting *Paragonimus* infection has also been reported (Kusner and King, 1993). Thus, an integrated approach combining surgery and chemotherapy is indicated. Triclabendazole is currently recommended for NP but praziquantel and bithionol had also been successfully used (Moon et al., 1964; Oh, 1968a). There is evidence indicating that therapy results in worsened symptoms due to the death of parasites and increased local inflammation. Therefore, corticosteroids may be required during treatment to decrease inflammation and oedema formation at the site of the lesion (Kusner and King, 1993).

12.6.5. Geographical distribution and epidemiology

Recent estimates put the number of people at risk of paragonimiasis at 293 million, and the number of infections at more than 20 million (Keiser and Utzinger, 2005, 2009). Approximately two-thirds of the infections are concentrated in P.R. China. A systematic literature review identified 23,703 cases in P.R. China before 1999, and a prevalence of 4.2% (452/10,692) for NP (Xu et al., 1999b). The recent national parasitological survey found a seroprevalence of 1.7% (Wang, 2008). In the 1950s, paragonimiasis was highly endemic in Japan; an extensive seroepidemiological survey indicated that the disease was endemic throughout the country with the exception of Hokkaido, the northernmost island. In subsequent decades, the seroprevalence steadily declined but the parasite has re-emerged in recent years (Nawa and Nakamura-Uchiyama, 2005). A similar situation is reported from Korea. It was estimated that more than 2 million people were infected in the late 1960s, as determined by intradermal tests, and about 40% of them were egg-positive (Cho et al., 1997). Along with socioeconomic development and environmental changes, the prevalence sharply declined in the 1990s. In recent years, approximately 100 cases were diagnosed annually by an ELISA test undertaken for clinical differentiation from tuberculosis.

Several studies have confirmed that paragonimiasis is endemic in at least seven provinces in northwest Vietnam (De et al., 2000; Doanh et al., 2005; Queuche et al., 1997; Vien et al., 1997). The prevalence among residents ranged from 0.2% to 15% (De et al., 2000; Doanh et al., 2005; Queuche et al., 1997). The egg-positive rate in sputum was as high as 28.4% among individuals reporting chronic coughing (Queuche et al., 1997). In Thailand, the prevalence of paragonimiasis has decreased over the past 2–3 decades. A recent study found that the egg-positive rate in sputum and stool declined from 6% and 1% in 1985 respectively to zero in 2005 (Yoonuan et al., 2008). However, the parasite infection among mountain crabs increased from 21.0% in 1985 to 35.9% in 2005 (Yoonuan et al., 2008). In the Philippines, the endemicity of paragonimiasis is currently unknown (de Leon and Piad, 2005). Previous studies showed that the parasite is endemic in the south of the country; eggs of *P. westermani* were frequently detected in sputum samples of "tuberculosis" patients, especially among "drug resistant" cases. Between 11.6% and 45% of all tuberculosis patients or residents with chronic cough excreted *Paragonimus* eggs (Belizario et al., 1997; de Leon and Piad, 2005).

NP accounts for a small fraction of all *Paragonimus* infections. The recent national sampling survey in P.R. China identified 215 paragonimiasis cases from sampled hospitals among whom 24 showed CNS involvement (Wang, 2008). The percentage can reach 33.7% among hospitalised paragonimiasis cases in highly endemic areas; between 1979 and 1994, a total of 315 cases with paragonimiasis were found in three hospitals in Zhejiang province, and 106 patients suffered from CNS involvement (Li et al., 1996). A review of all 164 children hospitalised with paragonimiasis between 1975 and 1989 in a mountainous area of Hubei province found that 23.1% of them had developed NP (Zhang, 1990). In a similar study, 21.8% of 280 paediatric patients hospitalised between 1986 and 2006 suffered from CNS involvement (Li et al., 2008). In Vietnam, cerebrospinal involvement in human paragonimiasis occurred at a frequency of 1.3–8% (De et al., 2000; Queuche et al., 1997). Following the decline in *Paragonimus* infections, NP now is rare in Korea and Japan, while at the beginning of 1966 it had been estimated that about 5000 cases of NP existed in Korea (Oh, 1968a).

In P.R. China, *P. westermani* and *P. skrjabini* are the two most common pathogens causing paragonimiasis. Whilst *P. westermani* is the predominant species in the northeast and east of the country, *P. skrjabini* is endemic in the centre and south (Wu, 2005). The difference between *P. westermani* and *P. skrjabini* with regard to CNS involvement is not known, but it has been suggested that since the latter species usually migrates in subcutaneous tissue and viscera, it is more likely to involve the CNS (Wu, 2005). In Vietnam, at least four species have been found, but *P. heterotremus* was the most common one (Doanh et al., 2005, 2008). Although adult worms have never been isolated from patients thus far, human paragonimiasis in the country is assumed to be caused by *P. heterotremus*, since the morphology of the eggs in the sputum of some patients was suggestive of this species and metacercariae of this species are most frequently found in crabs commonly eaten in some areas (Doanh et al., 2005). In Thailand, six species have been identified in at least 23 provinces, but only *P. heterotremus* has been confirmed in humans (Waikagul and Yoonuan, 2005). In the Philippines, *P. westermani* is the predominant species (de Leon and Piad, 2005).

The prevalence of paragonimiasis is generally declining in the Far East and Southeast Asia. However, several factors potentially complicate the current situation. First, international travel, population movement and trade were linked to case reports outside traditional endemic areas. This is particularly obvious in P.R. China where many infections are diagnosed in non-endemic areas among migrant labour communities. An outbreak due to the consumption of raw crabs imported from Korea affected more than 600 individuals in a Chinese border city (Kang et al., 2002). Second, additional paratenic animals are recognised as a source of infection. For example, paragonimiasis is re-emerging in Japan due to the consumption of raw wild boar meat (Uchiyama et al., 1999). Traditional eating habits are difficult to change. Barbecued crabs are believed to be an important source of infection for children in rural areas, especially in Vietnam and P.R. China (Doanh et al., 2005). Dishes such as drunk crab (P.R. China), soybean sauce-soaked crabs (Korea and P.R. China) and crab juice (Japan and Vietnam) are common routes of infection for adults. Health education targeting eating habits plays an important role in the control of this infection but struggles to succeed wherever people are accustomed to these dishes. Environmental change has been highlighted as an alternative way to decrease the prevalence of paragonimiasis. Many surveys documented a decline in intermediate host densities and in their prevalence of infection (Cho et al., 1997; Xu and Mao, 2002).

12.7. SCHISTOSOMIASIS

12.7.1. Pathogen

Human schistosomiasis is caused by five different *Schistosoma* species, namely *S. haematobium*, *S. intercalatum*, *S. japonicum*, *S. mansoni* and *S. mekongi*. The two species that are endemic in Southeast Asia and the Far East are *S. japonicum* and *S. mekongi*. Detailed reviews are available elsewhere in this thematic volume of the *Advances in Parasitology* (Muth et al., 2010; Zhou et al., 2010). In brief, *S. japonicum* in P.R. China has a documented history of over two millennia. The first parasitologically diagnosed case was described in 1888 in Japan (Grove, 1990). *S. mekongi*, previously considered an *S. japonicum*-like parasite, was first described in 1957 and firmly established in 1978 (Grove, 1990). Neuroschistosomiasis (NS) occurs when eggs end up in the CNS. The first report of NS was provided in an autopsy report by Yamagiwa in 1889 (Mitsuno, 1955). Approximately 2% of all patients with acute schistosomiasis japonica have CNS complications (Jaureguiberry and Caumes, 2008), but a higher percentage is observed in chronic and advanced stages with portal hypertension (Liu, 1993; Pittella, 1997). Only few NS cases due to *S. mekongi* have been reported (Carmody et al., 2008; Houston et al., 2004).

For a detailed description of the life cycle of *S. japonicum* and *S. mekongi*, the reader is referred to recent reviews (Ross et al., 2002; Utzinger et al., 2005; Zhou et al., 2010). In brief, male and female schistosomes pair, with the male holding the longer and thinner female in its body groove, and live in the mesenteric venous plexus of humans and mammals. Eggs must cross the intestinal wall and 25–30% of all eggs are excreted in faeces while the others are trapped in the intestinal and vesical walls or carried to the liver and other organs via the portal circulation (Pittella, 1997). Larvae hatch when eggs reach freshwater bodies, releasing miracidia that penetrate the intermediate host snail, *Oncomelania* spp. for *S. japonicum* and *Neotricula aperta* for *S. mekongi*. Within 4–6 weeks, cercariae are released by the snail and actively seek a suitable definitive host (Gryseels et al., 2006). Immediately after skin penetration, the cercariae transform into schistosomula and reach the lungs via the circulation system. The schistosomula pass through the lungs and finally enter the portal system via the left heart. The adult worms pair and reach the mucosal branches of the inferior mesenteric and superior haemorrhoidal veins where the females start oviposition. The latent period in humans varies between 29 and 42 days for *S. japonicum* (Pittella, 1997).

Humans are permissive definitive hosts for both *S. japonicum* and *S. mekongi*. Eggs can accidentally end up in the CNS, but the route by which eggs enter the CNS is not clear. The most plausible route is via the retrograde abdominal venous flow to the veins of the spinal cord and brain through the valveless venous plexus of Batson (Liu, 1993). Alternatively, the eggs might enter the pulmonary or portal-pulmonary arteriovenous shunts in advanced hepatosplenic and cardiopulmonary schistosomiasis and then be carried to the CNS via the arterial system. Clusters of eggs in the brain parenchyma suggest that migration of adult worms to the spinal cord or cerebral veins followed by direct oviposition is another possible route, although adult worms have seldom been found in close proximity to the brain and spinal cord.

12.7.2. Clinical manifestations

The clinical manifestations of schistosomiasis vary depending on the developmental stage of the parasite. The typical signs and symptoms consistent with Katayama syndrome usually appear 2–12 weeks post-infection (Ross et al., 2007). The syndrome is characterised by non-specific signs and symptoms, such as fever, fatigue, myalgia, malaise, urticaria and non-productive cough. Eosinophilia in peripheral blood and patchy pulmonary infiltrates on chest radiographs are frequently detected. The symptoms of schistosomiasis japonica usually appear about 42 days after the first exposure or a re-infection or superinfection (Ross et al., 2001). The incubation period of neurological symptoms among a series of 42 patients with cerebral schistosomiasis japonica varied from 6 months to 9 years with an average of 2.3 years (Torres, 1965).

CNS involvement in schistosomiasis japonica can occur during or immediately after the acute phase of Katayama syndrome, or in an inapparent acute form without obvious systemic manifestations (Pittella, 1997). On the first occasion, usually accompanied by cerebral vasculitis

(Carod-Artal, 2008; Jaureguiberry and Caumes, 2008), the main neurological features are diffuse encephalitis and/or meningitis including headache, vomiting, speech disturbances, disorientation, visual abnormality, urinary incontinence, ataxia, motor deficit usually manifested as hemiplegia, hemiparesis or quadriplegia and even coma (Pittella, 1997). Some of these symptoms are transient and disappear within a few days or weeks. The tumoral form occurs more insidiously (Pittella, 1997). The resulting symptoms are related to increased intracranial pressure and a focal mass effect. Seizures accompanied by the loss of consciousness are the most frequently observed neurological symptoms in this form (Jing et al., 2007; Pittella, 1997). Additionally, headache, visual abnormality, sensory disturbance, papilloedema, hemiparesis and dysphasia are commonly observed (Jing et al., 2007).

The location of schistosome eggs in the CNS depends on the species. While the eggs of *S. japonicum* tend to accumulate in the brain, those of *S. mansoni* and *S. haematobium* usually reach the lower spinal cord (Liu, 1993). Therefore, the spinal form is relatively rare in Eastern Asia. Myelopathy includes granulomatous masses and transverse myelitis, which mainly involve the lower spinal cord (Jiang et al., 2008; Wan et al., 2006; Wang, 1984). The characteristic clinical picture is an initial burning pain radiating from the thoracolumbar region towards the lower extremities, followed by progressive weakness of the lower limbs, flaccid paraplegia, urinary incontinence, sphincter dysfunction and sensory disturbance from the pelvic girdle downwards. Schistosome myelitis has a similar spectrum of neurologic symptoms as those caused by granulomatous masses. It tends to result in a more acute systemic illness with a shorter incubation period than patients with schistosomal mass lesions. The onset is characterised by back or leg pain, followed by leg weakness or paralysis and sensory loss.

12.7.3. Diagnosis

The definitive diagnosis of NS relies on demonstrating schistosome eggs in granulomas in neural tissues. However, a preoperative diagnosis can often be established based on a set of criteria, but there is no single specific and sensitive indicator for NS. The appearance of typical neurological symptoms in patients who live in or travel to schistosomiasis-endemic areas should be considered as suspected NS cases. A diagnosis is then reached after ruling out other possibilities, especially other helminth infections and intracranial tumours. Clinical symptoms, immunological tests, imaging and laboratory findings should be considered in differential diagnosis. The clinical features of the tumoral form of NS are usually indistinguishable from those resulting from other slow-expanding intracranial lesions. Spinal cord NS, on the other hand, may be suspected whenever a patient from an endemic area presents with rapidly progressing signs and symptoms of transverse myelitis involving the lumbosacral segments of the spinal cord (conus medullaris). Clinical diagnosis is difficult whenever higher segments of the spinal cord are involved and if neurological symptoms progress slowly.

Eosinophil cells are often found in the blood or CSF, especially at an early stage. Steroid treatment strongly influences this indicator and eosinophil counts are usually normal if the patient was given anti-inflammatory drugs (Ferrari et al., 2004). The presence of eggs in the faeces is a suggestive finding. When faeces examination is repeatedly negative, rectal biopsy is recommended to boost sensitivity (Ferrari et al., 2004; Watt et al., 1986). The role of CT and MRI for diagnosing NS is still controversial. Imaging can show non-specific abnormalities in the CNS at a later stage or in seriously affected patients (Pittella, 1997). A recent study of cerebral schistosomiasis japonica showed multiple clustered, 1–3 mm sized enhanced nodules in the T1-weighted MRI (Liu et al., 2008). In spinal schistosomiasis, MRI may reveal an enlarged spinal cord (usually of the conus medullaris) with spotty enhancement after gadolinium injection, but atrophy may be demonstrated on CT and MRI several months after the initial signs (Pittella, 1997). Many immunoserological assays have been used to detect schistosome infections in patients with CNS involvement (Pammenter et al., 1991; Scrimgeour and Gajdusek, 1985), but none achieved sufficiently high levels of sensitivity and specificity. Monoclonal antibodies of various immunoglobulin isotypes have been tested for their ability to detect antibodies against soluble egg antigen of *S. mansoni* in CSF, and IgG1 were considered the most discriminating isotype marker for the diagnosis of NS (Ferrari et al., 1999; Magalhaes-Santos et al., 2003).

The extent of NS is probably underestimated since it is difficult to diagnose due to a lack of sensitive and specific diagnostic tools. It may be particularly neglected in patients with advanced schistosomiasis, often characterised by induced hydroperitoneum, since elevated intra-abdominal pressure increases the CNS invasion of eggs (Liu, 1993). In this case, the CNS involvement may be misdiagnosed as a secondary symptom of hepatosplenic and cardiopulmonary lesions. Diagnosis is especially challenging in patients without gastrointestinal symptoms and egg-negative stool examination (Zhou et al., 2009).

12.7.4. Treatment and clinical management

Comprehensive reviews are available for the treatment and community-based control of schistosomiasis (Chen, 2005; Utzinger and Keiser, 2004), and the discovery and development of antischistosomal drugs in P.R. China are reviewed elsewhere (Xiao et al., 2010). At present, praziquantel is the only effective drug against all forms of schistosomiasis. It has only few and transient side effects and has been widely and effectively used in population-based control programmes, usually with a regimen of 40–60 mg/kg in single or divided doses (Chen, 2005; WHO, 2002). For the management of NS, a series of studies and clinical observations indicated good efficacy of praziquantel (Watt et al., 1986). It was observed that praziquantel tends to aggravate the condition at the early stage when steroid therapy is required (Jaureguiberry et al., 2007). Since other helminth infections in the CNS such as NC can be present simultaneously, a combination of praziquantel and steroids is recommended for all treatments of NS (Ferrari et al., 2008). The necessary duration of anti-inflammatory and anthelminthic treatment varies between individuals. Surgery to confirm the presence of schistosome eggs and granulomas is rarely used today. However, surgery is required for cases with medullary compression whenever chemotherapy is not successful (Jiang et al., 2008).

12.7.5. Geographical distribution and epidemiology

Schistosomiasis japonica is currently endemic in P.R. China, the Philippines and Indonesia. Schistosomiasis mekongi occurs in Lao PDR and Cambodia. For detailed information about the epidemiology of Asian schistosomiasis, the reader is referred to two accompanying reviews in this thematic issue of the *Advances in Parasitology* (Muth et al., 2010; Zhou et al., 2010). In brief, an estimated 726,000 people in seven provinces are infected with *S. japonicum* in P.R. China (Zhou et al., 2007). In the Philippines, an estimated 100,000 people are infected in three regions, namely Mindanao, Visayas and Luzon (Zhou et al., 2010). In Indonesia, less than 3000 people are infected in a few isolated villages. The total population at risk of schistosomiasis mekongi is estimated at 60,000 in Lao PDR and 80,000 in Cambodia (Urbani et al., 2002).

NS caused by *S. japonicum* occurs in about 2% of all patients with acute infections (Jaureguiberry and Caumes, 2008). The proportion can reach 4.3% among hospitalised adult schistosomiasis patients in P.R. China (Ross et al., 2001). Two cases with CNS involvement due to *S. mekongi* have been reported (Carmody et al., 2008; Houston et al., 2004). No population-representative data on NS exist, but data from single hospitals indicate that NS is a considerable problem in schistosomiasis-endemic areas. For example, 67 patients with NS were reported by the affiliated hospital of the Hunan Provincial Institute of Parasitic Diseases between 1994 and 2006 (Jing et al., 2007). Sixty-two cases were reported from a hospital in Jianli city in Hubei province between 2000 and 2004 (Liu et al., 2005). A retrospective survey covering 13 endemic counties in Anhui province documented 62 NS cases between 1997 and 2004 (Huang et al., 2008). No difference in risk factors for intestinal or CNS location of schistosomes could be established; young male farmers and fishermen were at particular risk.

The number of NS cases is expected to decline in line with further progress made in the control of schistosomiasis. However, the advent of improved diagnostic techniques may increase the number of diagnosed cases. For example, wider availability of neuroimaging techniques such as CT and MRI facilitates an accurate diagnosis of NS. Some studies also indicated that NS caused by *S. mansoni* were associated with light infections and is primarily found in travellers from non-endemic areas as well as young immunologically naïve locals (Ferrari et al., 2008; Graeff-Teixeira et al., 2009). If the same situation were to exist for schistosomiasis japonica, the number of NS cases could be expected to increase as the prevalence further declines.

12.8. CONCLUDING REMARKS AND RESEARCH NEEDS

The major cerebrospinal helminthiases occurring in Southeast Asia and the Far East have been reviewed here, with key features summarised in Table 12.1. While NC is a well-known disease with a long history, other helminth infections involving the CNS are emerging, such as angiostrongyliasis. A general feature of helminthiases of the CNS is that their neurological manifestations are non-specific, and hence they are often missed or misdiagnosed in clinical practice. It is therefore recommended that a set of diagnostic criteria, including epidemiological history, clinical manifestations, results from physical examinations and laboratory findings were employed to improve diagnostic outcomes. The eosinophil cell count in the CSF or peripheral blood is an important indicator of helminth infection in general, but is often normal, especially in the chronic stages of infection. Neuroimaging techniques, including MRI and CT, have revolutionised the diagnosis of intracranial infections, although the images may not be specific. Immunological assays have been developed for many helminth infections, but their sensitivity and specificity are generally questionable. Chemotherapy proved effective for patient management but is still controversial for most infections. Anti-inflammatory drugs such as corticosteroids are often needed to suppress inflammation resulting from the degeneration of worms. Surgery is the treatment of last resort if chemotherapy is not available or ineffective and if patients present severe complications.

There are several important issues emerging in connection with helminth infections involving the CNS. First, the production and consumption of pork and aquatic products are rapidly increasing in Asia and put more people at risk of food-borne parasitic diseases such as cysticercosis, gnathostomiasis and paragonimiasis. The spread of exotic snail species has contributed to the emergence of angiostrongyliasis in the mainland of P.R. China. Second, tourism and large population movements put people from non-endemic areas at risk. Third, the transportation and trade of food within and across countries may facilitate transmission beyond the known endemic areas. Fourth, other more traditional risk factors persist, e.g. special eating habits. For example, angiostrongyliasis is associated with the consumption of snails or slugs, sparganosis with that of frogs and snakes, or drinking snake bile and blood, and paragonimiasis with raw crab dishes. Although cysticercosis is not directly related to the consumption of raw pork, *Taenia* spp. infections may increase the risk of cysticercosis and help to sustain transmission.

Except for NC and angiostrongyliasis, cerebrospinal helminth infections are accidental. Reducing the overall prevalence of these parasites is therefore the most effective measure to control cerebrospinal helminthiases. For paragonimiasis, taeniasis and schistosomiasis, early treatment of infection is an important measure to prevent cerebrospinal involvement and other long-term sequelae. Health education and changing human behaviour is, in principle, effective to prevent all of these diseases, but is easier said than done. Food safety and hygiene is the basic issue for the control of food-borne diseases, whereas better access to clean water and adequate sanitation plays an important role for schistosomiasis prevention and control. Commercial farming in enclosed settings and using safe feed may be a way to guarantee food safety. However, its feasibility is questionable in low-income areas. Supervision and inspection are also required. Parallel to reducing the risk of infection, strengthening the awareness and diagnostic ability of clinicians plays an important role. Understanding the epidemic situation may be the first step to propose a robust control policy. Unfortunately, the cerebrospinal form of most helminthiases is frequently neglected or misdiagnosed, and hence the available data probably fail to reflect their real status. The establishment of rigorous surveillance systems focusing on combinations of symptoms rather than parasitological diagnoses alone and thus referring to a group of diseases sharing similar indicators is a measure of potential value.

Cerebrospinal helminth infections are a rare clinical entity, but an emerging public health issue. Several research priorities are highlighted here. First, effective diagnostic tools are needed. With regard to immunological assays against gnathostomiasis, for example, the immunoblot technique is now widely and effectively used for its diagnosis in Thailand (Rojekittikhun, 2005) and Japan (Ando, 2005). However, almost all gnathostomiasis cases in P.R. China are parasitologically diagnosed by biopsy, which is not feasible for cerebrospinal infections. The lack of immunological assays is an important explanation for the current underestimation of gnathostomiasis, and hence NG, in P.R. China. There is therefore a need to develop and validate immunological assays against gnathostomiasis or to make existing ones readily available. Second, although mechanisms of CNS involvement are difficult to reveal, such information is necessary for enhanced patient management. For example, humans may take the place of the second intermediate hosts for *Gnathostoma* and *Spirometra* when they ingest infected copepods. Drinking untreated freshwater has been suggested as a route for human infection (Holodniy et al., 1991; Punyagupta et al., 1990), but whether the unusual role of humans increases the chance for parasites to enter the CNS is still a matter of debate. Third, concerted efforts are needed to evaluate existing anthelminthic drugs for the treatment of helminthiases affecting the CNS, including dose-finding studies and combination chemotherapy. For diseases where there is currently no effective drug available (e.g. sparganosis), there is an urgent need to develop such drugs. Although surgery can improve conditions of patients, infections with multiple worms call for chemotherapy. For existing drugs, a main problem affecting the evaluation of treatment efficacies for cerebrospinal helminth infections is the small number of potential participants. Collaboration among hospitals and disease outbreaks with sufficient numbers of people affected may provide opportunities to address this issue. Fourth, investigations on the burden of disease due to helminths invading the CNS are necessary. Indeed, neurohelminthiasis can result in epilepsy, paralysis, and hence loss of labour capacity. Surveillance networks on helminth infections of the CNS, facilitated by collaborations among different hospitals and disease control institutions in highly endemic regions, holds promise to reveal the true public health burden. Hospital-based surveillance systems potentially increase the capacity of detecting rare or neglected diseases, including neurohelminthiases.

Concluding, it is clear that helminth infections of the CNS in Southeast Asia and the Far East are an emerging public health problem, and concerted efforts are necessary to raise awareness of the public and clinicians to improve diagnosis and patient management. Special emphasis on the prevention of these infections through surveillance networks is needed, and decision-makers in the region are invited to engage actively in addressing this challenge.

ACKNOWLEDGEMENTS

We thank Kathrin Ziegelbauer from the Swiss Tropical and Public Health Institute for her helpful comments on an earlier version of this manuscript. S.Lv is grateful to the "Stipendienkommission für Nachwuchskräfte aus Entwicklungsländern" from the Canton of Basel-Stadt, Switzerland, for a Ph.D. fellowship, P. Steinmann to the Swiss National Science Foundation (project no. PBBSP3-123193) and the Novartis Foundation, X.N. Zhou to the Chinese Important Scientific Research Project on Infectious Diseases (grant no. 2008ZX10004-011) and J. Utzinger to the Swiss National Science Foundation (project no. PPOOB-102883, PPOOB-119129).

REFERENCES

Anantaphruti, M.T., 2002. Immunodiagnosis of gnathostomiasis. J. Trop. Med. Parasitol. 25, 83–90.

Anderson, R.C., 2000. Nematode Parasites of Vertebrates: Their Development and Transmission. CABI, Wallingford.

Ando, K., 2005. Gnathostomiasis in Japan. In: Arizono, N., Chai, J.Y., Nawa, Y., Takahashi, Y. (Eds.), Asian Parasitology: Food-Borne Helminthiasis in Asia. Vol. 1. The Federation of Asian Parasitologists, Chuo-ku, pp. 231–239.

Belizario, V., Guan, M., Borja, L., Ortega, A., Leonardia, W., 1997. Pulmonary paragonimiasis and tuberculosis in Sorsogon, Philippines. Southeast Asian J. Trop. Med. Public Health 28 (Suppl. 1), 37–45.

Bergsneider, M., 1999. Endoscopic removal of cysticercal cysts within the fourth ventricle. Technical note. J. Neurosurg. 91, 340–345.

Bergsneider, M., Holly, L.T., Lee, J.H., King, W.A., Frazee, J.G., 2000. Endoscopic management of cysticercal cysts within the lateral and third ventricles. J. Neurosurg. 92, 14–23.

Bethony, J., Brooker, S., Albonico, M., Geiger, S.M., Loukas, A., Diemert, D., et al., 2006. Soil-transmitted helminth infections: ascariasis, trichuriasis, and hookworm. Lancet 367, 1521–1532.

Bittencourt, P.R., Gracia, C.M., Gorz, A.M., Mazer, S., Oliveira, T.V., 1990. High-dose praziquantel for neurocysticercosis: efficacy and tolerability. Eur. Neurol. 30, 229–234.

Blair, D., Xu, Z.B., Agatsuma, T., 1999. Paragonimiasis and the genus *Paragonimus*. Adv. Parasitol. 42, 113–222.

Boongird, P., Phuapradit, P., Siridej, N., Chirachariyavej, T., Chuahirun, S., Vejjajiva, A., 1977. Neurological manifestations of gnathostomiasis. J. Neurol. Sci. 31, 279–291.

Bowden, D.K., 1981. Eosinophilic meningitis in the New Hebrides: two outbreaks and two deaths. Am. J. Trop. Med. Hyg. 30, 1141–1143.

Bunnag, T., Comer, D.S., Punyagupta, S., 1970. Eosinophilic myeloencephalitis caused by *Gnathostoma spinigerum*. Neuropathology of nine cases. J. Neurol. Sci. 10, 419–434.

Bunyaratavej, K., Pongpunlert, W., Jongwutiwes, S., Likitnukul, S., 2008. Spinal gnathostomiasis resembling an intrinsic cord tumor/myelitis in a 4-year-old boy. Southeast Asian J. Trop. Med. Public Health 39, 800–803.

Carmody, D., Nolan, C., Allcutt, D., 2008. Intracranial *Schistosoma mekongi* infection. Ir. Med. J. 101, 315.

Carod-Artal, F.J., 2008. Neurological complications of *Schistosoma* infection. Trans. R. Soc. Trop. Med. Hyg. 102, 107–116.

Carpio, A., 2002. Neurocysticercosis: an update. Lancet Infect. Dis. 2, 751–762.

Cha, S.H., Chang, K.H., Cho, S.Y., Han, M.H., Kong, Y., Suh, D.C., et al., 1994. Cerebral paragonimiasis in early active stage: CT and MR features. Am. J. Roentgenol. 162, 141–145.

Chai, J.Y., Han, E.T., Shin, E.H., Park, J.H., Chu, J.P., Hirota, M., et al., 2003. An outbreak of gnathostomiasis among Korean emigrants in Myanmar. Am. J. Trop. Med. Hyg. 69, 67–73.

Chang, K.H., Cho, S.Y., Chi, J.G., Kim, W.S., Han, M.C., Kim, C.W., et al., 1987. Cerebral sparganosis: CT characteristics. Radiology 165, 505–510.

Chang, K.H., Chi, J.G., Cho, S.Y., Han, M.H., Han, D.H., Han, M.C., 1992. Cerebral sparganosis: analysis of 34 cases with emphasis on CT features. Neuroradiology 34, 1–8.

Chen, H.T., 1935. Un nouveau nematode Pulmonaire, *Pulmonema cantonensis*, n. g., n. sp. des rats de Canton. Ann. Parasitol. 13, 312–317.

Chen, J.Q., 1983. A neonatal case of sparganosis. Chin. J. Pediatr. 21, 77.

Chen, M.G., 2005. Use of praziquantel for clinical treatment and morbidity control of schistosomiasis japonica in China: a review of 30 years' experience. Acta Trop. 96, 168–176.

Chen, M.G., Chang, Z.S., Shao, X.Y., Liu, M.D., Blair, D., Chen, S.H., et al., 2001. Paragonimiasis in Yongjia county, Zhejiang province, China: clinical, parasitological and karyotypic studies on *Paragonimus westermani*. Southeast Asian J. Trop. Med. Public Health 32, 760–769.

Chen, H.L., Lei, C.Q., Chen, Y., Huang, X.M., Yu, K.G., Yao, L.N., 2002. Case report: sparganosis after eating raw frogs. J. Pract. Parasit. Dis. 10, 134.

Chen, Y.D., Xu, L.Q., Zhou, X.N., 2004. Distribution and disease burden of cysticercosis in China. Southeast Asian J. Trop. Med. Public Health 35, 231–239.

Cheng, Y.F., 2004. Diagnosis and treatment of 50 pediatric patients with cerebral paragonimiasis. Shanxi Med. J. 33, 656–658.

Chitanondh, H., Rosen, L., 1967. Fatal eosinophilic encephalomyelitis caused by the nematode *Gnathostoma spinigerum*. Am. J. Trop. Med. Hyg. 16, 638–645.

Cho, S.Y., Bae, J.H., Seo, B.S., 1975. Some aspects of human sparganosis in Korea. Kisaengchunghak Chapchi 13, 60–77.

Cho, S.Y., Kong, Y., Kang, S.Y., 1997. Epidemiology of paragonimiasis in Korea. Southeast Asian J. Trop. Med. Public Health 28 (Suppl. 1), 32–36.

Chotmongkol, V., Sawanyawisuth, K., Thavornpitak, Y., 2000. Corticosteroid treatment of eosinophilic meningitis. Clin. Infect. Dis. 31, 660–662.

Chotmongkol, V., Wongjitrat, C., Sawadpanit, K., Sawanyawisuth, K., 2004. Treatment of eosinophilic meningitis with a combination of albendazole and corticosteroid. Southeast Asian J. Trop. Med. Public Health 35, 172–174.

Chotmongkol, V., Sawadpanitch, K., Sawanyawisuth, K., Louhawilai, S., Limpawattana, P., 2006. Treatment of eosinophilic meningitis with a combination of prednisolone and mebendazole. Am. J. Trop. Med. Hyg. 74, 1122–1124.

Colli, B.O., Martelli, N., Assirati, J.A., Jr., Machado, H.R., de Vergueiro Forjaz, S., 1986. Results of surgical treatment of neurocysticercosis in 69 cases. J. Neurosurg. 65, 309–315.

Colli, B.O., Carlotti, C.G., Jr., Assirati, J.A., Jr., Machado, H.R., Valenca, M., Amato, M.C., 2002. Surgical treatment of cerebral cysticercosis: long-term results and prognostic factors. Neurosurg. Focus 12, e3.

Conlan, J., Khounsy, S., Inthavong, P., Fenwick, S., Blacksell, S., Thompson, R.C., 2008. A review of taeniasis and cysticercosis in the Lao People's Democratic Republic. Parasitol. Int. 57, 252–255.

Cox, F.E.G., 2002. History of human parasitology. Clin. Microbiol. Rev. 15, 595–612.

Crompton, D.W.T., 1999. How much human helminthiasis is there in the world? J. Parasitol. 85, 397–403.

Cross, J.H., 1987. Public health importance of *Angiostrongylus cantonensis* and its relatives. Parasitol. Today 3, 367–369.

Cudlip, S.A., Wilkins, P.R., Marsh, H.T., 1998. Endoscopic removal of a third ventricular cysticercal cyst. Br. J. Neurosurg. 12, 452–454.

Cui, J., Wang, Z.Q., Wu, F., Jin, X.X., 1998. An outbreak of paragonimiosis in Zhengzhou city, China. Acta Trop. 70, 211–216.

Dai, Y.Q., 1997. Clinical analysis of 28 pediatric patients with cerebral paragonimiasis. Central China Med. J. 21, 271–272.

de Leon, W.U., Piad, J.N.C., 2005. Paragonimiasis in the Philippines. In: Arizono, N., Chai, J. Y., Nawa, Y., Takahashi, Y. (Eds.), Asian Parasitology: Food-Borne Helminthiasis in Asia. Vol. 1. The Federation of Asian Parasitologists, Chuo-ku, pp. 133–137.

de Silva, N.R., Brooker, S., Hotez, P.J., Montresor, A., Engels, D., Savioli, L., 2003. Soil-transmitted helminth infections: updating the global picture. Trends Parasitol. 19, 547–551.

De, N.V., Cong, L.D., Kino, H., Son, D.T., Vien, H.V., 2000. Epidemiology, symptoms and treatment of paragonimiasis in Sin Ho district, Lai Chau province, Vietnam. Southeast Asian J. Trop. Med. Public Health 31 (Suppl. 1), 26–30.

Del Brutto, O.H., 1994. Prognostic factors for seizure recurrence after withdrawal of antiepileptic drugs in patients with neurocysticercosis. Neurology 44, 1706–1709.

Del Brutto, O.H., Sotelo, J., 1990. Albendazole therapy for subarachnoid and ventricular cysticercosis. Case report. J. Neurosurg. 72, 816–817.

Del Brutto, O.H., Santibanez, R., Noboa, C.A., Aguirre, R., Diaz, E., Alarcon, T.A., 1992. Epilepsy due to neurocysticercosis: analysis of 203 patients. Neurology 42, 389–392.

Del Brutto, O.H., Sotelo, J., Roman, G.C., 1998. Neurocysticercosis: A Clinical Handbook. Swets and Zeitlinger, Lisse.

Del Brutto, O.H., Rajshekhar, V., White, A.C., Jr., Tsang, V.C., Nash, T.E., Takayanagui, O.M., et al., 2001. Proposed diagnostic criteria for neurocysticercosis. Neurology 57, 177–183.

Del Brutto, O.H., Roos, K.L., Coffey, C.S., García, H.H., 2006. Meta-analysis: cysticidal drugs for neurocysticercosis: albendazole and praziquantel. Ann. Intern. Med. 145, 43–51.

Deng, Z.H., Cai, J.S., Lin, R.X., Pei, F.Q., Cui, H.E., Ou, Y., et al., 2007. The first local outbreak of *Angiostrongylus cantonensis* infection in Guangdong province. South China J. Prev. Med. 33, 17–20.

Díaz Camacho, S.P., Willms, K., de la Cruz Otero Mdel, C., Zazueta Ramos, M.L., Bayliss Gaxiola, R., Castro Velázquez, R., et al., 2003. Acute outbreak of gnathostomiasis in a fishing community in Sinaloa, Mexico. Parasitol. Int. 52, 133–140.

Diaz, F., García, H.H., Gilman, R.H., Gonzales, A.E., Castro, M., Tsang, V.C., et al., 1992. Epidemiology of taeniasis and cysticercosis in a Peruvian village. The Cysticercosis Working Group in Peru. Am. J. Epidemiol. 135, 875–882.

Doanh, P.N., Le, N.T., The, D.T., 2005. *Paragonimus* and paragonimiasis in Vietnam. In: Arizono, J.Y., Chai, J.Y., Nawa, Y., Takahashi, Y. (Eds.), Asian Parasitology: Food-Borne Helminthiasis in Asia. Vol. 1. The Federation of Asian Parasitologists, Chuo-ku, pp. 149–153.

Doanh, P.N., Shinohara, A., Horii, Y., Habe, S., Nawa, Y., Le, N.T., 2008. Discovery of *Paragonimus proliferus* in Northern Vietnam and their molecular phylogenetic status among genus *Paragonimus*. Parasitol. Res. 102, 677–683.

Dorny, P., Somers, R., Dang, T., Nguyen, V.K., Vercruysse, J., 2004. Cysticercosis in Cambodia. Lao PDR and Vietnam. Southeast Asian J. Trop. Med. Public Health 35, 223–226.

Dorta-Contreras, A.J., Noris-García, E., Escobar-Perez, X., Padilla Docal, B., 2005. IgG1, IgG2 and IgE intrathecal synthesis in *Angiostrongylus cantonensis* meningoencephalitis. J. Neurol. Sci. 238, 65–70.

Eamsobhana, P., Tungtrongchitr, A., 2005. Angiostrongyliasis in Thailand. In: Arizono, N., Chai, J.Y., Nawa, Y., Takahashi, Y. (Eds.), Asian Parasitology: Food-Borne Helminthiasis in Asia. Vol. 1. The Federation of Asian Parasitologists, Chuo-ku, pp. 183–197.

Eom, K.S., Kim, T.Y., 2009. Migration of cerebral sparganosis to the ipsilateral cerebellar hemisphere. Acta Parasitol. 54, 276–280.

Erhart, A., Dorny, P., Van De, N., Vien, H.V., Thach, D.C., Toan, N.D., et al., 2002. *Taenia solium* cysticercosis in a village in northern Viet Nam: seroprevalence study using an ELISA for detecting circulating antigen. Trans. R. Soc. Trop. Med. Hyg. 96, 270–272.

Fang, W., 2002. Clinical and epidemiological analysis of 410 pediatric cases with neurocysticercosis. Chin. J. Zoonoses 18, 132–133.

Fang, W., Lian, Z.Q., Fang, C., 1995. A survey on epidemiological factors of taeniasis/cysticercosis in a Bai minority village, Dali. Chin. J. Parasitic Dis. Control 8, 199.

Faust, E.C., Campbell, H.E., Kellogg, C.R., 1929. Morphological and biological studies on the species of *Diphyllobothrium* in China. Am. J. Hyg. 9, 560–583.

Ferrari, T.C., Correa-Oliveira, R., Xavier, M.A., Gazzinelli, G., Cunha, A.S., 1999. Estimation of the local synthesis of immunoglobulin G (IgG) in the central nervous system of patients with spinal cord schistosomiasis by the IgG index. Trans. R. Soc. Trop. Med. Hyg. 93, 558–559.

Ferrari, T.C., Moreira, P.R., Cunha, A.S., 2004. Spinal cord schistosomiasis: a prospective study of 63 cases emphasizing clinical and therapeutic aspects. J. Clin. Neurosci. 11, 246–253.

Ferrari, T.C., Moreira, P.R., Cunha, A.S., 2008. Clinical characterization of neuroschistosomiasis due to *Schistosoma mansoni* and its treatment. Acta Trop. 108, 89–97.

Fleury, A., Gomez, T., Alvarez, I., Meza, D., Huerta, M., Chavarria, A., et al., 2003. High prevalence of calcified silent neurocysticercosis in a rural village of Mexico. Neuroepidemiology 22, 139–145.

Fleury, A., Morales, J., Bobes, R.J., Dumas, M., Yanez, O., Pina, J., et al., 2006. An epidemiological study of familial neurocysticercosis in an endemic Mexican community. Trans. R. Soc. Trop. Med. Hyg. 100, 551–558.

Fung, C.F., Ng, T.H., Wong, W.T., 1989. Sparganosis of the spinal cord. Case report. J. Neurosurg. 71, 290–292.

Furugen, M., Yamashiro, S., Tamayose, M., Naha, Y., Miyagi, K., Nakasone, C., et al., 2006. Elsberg syndrome with eosinophilic meningoencephalitis caused by *Angiostrongylus cantonensis*. Intern. Med. 45, 1333–1336.

García, H.H., Del Brutto, O.H., 2005. Neurocysticercosis: updated concepts about an old disease. Lancet Neurol. 4, 653–661.

García, H.H., Martinez, M., Gilman, R., Herrera, G., Tsang, V.C., Pilcher, J.B., et al., 1991. Diagnosis of cysticercosis in endemic regions. The Cysticercosis Working Group in Peru. Lancet 338, 549–551.

García, H.H., Araoz, R., Gilman, R.H., Valdez, J., Gonzalez, A.E., Gavidia, C., et al., 1998. Increased prevalence of cysticercosis and taeniasis among professional fried pork vendors and the general population of a village in the Peruvian highlands. Cysticercosis Working Group in Peru. Am. J. Trop. Med. Hyg. 59, 902–905.

García, H.H., Evans, C.A., Nash, T.E., Takayanagui, O.M., White, A.C., Jr., Botero, D., et al., 2002. Current consensus guidelines for treatment of neurocysticercosis. Clin. Microbiol. Rev. 15, 747–756.

García, H.H., Pretell, E.J., Gilman, R.H., Martinez, S.M., Moulton, L.H., Del Brutto, O.H., et al., 2004. A trial of antiparasitic treatment to reduce the rate of seizures due to cerebral cysticercosis. N. Engl. J. Med. 350, 249–258.

Germann, R., Schächtele, M., Neßler, G., Seitz, U., Kniehl, E., 2003. Cerebral gnathostomiasis as a cause of an extended intracranial bleeding. Klin. Pädiatr. 215, 223–225.

Gilman, R.H., Del Brutto, O.H., García, H.H., Martinez, M., 2000. Prevalence of taeniosis among patients with neurocysticercosis is related to severity of infection. The Cysticercosis Working Group in Peru. Neurology 55, 1062.

Gogia, S., Talukdar, B., Choudhury, V., Arora, B.S., 2003. Neurocysticercosis in children: clinical findings and response to albendazole therapy in a randomized, double-blind, placebo-controlled trial in newly diagnosed cases. Trans. R. Soc. Trop. Med. Hyg. 97, 416–421.

Gorgolas, M., Santos-O'Connor, F., Unzu, A.L., Fernandez-Guerrero, M.L., Garate, T., Troyas Guarch, R.M., et al., 2003. Cutaneous and medullar gnathostomiasis in travelers to Mexico and Thailand. J. Travel Med. 10, 358–361.

Graeff-Teixeira, C., da Silva, A.C., Yoshimura, K., 2009. Update on eosinophilic meningoencephalitis and its clinical relevance. Clin. Microbiol. Rev. 22, 322–348.

Grove, D.I., 1990. A History of Human Helminthology. CABI, Wallingford.

Gryseels, B., Polman, K., Clerinx, J., Kestens, L., 2006. Human schistosomiasis. Lancet 368, 1106–1118.

Guo, D.M., Xie, S.P., Liu, A.H., 2001. Classification of neurocysticercosis and mechanism of headache: 6585 cases report. J. Capital Univ. Med. Sci. 22, 349–350.

Gushulak, B.D., MacPherson, D.W., 2004. Globalization of infectious diseases: the impact of migration. Clin. Infect. Dis. 38, 1742–1748.

He, Z.Y., Jia, L., Huang, F., Liu, G.R., Li, J., Dou, X.F., et al., 2007. Investigation on outbreak of angiostrongyliasis cantonensis in Beijing. Chin. J. Public Health 23, 1241–1242.

Herman, J.S., Chiodini, P.L., 2009. Gnathostomiasis, another emerging imported disease. Clin. Microbiol. Rev. 22, 484–492.

Hidelaratchi, M.D., Riffsy, M.T., Wijesekera, J.C., 2005. A case of eosinophilic meningitis following monitor lizard meat consumption, exacerbated by anthelminthics. Ceylon Med. J. 50, 84–86.

Higashi, K., Aoki, H., Tatebayashi, K., Morioka, H., Sakata, Y., 1971. Cerebral paragonimiasis. J. Neurosurg. 34, 515–527.

Holodniy, M., Almenoff, J., Loutit, J., Steinberg, G.K., 1991. Cerebral sparganosis: case report and review. Rev. Infect. Dis. 13, 155–159.

Hotez, P.J., Molyneux, D.H., Fenwick, A., Kumaresan, J., Ehrlich Sachs, S., Sachs, J.D., et al., 2007. Control of neglected tropical diseases. N. Engl. J. Med. 357, 1018–1027.

Houston, S., Kowalewska-Grochowska, K., Naik, S., McKean, J., Johnson, E.S., Warren, K., 2004. First report of *Schistosoma mekongi* infection with brain involvement. Clin. Infect. Dis. 38, e1–e6.

Huang, A.Q., 2000. Clinical analysis of 41 cases with cerebral paragonimiasis. Chin. J. Zoonoses 16, 115.

Huang, J.M., 2003. Two cases of sparganosis due to treating dermatitis with raw frog skin. Xin Yi Xue 34 (Suppl.), 137–138.

Huang, W.D., Liu, Y.Q., Zhong, H., 1990. The primary investigation on *Spirometra mansoni* among snakes in Zhanjiang, China. J. Guangdong Med. Coll. 8, 178–179.

Huang, Y.E., Wang, T.P., Zhang, S.Q., 2008. Clinical analysis of 62 neuroschistosomiasis cases and an proposed diagnosis criteria. J. Trop. Dis. Parasitol. 6, 15–17.

Hwang, K.P., 1997. Anthelmintics in the treatment of eosinophilic meningitis. Acta Paed. Sin. 38 (Suppl.), 1–6.

Hwang, K.P., Chen, E.R., 1991. Clinical studies on angiostrongyliasis cantonensis among children in Taiwan. Southeast Asian J. Trop. Med. Public Health 22 (Suppl.), 194–199.

Ito, A., Urbani, C., Qiu, J.M., Vuitton, D.A., Qiu, D.C., Heath, D.D., et al., 2003. Control of echinococcosis and cysticercosis: a public health challenge to international cooperation in China. Acta Trop. 86, 3–17.

Ito, A., Nakao, M., Wandra, T., Suroso, T., Okamoto, M., Yamasaki, H., et al., 2005. Taeniasis and cysticercosis in Asia and the Pacific: present state of knowledge and perspectives. Southeast Asian J. Trop. Med. Public Health 36 (Suppl. 4), 123–130.

Jaureguiberry, S., Caumes, E., 2008. Neurological involvement during Katayama syndrome. Lancet Infect. Dis. 8, 9–10.

Jaureguiberry, S., Ansart, S., Perez, L., Danis, M., Bricaire, F., Caumes, E., 2007. Acute neuroschistosomiasis: two cases associated with cerebral vasculitis. Am. J. Trop. Med. Hyg. 76, 964–966.

Jiang, Y.G., Zhang, M.M., Xiang, J., 2008. Spinal cord schistosomiasis japonica: a report of 4 cases. Surg. Neurol. 69, 392–397.

Jing, Q.S., Luo, L.X., Chen, Z., Wang, H.B., Zheng, N., 2007. Analysis of clinical manifestation of cerebral schistosomiasis. J. Trop. Med. 7, 435–437.

Jitpimolmard, S., Sawanyawisuth, K., Morakote, N., Vejjajiva, A., Puntumetakul, M., Sanchaisuriya, K., et al., 2007. Albendazole therapy for eosinophilic meningitis caused by *Angiostrongylus cantonensis*. Parasitol. Res. 100, 1293–1296.

Kang, Y., Gong, Z.J., Yi, C.C., 2002. An outbreak of paragonimiasis due to imported crabs. Chin. J. Parasitol. Parasit. Dis. 18, 175.

Keiser, J., Utzinger, J., 2005. Emerging foodborne trematodiasis. Emerg. Infect. Dis. 11, 1507–1514.

Keiser, J., Utzinger, J., 2009. Food-borne trematodiases. Clin. Microbiol. Rev. 22, 466–483.

Keiser, J., Utzinger, J., 2010. The drugs we have and the drugs we need against major helminth infections. Adv. Parasitol. 73, 197–230.

Kim, H., Kim, S.I., Cho, S.Y., 1984. Serological diagnosis of human sparganosis by means of micro-ELISA. Kisaengchunghak Chapchi 22, 222–228.

Kim, D.G., Paek, S.H., Chang, K.H., Wang, K.C., Jung, H.W., Kim, H.J., et al., 1996. Cerebral sparganosis: clinical manifestations, treatment, and outcome. J. Neurosurg. 85, 1066–1071.

Kim, I.Y., Jung, S., Jung, T.Y., Kang, S.S., Chung, T.W., 2007. Contralateral migration of cerebral sparganosis through the splenium. Clin. Neurol. Neurosurg. 109, 720–724.

Kimura, S., Kashima, M., Kawa, Y., Nakamura, F., Nawa, Y., Takai, K., et al., 2003. A case of subcutaneous sparganosis: therapeutic assessment by an indirect immunofluorescence antibody titration using sections of the worm body obtained from the patient. Br. J. Dermatol. 148, 369–371.

Kliks, M.M., Palumbo, N.E., 1992. Eosinophilic meningitis beyond the Pacific Basin: the global dispersal of a peridomestic zoonosis caused by *Angiostrongylus cantonensis*, the nematode lungworm of rats. Soc. Sci. Med. 34, 199–212.

Kliks, M.M., Kroenke, K., Hardman, J.M., 1982. Eosinophilic radiculomyeloencephalitis: an angiostrongyliasis outbreak in American Samoa related to ingestion of *Achatina fulica* snails. Am. J. Trop. Med. Hyg. 31, 1114–1122.

Kozan, E., Gonenc, B., Sarimehmetoglu, O., Aycicek, H., 2005. Prevalence of helminth eggs on raw vegetables used for salads. Food Control 16, 239–242.

Kraivichian, P., Kulkumthorn, M., Yingyourd, P., Akarabovorn, P., Paireepai, C.C., 1992. Albendazole for the treatment of human gnathostomiasis. Trans. R. Soc. Trop. Med. Hyg. 86, 418–421.

Kraivichian, K., Nuchprayoon, S., Sitichalernchai, P., Chaicumpa, W., Yentakam, S., 2004. Treatment of cutaneous gnathostomiasis with ivermectin. Am. J. Trop. Med. Hyg. 71, 623–628.

Kudesia, S., Indira, D.B., Sarala, D., Vani, S., Yasha, T.C., Jayakumar, P.N., et al., 1998. Sparganosis of brain and spinal cord: unusual tapeworm infestation (report of two cases). Clin. Neurol. Neurosurg. 100, 148–152.

Kumar, V., Kyprianou, I., Keenan, J.M., 2005. Ocular angiostrongyliasis: removal of a live nematode from the anterior chamber. Eye 19, 229–230.

Kusner, D.J., King, C.H., 1993. Cerebral paragonimiasis. Semin. Neurol. 13, 201–208.

Le, T.X., Rojekittikhun, W., 2000. A survey of infective larvae of *Gnathostoma* in eels sold in Ho Chi Minh city. Southeast Asian J. Trop. Med. Public Health 31, 133–137.

Leon, L.A., Almeida, R., Mueller, J.F., 1972. A case of ocular sparganosis in Ecuador. J. Parasitol. 58, 184–185.

Lescano, A.G., García, H.H., Gilman, R.H., Gavidia, C.M., Tsang, V.C., Rodriguez, S., et al., 2009. *Taenia solium* cysticercosis hotspots surrounding tapeworm carriers: clustering on human seroprevalence but not on seizures. PLoS Negl. Trop. Dis. 3, e371.

Li, D.J., Liao, Y.F., Zhu, X.R., Liu, S.X., 1996. Electroencephalogram analysis of 106 cases with cerebral paragonimiasis. J. Wenzhou Med. Coll. 26, 22–24.

Li, D.N., He, A., Wang, Q., Liang, Y., Li, Z.Y., Meng, J.X., et al., 2001. Three lethal cases of angiostrongyliasis cantonensis infected children. Chin. J. Parasitol. Parasit. Dis. 19, 310–311.

Li, L.S., Lin, J.X., Zhang, R.Y., Fang, Y.Y., Lin, K.Q., 2006a. A severe case of angiostrongyliasis due to eating raw slugs. Chin. J. Parasitol. Parasit. Dis. 24, 460.

Li, L.S., Zhou, X.N., Lin, J.X., Zhang, Y., Chen, Y.Z., Zhang, R.Y., et al., 2006b. Discovery of six new host species of *Angiostrongylus cantonensis* and investigation on the epidemic foci in Fujian province. Chin. J. Zoonoses 22, 533–537.

Li, P., Fu, P., He, J.C., 2008. Analysis of the clinical type and therapeutic efficiency of 280 children cases with paragonimiasis. J. Path. Biol. 3, 2–3.

Li, M.W., Lin, H.Y., Xie, W.T., Gao, M.J., Huang, Z.W., Wu, J.P., et al., 2009. Enzootic sparganosis in Guangdong, People's Republic of China. Emerg. Infect. Dis. 15, 1317–1318.

Lin, J.X., Zhu, K., Chen, B.J., Zhang, R.Y., Ni, Y.Q., Ding, F., 2002. Sparganosis due to application of frog flesh: one case. J. Trop. Med. 2, 167–168.

Lin, B.L., Chen, L.B., Zhang, X.H., Lin, C.S., Yang, S.J., 2003a. Clinical analysis of 11 cases of sparganosis in Guangdong province. J. Sun Yat-Sen Univ. (Med. Sci.) 24, 79–80.

Lin, J.X., Li, Y.S., Zhu, K., Chen, B.J., Cheng, Y.Z., Lin, J.C., et al., 2003b. Epidemiological study on group infection of *Angiostrongylus cantonensis* in Changle city. Chin. J. Parasitol. Parasit. Dis. 21, 110–112.

Lin, X.M., Liu, C.J., Yan, Q.Y., He, L.J., Zhang, H.W., Zhang, Q., et al., 2008. Investigation and analysis on infection of *Sparganum mansoni* by eating alive tadpole. Chin. J. Zoonoses 24, 1173–1175.

Lindo, J.F., Escoffery, C.T., Reid, B., Codrington, G., Cunningham-Myrie, C., Eberhard, M.L., 2004. Fatal autochthonous eosinophilic meningitis in a Jamaican child caused by *Angiostrongylus cantonensis*. Am. J. Trop. Med. Hyg. 70, 425–428.

Liu, L.X., 1993. Spinal and cerebral schistosomiasis. Semin. Neurol. 13, 189–200.

Liu, Y.J., 2006. Sparganosis in spinal cord: two cases report. Chin. J. Spine Spinal Cord 16, 137–138.

Liu, P.M., An, G.Z., 2000. A case report: rare nasal angiostrongyliasis. Chin. J. Zoonoses 16, 116.

Liu, M., Boireau, P., 2002. Trichinellosis in China: epidemiology and control. Trends Parasitol. 18, 553–556.

Liu, Z.M., Zeng, M., Li, J.Z., Yang, D.M., 2005. Diagnosis and treatment of brain schistosomiasis: a report on 62 cases. Mod. Diagn. Treat. 16, 369–370.

Liu, Z.R., Zhou, F.Y., Zeng, X.P., Shen, L.Y., Wang, P.Z., Ding, L.P., et al., 2006. Clinical analysis of three cases of eosinophilic meningitis due to eating raw slugs. Zhejiang Prev. Med. 18, 63–64.

Liu, H., Lim, C.C., Feng, X., Yao, Z., Chen, Y., Sun, H., et al., 2008. MRI in cerebral schistosomiasis: characteristic nodular enhancement in 33 patients. Am. J. Roentgenol. 191, 582–588.

Lo, Y.K., Chao, D., Yan, S.H., Liu, H.C., Chu, F.L., Huang, C.I., et al., 1987. Spinal cord proliferative sparganosis in Taiwan: a case report. Neurosurgery 21, 235–238.

Loria-Cortes, R., Lobo-Sanahuja, J.F., 1980. Clinical abdominal angiostrongylosis. A study of 116 children with intestinal eosinophilic granuloma caused by *Angiostrongylus costaricensis*. Am. J. Trop. Med. Hyg. 29, 538–544.

Lv, S., Zhang, Y., Steinmann, P., Zhou, X.N., 2008. Emerging angiostrongyliasis in mainland China. Emerg. Infect. Dis. 14, 161–164.

Lv, S., Zhang, Y., Chen, S.R., Wang, L.B., Fang, W., Chen, F., et al., 2009a. Human angiostrongyliasis outbreak in Dali, China. PLoS Negl. Trop. Dis. 3, e520.

Lv, S., Zhang, Y., Liu, H.X., Hu, L., Yang, K., Steinmann, P., et al., 2009b. Invasive snails and an emerging infectious disease: results from the first national survey on *Angiostrongylus cantonensis* in China. PLoS Negl. Trop. Dis. 3, e368.

Mac Arthur, W.P., 1934. Cysticercosis as seen in the British Army, with special reference to the production of epilepsy. Trans. R. Soc. Trop. Med. Hyg. 27, 343–357.

Magalhaes-Santos, I.F., Lemaire, D.C., Andrade-Filho, A.S., Queiroz, A.C., Carvalho, O.M., Carmo, T.M., et al., 2003. Antibodies to *Schistosoma mansoni* in human cerebrospinal fluid. Am. J. Trop. Med. Hyg. 68, 294–298.

Maleewong, W., 1997. Recent advances in diagnosis of paragonimiasis. Southeast Asian J. Trop. Med. Public Health 28 (Suppl. 1), 134–138.

Maleewong, W., Pariyanonda, S., Sitthithaworn, P., Daenseegaew, W., Pipitgool, V., Tesana, S., et al., 1992. Seasonal variation in the prevalence and intensity of canine *Gnathostoma spinigerum* infection in northeastern Thailand. J. Helminthol. 66, 72–74.

Malhotra, S., Mehta, D.K., Arora, R., Chauhan, D., Ray, S., Jain, M., 2006. Ocular angiostrongyliasis in a child—first case report from India. J. Trop. Pediatr. 52, 223–225.

Malvy, D., Ezzedine, K., Receveur, M.C., Pistone, T., Crevon, L., Lemardeley, P., et al., 2008. Cluster of eosinophilic meningitis attributable to *Angiostrongylus cantonensis* infection in French policemen troop returning from the Pacific Islands. Travel Med. Infect. Dis. 6, 301–304.

Maretic, T., Perovic, M., Vince, A., Lukas, D., Dekumyoy, P., Begovac, J., 2009. Meningitis and radiculomyelitis caused by *Angiostrongylus cantonensis*. Emerg. Infect. Dis. 15, 996–998.

Margono, S.S., Ito, A., Sato, M.O., Okamoto, M., Subahar, R., Yamasaki, H., et al., 2003. *Taenia solium* taeniasis/cysticercosis in Papua, Indonesia in 2001: detection of human worm carriers. J. Helminthol. 77, 39–42.

Margono, S.S., Sutjahyono, R.W., Kurniawan, A., Nakao, M., Mulyani, T., Wandra, T., et al., 2007. Diphyllobothriasis and sparganosis in Indonesia. Trop. Med. Health 35, 301–305.

Martinez, H.R., Rangel-Guerra, R., Arredondo-Estrada, J.H., Marfil, A., Onofre, J., 1995. Medical and surgical treatment in neurocysticercosis a magnetic resonance study of 161 cases. J. Neurol. Sci. 130, 25–34.

Mitsuno, T., 1955. Cerebral granuloma caused by *Schistosoma japonicum*. J. Neurosurg. 12, 291–299.

Miyazaki, I., 1960. On the genus *Gnathostoma* and human gnathostomiasis, with special reference to Japan. Exp. Parasitol. 9, 338–370.

Moon, T.J., Yoon, B.Y., Hahn, Y.S., 1964. Spinal paragonimiasis. Yonsei Med. J. 5, 55–61.

Moore, D.A., McCroddan, J., Dekumyoy, P., Chiodini, P.L., 2003. Gnathostomiasis: an emerging imported disease. Emerg. Infect. Dis. 9, 647–650.

Mueller, J.F., 1935. A *Diphyllobothrium* from cats and dogs in the Syracuse region. J. Parasitol. 21, 114–121.

Mueller, J.F., 1974. The biology of *Spirometra*. J. Parasitol. 60, 3–14.

Muller, R., 2002. Worms and Human Disease. CABI, Wallingford.

Murrell, K.D., Fried, B., 2007. Food-Borne Parasitic Zoonoses: Fish and Plant-Borne Parasites. Springer, New York.

Murthy, J.M., Yangala, R., 2000. Etiological spectrum of localization-related epilepsies in childhood and the need for CT scan in children with partial seizures with no obvious causation—a study from south India. J. Trop. Pediatr. 46, 202–206.

Muth, S., Sayasone, S., Odermatt-Biays, S., Phompida, S., Duong, S., Odermatt, P., 2010. *Schistosoma mekongi* in Cambodia and Lao People's Democratic Republic. Adv. Parasitol. 72, 179–203.

Nash, T.E., Del Brutto, O.H., Butman, J.A., Corona, T., Delgado-Escueta, A., Duron, R.M., et al., 2004. Calcific neurocysticercosis and epileptogenesis. Neurology 62, 1934–1938.

Nash, T.E., Singh, G., White, A.C., Rajshekhar, V., Loeb, J.A., Proano, J.V., et al., 2006. Treatment of neurocysticercosis: current status and future research needs. Neurology 67, 1120–1127.

Nawa, Y., Nakamura-Uchiyama, F., 2005. *Paragonimus* and paragonimiasis in Japan. In: Arizono, J.Y., Chai, J.Y., Nawa, Y., Takahashi, Y. (Eds.), Asian Parasitology: Food-Borne Helminthiasis in Asia. Vol. 1. The Federation of Asian Parasitologists, Chuo-ku, pp. 125–131.

Nawa, Y., Tungtrongchitr, A., 2005. Angiostrongyliasis in Japan. In: Arizono, N., Chai, J.Y., Nawa, Y., Takahashi, Y. (Eds.), Asian Parasitology: Food-Borne Helminthiasis in Asia. Vol. 1. The Federation of Asian Parasitologists, Chuo-ku, pp. 213–216.

Neal, J.H., 1995. An endoscopic approach to cysticercosis cysts of the posterior third ventricle. Neurosurgery 36, 1040–1043.

Nomura, Y., Nagakura, K., Kagei, N., Tsutsumi, Y., Araki, K., Sugawara, M., 2000. Gnathostomiasis possibly caused by *Gnathostoma malaysiae*. Tokai J. Exp. Clin. Med. 25, 1–6.

Nontasut, P., Bussaratid, V., Chullawichit, S., Charoensook, N., Visetsuk, K., 2000. Comparison of ivermectin and albendazole treatment for gnathostomiasis. Southeast Asian J. Trop. Med. Public Health 31, 374–377.

Nontasut, P., Claesson, B.A., Dekumyoy, P., Pakdee, W., Chullawichit, S., 2005. Double-dose ivermectin vs albendazole for the treatment of gnathostomiasis. Southeast Asian J. Trop. Med. Public Health 36, 650–652.

Noor Azian, M.Y., Hakim, S.L., Sumiati, A., Norhafizah, M., 2006. Seroprevalence of cysticercosis in a rural village of Ranau, Sabah, Malaysia. Southeast Asian J. Trop. Med. Public Health 37, 58–61.

Ogata, K., Nawa, Y., Akahane, H., Diaz Camacho, S.P., Lamothe-Argumedo, R., Cruz-Reyes, A., 1998. Gnathostomiasis in Mexico. Am. J. Trop. Med. Hyg. 58, 316–318.

Oh, S.J., 1968a. Cerebral paragonimiasis. J. Neurol. Sci. 8, 27–48.

Oh, S.J., 1968b. Spinal paragonimiasis. J. Neurol. Sci. 6, 125–140.

Oh, S.J., 1969. Cerebral and spinal paragonimiasis. A histopathological study. J. Neurol. Sci. 9, 205–236.

Owatari, S., Yukitake, M., Sugawara, K., Sakai, J., Yamamoto, H., 1994. Two cases of *Paragonimus westermani* in one family. Nihon Kyobu Shikkan Gakkai Zasshi 32, 476–479.

PAHO, 2003. Zoonoses and Communicable Diseases Common to Man and Animals: Parasitoses. Pan American Health Organization, Washington, DC.

Pammenter, M.D., Haribhai, H.C., Epstein, S.R., Rossouw, E.J., Bhigjee, A.I., Bill, P.L., 1991. The value of immunological approaches to the diagnosis of schistosomal myelopathy. Am. J. Trop. Med. Hyg. 44, 329–335.

Parameswaran, K., 2006. Case series of eosinophilic meningoencephalitis from South India. Ann. Indian Acad. Neurol. 9, 217–222.

Pawlowski, Z., Allan, J., Sarti, E., 2005. Control of *Taenia solium* taeniasis/cysticercosis: from research towards implementation. Int. J. Parasitol. 35, 1221–1232.

Pittella, J.E., 1997. Neuroschistosomiasis. Brain Pathol. 7, 649–662.

Prabhakaran, V., Rajshekhar, V., Murrell, K.D., Oommen, A., 2004. *Taenia solium* metacestode glycoproteins as diagnostic antigens for solitary cysticercus granuloma in Indian patients. Trans. R. Soc. Trop. Med. Hyg. 98, 478–484.

Prociv, P., Spratt, D.M., Carlisle, M.S., 2000. Neuro-angiostrongyliasis: unresolved issues. Int. J. Parasitol. 30, 1295–1303.

Punyagupta, S., Bunnag, T., Juttijudata, P., Rosen, L., 1970. Eosinophilic meningitis in Thailand. Epidemiologic studies of 484 typical cases and the etiologic role of *Angiostrongylus cantonensis*. Am. J. Trop. Med. Hyg. 19, 950–958.

Punyagupta, S., Juttijudata, P., Bunnag, T., 1975. Eosinophilic meningitis in Thailand. Clinical studies of 484 typical cases probably caused by *Angiostrongylus cantonensis*. Am. J. Trop. Med. Hyg. 24, 921–931.

Punyagupta, S., Bunnag, T., Juttijudata, P., 1990. Eosinophilic meningitis in Thailand. Clinical and epidemiological characteristics of 162 patients with myeloencephalitis probably caused by *Gnathostoma spinigerum*. J. Neurol. Sci. 96, 241–256.

Qi, R.L., Liu, Y.F., Wang, H., Liang, S.J., Shen, H.X., Li, X.M., et al., 2008. An investigation on infection of sparganum of *Spirometra mansoni* in frogs from Guangzhou city from 2004 to 2007. J. Trop. Med. 8, 1178–1179.

Qiu, M.H., Qiu, M.D., 2009. Human plerocercoidosis and sparganosis: II. a historical review on pathology, clinics, epidemiology and control. Chin. J. Parasitol. Parasit. Dis. 27, 251–260.

Queuche, F., Cao Van, V., Le Dang, H., 1997. Endemic area of paragonimiasis in Vietnam. Santé 7, 155–159.

Ramirez-Avila, L., Slome, S., Schuster, F.L., Gavali, S., Schantz, P.M., Sejvar, J., et al., 2009. Eosinophilic meningitis due to *Angiostrongylus* and *Gnathostoma* species. Clin. Infect. Dis. 48, 322–327.

Rojekittikhun, W., 2002a. Current status of *Gnathostoma* infection in Thailand. J. Trop. Med. Parasitol. 25, 47–52.

Rojekittikhun, W., 2002b. On the biology of *Gnathostoma spinigerum*. J. Trop. Med. Parasitol. 25, 91–98.

Rojekittikhun, W., 2005. Gnathostomiasis in Thailand. In: Arizono, N., Chai, J.Y., Nawa, Y., Takahashi, Y. (Eds.), Asian Parasitology: Food-Borne Helminthiasis in Asia. Vol. 1. The Federation of Asian Parasitologists, Chuo-ku, pp. 241–259.

Rojekittikhun, W., Chaiyasith, T., Nuamtanong, S., Pubampen, S., Maipanich, W., Tungtrongchitr, R., 2002. *Gnathostoma* infection in Nakhon Nayok and Prachin Buri, Central Thailand. Southeast Asian J. Trop. Med. Public Health 33, 474–484.

Rojekittikhun, W., Chaiyasith, T., Nuamtanong, S., Komalamisra, C., 2004. *Gnathostoma* infection in fish caught for local consumption in Nakhon Nayok province, Thailand I. Prevalence and fish species. Southeast Asian J. Trop. Med. Public Health 35, 523–530.

Roman, G., Sotelo, J., Del Brutto, O., Flisser, A., Dumas, M., Wadia, N., et al., 2000. A proposal to declare neurocysticercosis an international reportable disease. Bull. World Health Organ. 78, 399–406.

Rosen, L., Chappell, R., Laqueur, G.L., Wallace, G.D., Weinstein, P.P., 1962. Eosinophilic meningoencephalitis caused by a metastrongylid lung-worm of rats. JAMA 179, 620–624.

Rosen, L., Loison, G., Laigret, J., Wallace, G.D., 1967. Studies on eosinophilic meningitis. 3. Epidemiologic and clinical observations on Pacific islands and the possible etiologic role of *Angiostrongylus cantonensis*. Am. J. Epidemiol. 85, 17–44.

Rosenfeld, E.A., Byrd, S.E., Shulman, S.T., 1996. Neurocysticercosis among children in Chicago. Clin. Infect. Dis. 23, 262–268.

Ross, A.G.P., Sleigh, A.C., Li, Y., Davis, G.M., Williams, G.M., Jiang, Z., et al., 2001. Schistosomiasis in the People's Republic of China: prospects and challenges for the 21st century. Clin. Microbiol. Rev. 14, 270–295.

Ross, A.G.P., Bartley, P.B., Sleigh, A.C., Olds, G.R., Li, Y., Williams, G.M., et al., 2002. Schistosomiasis. N. Engl. J. Med. 346, 1212–1220.

Ross, A.G., Vickers, D., Olds, G.R., Shah, S.M., McManus, D.P., 2007. Katayama syndrome. Lancet Infect. Dis. 7, 218–224.

Ruiz-García, M., Gonzalez-Astiazaran, A., Rueda-Franco, F., 1997. Neurocysticercosis in children. Clinical experience in 122 patients. Childs Nerv. Syst. 13, 608–612.

Rusnak, J.M., Lucey, D.R., 1993. Clinical gnathostomiasis: case report and review of the English-language literature. Clin. Infect. Dis. 16, 33–50.

Sáenz, B., Ruíz-García, M., Jiménez, E., Hernández-Aguilar, J., Suastegui, R., Larralde, C., et al., 2006. Neurocysticercosis: clinical, radiologic, and inflammatory differences between children and adults. Pediatr. Infect. Dis. J. 25, 801–803.

Saksirisampant, W., Kulkaew, K., Nuchprayoon, S., Yentakham, S., Wiwanitkit, V., 2002. A survey of the infective larvae of *Gnathostoma spinigerum* in swamp eels bought in a local market in Bangkok, Thailand. Ann. Trop. Med. Parasitol. 96, 191–195.

Samarasinghe, S., Perera, B.J., Ratnasena, B.G., 2002. First two cases of gnathostomiasis in Sri Lanka. Ceylon Med. J. 47, 96–97.

Sanchez, A.L., Lindback, J., Schantz, P.M., Sone, M., Sakai, H., Medina, M.T., et al., 1999. A population-based, case-control study of *Taenia solium* taeniasis and cysticercosis. Ann. Trop. Med. Parasitol. 93, 247–258.

Sarti, E., Schantz, P.M., Plancarte, A., Wilson, M., Gutierrez, O.I., Aguilera, J., et al., 1994. Epidemiological investigation of *Taenia solium* taeniasis and cysticercosis in a rural village of Michoacan state, Mexico. Trans. R. Soc. Trop. Med. Hyg. 88, 49–52.

Sawanyawisuth, K., Sawanyawisuth, K., 2008. Treatment of angiostrongyliasis. Trans. R. Soc. Trop. Med. Hyg. 102, 990–996.

Sawanyawisuth, K., Limpawattana, P., Busaracome, P., Ninpaitoon, B., Chotmongkol, V., Intapan, P.M., et al., 2004a. A 1-week course of corticosteroids in the treatment of eosinophilic meningitis. Am. J. Med. 117, 802–803.

Sawanyawisuth, K., Tiamkao, S., Kanpittaya, J., Dekumyoy, P., Jitpimolmard, S., 2004b. MR imaging findings in cerebrospinal gnathostomiasis. Am. J. Neuroradiol. 25, 446–449.

Sawanyawisuth, K., Chlebicki, M.P., Pratt, E., Kanpittaya, J., Intapan, P.M., 2009. Sequential imaging studies of cerebral gnathostomiasis with subdural hemorrhage as its complication. Trans. R. Soc. Trop. Med. Hyg. 103, 102–104.

Schantz, P.M., Sarti, E., Plancarte, A., Wilson, M., Criales, J.L., Roberts, J., et al., 1994. Community-based epidemiological investigations of cysticercosis due to *Taenia solium*: comparison of serological screening tests and clinical findings in two populations in Mexico. Clin. Infect. Dis. 18, 879–885.

Scharf, D., 1988. Neurocysticercosis. Two hundred thirty-eight cases from a California hospital. Arch. Neurol. 45, 777–780.

Schmutzhard, E., Boongird, P., Vejjajiva, A., 1988. Eosinophilic meningitis and radiculomyelitis in Thailand, caused by CNS invasion of *Gnathostoma spinigerum* and *Angiostrongylus cantonensis*. J. Neurol. Neurosurg. Psychiatry 51, 80–87.

Scrimgeour, E.M., Gajdusek, D.C., 1985. Involvement of the central nervous system in *Schistosoma mansoni* and *S. haematobium* infection. A review. Brain 108, 1023–1038.

Senanayake, N., Roman, G.C., 1993. Epidemiology of epilepsy in developing countries. Bull. World Health Organ. 71, 247–258.

Sharma, D.C., 2005. Paragonimiasis causing diagnostic confusion with tuberculosis. Lancet Infect. Dis. 5, 538.

Sieu, T.P., Dung, T.T., Nga, N.T., Hien, T.V., Dalsgaard, A., Waikagul, J., et al., 2009. Prevalence of *Gnathostoma spinigerum* infection in wild and cultured swamp eels in Vietnam. J. Parasitol. 95, 246–248.

Simanjuntak, G.M., Margono, S.S., Okamoto, M., Ito, A., 1997. Taeniasis/cysticercosis in Indonesia as an emerging disease. Parasitol. Today 13, 321–322.

Sinawat, S., Sanguansak, T., Angkawinijwong, T., Ratanapakorn, T., Intapan, P.M., Sinawat, S., et al., 2008. Ocular angiostrongyliasis: clinical study of three cases. Eye (London) 22, 1446–1448.

Singhi, P., Singhi, S., 2009. Neurocysticercosis in children. Indian J. Pediatr. 76, 537–545.

Singhi, P., Ray, M., Singhi, S., Khandelwal, N., 2000. Clinical spectrum of 500 children with neurocysticercosis and response to albendazole therapy. J. Child Neurol. 15, 207–213.

Slom, T.J., Cortese, M.M., Gerber, S.I., Jones, R.C., Holtz, T.H., Lopez, A.S., et al., 2002. An outbreak of eosinophilic meningitis caused by *Angiostrongylus cantonensis* in travelers returning from the Caribbean. N. Engl. J. Med. 346, 668–675.

Somers, R., Dorny, P., Nguyen, V.K., Dang, T.C., Goddeeris, B., Craig, P.S., et al., 2006. *Taenia solium* taeniasis and cysticercosis in three communities in north Vietnam. Trop. Med. Int. Health 11, 65–72.

Song, T., Wang, W.S., Zhou, B.R., Mai, W.W., Li, Z.Z., Guo, H.C., et al., 2007. CT and MR characteristics of cerebral sparganosis. Am. J. Neuroradiol. 28, 1700–1705.

Sotelo, J., Guerrero, V., Rubio, F., 1985. Neurocysticercosis: a new classification based on active and inactive forms. A study of 753 cases. Arch. Intern. Med. 145, 442–445.

Sotelo, J., Penagos, P., Escobedo, F., Del Brutto, O.H., 1988. Short course of albendazole therapy for neurocysticercosis. Arch. Neurol. 45, 1130–1133.

Sotelo, J., del Brutto, O.H., Penagos, P., Escobedo, F., Torres, B., Rodriguez-Carbajal, J., et al., 1990. Comparison of therapeutic regimen of anticysticercal drugs for parenchymal brain cysticercosis. J. Neurol. 237, 69–72.

Sripa, B., Kaewkes, S., Intapan, P.M., Maleewong, W., Brindley, P.J., 2010. Food-borne trematodiases: epidemiology, pathology, clinical manifestation and control. Adv. Parasitol. 72, 305–350.

Steinmann, P., Zhou, X.N., Li, Y.L., Li, H.J., Chen, S.R., Yang, Z., et al., 2007. Helminth infections and risk factor analysis among residents in Eryuan county, Yunnan province, China. Acta Trop. 104, 38–51.

Steinmann, P., Du, Z.W., Wang, L.B., Wang, X.Z., Jiang, J.Y., Li, L.H., et al., 2008. Extensive multiparasitism in a village of Yunnan province, People's Republic of China, revealed by a suite of diagnostic methods. Am. J. Trop. Med. Hyg. 78, 760–769.

Suankratay, C., Wilde, H., Berger, S., 2001. Thailand: country survey of infectious diseases. J. Travel Med. 8, 192–203.

Suastegui Roman, R.A., Soto-Hernandez, J.L., Sotelo, J., 1996. Effects of prednisone on ventriculoperitoneal shunt function in hydrocephalus secondary to cysticercosis: a preliminary study. J. Neurosurg. 84, 629–633.

Sugaroon, S., Wiwanitkit, V., 2003. *Gnathostoma* infective stage larvae in swamp eels (*Fluta alba*) at a metropolitan market in Bangkok, Thailand. Ann. Clin. Lab. Sci. 33, 94–96.

Takeuchi, K., 1918. A case with plerocercoid which is parasitic in the brain. Nippon Byori Gakkai Kaishi. 7, 611–620.

Tapchaisri, P., Nopparatana, C., Chaicumpa, W., Setasuban, P., 1991. Specific antigen of *Gnathostoma spinigerum* for immunodiagnosis of human gnathostomiasis. Int. J. Parasitol. 21, 315–319.

Tesana, S., Srisawangwong, T., Sithithaworn, P., Laha, T., 2008. *Angiostrongylus cantonensis*: experimental study on the susceptibility of apple snails, *Pomacea canaliculata* compared to *Pila polita*. Exp. Parasitol. 118, 531–535.

Toma, H., Matsumura, S., Oshiro, C., Hidaka, T., Sato, Y., 2002. Ocular angiostrongyliasis without meningitis symptoms in Okinawa, Japan. J. Parasitol. 88, 211–213.

Torres, M.L., 1965. Cerebral schistosomiasis: clinical report of a proven cerebral granuloma and review of 41 other proven cases in the literature. Philipp. J. Surg. Surg. Spec. 20, 289–307.

Tsai, H.C., Liu, Y.C., Kunin, C.M., Lee, S.S., Chen, Y.S., Lin, H.H., et al., 2001a. Eosinophilic meningitis caused by *Angiostrongylus cantonensis*: report of 17 cases. Am. J. Med. 111, 109–114.

Tsai, T.H., Liu, Y.C., Wann, S.R., Lin, W.R., Lee, S.J., Lin, H.H., et al., 2001b. An outbreak of meningitis caused by *Angiostrongylus cantonensis* in Kaohsiung. J. Microbiol. Immunol. Infect. 34, 50–56.

Tsai, H.C., Lee, S.S., Huang, C.K., Yen, C.M., Chen, E.R., Liu, Y.C., 2004. Outbreak of eosinophilic meningitis associated with drinking raw vegetable juice in southern Taiwan. Am. J. Trop. Med. Hyg. 71, 222–226.

Tsang, V.C., Brand, J.A., Boyer, A.E., 1989. An enzyme-linked immunoelectrotransfer blot assay and glycoprotein antigens for diagnosing human cysticercosis (*Taenia solium*). J. Infect. Dis. 159, 50–59.

Uchiyama, F., Morimoto, Y., Nawa, Y., 1999. Re-emergence of paragonimiasis in Kyushu, Japan. Southeast Asian J. Trop. Med. Public Health 30, 686–691.

Urbani, C., Sinoun, M., Socheat, D., Pholsena, K., Strandgaard, H., Odermatt, P., et al., 2002. Epidemiology and control of mekongi schistosomiasis. Acta Trop. 82, 157–168.

Utzinger, J., Keiser, J., 2004. Schistosomiasis and soil-transmitted helminthiasis: common drugs for treatment and control. Expert Opin. Pharmacother. 5, 263–285.

Utzinger, J., Zhou, X.N., Chen, M.G., Bergquist, R., 2005. Conquering schistosomiasis in China: the long march. Acta Trop. 96, 69–96.

Vien, C.V., Phue, N.C., Ha, L.D., Tuan, L.M., Van, N.T., Pao, T.C., et al., 1997. Paragonimiasis in Sin Ho district, Lai Chau province, Viet Nam. Southeast Asian J. Trop. Med. Public Health 28 (Suppl. 1), 46.

Vortel, V., Pur, J., Halberstadt, P., Valkounova, J., 1995. Human sparganosis. Cesk. Patol. 31, 3–8.

Wadia, N.H., Singh, G., 2002. *Taenia solium*: a historical note. In: Singh, Prabhakar (Ed.), *Taenia solium* Cysticercosis: From Basic to Clinical Science. CABI, Wallingford, pp. 157–168.

Waikagul, J., Yoonuan, T., 2005. *Paragonimus* and paragonimiasis in Thailand. In: Arizono, J.Y., Chai, J.Y., Nawa, Y., Takahashi, Y. (Eds.), Asian Parasitology: Food-Borne Helminthiasis in Asia. Vol. 1. The Federation of Asian Parasitologists, Chuo-ku, pp. 139–148.

Waikagul, J., Dekumyoy, P., Anantaphruti, M.T., 2006. Taeniasis, cysticercosis and echinococcosis in Thailand. Parasitol. Int. 55 (Suppl.), 175–180.

Walker, M., Zunt, J.R., 2005. Parasitic central nervous system infections in immunocompromised hosts. Clin. Infect. Dis. 40, 1005–1015.

Wallace, G.D., Rosen, L., 1966. Studies on eosinophilic meningitis. 2. Experimental infection of shrimp and crabs with *Angiostrongylus cantonensis*. Am. J. Epidemiol. 84, 120–131.

Wallace, G.D., Rosen, L., 1967. Studies on eosinophilic meningitis. IV. Experimental infection of fresh-water and marine fish with *Angiostrongylus cantonensis*. Am. J. Epidemiol. 85, 395–402.

Wan, F., Chen, J.C., Chen, J., Lei, T., Xue, D.L., Li, L., et al., 2006. Report of six cases with spinal schistosomiasis. Chin. J. Neurosurg. Dis. Res. 5, 83–84.

Wang, D.Z., 1984. Case report: an acute schistosomiasis with dysfunction of spinal cord. Chin. J. Parasitol. Parasit. Dis. 2, 205.

Wang, L.D., 2008. Report on the national survey of current status of major human parasitic diseases in China. People's Medical Publishing House, Beijing.

Wang, Q.P., Lai, D.H., Zhu, X.Q., Chen, X.G., Lun, Z.R., 2008. Human angiostrongyliasis. Lancet Infect. Dis. 8, 621–630.

Watt, G., Adapon, B., Long, G.W., Fernando, M.T., Ranoa, C.P., Cross, J.H., 1986. Praziquantel in treatment of cerebral schistosomiasis. Lancet 328, 529–532.

Wei, G.Z., Li, C.J., Meng, J.M., Ding, M.C., 1988. Cysticercosis of the central nervous system. A clinical study of 1, 400 cases. Chin. Med. J. (Engl.) 101, 493–500.

White, A.C., 2000. Neurocysticercosis: updates on epidemiology, pathogenesis, diagnosis, and management. Annu. Rev. Med. 51, 187–206.

WHO, 2002. Prevention and Control of Schistosomiasis and Soil-Transmitted Helminthiasis: Report of a WHO Expert Committee. WHO Technical Report Series 912. World Health Organisation, Geneva.

Willingham, A.L., III, Wu, H.W., Coulan, J., Strija, F., 2010. Combating *Taenia solium* cysticercosis in Southeast Asia: an opportunity for improving human health and livestock production. Adv. Parasitol. 72, 235–266.

Willingham, A.L., III, De, N.V., Doanh, N.Q., Cong le, D., Dung, T.V., Dorny, P., et al., 2003. Current status of cysticercosis in Vietnam. Southeast Asian J. Trop. Med. Public Health 34 (Suppl. 1), 35–50.

Wilson, M., Bryan, R.T., Fried, J.A., Ware, D.A., Schantz, P.M., Pilcher, J.B., et al., 1991. Clinical evaluation of the cysticercosis enzyme-linked immunoelectrotransfer blot in patients with neurocysticercosis. J. Infect. Dis. 164, 1007–1009.

Wiwanitkit, V., 2004. A note on the correlation between rainfall and the prevalence of *Gnathostoma* spp. infective stage larvae in swamp eels in Thailand. Parasite 11, 401–404.

Wiwanitkit, V., 2005. A review of human sparganosis in Thailand. Int. J. Infect. Dis. 9, 312–316.

Wu, G.L., 2005. Human Parasitology. People's Medical Publishing House, Beijing.

Wu, K.H., Lin, W.S., 2001. A survey on *Spirometra mansoni* among frogs in Qingkou and Ganzhe townships, Minhou county. Fujian Med. J. 23, 102–103.

Wu, G.Y., Yang, Y.M., Zheng, K.P., 1990. Sparganosis in cerebral and lumbar cord: one case report. Chin. J. Parasitol. Parasit. Dis. 8, 126.

Wu, J.H., Lin, L.Q., Wang, H.M., Zhang, L.D., 1997. A survey on *Sparganum* infection of frogs sold in Guangzhou markets. J. Guangzhou Chin. Med. Coll. 14, 193–194.

Wu, Z.J., Chen, Y., Qiu, X.L., Jiang, H.T., 2007. An investigation of plerocercoid infection of frogs in Guiyang city and an analysis on clinical characteristics of 104 cases. J. Guiyang Med. Coll. 32, 140–141.

Xiao, S.H., Keiser, J., Chen, M.G., Tanner, M., Utzinger, J., 2010. Research and development of antischistosomal drugs in People's Republic of China: a 60-year review. Adv. Parasitol. 73, 231–295.

Xu, J.T., Mao, L.L., 2002. Surveillance of paragonimiasis in Liaoning province during 1990-2001. Chin. J. Parasitic Dis. Control 15, 3.

Xu, L.Q., Jiang, Z.X., Zhou, C.H., Zhang, X.Q., Ren, Z.X., Chang, J., et al., 1999a. Distribution of cysticercosis in China. Chin. J. Parasitic Dis. Control 12, 30–32.

Xu, L.Q., Yu, S.H., Xu, S.M., 1999b. Distribution and Pathogenic Impact of Human Parasites in China. People's Medical Publishing House, Beijing.

Ye, L.P., Sun, Y.W., Xu, G.Z., Lu, D., Zhang, J.N., 2005. An investigation on *Spirometra mansoni* infection among frogs sold on markets in Ningbo city. Chin. J. Zoonoses 21, 443.

Yii, C.Y., 1976. Clinical observations on eosinophilic meningitis and meningoencephalitis caused by *Angiostrongylus cantonensis* on Taiwan. Am. J. Trop. Med. Hyg. 25, 233–249.

Yii, C.Y., Chen, C.Y., Chen, E.R., Hsieh, H.C., Shih, C.C., 1975. Epidemiologic studies of eosinophilic meningitis in southern Taiwan. Am. J. Trop. Med. Hyg. 24, 447–454.

Yin, H.J., 1997. Clinical analysis of 36 pediatric patients with cerebral paragonimiasis. Chongqing Med. J. 26, 338–339.

Yoonuan, T., Vanvanitchai, Y., Dekumyoy, P., Komalamisra, C., Kojima, S., Waikagul, J., 2008. Paragonimiasis prevalences in Saraburi province, Thailand, measured 20 years apart. Southeast Asian J. Trop. Med. Public Health 39, 593–600.

Zhang, E.X., 1990. Clinical analysis of 38 pediatric cases with cerebral paragonimiasis in the west mountainous area of Hubei province. Clin. Pediatr. J. 8, 177–179.

Zhang, E.D., Li, M.L., 1999. Clinical and CT characteristics of 1062 cases of neurocysticercosis. Henan J. Prev. Med. 10, 252–253.

Zhao, W.X., 1994. Human Parasitology. People's Medical Publishing House, Beijing.

Zhao, H.M., Zhou, S.C., Chen, X.L., Ji, X.R., Li, Y.J., Han, M., 1998. Spinal sparganosis: one case. Chin. J. Zoonoses 14, 49.

Zhou, X.N., Guo, J.G., Wu, X.H., Jiang, Q.W., Zheng, J., Dang, H., et al., 2007. Epidemiology of schistosomiasis in the People's Republic of China, 2004. Emerg. Infect. Dis. 13, 1470–1476.

Zhou, J., Li, G., Xia, J., Xiao, B., Bi, F., Liu, D., et al., 2009. Cerebral schistosomiasis japonica without gastrointestinal system involvement. Surg. Neurol. 71, 481–486.

Zhou, X.N., Bergquist, R., Leonardo, L., Yang, G.J., Yang, K., Sudomo, M., et al., 2010. Schistosomiasis japonica: research and control. Adv. Parasitol. 72, 145–178.

CHAPTER 13

Less Common Parasitic Infections in Southeast Asia that can Produce Outbreaks

Peter Odermatt,[*,†] **Shan Lv,**[*,†,‡] and **Somphou Sayasone**[*,†,§]

Contents

* Department of Epidemiology and Public Health, Swiss Tropical and Public Health Institute, Basel, Switzerland
† University of Basel, Basel, Switzerland
‡ National Institute of Parasitic Diseases, Chinese Center for Disease Control and Prevention, Shanghai, People's Republic of China
§ National Institute of Public Health, Ministry of Health, Vientiane, Lao People's Democratic Republic

Advances in Parasitology, Volume 72
ISSN 0065-308X, DOI: 10.1016/S0065-308X(10)72013-3

Abstract

The culturally deeply rooted habit of eating raw or undercooked foodstuffs, coupled with inadequate hygiene practices and lack of separation between foodstuff and wildlife in parts of Southeast Asia have repeatedly led to outbreaks due to rare parasitic infections. Trichinellosis, capillariasis and angiostrongyliasis are the three prime examples of such outbreaks occurring in Southeast Asia. We review the current knowledge of trichinellosis, capillariasis and angiostrongyliasis. Whilst infections—caused by nematodes—are rarely reported, their public health importance is considerable. Regarding trichinellosis, the large body of literature arises from a few countries only, indicating that available information underestimates the true extent and burden of this disease. Changes in socio-economic conditions in Southeast Asia and control efforts at the animal–human interface resulted in changing patterns of transmission and outbreaks of trichinellosis. Capillariasis is mainly found in the Philippines and Thailand. However, health service providers are mostly unaware of this disease due to its sporadic occurrence, delaying its diagnosis and commonly leading to inappropriate treatment and control. Angiostrongyliasis is an emerging parasitic infection with a number of significant outbreaks reported recently, particularly in the People's Republic of China. Angiostrongyliasis causes severe neurological disease and specialised health services are required for prompt diagnosis and adequate patient management. There is a need to improve preventive measures, stronger collaboration between veterinary and public health cadres and rigorous surveillance to adequately tackle trichinellosis, capillariasis, angiostrongyliasis and other uncommon parasitic diseases that have been linked to outbreaks.

13.1. INTRODUCTION

The occurrence of parasitic infections and their public health impact are often determined by the endemicity level in a population. Typical indicators are prevalence or intensity of infection in a population sample or a specific subgroup, for example, prevalence of soil-transmitted helminth or schistosome infections among school-aged children or entire communities in a single village, county or province (Steinmann et al., 2007, 2008; Zhou et al., 2007). Risk factors for infection, morbidity and mortality are obtained as a means to estimate the public health burden. Parasitic infections such as *Plasmodium* typically show seasonal patterns, which are governed by climatic factors and human behaviour (Childs et al., 2006). An important feature of parasitic infections in Southeast Asia is that they often occur in outbreaks. An outbreak is a term used in epidemiology to describe an occurrence (incidence) of a disease greater than what is expected over a particular time span and in a geographically confined area. It may be a small and localised event or involve thousands of people across an entire continent over several months. Formally, two linked cases of a rare infectious disease may be sufficient to constitute an outbreak.

This chapter focuses on three parasitic diseases that are quite rare, but have the potential to cause outbreaks, namely trichinellosis, capillariasis and angiostrongyliasis. These diseases particularly affect Southeast Asia, which includes 12 countries (i.e. Brunei, Cambodia, Timor-Leste, Indonesia, Lao People's Democratic Republic (Lao PDR), Malaysia, Myanmar, Papua New Guinea, Philippines, Singapore, Thailand and Vietnam). The People's Republic of China (P.R. China), which does not formally belong to the Southeast Asian region, is also included, because the south P.R. China shares similar eco-epidemiological and socio-cultural features with other settings of Southeast Asia. In a companion piece discussing the so-called neglected tropical diseases in Southeast Asia, P.R. China is also included (Hotez and Ehrenberg, 2010).

Our chapter is structured as follows. First, we focus on trichinellosis, a cosmopolite nematode infection, comprising of several parasite species of different regions of the world and in a variety of hosts. This parasite leads to epidemics, which vary greatly in size, affected number of people and area, and morbidity and mortality. Second, information on outbreaks of capillariasis is summarised. *Capillaria* is the least known outbreak-producing nematode. It has been discovered in Southeast Asia (Philippines), is thought to have the highest public health burden in this region, although transmission has been reported from other parts of the world. Third, we discuss angiostrongyliasis, an emerging zoonotic nematode infection with a host of recent outbreaks occurring in P.R. China. As human infection leads to cerebral disease (Lv et al., 2010), it is a most perilous infection. We conclude our review by summarising key features of the three parasites and their role in producing outbreaks, and propose ways in which their public health impact might be addressed in the Southeast Asian region.

13.2. TRICHINELLOSIS

Trichinellosis is a zoonosis with a worldwide occurrence (Dupouy-Camet, 2000; Gottstein et al., 2009). Today, eight species of the genus *Trichinella* (i.e. *T. spiralis*, *T. nativa*, *T. britovi*, *T. murrelli*, *T. nelsoni*,

T. pseudospiralis, *T. papuae* and *T. zimbabwensis*) are known, and they display different geographical distributions (Gottstein et al., 2009). Over the past 50 years, *Trichinella* infections have only rarely been reported, most often in countries of Southeast Asia.

13.2.1. Life cycle, mode of transmission, clinical aspects and treatment

A domestic and a sylvatic transmission cycle must be distinguished. Predators such as larger mammals become infected when consuming their prey, mainly rodents. The consumption of their carcasses by rodents closes the transmission cycle. The infection of *Trichinella* parasites weakens the host, which in turn enhances the force of transmission. Infected rodents play a major role in introducing the parasite to household-bred pigs, leading to domestic transmission. At the household level, *Trichinella* is transmitted to humans by consumption of raw or insufficiently cooked infected pork meat; while unsafe pig feeding practices or exposure to roaming rodents lead to infections in pigs.

Human trichinellosis is most commonly acquired through the ingestion of raw or undercooked pork containing encysted *Trichinella* larvae (Pozio, 2001a). However, trichinellosis has also been reported after ingestion of meat from bear, walrus, boar, cougar and other wild animals. In the human host, encysted larvae excyst and penetrate the small intestinal wall. During the acute enteric phase, humans experience nausea, vomiting, diarrhoea and abdominal pain. Following maturation and mating, the female worm resides in the intestine where it produces larvae, which migrate into the lymphatic and blood vessels to finally end up and encyst in striated muscles. The migratory phase may last several weeks up to 3 months. The parasite induces the transformation of its surroundings into a nurse cell, which sustains the encysted larva. Cysts calcify over a period of many years. The encystment is specific for the skeletal muscle, and does not occur in other muscles, for example, cardiac tissue. A similar development occurs in other suitable hosts. Thus, the consumption of insufficiently cooked and larvae-containing meat leads to new infections.

The signs and symptoms of trichinellosis are directly related to the number of larvae ingested (Dupouy-Camet et al., 2002). Though the majority of infections are asymptomatic, typical symptoms of the migratory phase include fever, severe myalgia, periorbital oedema, conjunctivitis and muscle tenderness. Usually, an infection is associated with eosinophilia and increased muscle-related enzyme levels. If two or more epidemiologically interconnected individuals (e.g. from the same household or sharing the same dishes) have high fever, periorbital or facial oedema and myalgia, trichinellosis should be suspected (Dupouy-Camet et al., 2002; Gottstein et al., 2009).

Additional diagnostic arguments are based on serological tools, which become positive 2–3 weeks post-infection. Muscle biopsies provide specific diagnosis but have low sensitivity (around 50% of infections are detected). Biopsy is of particular value in large outbreaks, as the *Trichinella* species can be determined based on morphological and molecular characteristics of the encysted muscle larvae (Dupouy-Camet et al., 2002; Gottstein et al., 2009).

Severe morbidity such as pneumonitis, encephalitis and myocarditis with sometimes fatal outcome may be caused by the larvae during their migration, in combination with the inflammatory response of the affected organ. However, in most cases trichinellosis is a self-limiting disease. Alternatively, it can be treated with benzimidazoles, albendzole and mebendazole (Dupouy-Camet et al., 2002).

13.2.2. Trichinellosis outbreak in Southeast Asia and P.R. China

Most information on trichinellosis outbreaks in the Southeast Asian region is available from P.R. China and Thailand. The parasite has also been shown to be endemic in Cambodia, Indonesia, Lao PDR, Malaysia, Myanmar and Papua New Guinea either in humans or in animal hosts (Pozio, 2001b). However, descriptions and analyses of outbreaks in the peer-reviewed international literature are scarce for many countries in this region.

13.2.2.1. P.R. China

There is a wealth of information on trichinellosis outbreaks in Chinese journals, documenting both the local epidemiology and the public health burden of this disease. The first official report regards a case of trichinellosis in Tibet in 1964 (Huang, 1965). From this observation until 1999, reports of 548 outbreaks are available (Wang and Cui, 2001b). They involved more than 23,000 individuals and 236 deaths. These 35 years can be stratified into three main periods (Liu and Boireau, 2002): (i) 1964–1979 with outbreaks mainly occurring in areas where local residents, often ethnic minorities, customarily consume raw meat; (ii) 1980–1989 characterised by a rapid increase in meat consumption going hand-in-hand with economic development and growth in 20 provinces; and (iii) 1990–1999 marked by a decreasing incidence of human trichinellosis in traditional endemic areas, but an increase in other regions, indicating weak food hygiene conditions.

In the new millennium, additional trichinellosis outbreaks have been recorded. We made an attempt to systematically review the literature (both English and Chinese) and identified 16 reports, involving 1623 patients of whom eight died (Table 13.1). The largest outbreak involved 841 patients. Most cases occurred in the northeastern, central and southwestern provinces of P.R. China. The consumption of infected pork meat

TABLE 13.1 Trichinellosis outbreaks in P.R. China, 2000–2009

Year	Location	Exposed (*n*)	Cases (*n*)	Population	Source of infection	Mean incubation period (days)	Parasitological diagnosis (%)[c]	Supplementary diagnosis	Outcome (case-fatality rate %)	Reference(s)
2000	Yongning, Guangxi province	25	23	Villagers	Pickled pork	Unknown	2 (100)	—	No death (0)	Yao et al. (2002)
2000	Jianshui, Yunnan province	6	6	Road building workers	Raw pork	2–4	2 (100)	—	1 death (16.7)	Xu (2002)
2001	Dazi, Tibet	115	46	Villagers	Raw pork	5–15	2 (100)	Larvae in pork meat	1 death (2.2)	Su et al. (2002)
2001	Nandan, Guangxi province	68	36	Yao ethnic minority	Pickled pork	8–23 (13.5)	1 (100)	Larvae in pork meat	No death (0)	Tian et al. (2001); Yao (2008)
2002	Baiyu, Sichuan province	63 (25 due to undercooked boar)	23	Tibet herdsman	Raw boar	5–20 (13)	2 (100)	—	1 death (4.3)	Ye et al. (2003)
2002	Suifenghe, Heilongjiang province	Unknown	7	Family and relatives	Raw dog meat	Unknown	Unknown	Larvae in dog meat	No death (0)	Yuan and Zhang (2002)
2002	Milin, Tibet	Unknown	3	Villagers	Raw pork	10	1 (100)	—	3 deaths (100)	Ci et al. (2003)
2002	Dali, Yunnan province	Unknown	127	Bai ethnic minority	Raw pork	Unknown	Unknown	—	No death (0)	Dai (2003)
2003	Eryuan, Yunnan province	Unknown	168	Bai ethnic minority	Raw pork	1–7	Unknown	—	No death (0)	Luo et al. (2004)

2004	Dali, Yunnan province	1920	132[a]	Bai ethnic minority	Raw pork	11–30	Unknown	—	No death (0)	Zhang et al. (2007)
2005	Xiangyun, Yunnan province	unknown	24	Yi ethnic minority	Raw pork	2–25	Unknown	—	No death (0)	Wang and Liu (2006); Zhang et al. (2007)
2006	Puer, Yunnan province	57	49	Travellers to Lao PDR	Unknown	1–20 (17)	5 (100)[d]	—	No death (0)	Yao (2008)
2006	Dali, Yunnan province	120	103	Villagers	Raw pork	7–24	Unknown	—	No death (0)	Ke et al. (2007)
2007	Dali, Yunnan province	unknown	841[b]	Villagers	Raw pork	Unknown	Unknown	—	No death (0)	Ma (2008)
2007	Gongbujiangda, Tibet	10	9	Tibet migrant worker	Raw pork	1	4 (75%)	Larvae in pork meat	2 deaths (22.2)	Hong et al. (2008)
2008	Mengla, Yunnan province	26	26	Hani ethnic minority	Raw boar	4–12 (7)	2 (0)	Larvae in pork meat	No death (0)	Wang et al. (2009)

[a] The number of cases includes those identified within one month of exposure.
[b] Number of cases in a hospital.
[c] Biopsy of *gastrocnemius*, only taking samples from patients with typical manifestations.
[d] Total number of individuals who were examined is unknown.

is responsible for the majority of the outbreaks, with mutton and game meat involved in a few cases (Wang and Cui, 2001b; Wang et al., 2006). Dog meat has also been identified as a possible source of infections (Cui and Wang, 2001).

The trichinellosis prevalence in pigs and rats is considerable. For example, in Hubei province in 1998 it amounted to 5.6% and 10.5%, respectively. The high infection rates in pork are explained by unsafe pig feeding practices and utilisation of raw or undercooked meat from food scraps for feeding pigs (Liu and Boireau, 2002; Wang and Cui, 2001a; Wang et al., 2007). Pork consumption has considerably increased over the last decades, particularly in Southeast Asia (Erlanger et al., 2009; Keiser et al., 2005). Especially the consumption of scalded pork and mutton cubes as well as dumplings during the winter months has increased, but cooking practices are not always adequate. Therefore, trichinellosis outbreaks have also increasingly occurred in central and northwestern P.R. China where raw meat consumption is not customarily prevalent (Wang and Cui, 2001a).

The complex and changing interplay of factors related to pork meat production and hygiene, and food consumption behaviour is responsible that today trichinellosis is still a public health concern, although substantial efforts and progress in control have been made (Cui et al., 2006).

13.2.2.2. Thailand and Lao PDR

Abundant information is available on trichinellosis outbreaks in Thailand. For example, Kaewpitoon et al. (2008) reviewed the available information on outbreaks since the start of records keeping on trichinellosis in 1962. Overall, 135 outbreaks were documented including 7340 individuals and 97 deaths. Between 1962 and 1971, 10 outbreaks with a total of 764 patients were counted and 54 deaths were recorded (Khamboonruang and Nateewatana, 1975; Suriyanon and Klunklin, 1972). All outbreaks occurred in northwestern Thailand at the border to Myanmar (Mae Hong Son province) and Lao PDR (Chiang Mai and Non provinces). In eight of these outbreaks, the source of infection was linked to pork consumption. The consumption of a wild boar was found to be responsible for one outbreak and that of a jackal for the tenth outbreak. The consumption of raw meat is widespread in local ethnic minority populations, for example, the "labh" dishes which contain raw or insufficiently cooked minced meat (Khamboonruang and Nateewatana, 1975), which underscores that new research is warranted to further explore the links between ethnic minority groups and the so-called neglected tropical diseases (Schratz et al., 2010). The authors of the above-mentioned review of 10 trichinellosis outbreaks concluded that the number of outbreaks underestimated the true number of infections. Indeed, the three major outbreaks went unreported before an epidemic was documented in 1971 (Khamboonruang and Nateewatana, 1975).

Until the late 1980s, more than 100 trichinellosis outbreaks were recorded (Pozio and Khamboonruang, 1989), most of them in north Thailand. By the end of 1975, the Ministry of Public Health had recorded more than 118 distinct outbreaks, involving 5400 patients and 95 deaths (Khamboonruang, 1991). Based on the examination of pigs and rats, *T. spiralis* was identified as the aetiologic agent. This species could later be identified with isoenzymatic typing of parasite material isolated from a patient (Pozio and Khamboonruang, 1989). In north Thailand, the consumption of raw or insufficiently cooked foodstuffs is a deeply culturally rooted habit. Hill-tribe pigs, wild boars and jackals were identified as common reservoirs of an infection (Khamboonruang, 1991).

Case confirmation based on muscle biopsy was initially used. However, later on, this approach was replaced by serological testing (IgG ELISA) (Morakote et al., 1991), which was shown to have 100% sensitivity from 50 to 411 days post-infection (Morakote et al., 1992). The clinical picture followed the typical symptoms, where almost all patients suffered from severe myalgia, fever and facial oedema (Limsuwan and Siriprasert, 1994). In-depth analysis of the outbreaks in 1994–1995 and 2006 revealed *T. pseudospiralis* (Jongwutiwes et al., 1998) and *T. papuae* (Khumjui et al., 2008) as the responsible species. Hence, molecular diagnostic techniques clearly showed that trichinellosis is caused by a higher diversity of circulating parasites than previously anticipated.

In neighbouring Lao PDR, cases of trichinellosis are occasionally diagnosed in the central hospitals. However, the infection is largely unknown to health professionals. So far, only three reports of outbreaks have been documented in the peer-reviewed literature. The first publication dates back to 1976 and reports an epidemic in the capital Vientiane in which 32 individuals were affected after consumption of pork meat (Sicard et al., 1976). Some 30 years later, in 2004, the observation of three cases of suspected trichinellosis at the same central hospital led to a village-based follow-up investigation of a potential outbreak in Borikamsay province. In two villages, 22 further patients with a typical history were identified (Sayasone et al., 2006). Among them, 21 patients were seropositive (confirmed by Western blot). In June 2005, a large-scale outbreak occurred in the northern province of Oudomxay where at least 650 persons were affected (Barennes et al., 2008). Pork meat samples from 11 pigs showed that one pig was infected with *T. spiralis*.

In all three outbreaks, Lao-Loum (low-land dwellers) group was affected and pork meat, consumed during festive events (e.g. New Year, marriages and funeral gatherings), was identified as the source of infection. The majority of the Lao population is Lao-Loum and has a culturally deeply rooted fondness for raw food consumption, including pork meat. This also results in high rates of other food-borne infectious diseases, for example, food-borne trematodiasis (Keiser and Utzinger, 2009; Odermatt et al., 2007; Sayasone et al., 2007; Sripa et al., 2010). The issue that food preferences and consumption habits are often maintained abroad is illustrated by trichinellosis outbreaks in Lao communities in the United States (CDC, 1984; McAuley et al., 1992).

The Lao population is scattered and the majority live from subsistence farming. Pig rearing is widespread. Traditionally, animals are either roaming freely around the household or only loosely attached. Contact with wild animals, in particular rodents, is possible. Most pigs are slaughtered at the household, and meat control is only performed on a very small proportion of the animals.

13.2.3. Conclusions

Trichinellosis is a food-borne parasitic infection, and numerous outbreaks have occurred in Southeast Asian countries. The published reports, however, relate only to a few countries and it is most likely that the true extent of the public health importance of trichinellosis is much larger. The habit of eating insufficiently cooked meat is common throughout Southeast Asia, and hence outbreaks of trichinellosis are likely to occur. Sporadic human trichinellosis cases are also seen in countries where no outbreaks have been found, for example, in Vietnam (Taylor et al., 2009). More accurate documentation of these infections is essential, as this information will provide new evidence on circulating parasites, which may be transmitted to humans. Hence, there is a need to sensitise health services and to strengthen surveillance systems so that cases and outbreaks of trichinellosis can be more readily documented and prevention and control implemented more rigorously.

13.3. CAPILLARIASIS

Capillaria belongs to the nematode superfamily Trichinelloidae. More than 250 species are known to infect vertebrates. Three species, *C. aeruginosa*, *C. hepatica* and *C. philippinensis*, cause human capillariasis. Of these, *C. philippinensis* is of medical concern (Cross, 1992; Saichua et al., 2008). It causes a severe intestinal disease and death may occur if it is not treated correctly and timely. In the last decade, *C. philippinensis* outbreaks have been identified in several countries of Southeast Asia (Bair et al., 2004; Cross, 1992; el-Dib and Doss, 2002; Saichua et al., 2008).

13.3.1. Life cycle, mode of transmission, clinical consequences and treatment

C. philippinensis has a complex life cycle. Small freshwater fish act as intermediate hosts and fish-eating birds are the natural definitive hosts (Cross, 1992; Saichua et al., 2008). Parasite eggs excreted via faeces of infected animals reach water bodies where they are ingested by small fresh- and brackish water fish. The larvae hatch in the fish intestine and migrate to the mesenteries where they develop into infective forms 1–2 weeks post-infection (Cross, 1992). Humans acquire an infection when they consume such fish raw or insufficiently cooked. Handling fish under poor sanitary conditions may also contaminate other food or kitchen instruments (Soukhathammavong et al., 2008). In humans, the larvae are restricted to the intestinal mucus where they mature within 2 weeks. Female worms start producing eggs 3 weeks after infection. Eggs may also develop into infective larvae in the human intestine. This auto-infection results in overwhelming parasite loads, which may lead to a fatal outcome (Cross, 1992).

Patients with intestinal capillariasis suffer from various gastrointestinal symptoms, such as watery diarrhoea, weight loss, muscle wasting, borborygmus, abdominal pain, pedal oedema and fluid loss (Bair et al., 2004; Cross, 1992; Soukhathammavong et al., 2008). Biochemical tests of the blood show a low level of plasma proteins and an electrolyte imbalance, that is hypokalaemia, which may cause death due to heart failure (Cross, 1992).

C. philippinensis is diagnosed by identifying the parasite eggs in the stool, which may also contain larvae and adult worms. The peanut-shaped egg with flattened bipolar plugs is often confused with eggs of the soil-transmitted helminth *Trichuris trichiura* (Figs. 13.1 and 13.2). Female *C. philippinensis* worms only sporadically produce eggs (Saichua et al., 2008). Therefore, examining a single stool sample is an unreliable

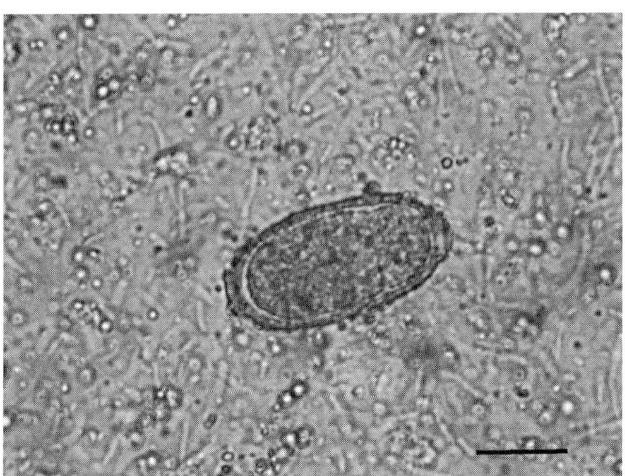

FIGURE 13.1 Elongated peanut-shaped *C. philippinensis* egg (size 46.1 × 22.1 μm) with flattened bipolar plugs and striated shell (bar 22 μm).

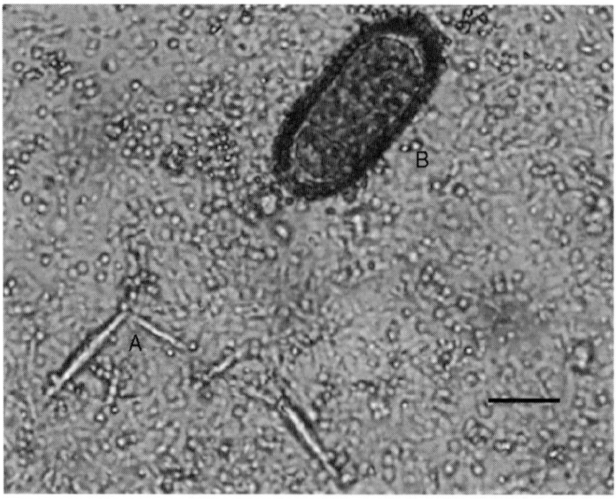

FIGURE 13.2 Stool examination with Charcot-Leyden Crystals (A) and *C. philippinensis* eggs (B), (bar 22 μm).

diagnostic approach, and repeated stool sampling is required to enhance diagnostic sensitivity. Early diagnosis and treatment prevents patients from fatal complications (Saichua et al., 2008).

Several anthelminthic drugs are efficacious against capillariasis (Bair et al., 2004; Cross, 1992; Hong et al., 1994; Soukhathammavong et al., 2008). Particularly albendazole and mebendazole are used. Albendazole 400 mg or mebendazole 200 mg over at least 3 weeks are required for parasite clearance. Relapses occur if the treatment duration is inadequate (Cross and Basaca-Sevilla, 1987; Soukhathammavong et al., 2008).

13.3.2. First observations and outbreaks

The first human case of intestinal capillariasis was diagnosed in 1963 by Chitwood et al. (1968) during an autopsy of a male patient from Ilocos Norte province, northern Luzon in the Philippines. The patient died from intractable 3-week lasting diarrhoea and malabsorption 3 days after admission to a hospital in Manila (Chitwood et al., 1968; Cross, 1992; Saichua et al., 2008). The public health significance of this parasite was recognised 3 years later (1967), when a capillariasis outbreak was identified. Between 1995 and 1997, more than 1000 people were diagnosed with capillariasis in Pudoc West village, 77 cases manifested significant symptoms. From 1967 to 1990, the parasite was frequently diagnosed in the northern Luzon. A total of 1884 cases were confirmed, of whom 110 patients died (Cross, 1992; Saichua et al., 2008).

C. philippinensis infections were also reported from other Southeast Asian countries. In Thailand, the first report of intestinal capillariasis dates back to 1973, when an 18-month-old girl suffering from diarrhoea and malabsorption was diagnosed with this infection (Pradatsundarasar et al., 1973). In 1981, a capillariasis outbreak occurred in the northeastern province of Sisaket (Table 13.2). More than 20 patients were found, almost half of whom ($n = 9$) died (Saichua et al., 2008). Between 1979 and 1981, 15 of approximately 100 capillariasis patients admitted to hospitals in Thailand died (Kunaratanapruk et al., 1983). Subsequently, another 82 cases were reported from other provinces of Thailand (Saichua et al., 2008).

Sporadic cases have also been reported from Indonesia (Bangs et al., 1994). In Lao PDR, the first three cases have been documented recently. Among them, two patients had acquired the infection in Thailand, while the third one had no history of travelling abroad confirming that parasite transmission occurred in Lao PDR (Soukhathammavong et al., 2008), and therefore, outbreaks are potentially possible.

Infections were also diagnosed in India, the Islamic Republic of Iran, Korea, Japan, Taiwan and the United Arab Emirates (el Hassan and Mikhail, 1992; Hoghooghi-Rad et al., 1987; Lu et al., 2006), in Africa (Egypt) (Ahmed et al., 1999; el-Dib and Doss, 2002; el-Dib et al., 1999) and two imported cases in Europe (Italy and Spain) (Chichino et al., 1992; Dronda et al., 1993; onso-Sanz et al., 1995). The latter two infections have been acquired in Indonesia and South America (Chichino et al., 1992; Dronda et al., 1993). However, based on current information, epidemic occurrence of *Capillaria* is restricted to Southeast Asia.

13.3.3. Conclusions

Capillariasis was discovered in Southeast Asia where outbreaks have led to deaths. The similarity between *Capillaria* and *T. trichiura* eggs often results in confusion, late diagnosis and inappropriate treatment. Although outbreaks in Southeast Asia have only been reported from the Philippines and Thailand, occasional cases in many other countries indicate that the parasite is widely circulating in the environment (fish and birds). Outbreaks due to this parasite can thus not be ruled out and vigilance is recommended.

13.4. ANGIOSTRONGYLIASIS

Detailed descriptions of the nematode *Angiostrongylus cantonensis* and its clinical importance are provided elsewhere, including a chapter by Lv and colleagues published in this special thematic volume of the *Advances in Parasitology* (Lv et al., 2010; Wang et al., 2008). Here, we briefly

TABLE 13.2 *Capillaria philippinensis* outbreaks in Thailand and the Philippines

Country	Location	Year	No. of cases	Outcome (case–fatality rate %)	Reference
Thailand	Sisaket province village hospital	1981	20	9 deaths (45.0)	Saichua et al. (2008)
		1979–1981	100	15 deaths (15.0)	Kunaratanapruk et al. (1983)
	All provinces	1994–2006	82	1 death (1.2)	Saichua et al. (2008)
Philippines	Pudoc West village	1965–1967	1000	77 deaths (7.7)	Cross (1992)
	Northern Luzon	1967–1990	1884	110 deaths (5.8)	Cross (1992)
	Compostela Valley province	2000	17	No death (0)	Belizario et al. (2000)

summarise the epidemiology of angiostrongyliasis and then focus on the phenomenon of outbreaks, which is the common form of how angiostrongyliasis occurs in Southeast Asia and particularly in P.R. China.

13.4.1. Life cycle, clinical aspects and treatment

Human angiostrongyliasis, typically characterised by eosinophilic meningitis, is caused by the rat lungworm, *A. cantonensis* (Chen 1935). Adult worms parasitise the pulmonary arteries and right heart in rats. Released eggs hatch in capillaries of the lung tissue and the first-stage larvae (L_1) penetrate through the capillary walls to enter the airways. The L_1 are then swallowed and passed with the faeces. After ingesting by molluscs, the larvae invade tissues (e.g. the gut wall, muscle and mantle) and further develop. The developmental time is governed by temperature. A linear relationship between development and temperature has been estimated for the range between 19 °C and 31 °C (Ishii, 1984; Lv et al., 2006). The L_1 develop into infective third-stage larvae (L_3) after two moults. The development continues if molluscs with L_3 are ingested by the rat definitive host. L_3 then enter the bloodstream by penetrating the intestinal wall. The larvae experience two further moults in the central nervous system (CNS) and then enter the pulmonary arteries where they mature (Murrell and Fried, 2007). Paratenic hosts (e.g. frogs, lizards, crabs, shrimps and fish) can host infective L_3 for several days or weeks (Wallace and Rosen, 1966, 1967).

Humans acquire an infection when they ingest mollusc intermediate hosts, which harbour L_3. Common sources of infection include terrestrial and freshwater snails and contaminated vegetables. Other known infection routes are the ingestion of terrestrial slugs, frogs, lizards and shrimps. Humans are accidental hosts of *A. cantonensis*. L_3 develop to the fourth or fifth stage in the CNS, but rarely reach sexual maturity in the human pulmonary arteries. Therefore, typical manifestations induced by this parasite occur in the CNS and occasionally other organs such as the eyes and nose. The incubation period varies between 1 and 54 days, depending on the source of infection and the number of larvae ingested (Lv et al., 2010). The most common symptoms include severe headache, neck stiffness, paraesthesia, nausea and vomiting. Fever is common in paediatric patients (Hwang and Chen, 1991). An elevated eosinophilic cell count in cerebrospinal fluid (CSF) is an important indicator for *A. cantonensis* infections. Due to the possibility of other pathogens inducing eosinophilic meningitis, differential diagnosis is necessary (Graeff-Teixeira et al., 2009; Lv et al., 2010).

Presence of *A. cantonensis* larvae in CSF leads to definitive diagnosis. Increase of internal diameter of spinal needle or CSF aspiration with a syringe was proposed to favour the detection rate of parasite. Indeed, discovery rate could reach as high as 41.5% in 82 cases

(Hwang and Chen, 1991) and 61.5% in 13 spinal taps (Yii, 1976) when aspirating CSF with a syringe with a negative pressure or lumbar puncture using tap needles with internal diameters of 0.4–0.8 mm, much wider than the needles with $\leq$0.3 mm, which are routinely used for lumbar puncture.

Albendazole and mebendazole are commonly used to treat angiostrongyliasis patients (Sawanyawisuth and Sawanyawisuth, 2008). Levamisole has been used to treat paediatric patients with reportedly good efficacy (Hwang, 1997). Corticosteroids are useful by modulating the inflammatory response but a considerable number of relapses have been reported (Sawanyawisuth et al., 2004; Tsai et al., 2004). Currently, a combination of anthelminthic drugs and corticosteroids is recommended for the treatment of angiostrongyliasis (Chotmongkol et al., 2004, 2006). The recommended regime is albendazole 15 mg/kg/day (or mebendazole 10 mg/kg/day) with prednisolone 60 mg/day for 14 days. The regime of albendazole 200 mg/day for 5 days and 400 mg/day for 5 more days, accompanied with dexamethasone 5–10 mg/day is also recommended (Wang et al., 2002). Supportive measures, such as repeated lumbar puncture and mannitol transfusion can relieve symptoms (Chotmongkol et al., 2000; Lv et al., 2009a). Removal of worms by surgery from the eye chamber is an effective measure to treat ocular angiostrongyliasis.

13.4.2. Outbreak: The common form of angiostrongyliasis occurrence

Angiostrongyliasis epidemics occur due to specific behaviours and risk factors. A 2-year study (1968–1969) identified 125 cases in southern Taiwan and demonstrated the consumption of the giant African land snail, *Achatina fulica*, as the main source of infection (Yii et al., 1975). Similarly, a study conducted between 1965 and 1968 identified 484 cases of *A. cantonensis* infections in Thailand (Punyagupta et al., 1975). The principal source of infection was consumption of freshwater snails belonging to the genus of *Pila*. It has been estimated that thousands of human cases occurred each year at that time. Even at present, several hundred suspected angiostrongyliasis cases are admitted annually to hospitals in Thailand (Eamsobhana and Tungtrongchitr, 2005).

The known angiostrongyliasis outbreaks in Southeast Asia and the Far East are summarised in Table 13.3. The frequency of outbreaks increased in the last decade, especially in P.R. China. The rise has been attributed to the spread of the snail *Pomacea canaliculata* (Lv et al., 2008, 2009b). Except for two outbreaks, which occurred in Okinawa and Taiwan, most were related to the invasive terrestrial snail *A. fulica*, introduced into Southeast Asia around 1930 (Mead, 1961) and the invasive freshwater

TABLE 13.3 Angiostrongyliasis outbreaks in Southeast Asia and the Far East

Year	Location	Exposed (*n*)	Case (*n*)	Population	Source of infection	Mean incubation period (days)	Parasitological diagnosis (%)	Outcome (case-fatality rate %)	Reference(s)
1985	Taoyuan	Unknown	9	A local family, 1 child	*A. fulica*	Unknown	1, spinal taps (11.1)	Four deaths (44.4)	Hwang and Chen (1986)
1985	Kaohsiung	5	4	Local residents, 4 children	*P. canaliculata*	Unknown	1, spinal taps (25.0)	No death (0)	Hwang and Chen (1986)
1997	Wenzhou	Unknown	65	Local residents	*P. canaliculata*	1–20 (10.3)[a]	0 (0)	No death (0)	Zheng et al. (2001)
1998	Kaohsiung	Unknown	8	Group of Thai migrant workers	*P. canaliculata*	5–12 (7.6)[b]	0 (0)	No death (0)	Tsai et al. (2001b)
1999	Kaohsiung	Unknown	9	Group of Thai migrant workers	*P. canaliculata*	13 ± 7	2, spinal taps (22.2)	No death (0)	Tsai et al. (2001a)
2000[c]	Okinawa, Japan	Unknown	7	Local residents	Contaminated vegetable	Unknown	1, spinal taps (14.3)	No death (0)	Asato et al. (2004); Nawa (2005)
2001	Kaohsiung	Unknown	5	A local family	Vegetable juice	54 ± 30	0 (0)	No death (0)	Tsai et al. (2004)
2002	Changle	8	8	Local residents, 8 children	*P. canaliculata*	5–7 (6)	1, spinal taps (12.5)	No death (0)	Lin et al. (2003)
2002	Fuzhou	10	9	Staff from the same institute	*P. canaliculata*	Unknown	0 (0)	No death (0)	Wu and Yan (2004)
2002	Fuzhou	20	13	Staff from the same institute	*A. fulica*	2–19 (10.2)	0 (0)	No death (0)	Yang et al. (2004)
2004	Kunming	Unknown	25	Local residents	*P. canaliculata*	2–20	0 (0)	No death (0)	Han et al. (2005)

(*continued*)

TABLE 13.3 *(continued)*

Year	Location	Exposed (*n*)	Case (*n*)	Population	Source of infection	Mean incubation period (days)	Parasitological diagnosis (%)	Outcome (case-fatality rate %)	Reference(s)
2005	Kunming	Unknown	9	Local residents	*P. canaliculata*	Unknown	0 (0)	No death (0)	Wei et al. (2005)
2006	Beijing	Unknown	160	Local residents	*P. canaliculata*	1–41 (14)	0 (0)	No death (0)	He et al. (2007)
2007	Guangning	14 to raw or undercooked snails, 3 to insufficiently cooked snails	6	Group of Bai migrant workers	*P. canaliculata*	3–19 (10.7)	0 (0)	No death (0)	Deng et al. (2007)
2008	Dali	Unknown	41	Local residents	*P. canaliculata*	3–50 days (16)	0 (0)	No death (0)	Lv et al. (2009a)

[a] Assessed in 47 cases (Xue et al., 2000).
[b] Assessed in 5 cases.
[c] Original article in Japanese; the important information is available in other articles.

snail *P. canaliculata*, introduced into this region around 1980 (Joshi and Sebastian, 2006). Recently, the transmission pattern has shifted from *A. fulica* to *P. canaliculata* as the main source of infection. The lower intensity of infection due to the latter species probably also explains the lower parasite recovery rate and the lower case-fatality rate in recent outbreaks (see Table 13.3).

Most outbreaks occurred when snails were collected and prepared for consumption by individuals. However, several outbreaks, such as the one in Wenzhou in 1997 (Zheng et al., 2001), the large 2006 outbreak in Beijing (He et al., 2007) and the most recent outbreak in Dali in 2008 (Lv et al., 2009a) were traced back to restaurants. This shows that the increasing diversification of the diet and convenient long-distance transportation of foodstuffs now also puts urban consumers at risk of angiostrongyliasis. In such cases, more individuals are involved and the epidemiological picture is more complex.

Migrants and children are at the highest risk of angiostrongyliasis. In four outbreaks pertaining to migrant workers (Deng et al., 2007; Kliks et al., 1982; Tsai et al., 2001), all individuals reported eating snails regularly and not being aware of the parasite. Snails collected and barbecued by children were the source of infection in at least two outbreaks (Hwang and Chen, 1986; Lin et al., 2003). Specific behaviours and eating habits are important determinants in outbreaks. Eating raw *A. fulica*, the source of infection for an outbreak in Taoyuan in 1985 (Hwang and Chen, 1986) and drinking raw vegetable juice in Kaohsiung in 2001 (Tsai et al., 2004), were identified as additional sources of infection. Terrestrial slugs are still used in traditional medicine to treat some illnesses in certain areas which can result in angiostrongyliasis (Li et al., 2006; Liu et al., 2006). The outbreaks in Guangning in 2007 (Deng et al., 2007) and Dali in 2008 (Lv et al., 2009a) affected the Bai ethnic minority in Yunnan province, for which snails are a favourite dish. Traditionally, snail food is prepared from native species, namely *Cipangopaludina* spp. (Lv et al., 2009a), but *P. canaliculata*, which has a similar appearance, is now often used as an alternative.

13.4.3. Challenges: Outbreak identification and behaviour change

Outbreak identification differs from individual diagnosis because additional information regarding exposure history and shared clinical manifestations can help shedding additional light (Lv et al., 2009a). However, prompt and accurate diagnosis of index patients is a challenge in angiostrongyliasis outbreaks. Parasitological diagnosis is generally absent, especially in outbreaks (Table 13.3), although the patient's position before lumbar puncture and the technique employed in spinal tap may affect the parasite recovery rate (Tsai et al., 2001; Yii, 1976). Immunological assays are important alternatives but their sensitivity and specificity need to be further improved. Recently, a set of stratified diagnostic criteria has been proposed (Lv et al., 2009a). Three stratifications, that is suspected, clinically diagnosed and parasitologically confirmed, are considered according to the strength of the available evidence. These criteria can direct clinicians towards a diagnosis, but improved diagnostic techniques are urgently needed.

The variable and long incubation period (see Table 13.3) primarily accounts for the spatio-temporal scattering of cases, which further obscures outbreaks. In several major outbreaks the exact number of exposed individuals and involved patients were difficult to determine. For example, potential cases might travel to different places during the incubation period (Slom et al., 2002; Zheng et al., 2009). The identification of the source of infection is important but challenging. Few outbreak reports managed to identify the exact source of infection because foodstuffs are unlikely to be still available 2 weeks (the average incubation period of angiostrongyliasis) after the event in question. Instead, molluscs obtained from local markets or in the field can be examined for supplementary evidence. However, the source of snails sold in food markets changes constantly (He et al., 2007; Lv et al., 2009a). Therefore, long-time surveillance was proposed in order to investigate the safety of foodstuffs sold in local markets (Lv et al., 2009a). Although the evidence from food investigation may be weak for confirming specific outbreaks, positive findings imply generally unsafe food conditions.

Most *A. cantonensis* infections are moderate, and hence symptoms are mild or transient (Malvy et al., 2008; Punyagupta et al., 1975). Severe infections due to heavier worm burdens are usually related to the consumption of terrestrial molluscs, for example, *A. fulica* and slugs. In recent years, *P. canaliculata* has become the key vector of *A. cantonensis* in some areas and the resulting lower infection intensity is an additional challenge for outbreak identification. In an outbreak occurring in Guangning in 2007, 14 individuals had consumed raw *P. canaliculata*, but less than half of them ($n = 6$) reported relevant symptoms and only two sought medical assistance in a hospital (Deng et al., 2007).

Traditional habits such as the consumption of snails and slugs are difficult to change. Although the majority of the identified angiostrongyliasis outbreaks are related to the consumption of raw snails, slugs and paratenic hosts, risks extend also beyond consumption itself. For example, eating raw *A. fulica*, slugs, frogs and lizards may be considered a way to actually improve health (Hwang and Chen, 1986; Lai, 2006; Li et al., 2006; Liu et al., 2006; Parameswaran, 2006) and releasing snails may be an aspect of local culture (Chen et al., 2008) but also contributes to the spread of the parasite.

13.5. CONCLUDING REMARKS

Outbreaks due to trichinellosis, capillariasis and angiostrongyliasis are rare but when they occur, they cause considerable morbidity and even mortality, and hence often strain already weak health systems in affected countries of Southeast Asia. We reviewed outbreaks of three helminthiases, all caused by nematodes and discussed their public health significance. Importantly, the three diseases are food-borne zoonotic infections. Hence, the habit of eating raw or insufficiently cooked foodstuff (e.g. pork, fish and snails) is the underlying risk factor. Therefore, raising awareness and setting-specific health information, education and communication (IEC) in endemic areas is an important measure to prevent infection and outbreak occurrence. However, since consumption of raw foodstuffs is often deeply rooted culturally, changing such behaviours is a formidable challenge (Keiser and Utzinger, 2009; Lv et al., 2010; Sripa et al., 2010).

Enhancing food safety, particularly in areas where humans eat raw, is a key feature to reduce food-borne infectious diseases. Hence, food inspection systems should be developed and implemented in local markets in order to prevent the distribution of unsafe pork meat, fish and snails. Unsafe production of pork meat, such as unsafe feeding practices, introduces the parasite into the animal food chain. However, pigs raised and slaughtered under traditional husbandry practices, and small-holder fish or snail farming and local consumption, is common in some rural areas of Southeast Asia, and might be particularly widespread among ethnic minority groups (Schratz et al., 2010). Hence, it will be extremely difficult to change these behaviours to make a lasting impact. Furthermore, the causative agents may infect a variety of hosts, some of which may become carriers unexpected for humans. For example, paratenic infections of wild animals can lead to sporadic or outbreaks in human populations.

In recent years, improved diagnosis in humans and detection of infections in intermediate hosts and reservoir animals have provided new tools for prevention and control. Strengthening of surveillance systems and human and animal health services alike by introducing this information is assuring early and adequate response activities. Outbreaks of uncommon parasitic zoonosis are preventable. The close collaboration of human and animal preventive and curative health services is essential.

ACKNOWLEDGEMENTS

We thank the guest editors for inviting us to prepare this manuscript. Comments and suggestions by an anonymous reviewer and careful editing done by Dr. P. Steinmann are highly appreciated.

REFERENCES

Ahmed, L., el-Dib, N.A., el-Boraey, Y., Ibrahim, M., 1999. *Capillaria philippinensis*: an emerging parasite causing severe diarrhoea in Egypt. J. Egypt. Soc. Parasitol. 29, 483–493.

Asato, R., Taira, K., Nakamura, M., Kudaka, J., Itokazu, K., Kawanaka, M., 2004. Changing epidemiology of angiostrongyliasis cantonensis in Okinawa prefecture, Japan. Jpn. J. Infect. Dis. 57, 184–186.

Bair, M.J., Hwang, K.P., Wang, T.E., Liou, T.C., Lin, S.C., Kao, C.R., et al., 2004. Clinical features of human intestinal capillariasis in Taiwan. World J. Gastroenterol. 10, 2391–2393.

Bangs, M.J., Purnomo, Andersen, E.M., 1994. A case of capillariasis in a highland community of Irian Jaya, Indonesia. Ann. Trop. Med. Parasitol. 88, 685–687.

Barennes, H., Sayasone, S., Odermatt, P., De, B.A., Hongsakhone, S., Newton, P.N., et al., 2008. A major trichinellosis outbreak suggesting a high endemicity of *trichinella* infection in Northern Laos. Am. J. Trop. Med. Hyg. 78, 40–44.

Belizario, V.Y., de Leon, W.U., Esparar, D.G., Galang, J.M., Fantone, J., Verdadero, C., 2000. Compostela valley: a new endemic focus for capillariasis philippinensis. Southeast Asian J. Trop. Med. Public Health 31, 478–481.

CDC, 1984. Trichinosis–Texas. MMWR Morb. Mortal. Wkly. Rep. 33, 517–518.

Chen, S.R., Lv, S., Wang, L.B., Fang, W., Chen, F., Li, K.R., et al., 2008. Epidemiological investigation of first angiostrongyliasis outbreak in Dali prefecture, Yunnan province. Parasit. Infect. Dis. 16, 137–138.

Chichino, G., Bernuzzi, A.M., Bruno, A., Cevini, C., Atzori, C., Malfitano, A., et al., 1992. Intestinal capillariasis (*Capillaria philippinensis*) acquired in Indonesia: a case report. Am. J. Trop. Med. Hyg. 47, 10–12.

Childs, D.Z., Cattadori, I.M., Suwonkerd, W., Prajakwong, S., Boots, M., 2006. Spatiotemporal patterns of malaria incidence in northern Thailand. Trans. R. Soc. Trop. Med. Hyg. 100, 623–631.

Chitwood, M.B., Valesquez, C., Salazar, N.G., 1968. *Capillaria philippinensis* sp. n. (Nematoda: Trichinellida), from the intestine of man in the Philippines. J. Parasitol. 54, 368–371.

Chotmongkol, V., Sawanyawisuth, K., Thavornpitak, Y., 2000. Corticosteroid treatment of eosinophilic meningitis. Clin. Infect. Dis. 31, 660–662.

Chotmongkol, V., Wongjitrat, C., Sawadpanit, K., Sawanyawisuth, K., 2004. Treatment of eosinophilic meningitis with a combination of albendazole and corticosteroid. Southeast Asian J. Trop. Med. Public Health 35, 172–174.

Chotmongkol, V., Sawadpanitch, K., Sawanyawisuth, K., Louhawilai, S., Limpawattana, P., 2006. Treatment of eosinophilic meningitis with a combination of prednisolone and mebendazole. Am. J. Trop. Med. Hyg. 74, 1122–1124.

Ci, R., Si, T., Wang, H.J., Ma, P.C., Ge, M.C.R., 2003. An outbreak of trichinellosis in Milin county, Tibet. Chin. J. Parasitol. Parasit. Dis. 21, 60.

Cross, J.H., 1992. Intestinal capillariasis. Clin. Microbiol. Rev. 5, 120–129.

Cross, J.H., Basaca-Sevilla, V., 1987. Albendazole in the treatment of intestinal capillariasis. Southeast Asian J. Trop. Med. Public Health 18, 507–510.

Cui, J., Wang, Z.Q., 2001. Outbreaks of human trichinellosis caused by consumption of dog meat in China. Parasite 8, S74–S77.

Cui, J., Wang, Z.Q., Kennedy, M.W., 2006. The re-emergence of trichinellosis in China? Trends Parasitol. 22, 54–55.

Dai, L.H., 2003. Investigation report of a trichinellosis outbreak. Chin. J. Parasit. Dis. Control 16, 68.

Deng, Z.H., Cai, J.S., Lin, R.X., Pei, F.Q., Cui, H.E., Ou, Y., et al., 2007. The first local outbreak of *Angiostrongylus cantonensis* infection in Guangdong province. South China J. Prev. Med. 33, 17–20.

Dronda, F., Chaves, F., Sanz, A., Lopez-Velez, R., 1993. Human intestinal capillariasis in an area of nonendemicity: case report and review. Clin. Infect. Dis. 17, 909–912.

Dupouy-Camet, J., 2000. Trichinellosis: a worldwide zoonosis. Vet. Parasitol. 93, 191–200.

Dupouy-Camet, J., Kociecka, W., Bruschi, F., Bolas-Fernandez, F., Pozio, E., 2002. Opinion on the diagnosis and treatment of human trichinellosis. Expert Opin. Pharmacother. 3, 1117–1130.

Eamsobhana, P., Tungtrongchitr, A., 2005. Angiostrongyliasis in Thailand. Asian Parasitology: Food-Borne Helminthiasis in Asia. The Federation of Asian Parasitologist, Chuo-Ku pp. 183–197.

el Hassan, E.H., Mikhail, W.E., 1992. Malabsorption due to *Capillaria philippinensis* in an Egyptian woman living in Dubai, United Arab Emirates. Trans. R. Soc. Trop. Med. Hyg. 86, 79.

el-Dib, N.A., Ahmed, J.A., El-Arousy, M., Mahmoud, M.A., Garo, K., 1999. Parasitological aspects of *Capillaria philippinensis* recovered from Egyptian patients. J. Egypt. Soc. Parasitol. 29, 139–147.

el-Dib, N.A., Doss, W.H., 2002. Intestinal capillariasis in Egypt epidemiological background. J. Egypt. Soc. Parasitol. 32, 145–154.

Erlanger, T.E., Weiss, S., Keiser, J., Utzinger, J., Wiedenmayer, K., 2009. Past, present, and future of Japanese encephalitis. Emerg. Infect. Dis. 15, 1–7.

Gottstein, B., Pozio, E., Nockler, K., 2009. Epidemiology, diagnosis, treatment, and control of trichinellosis. Clin. Microbiol. Rev. 22, 127–145.

Graeff-Teixeira, C., da Silva, A.C., Yoshimura, K., 2009. Update on eosinophilic meningoencephalitis and its clinical relevance. Clin. Microbiol. Rev. 22, 322–348.

Han, J.F., Zhu, Y.H., Ji, W.Z., Li, Y., Yan, Y., Yin, M., et al., 2005. Clinical analysis of 25 cases with eosinophilic meningitis. Chin. J. Epidemiol. 26, 679.

He, Z.Y., Jia, L., Huang, F., Liu, G.R., Li, J., Dou, X.F., et al., 2007. Investigation on outbreak of angiostrongyliasis cantonensis in Beijing. Chin. J. Public Health 23, 1241–1242.

Hoghooghi-Rad, N., Maraghi, S., Narenj-Zadeh, A., 1987. *Capillaria philippinensis* infection in Khoozestan Province, Iran: case report. Am. J. Trop. Med. Hyg. 37, 135–137.

Hong, S.T., Kim, Y.T., Choe, G., Min, Y.I., Cho, S.H., Kim, J.K., et al., 1994. Two cases of intestinal capillariasis in Korea. Korean J. Parasitol. 32, 43–48.

Hong, X.H., Guo, Z.M., Ci, R.D.Z., Long, E.K., Ma, Y., Bian, B.Z.M., et al., 2008. Investigation and clinical analysis of an outbreak of trichinellosis. Chin. J. Parasitol. Parasit. Dis. 26, 79–80.

Hotez, P.J., Ehrenberg, J.P., 2010. Escalating the global fight against neglected tropical diseases through interventions in the Asia Pacific Region. Adv. Parasitol. 72, 31–53.

Huang, F.C., 1965. Report of one case of human trichinellosis. Chin. J. Int. Med. 13, 392.

Hwang, K.P., 1997. Anthelmintics in the treatment of eosinophilic meningitis. Acta Paed. Sin. 38 (Suppl), 1–6.

Hwang, K.P., Chen, E.R., 1986. Eosinophilic meningitis due to *Angiostrongylus cantonensis*. Epidemiol. Bull. 2, 21–36.

Hwang, K.P., Chen, E.R., 1991. Clinical studies on angiostrongyliasis cantonensis among children in Taiwan. Southeast Asian J. Trop. Med. Public Health 22 (Suppl), 194–199.

Ishii, A.I., 1984. Effects of temperature on the larval development of *Angiostrongylus cantonensis* in the intermediate host, *Biomphalaria glabrata*. Parasitol. Res. 70, 375–379.

Jongwutiwes, S., Chantachum, N., Kraivichian, P., Siriyasatien, P., Putaporntip, C., Tamburrini, A., et al., 1998. First outbreak of human trichinellosis caused by *Trichinella pseudospiralis*. Clin. Infect. Dis. 26, 111–115.

Joshi, R.C., Sebastian, L.S., 2006. Global Advances in Ecology and Management of Golden Apple Snails. PhilRice, Nueva Ecija.

Kaewpitoon, N., Kaewpitoon, S.J., Pengsaa, P., 2008. Food-borne parasitic zoonosis: distribution of trichinosis in Thailand. World J. Gastroenterol. 14, 3471–3475.

Ke, C.R., Li, Y.M., Liu, J.Z., Yi, S.S., Li, H.J., Yang, P.W., et al., 2007. A trichinellosis outbreak due to consumption of pigs treated with praziquantel before slaughter. Chin. J. Vector Biol. Control 18, 115.

Keiser, J., Maltese, M.F., Erlanger, T.E., Bos, R., Tanner, M., Singer, B.H., et al., 2005. Effect of irrigated rice agriculture on Japanese encephalitis, including challenges and opportunities for integrated vector management. Acta Trop. 95, 40–57.

Keiser, J., Utzinger, J., 2009. Food-borne trematodiases. Clin. Microbiol. Rev. 22, 466–483.

Khamboonruang, C., 1991. The present status of trichinellosis in Thailand. Southeast Asian J. Trop. Med. Public Health 22 (Suppl), 312–315.

Khamboonruang, C., Nateewatana, N., 1975. Trichinosis: a recent outbreak in Northern Thailand. Southeast Asian J. Trop. Med. Public Health 6, 74–78.

Khumjui, C., Choomkasien, P., Dekumyoy, P., Kusolsuk, T., Kongkaew, W., Chalamaat, M., et al., 2008. Outbreak of trichinellosis caused by *Trichinella papuae*, Thailand, 2006. Emerg. Infect. Dis. 14, 1913–1915.

Kliks, M.M., Kroenke, K., Hardman, J.M., 1982. Eosinophilic radiculomyeloencephalitis: an angiostrongyliasis outbreak in American Samoa related to ingestion of *Achatina fulica* snails. Am. J. Trop. Med. Hyg. 31, 1114–1122.

Kunaratanapruk, S., Lam-Ong, S., Chatsirimongkol, C., Dhirasut, C., Laohanuwat, C., 1983. Intestinal capillariasis in the province: a report of 100 cases. Ramathibodi Med. J. 6, 253–258.

Lai, S.C., 2006. Chinese herbal medicine Yin-Chen-Extract as an adjunct to anthelmintic albendazole used against *Angiostrongylus cantonensis*-induced eosinophilic meningitis or meningoencephalitis. Am. J. Trop. Med. Hyg. 75, 556–562.

Li, L.S., Lin, J.X., Zhang, R.Y., Fang, Y.Y., Lin, K.Q., 2006. A severe case of angiostrongyliasis due to eating raw slugs. Chin. J. Parasitol. Parasit. Dis. 24, 460.

Limsuwan, S., Siriprasert, V., 1994. A clinical study on trichinosis in Changwat Phayao, Thailand. Southeast Asian J. Trop. Med. Public Health 25, 305–308.

Lin, J.X., Li, Y.S., Zhu, K., Chen, B.J., Cheng, Y.Z., Lin, J.C., et al., 2003. Epidemiological study on group infection of *Angiostrongylus cantonensis* in Changle city. Chin. J. Parasitol. Parasit. Dis. 21, 110–112.

Liu, M., Boireau, P., 2002. Trichinellosis in China: epidemiology and control. Trends Parasitol. 18, 553–556.

Liu, Z.R., Zhou, F.Y., Zeng, X.P., Shen, L.Y., Wang, P.Z., Ding, L.P., et al., 2006. Clinical analysis of three cases of eosinophilic meningitis due to eating raw slugs. Zhejiang Prev. Med. 18, 63–64.

Lu, L.H., Lin, M.R., Choi, W.M., Hwang, K.P., Hsu, Y.H., Bair, M.J., et al., 2006. Human intestinal capillariasis (*Capillaria philippinensis*) in Taiwan. Am. J. Trop. Med. Hyg. 74, 810–813.

Luo, Z.Y., Li, W., Shen, L.J., 2004. An outbreak of trichinellosis. Chin. J. Zoonoses 20, 359.

Lv, S., Zhang, Y., Chen, S.R., Wang, L.B., Fang, W., Chen, F., et al., 2009a. Human angiostrongyliasis outbreak in Dali, China. PLoS Negl. Trop. Dis. 3, e520.

Lv, S., Zhang, Y., Liu, H.X., Hu, L., Yang, K., Steinmann, P., et al., 2009b. Invasive snails and an emerging infectious disease: results from the first national survey on *Angiostrongylus cantonensis* in China. PLoS Negl. Trop. Dis. 3, e368.

Lv, S., Zhang, Y., Steinmann, P., Zhou, X.N., 2008. Emerging angiostrongyliasis in mainland China. Emerg. Infect. Dis. 14, 161–164.

Lv, S., Zhang, Y., Steinmann, P., Zhou, X.N., Utzinger, J., 2010. Helminth infections of the central nervous system occurring in Southeast Asia and the Far East. Adv. Parasitol. 72, 351–408.

Lv, S., Zhou, X.N., Zhang, Y., Liu, H.X., Zhu, D., Yin, W.G., et al., 2006. The effect of temperature on the development of *Angiostrongylus cantonensis* (Chen 1935) in *Pomacea canaliculata* (Lamarck 1822). Parasitol. Res. 99, 583–587.

Ma, G.Y., 2008. An outbreak of acute trichinellosis in Dali prefecture. Parasit. Infect. Dis. 6, 55–56.

Malvy, D., Ezzedine, K., Receveur, M.C., Pistone, T., Crevon, L., Lemardeley, P., et al., 2008. Cluster of eosinophilic meningitis attributable to *Angiostrongylus cantonensis* infection in French policemen troop returning from the Pacific Islands. Travel Med. Infect. Dis. 6, 301–304.

McAuley, J.B., Michelson, M.K., Hightower, A.W., Engeran, S., Wintermeyer, L.A., Schantz, P.M., 1992. A trichinosis outbreak among Southeast Asian refugees. Am. J. Epidemiol. 135, 1404–1410.

Mead, A.R., 1961. The Giant African Snail: A Problem in Economic Malacology. University of Chicago Press, Chicago.

Morakote, N., Khamboonruang, C., Siriprasert, V., Suphawitayanukul, S., Marcanantachoti, W., Thamasonthi, W., 1991. The value of enzyme-linked immunosorbent assay (ELISA) for diagnosis of human trichinosis. Trop. Med. Parasitol. 42, 172–174.

Morakote, N., Sukhavat, K., Khamboonruang, C., Siriprasert, V., Suphawitayanukul, S., Thamasonthi, W., 1992. Persistence of IgG, IgM, and IgE antibodies in human trichinosis. Trop. Med. Parasitol. 43, 167–169.

Murrell, K.D., Fried, B., 2007. Food-Borne Parasitic Zoonoses: Fish and Plant-Borne Parasites. World Class Parasites 11. Springer, New York.

Nawa, Y., 2005. Angiostrongyliasis in Japan. In: Arizono, N., Chai, J.Y., Nawa, Y., Takahashi, Y. (Eds.), Asian Parasitology: Food-Borne Helminthiasis in Asia. Vol. 1. The Federation of Asian Parasitologists, Chuo-ku, pp. 213–216.

Odermatt, P., Habe, S., Manichanh, S., Tran, D.S., Duong, V., Zhang, W., et al., 2007. Paragonimiasis and its intermediate hosts in a transmission focus in Lao People's Democratic Republic. Acta Trop. 103, 108–115.

onso-Sanz, M., Chaves, F., Dronda, F., Catalan, S., Gonzalez-Lopez, A., 1995. Intestinal parasitoses in the prison population in the Madrid area (1991–1993). Enferm. Infecc. Microbiol. Clin. 13, 90–95.

Parameswaran, K., 2006. Case series of eosinophilic meningoencephalitis from South India. Ann. Indian Acad. Neurol. 9, 217–222.

Pozio, E., 2001a. New patterns of *Trichinella* infection. Vet. Parasitol. 98, 133–148.

Pozio, E., 2001b. Taxonomy of *Trichinella* and the epidemiology of infection in the Southeast Asia and Australian regions. Southeast Asian J. Trop. Med. Public Health 32 (Suppl 2), 129–132.

Pozio, E., Khamboonruang, C., 1989. Trichinellosis in Thailand: epidemiology and biochemical identification of the aethiological agent. Trop. Med. Parasitol. 40, 73–74.

Pradatsundarasar, A., Pecharanond, K., Chintanawongs, C., Ungthavorn, P., 1973. The first case of intestinal capillariasis in Thailand. Southeast Asian J. Trop. Med. Public Health 4, 131–134.

Punyagupta, S., Juttijudata, P., Bunnag, T., 1975. Eosinophilic meningitis in Thailand. Clinical studies of 484 typical cases probably caused by *Angiostrongylus cantonensis*. Am. J. Trop. Med. Hyg. 24, 921–931.

Saichua, P., Nithikathkul, C., Kaewpitoon, N., 2008. Human intestinal capillariasis in Thailand. World J. Gastroenterol. 14, 506–510.

Sawanyawisuth, K., Limpawattana, P., Busaracome, P., Ninpaitoon, B., Chotmongkol, V., Intapan, P.M., et al., 2004. A 1-week course of corticosteroids in the treatment of eosinophilic meningitis. Am. J. Med. 117, 802–803.

Sawanyawisuth, K., Sawanyawisuth, K., 2008. Treatment of angiostrongyliasis. Trans. R. Soc. Trop. Med. Hyg. 102, 990–996.

Sayasone, S., Odermatt, P., Vongphrachanh, P., Keoluangkot, V., Dupouy-Camet, J., Newton, P.N., et al., 2006. A trichinellosis outbreak in Borikhamxay Province, Lao PDR. Trans. R. Soc. Trop. Med. Hyg. 100, 1126–1129.

Sayasone, S., Odermatt, P., Phoumindr, N., Vongsaravane, X., Sensombath, V., Phetsouvanh, R., et al., 2007. Epidemiology of *Opisthorchis viverrini* in a rural district of southern Lao PDR. Trans. R. Soc. Trop. Med. Hyg. 101, 40–47.

Schratz, A., Fernanda Pineda, M., Reforma, L.G., Fox, N.M., Anh, T.L., Cavalli-Sforza, L.T., et al., 2010. Neglected diseases and ethnic minorities in the Western Pacific Region: exploring the links. Adv. Parasitol. 72, 79–107.

Sicard, D., Fontan, R., Richard-Lenoble, D., Gentilini, M., 1976. Human trichinosis. A recent epidemic in Vientiane (Laos) (apropos of 32 cases). Bull. Soc. Pathol. Exot. Filiales. 69, 521–525.

Slom, T.J., Cortese, M.M., Gerber, S.I., Jones, R.C., Holtz, T.H., Lopez, A.S., et al., 2002. An outbreak of eosinophilic meningitis caused by *Angiostrongylus cantonensis* in travelers returning from the Caribbean. N. Engl. J. Med. 346, 668–675.

Soukhathammavong, P., Sayasone, S., Harimanana, A.N., Akkhavong, A., Thammasack, S., Phoumindr, N., et al., 2008. Three cases of intestinal capillariasis in Lao People's Democratic Republic. Am. J. Trop. Med. Hyg. 79, 735–738.

Sripa, B., Kaewkes, S., Intapan, P.M., Maleewong, W., Brindley, P.J., 2010. Food-borne trematodiases in Southeast Asia: epidemiology, pathology, clinical manifestation and control. Adv. Parasitol. 72, 305–350.

Steinmann, P., Zhou, X.N., Li, Y.L., Li, H.J., Chen, S.R., Yang, Z., et al., 2007. Helminth infections and risk factor analysis among residents in Eryuan county, Yunnan province, China. Acta Trop. 104, 38–51.

Steinmann, P., Du, Z.W., Wang, L.B., Wang, X.Z., Jiang, J.Y., Li, L.H., et al., 2008. Extensive multiparasitism in a village of Yunnan province, People's Republic of China, revealed by a suite of diagnostic methods. Am. J. Trop. Med. Hyg. 78, 760–769.

Su, Z.L., Dan, Z.N.Z., Zhuo, M., Za, X.J.C., Wang, X.L., Ci, R., 2002. An outbreak of trichinellosis in Tibet. Chin. J. Parasitol. Parasit. Dis. 20, 363.

Suriyanon, V., Klunklin, K., 1972. Human trichinosis: analysis of cases during the tenth outbreak in North Thailand. Southeast Asian J. Trop. Med. Public Health 3, 390–396.

Taylor, W.R., Tran, G.V., Nguyen, T.Q., Dang, D.V., Nguyen, V.K., Nguyen, C.T., et al., 2009. Acute febrile myalgia in Vietnam due to trichinellosis following the consumption of raw pork. Clin. Infect. Dis. 49, e79–e83.

Tian, X.S., Yang, Y.C., Luo, S.G., He, W.T., 2001. An outbreak of trichinellosis caused by eating pickled pork. J. Youjiang Med. Coll. Natly. 23, 738–739.

Tsai, H.C., Lee, S.S., Huang, C.K., Yen, C.M., Chen, E.R., Liu, Y.C., 2004. Outbreak of eosinophilic meningitis associated with drinking raw vegetable juice in southern Taiwan. Am. J. Trop. Med. Hyg. 71, 222–226.

Tsai, H.C., Liu, Y.C., Kunin, C.M., Lee, S.S., Chen, Y.S., Lin, H.H., et al., 2001a. Eosinophilic meningitis caused by *Angiostrongylus cantonensis*: report of 17 cases. Am. J. Med. 111, 109–114.

Tsai, T.H., Liu, Y.C., Wann, S.R., Lin, W.R., Lee, S.S.J., Lin, H.H., et al., 2001b. An outbreak of meningitis caused by *Angiostrongylus cantonensis* in Kaohsiung. J. Microbiol. Immunol. Infect. 34, 50–56.

Wallace, G.D., Rosen, L., 1966. Studies on eosinophilic meningitis. 2. Experimental infection of shrimp and crabs with *Angiostrongylus cantonensis*. Am. J. Epidemiol. 84, 120–131.

Wallace, G.D., Rosen, L., 1967. Studies on eosinophilic meningitis IV. Experimental infection of fresh-water and marine fish with *Angiostrongylus cantonensis*. Am. J. Epidemiol. 85, 395–402.

Wang, L.B., Li, H.B., Wu, F.W., Che, Y., Zhu, J., Liu, J.Y., et al., 2009. Investigation report of a trichinellosis outbreak in Yunnan province, China. J. Pathogen Biol. 4, 156.

Wang, Q.P., Lai, D.H., Zhu, X.Q., Chen, X.G., Lun, Z.R., 2008. Human angiostrongyliasis. Lancet Infect. Dis. 8, 621–630.

Wang, X.T., Huang, H.J., Dong, Q.L., Lin, Y., Wang, Z.M., Li, F.Q., et al., 2002. A clinical study of eosinophilic meningitis caused by angiostrongyliasis. Chin. Med. J. 115, 1312–1315.

Wang, Y.Y., Liu, H.K., 2006. Diagnosis, treatment and nursing of cases from an outbreak of trichinellosis. J. Pathogen Biol. 1, 334.

Wang, Z.Q., Cui, J., 2001a. Epidemiology of swine trichinellosis in China. Parasite 8, S67–S70.

Wang, Z.Q., Cui, J., 2001b. The epidemiology of human trichinellosis in China during 1964–1999. Parasite 8, S63–S66.

Wang, Z.Q., Cui, J., Shen, L.J., 2007. The epidemiology of animal trichinellosis in China. Vet. J. 173, 391–398.

Wang, Z.Q., Cui, J., Xu, B.L., 2006. The epidemiology of human trichinellosis in China during 2000–2003. Acta Trop. 97, 247–251.

Wei, L.P., Zheng, K.W., Wei, Y., 2005. Clinical nursing of 9 cases with angiostrongyliasis. Chin. J. Clin. Nurs. 4, 21–22.

Wu, C.H., Yan, X.H., 2004. A mini-outbreak of angiostrongyliasis. Chin. J. Zoonoses 20, 454.

Xu, L., 2002. An outbreak of trichinosis in Jianshui county of Yunnan province, China. Chin. J. Parasitol. Parasit. Dis. 20, 56.

Xue, D.Y., Ruan, Y.Z., Lin, B.C., Zheng, R.Y., Fang, J.Q., Zhao, Q.Y., et al., 2000. Investigation of an outbreak of angiostrongyliasis in Wenzhou city. Chin. J. Parasitol. Parasit. Dis. 18, 176–178.

Yang, F.Z., Zhang, Y.Z., Tu, Z.P., Xu, L.S., 2004. Investigation of an outbreak of angiostrongyliasis presumably caused by consumption of snail meal. Strait J. Prev. Med. 10, 44–45.

Yao, Y., 2008. Clinical analysis of 49 cases with trichinellosis. Chin. Community Doc. 10, 157.

Yao, Y.F., Tang, J.R., Lu, L.Q., Yang, Y.C., Li, Q.F., 2002. Report of two outbreaks of trichinellosis caused by pickled pork in Guangxi province. Chin. J. Vet. Parasitol. 10, 46–47.

Ye, P., Huang, J.H., Zha, Z.K., Ge, D.C., Wang, H., 2003. Study on an outbreak of human trichinellosis resulted from eating wild boar. Chin. J. Zoonoses 19, 12.

Yii, C.Y., 1976. Clinical observations on eosinophilic meningitis and meningoencephalitis caused by *Angiostrongylus cantonensis* on Taiwan. Am. J. Trop. Med. Hyg. 25, 223–249.

Yii, C.Y., Chen, C.Y., Chen, E.R., Hsieh, H.C., Shih, C.C., 1975. Epidemiologic studies of eosinophilic meningitis in southern Taiwan. Am. J. Trop. Med. Hyg. 24, 447–454.

Yuan, S.F., Zhang, Y.L., 2002. A special food poisoning: trichinellosis. Chin. J. Pest Control 18, 50.

Zhang, L.L., Wang, Q.X., Liu, J.Z., Li, Y.M., 2007. An outbreak of food-borne *Trichinella* infection in Dali city. Chin. J. Pest Control 23, 352.

Zheng, D.F., Xiao, N., Tian, H.C., Chen, J.P., Chen, Y.L., Li, M.H., et al., 2009. The first case report of angiostrongyliasis caused by eating raw meal of *Ampularum crossean* in Sichuan province. Parasit. Infect. Dis. 7, 12–14.

Zheng, R.Y., Jin, R., Lin, B.C., Pan, C.W., Xue, D.Y., 2001. Probing and demonstrating etiological factors for the outbreak of angiostrongyliasis cantonensis in Wenzhou. Shanghai J. Prev. Med. 13, 105–107.

Zhou, X.N., Guo, J.G., Wu, X.H., Jiang, Q.W., Zheng, J., Dang, H., et al., 2007. Epidemiology of schistosomiasis in the People's Republic of China, 2004. Emerg. Infect. Dis. 13, 1470–1476.

INDEX

N

CONTENTS OF VOLUMES IN THIS SERIES

Volume 45

Volume 46

Volume 47

Volume 48

Volume 49

Volume 50

Volume 51

Volume 52

Volume 53

Volume 54

Volume 59

Volume 60

Volume 61

Volume 62

Volume 63

Volume 64

Volume 65

Volume 66

Volume 67

Volume 68

Volume 69

Volume 70

Volume 71

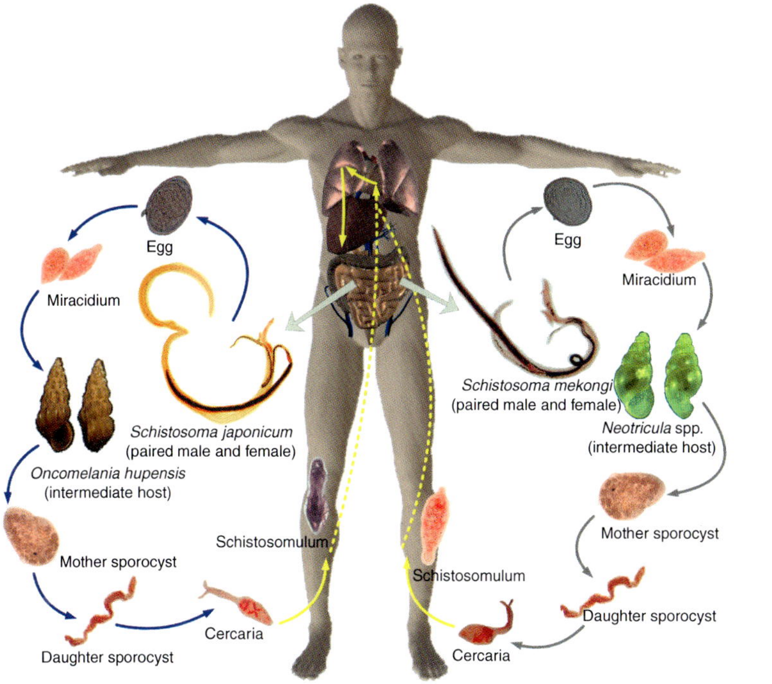

Humans are infected when cercariae, released from the intermediate host snail in water, penetrate the human skin, lose their forked tails and transform into schistosomula. While migrating via the lungs to the portal blood system of the liver, the schistosomula mature into adult male and female, 7–20 mm long worms, which pair up and take residence in the mesenteric venules, predominantly in the mesenteric veins draining the small intestine. Many of the eggs, deposited in the mesenteric veins by the female schistosomes follow the blood to the liver where they cause pathological lesions, but the majority penetrate the intestinal tissues and are eliminated with the faeces. If the eggs reach freshwater they hatch and release miracidia, which are attracted by specific snail species, which eventually become infected. The snail parasite stage includes two generations of sporocysts and ends with the production of cercariae which completes the life cycle.

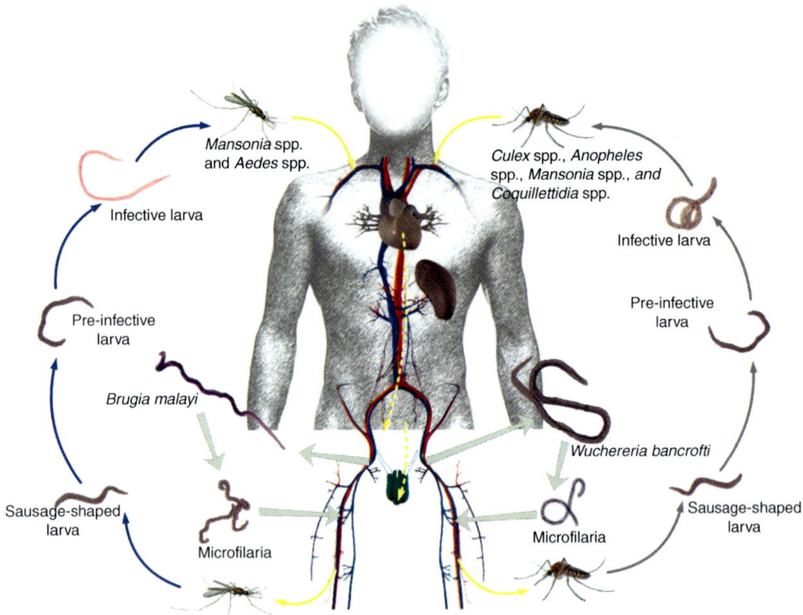

Humans act as the definitive host for the adult stages of *W. bancrofti* and *B. malayi*, which reside in the lymphatic system, predominantly in the lymph glands of the afferent lymphatic channels in the lower part of the body. The mature eggs (of first-stage microfilariae produced by the female worms) are found periodically in the peripheral blood. Mosquitoes serve as vectors and intermediate hosts. When infected through a blood meal from an infected human, the microfilariae from the human blood penetrate the insect midgut and migrate to the thoracic muscles where they increase in size, molt and develop through various stages, to finally migrate to the salivary glands of the third-stage larvae, which are infective for humans. They enter the insect proboscis and escape while the mosquito takes another blood meal 1 to 2 weeks later. The infective larvae penetrate the skin through the bite hole and develop into either male or female adults in the lymphatic system over a span of 6 months. There, the adult nematodes mate and produce large numbers of eggs, which enter the blood stream as microfilariae exhibiting the classic nocturnal periodicity, which means that the vector only gets infected when the microfilariae are in the peripheral blood which normally occurs at night.

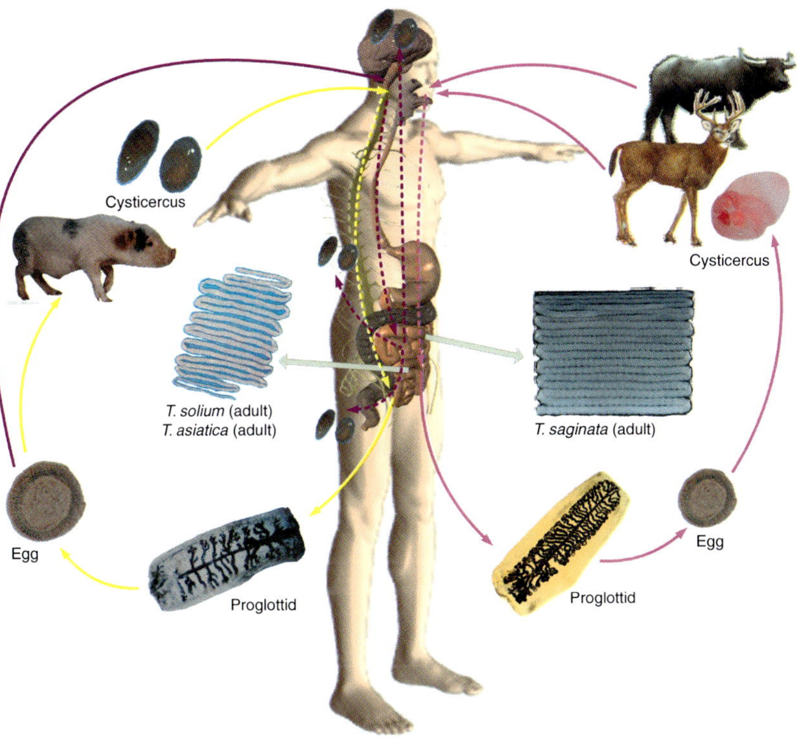

Humans act as the definitive host when consuming undercooked meat from infected animals, i.e. meat containing live tapeworm cysticerci. Ingested cysts evaginate and attach to the small intestine by their scolex and develop into adult tapeworms, which eventually produce eggs, which are released into the environment by the faecal route. The eggs develop into oncospheres when ingested by intermediate host animals susceptible to the infection The cycle completes when the onchospheres hatch and invade the intestinal wall to migrate to striated muscles, brain, liver and other tissues where they develop into cysticerci. The disease cysticercosis results from accidental swallowing of live eggs (dark purple arrows) and is commonly contracted by autoinfection (or transfer from one human to another), which is common in areas characterised by low-level sanitation.

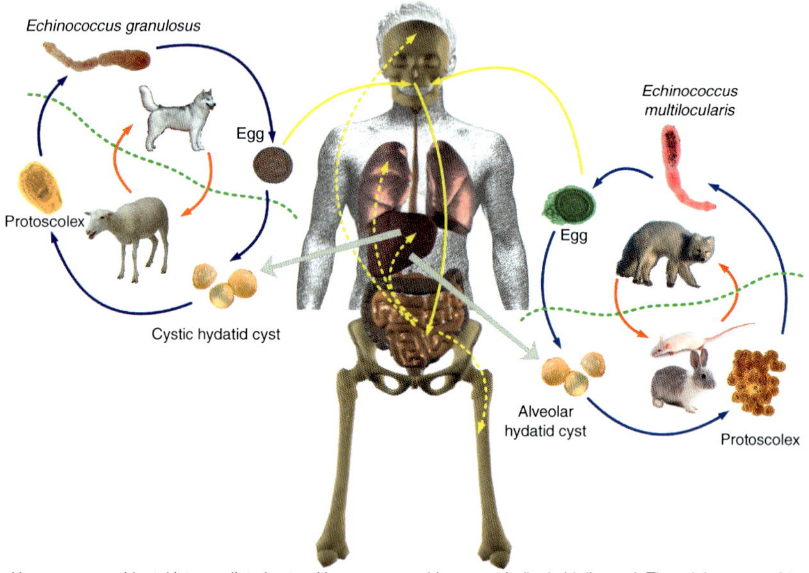

Humans are accidental intermediate hosts with respect to echinococcosis (hydatid disease). The adult worm resides in the small intestine of a canine definitive host, for example, the domestic dog. Gravid proglottids containing eggs are passed into the environment by the faecal route. Ingested by an intermediate host, for example, sheep (or humans as accidental hosts), the eggs hatch in the small intestine and release oncospheres that penetrate the intestinal wall and move through the circulatory system into different organs, in particular liver and lungs. Once an organ has been invaded, the oncospheres develop into cysts, which slowly enlarge, producing protoscolices and daughter cysts within each cyst. When the definitive host ingests cyst-containing organs of the infected intermediate host, protoscolices are released and attach to the intestine where they develop into adult worms.

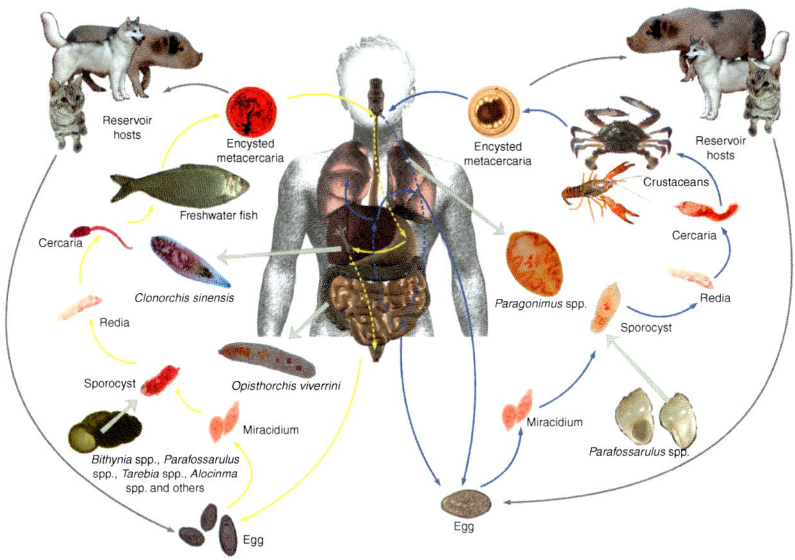

Embryonated eggs of the human liver flukes (*Clonorchis sinensis* and *Opisthorchis viverrini*) are discharged in the biliary ducts and excreted by the faecal route. Eggs which reach freshwater hatch and release miracidia that infect the intermediate host snail. Each miracidium develops into a sporocyst, which houses the asexual reproduction of rediae, which in turn house the asexual reproduction of cercariae. These eventually escape from the snail and parasitise fish of the Cyprinidae family by penetrating into the fish muscles and forming a protective metacercarial cyst encapsulating the parasite. Infection of humans occurs by ingestion of undercooked, salted, pickled or smoked freshwater fish. The cysts avoid digestion by the human gastric acids allowing metacercariae to reach the upper part of the small intestine (duodenum) and hatch there. The metacercariae then navigate towards their final habitat, the bile ducts of the liver, where they feed on bile and grow into sexually mature *Clonorchis* worms. The hermaphroditic adults produce numerous eggs, which are released into the intestine and the cycle completes when an egg hatches and again infects a snail. The cycle can also operate in various mammals, such as pigs, dogs, cats, etc., which therefore act as reservoirs of the infection.

In the case of *Paragonimus* spp., humans become infected when consuming inadequately cooked or pickled crustaceans containing metacercariae. The metacercariae excyst in the duodenum, penetrate the intestinal wall into the peritoneal cavity and from there pass through the diaphragm to end up in the lungs, where they encapsulate and develop into adults. The eggs are excreted unembryonated and are released into the environment when coughed up. Alternately, they are swallowed by the host and discharged via the faecal route. Eggs reaching freshwater embryonate and eventually release miracidia, which infect a specific snail which acts as the first intermediate host. From here the parasite develops in the same way as *Clonorchis* and *Opisthorchis* with the difference that the second intermediate host is not a fish but a small crustacean (crab or crayfish), in which it encysts and in which it is finally delivered to its mammalian hosts.

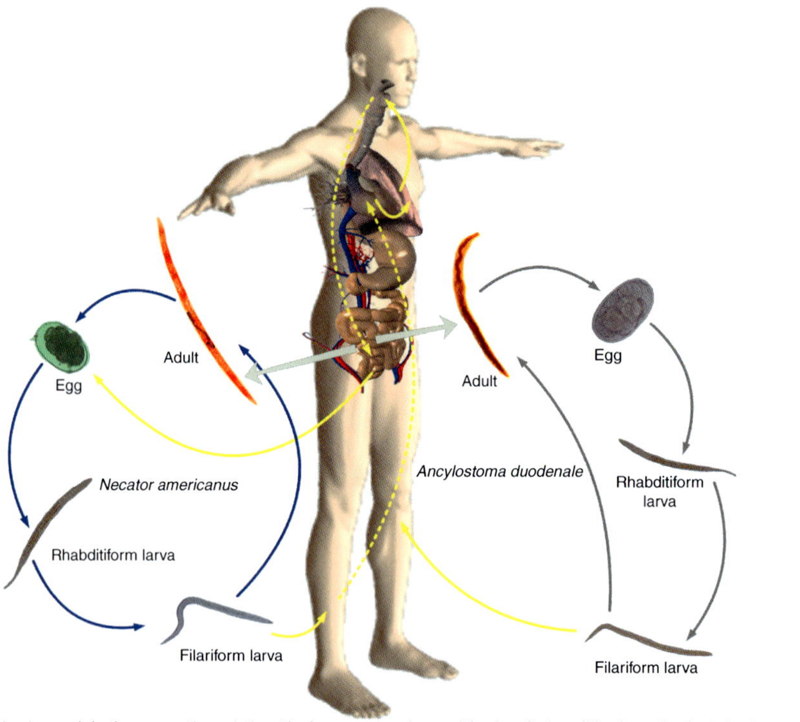

A hookworm infection occurs through the skin, for example, when walking barefoot or sitting in contaminated soil. Hookworm larvae penetrate the skin and enter the body, moving through the lymphatic system and blood vessels towards the lungs, where they penetrate into the pulmonary alveolae, ascend the bronchial tree to be coughed up into the troat and swallowed. Upon reaching the small intestine, they undergo two molts yielding fourth stage larvae that finally become adult male and female worms, which attach themselves to the lining of the upper parts of the small intestine and feed through sucking blood from the host. Eggs are continuously produced and passed with faeces to hatch in moist soil after a few days of incubation. The emerging larvae develop in the soil and, when fully developed, re-infect mammals, including humans.